Neurologic Emergencies

Editors

JOSEPH D. BURNS
ANNA M. CERVANTES-ARSLANIAN

NEUROLOGIC CLINICS

www.neurologic.theclinics.com

Consulting Editor
RANDOLPH W. EVANS

May 2021 • Volume 39 • Number 2

ELSEVIER

1600 John F. Kennedy Boulevard • Suite 1800 • Philadelphia, Pennsylvania, 19103-2899

http://www.theclinics.com

NEUROLOGIC CLINICS Volume 39, Number 2
May 2021 ISSN 0733-8619, ISBN-13: 978-0-323-83564-0

Editor: Stacy Eastman
Developmental Editor: Axell Ivan Jade Purificacion

Neurologic Clinics (ISSN 0733-8619) is published quarterly by Elsevier Inc., 360 Park Avenue South, New York, NY 10010–1710. Months of issue are February, May, August, and November. Periodicals postage paid at New York, NY, and additional mailing offices. Subscription prices are $333.00 per year for US individuals, $881.00 per year for US institutions, $100.00 per year for US students, $408.00 per year for Canadian individuals, $938.00 per year for Canadian institutions, $461.00 per year for international individuals, $938.00 per year for international institutions, $210.00 for foreign students/residents, and $100.00 for Canadian students/residents. To receive student/resident rate, orders must be accompanied by name of affiliated institution, date of term, and the *signature* of program/residency coordinator on institution letterhead. Orders will be billed at individual rate until proof of status is received. Foreign air speed delivery is included in all *Clinics* subscription prices. All prices are subject to change without notice. **POSTMASTER:** Send address changes to *Neurologic Clinics*, Elsevier Health Sciences Division, Subscription Customer Service, 3251 Riverport Lane, Maryland Heights, MO 63043. **Customer Service: Telephone: 1-800-654-2452 (U.S. and Canada); 314-447-8871 (outside U.S. and Canada). Fax: 314-447-8029. E-mail: journalscustomerservice-usa@elsevier.com (for print support); journalsonlinesupport-usa@elsevier.com (for online support).**

Reprints. For copies of 100 or more of articles in this publication, please contact the Commercial Reprints Department, Elsevier Inc., 360 Park Avenue South, New York, New York, 10010-1710; Tel.: +1-212-633-3874; Fax: +1-212-633-3820, and E-mail: reprints@elsevier.com.

Neurologic Clinics is also published in Spanish by Nueva Editorial Interamericana S.A., Mexico City, Mexico.

Neurologic Clinics is covered in *Current Contents/Clinical Medicine, MEDLINE/PubMed (Index Medicus), EMBASE/Excerpta Medica, and PsycINFO, and ISI/BIOMED.*

Contributors

CONSULTING EDITOR

RANDOLPH W. EVANS, MD
Clinical Professor, Department of Neurology, Baylor College of Medicine, Houston, Texas, USA

EDITORS

JOSEPH D. BURNS, MD
Director of Neurocritical Care, Division of Neurology, Lahey Hospital and Medical Center, Burlington, Massachusetts, USA; Associate Professor of Neurology and Neurosurgery, Tufts University School of Medicine, Boston, Massachusetts, USA

ANNA M. CERVANTES-ARSLANIAN, MD
Clinical Vice Chair of Neurology, Chief Division of Neurocritical Care, Boston Medical Center, Boston, Massachusetts, USA; Assistant Professor of Neurology, Neurosurgery, and Medicine, Boston University School of Medicine, Boston, Massachusetts, USA

AUTHORS

MOHAMAD ABDALKADER, MD
Departments of Neurology, Neurosurgery, and Radiology, Boston University School of Medicine, Boston Medical Center, Boston, Massachusetts

POUYA ALEXANDER AMELI, MD, MS
Departments of Neurology and Neurosurgery, University of Florida McKnight Brain Institute, Gainesville, Florida

ABDALLA A. AMMAR, PharmD, BCCCP, BCPS
Department of Pharmacy, Yale New Haven Health, New Haven, Connecticut

PRIA ANAND, MD
Assistant Professor of Neurology, Department of Neurology, Boston University School of Medicine, Boston Medical Center, Boston, Massachusetts

DIANA APETAUEROVA, MD
Division of Neurology, Lahey Hospital and Medical Center, Burlington, Massachusetts; Department of Neurology, Tufts University School of Medicine, Boston, Massachusetts

RAMANI BALU, MD, PhD
Assistant Professor, Department of Neurology, Hospital of the University of Pennsylvania, Perelman School of Medicine, University of Pennsylvania, Philadelphia, Pennsylvania

RACHEL BEEKMAN, MD
Assistant Professor, Department of Neurology, Yale School of Medicine, New Haven, Connecticut

JOSEPH D. BURNS, MD
Division of Neurology, Lahey Hospital and Medical Center, Burlington, Massachusetts; Departments of Neurology and Neurosurgery, Tufts University School of Medicine, Boston, Massachusetts

ANNA M. CERVANTES-ARSLANIAN, MD
Clinical Vice Chair, Chief of Neurocritical Care, Department of Neurology, Assistant Professor, Departments of Neurology, and Neurosurgery, and Medicine (Infectious Disease), Boston University School of Medicine, Boston Medical Center, Boston, Massachusetts

DAVID Y. CHUNG, MD, PhD
Division of Neurocritical Care, Department of Neurology, Boston Medical Center, Neurovascular Research Unit, Department of Radiology, Harvard Medical School, Massachusetts General Hospital, Boston, Massachusetts

CARLOS DAVID, MD
Associate Professor of Neurosurgery, Department of Neurosurgery, Tufts University School of Medicine, Boston, Massachusetts; Department of Neurosurgery, Lahey Hospital and Medical Center, Burlington, Massachusetts

RICHARD S. DOWD, MD
Department of Neurosurgery, Tufts University School of Medicine, Boston, Massachusetts

ILYAS ELI, MD
Department of Neurosurgery, Clinical Neurosciences Center, University of Utah, Salt Lake City, Utah; Department of Neurosurgery, Lahey Hospital and Medical Center, Burlington, Massachusetts

THOMAS FORD, MD
Department of Neurology, Boston University School of Medicine, Boston, Massachusetts

ZOHER GHOGAWALA, MD
Professor of Neurosurgery, Tufts University School of Medicine, Boston, Massachusetts; Department of Neurosurgery, Lahey Hospital and Medical Center, Burlington, Massachusetts

EMILY J. GILMORE, MD, MS
Associate Professor, Department of Neurology, Division of Neurocritical Care and Emergency Neurology, Yale School of Medicine, New Haven, Connecticut

DIANA GREENE-CHANDOS, MD, FNCS
Associate Professor of Neurology, Program Director, Neurosciences Critical Care Fellowship, Neurosciences Education Director, UNMH Adult Critical Care Center, University of New Mexico, Albuquerque, New Mexico

DAVID M. GREER, MD, MA
Chair, Department of Neurology, Boston University School of Medicine, Boston, Massachusetts

DANIEL F. HANLEY, MD
Professor of Neurology, Neurosurgery, and Anesthesia/Critical Care Medicine, Johns Hopkins University, Baltimore, Maryland

CARLOS S. KASE, MD
Professor of Neurology, Department of Neurology, Emory University School of Medicine, Atlanta, Georgia

DAVID KOPEL, MD
Department of Neurology, Boston, Massachusetts

JOSHUA KORNBLUTH, MD
Assistant Professor, Department of Neurology, Tufts University School of Medicine, Tufts Medical Center, Boston, Massachusetts

DAVID P. LERNER, MD
Division of Neurology, Lahey Hospital and Medical Center, Burlington, Massachusetts; Assistant Professor of Neurology, Department of Neurology, Tufts University School of Medicine, Boston, Massachusetts

CAROLINA B. MACIEL, MD, MSCR
Assistant Professor, Department of Neurology, UF Health Shands Hospital, University of Florida College of Medicine, Gainesville, Florida

ELIZABETH MACRI, MD
Assistant Professor of Neurology, Director of Neurohospitalists, Department of Neurology, University of New Mexico, Albuquerque, New Mexico

SOHAIL K. MAHBOOBI, MD
Department of Anesthesiology, Lahey Hospital and Medical Center, Burlington, Massachusetts; Clinical Assistant Professor of Anesthesiology and Perioperative Medicine, Tufts University School of Medicine, Boston, Massachusetts

CALEB R. S. MCENTIRE, MD
Clinical Fellow, Department of Neurology, Massachusetts General Hospital and Brigham and Women's Hospital, Harvard Medical School, Boston, Massachusetts

HEATHER E. MOSS, MD, PHD
Associate Professor, Department of Neurology and Neurological Sciences, Department of Ophthalmology, Stanford University, Stanford, California

THANH N. NGUYEN, MD
Departments of Neurology, Neurosurgery, and Radiology, Boston University School of Medicine, Boston Medical Center, Boston, Massachusetts

ALA NOZARI, MD, PhD
Professor of Anesthesiology, Boston University School of Medicine, Department of Anesthesiology, Boston Medical Center, Boston, Massachusetts

CHARLENE ONG, MD, MPHS
Assistant Professor, Department of Neurology, Boston University School of Medicine, Boston Medical Center, Boston, Massachusetts

EMANUELE ORRU', MD
Department of Radiology, Neurointerventional Radiology Division, Lahey Hospital and Medical Center, Burlington, Massachusetts

KENT A. OWUSU, PharmD, BCCCP, BCPS, FCCM
Department of Pharmacy, Care Signature, Yale New Haven Health, New Haven, Connecticut

PRITIKA A. PATEL, NP
Division of Neurology, Lahey Hospital and Medical Center, Burlington, Massachusetts

CRANDALL PEELER, MD
Assistant Professor, Department of Ophthalmology and Neurology, Boston, Massachusetts

ALEJANDRO A. RABINSTEIN, MD
Department of Neurology, Mayo Clinic, Rochester, Minnesota

POOJA RAIBAGKAR, MD
Concord Hospital Neurology Associates, Concord, New Hampshire

ANIL RAMINENI, MD
Clinical Assistant Professor of Neurology, Tufts University School of Medicine, Department of Neurology, Lahey Hospital and Medical Center, Burlington, Massachusetts

ERIK A. ROBERTS, BS
Boston University School of Medicine, Boston, Massachusetts

AMRA SAKUSIC, MD, PhD
Department of Neurology, Mayo Clinic, Jacksonville, Florida

BRIAN J. SCOTT, MD
Clinical Associate Professor, Neurology and Neurological Sciences, Division of Neurohospitalist Medicine, Department of Neurology, Stanford University School of Medicine, Stanford, California

SIDDHARTH SEHGAL, MD
Department of Neurology, Lahey Hospital and Medical Center, Assistant Professor of Neurology, Tufts University School of Medicine, Burlington, Massachusetts

KEVIN N. SHETH, MD
Associate Chair, Clinical Research, Department of Neurology, Yale School of Medicine, Professor of Neurology and Neurosurgery, Chief, Division of Neurocritical Care and Emergency Neurology, Yale School of Medicine, Yale New Haven Hospital, New Haven, Connecticut

JULIE G. SHULMAN, MD
Department of Neurology, Boston University School of Medicine, Boston, Massachusetts

TARUN D. SINGH, MBBS
Division of Critical Care Neurology, Mayo Clinic, Rochester, Minnesota

JUAN E. SMALL, MD
Department of Radiology, Neuroradiology Section, Lahey Hospital and Medical Center, Burlington, Massachusetts; Assistant Professor of Radiology, Tufts University School of Medicine, Boston, Massachusetts

SAMUEL J. SPIEGEL, MD
Resident Physician, Department of Neurology and Neurological Sciences, Stanford University, Stanford Healthcare, Palo Alto, California

ALEKSEY TADEVOSYAN, MD
Assistant Professor, Department of Neurology, Tufts University School of Medicine, Beth Israel Lahey Hospital and Medical Center, Burlington, Massachusetts

COURTNEY E. TAKAHASHI, MD, MCR
Assistant Professor, Department of Neurology, Boston University School of Medicine, Boston Medical Center, Boston, Massachusetts

ZACHARY D. THRELKELD, MD
Clinical Assistant Professor, Neurology and Neurological Sciences, Division of Neurocritical Care, Department of Neurology, Stanford University School of Medicine, Stanford, California

DEEPTI VIRMANI, MD
Neurology Resident, Department of Neurology, Boston University School of Medicine, Boston Medical Center, Boston, Massachusetts

BARBARA VOETSCH, MD, PhD, FAHA
Department of Neurology, Co-director of Comprehensive Stroke Center, Lahey Hospital and Medical Center, Assistant Professor of Neurology, Tufts University School of Medicine, Burlington, Massachusetts

MOLLY VORA, BS
Boston University School of Medicine, Boston, Massachusetts

EELCO F.M. WIJDICKS, MD, PhD
Division of Critical Care Neurology, Mayo Clinic, Rochester, Minnesota

SHUHAN ZHU, MD
Assistant Professor, Department of Neurology, Boston, Massachusetts

ADEEL S. ZUBAIR, MD
Department of Neurology, Yale School of Medicine, New Haven, Connecticut

Contents

An acutely comatose patient constitutes a medical emergency until proved otherwise. Managing these emergencies requires organized teamwork to recognize and treat life-threatening situations and reversible causes of coma. Once vital functions have been stabilized, information from the history and physical examination should be used to rationally guide subsequent testing. Identifying causes of coma for which emergency treatment is possible should be the priority. The treatment and prognosis depend on the cause.

Cardiac arrest survivors comprise a heterogeneous population, in which the etiology of arrest, systemic and neurologic comorbidities, and sequelae of post-cardiac arrest syndrome influence the severity of secondary brain injury. The degree of secondary neurologic injury can be modifiable and is influenced by factors that alter cerebral physiology. Neuromonitoring techniques provide tools for evaluating the evolution of physiologic variables over time. This article reviews the pathophysiology of hypoxic-ischemic brain injury, provides an overview of the neuromonitoring tools available to identify risk profiles for secondary brain injury, and highlights the importance of an individualized approach to post cardiac arrest care.

This article introduces the basic concepts of intracranial physiology and pressure dynamics. It also includes discussion of signs and symptoms and examination and radiographic findings of patients with acute cerebral herniation as a result of increased as well as decreased intracranial pressure. Current best practices regarding medical and surgical treatments and approaches to management of intracranial hypertension as well as future directions are reviewed. Lastly, there is discussion of some of the implications of critical medical illness (sepsis, liver failure, and renal failure) and treatments thereof on causation or worsening of cerebral edema, intracranial hypertension, and cerebral herniation.

Airway obstruction and respiratory failure are common complications of neurological emergencies. Anesthesia is often employed for airway management, surgical and endovascular interventions or in the intensive care units in patients with altered mental status or those requiring burst suppression. This article provides a summary of the unique airway management and anesthesia considerations and controversies for neurologic emergencies in general, as well as for specific commonly encountered conditions: elevated intracranial pressure, neuromuscular respiratory failure, acute ischemic stroke, and acute cervical spinal cord injury.

Neuromuscular respiratory failure can result from any disease that causes weakness of bulbar and/or respiratory muscles. Once compensatory mechanisms are overwhelmed, hypoxemic and hypercapnic respiratory failure ensues. The diagnosis of neuromuscular respiratory failure is primarily clinical, but arterial blood gases, bedside spirometry, and diaphragmatic ultrasonography can help in early assessment. Intensive care unit (ICU) admission is indicated for patients with severe bulbar weakness or rapidly progressing appendicular weakness. Intubation should be performed electively, particularly in patients with dysautonomia. Patients with an underlying treatable cause have the potential to regain functional independence with meticulous ICU care.

Headache is a common reason for seeking medical attention. Most cases are benign primary headache disorders; however, there is significant overlap between symptoms of these disorders and secondary headaches. Differentiating these clinical scenarios requires a careful history with attention to red flag symptoms and a neurologic examination. These details can identify dangerous disorders: subarachnoid hemorrhage, reversible cerebral vasoconstriction syndrome, elevated intracranial pressure, hydrocephalus, cerebral venous sinus thrombosis, arterial dissection, central nervous system infection, and inflammatory vasculitis. Older, pregnant, or immunocompromised patients have a higher risk for secondary disorders; clinicians should have a different threshold to conduct evaluations in such patients.

Vestibular symptoms, including dizziness, vertigo, and unsteadiness, are common presentations in the emergency department. Most cases have benign causes, such as vestibular apparatus dysfunction or orthostatic hypotension. However, dizziness can signal a more sinister condition, such as an acute cerebrovascular event or high-risk cardiac arrhythmia. A contemporary approach to clinical evaluation that emphasizes symptom duration and triggers along with a focused oculomotor and neurologic examination can differentiate peripheral causes from more serious central causes of vertigo. Patients with high-risk features should get brain MRI as the diagnostic investigation of choice.

centers, and provider expertise across multiple specialties. In the emergency department, patients should receive urgent intracranial imaging and consideration for tranexamic acid. Close observation in the intensive care unit environment helps identify problems, such as seizure, intracranial pressure crisis, and injury progression. In addition to traditional neurologic examination, patients benefit from use of intracranial monitors. Monitors gather physiologic data on intracranial and cerebral perfusion pressures to help guide therapy. Brain tissue oxygenation monitoring and cerebromicrodialysis show promise in studies.

pharmacologic therapies, and help determine if there is a role for immune modulation.

Zachary D. Threlkeld and Brian J. Scott

Cancer and cancer therapies have the potential to affect the nervous system in a host of different ways. Cerebral edema, increased intracranial pressure, cerebrovascular events, status epilepticus, and epidural spinal cord compression are among those most often presenting as emergencies. Neurologic side-effects of cancer therapies are often mild, but occasionally result in serious illness. Immunotherapies cause autoimmune-related neurologic side-effects that are generally responsive to immunosuppressive therapies. Emergency management of neuro-oncologic problems benefits from early identification and close collaboration among interdisciplinary team members and patients or surrogate decision-makers.

Caleb R.S. McEntire, Pria Anand, and Anna M. Cervantes-Arslanian

Neuroinfectious diseases can affect immunocompetent and immunosuppressed individuals and cause a variety of emergencies including meningitis, encephalitis, and abscess. Neurologic infections are frequently complicated by secondary injuries that also present emergently, such as cerebrovascular disease, acute obstructive hydrocephalus, and seizure. In most cases, timely recognition and early treatment of infection can improve the morbidity and mortality of infectious neurologic emergencies.

Pooja Raibagkar and Anil Ramineni

Over the past decade, understanding of autoimmune neurologic disorders has exponentially increased. Many patients present as a neurologic emergency and require timely evaluation with rapid management and intensive care. However, the diagnosis is often either missed or delayed, which may lead to a significant burden of disabling morbidity and even mortality. A high level of suspicion in the at-risk population should be maintained to facilitate more rapid diagnosis and prompt treatment. At present, there is no all-encompassing algorithm specifically applicable to the management of fulminant autoimmune neurologic disorders. This article discusses manifestations and management of various autoimmune neurologic emergencies.

Diana Apetauerova, Pritika A. Patel, Joseph D. Burns, and David P. Lerner

Acute presentation of new movement disorders and acute decompensation of chronic movement disorders are uncommon but potentially life-threatening. Inadvertent or purposeful overdose of many psychiatric medications can result in acute life-threatening movement disorders including serotonin syndrome, neuroleptic malignant syndrome, and malignant catatonia. Early withdrawal of potentiating medications, treatment with benzodiazepines and other diagnosis-specific drugs, and providing appropriate supportive care including airway and breathing management, hemodynamic stabilization, fluid resuscitation, and renal support including possible hemodialysis are the mainstays of acute management. Many of these conditions require admission to the neurologic intensive care unit.

NEUROLOGIC CLINICS

SERIES OF RELATED INTEREST

Neurosurgery Clinics
https://www.neurosurgery.theclinics.com/
Neuroimaging Clinics
www.neuroimaging.theclinics.com
Psychiatric Clinics
https://www.psych.theclinics.com/
Child and Adolescent Psychiatric Clinics
https://www.childpsych.theclinics.com/

THE CLINICS ARE AVAILABLE ONLINE!
Access your subscription at:
www.theclinics.com

Preface

Bringing Order to the Chaos of Neurologic Emergencies Amid the Chaos of a Pandemic

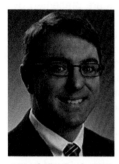 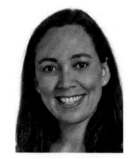

Joseph D. Burns, MD   Anna M. Cervantes-Arslanian, MD
Editors

Successfully caring for patients with neurologic emergencies presents significant challenges. The rapidity with which the emergency must be handled and the necessarily deliberate nature of the neurology involved are difficult to reconcile. The difficulty is compounded by the unforgiving nature of the injured nervous system and rapidly increasing body of knowledge about the conditions that cause these emergencies. Yet, the challenge is welcome. These patients are vulnerable, and our ability to meaningfully treat many previously devastating neurologic emergencies has improved dramatically in recent years. Accordingly, a well-informed, cognitively disciplined, pragmatically effective approach to patients with neurologic emergencies that successfully combines methodical neurologic problem solving with action-oriented emergency medicine and critical care is essential. In this issue of *Neurologic Clinics*, a group of expert authors skillfully combine lessons from both the scientific literature and their considerable clinical experience to help the reader achieve this goal for a wide range of neurologic emergencies, emphasizing the practical aspects of successfully managing these conditions in the "golden hour" of therapeutic opportunity.

By design, this issue of *Neurologic Clinics* starts with general clinical problems and then proceeds through disease-specific articles. Drs. Sakusic and Rabinstein provide a robust framework for assessing patients with acute coma, and Drs. Beekman and colleagues discuss cutting-edge advances in neuromonitoring following cardiac arrest. The next articles focus on management of specific aspects of neurologic emergencies: Drs. Tadevosyan and Kornbluth adeptly outline intracranial hypertension and brain herniation syndromes, while Dr. Ramineni and colleagues provide expert

Neurol Clin 39 (2021) xvii–xix
https://doi.org/10.1016/j.ncl.2021.03.001
0733-8619/21/© 2021 Published by Elsevier Inc.

guidance on anesthetic considerations in patients with neurologic emergencies, and Drs. Singh and Wijdicks provide an authoritative review of neuromuscular respiratory failure. Evaluation of emergent neurologic symptoms is considered next, with Dr. Kopel and colleagues presenting a comprehensive review of headache emergencies, and Drs. Sehgal and Voestch expertly outlining the evaluation of patients with dizziness and vertigo. Cerebrovascular emergencies follow with Drs. Zubair and Sheth reviewing acute ischemic stroke, renowned experts Drs. Kase and Hanley presenting the latest updates on early management of intracerebral hemorrhage, and Dr. Chung and colleagues covering the early management of aneurysmal subarachnoid hemorrhage. In the subsequent articles, severe traumatic injuries are presented by Dr. Takahashi and colleagues (severe blunt and penetrating traumatic brain injury) and Dr. Eli and colleagues (traumatic spinal cord injury). On the theme of spinal cord pathologic conditions, Dr. McEntire and colleagues next review nontraumatic myelopathy. Dr. Ameil and colleagues provide up-to-date guidance on the emergent management of status epilepticus. The articles that follow may be of particular interest to neurologic subspecialists: Neuro-oncologic emergencies are covered by Drs. Threlkeld and Scott, neuroinfectious diseases by Dr. McEntire and colleagues, neuro-immunology by Drs. Raibagkar and Ramineni, movement disorders by Dr. Apetauerova and colleagues, and neuroophthalmologic emergencies by Drs. Spiegel and Moss. Drs. Macari and Greene-Chandos provide a real tour de force in the next article on neurologic emergencies in pregnancy. Finally, we could not complete an issue covering neuroemergencies in 2020-2021 without specifically addressing the impact of the COVID-19 on neuroemergencies and special considerations for how to emergently manage patients suspected or confirmed to be infected with severe acute respiratory syndrome coronavirus 2, comprehensively covered here by Dr. Shulman and colleagues.

Over the past year, in line with their roles as experts in acute, emergency, and critical care, the authors of this issue have worked harder than ever before under conditions more challenging than previously imaginable, doing their part in emergency departments, intensive care units, and medical wards for the COVID-19 pandemic response while continuing their usual practice. And yet they spent time they did not have to share their expertise in world-class articles. William Osler notably said, "Humanity has but three great enemies: fever, famine, and war; of these by far the greatest, by far the most terrible, is fever." Fever did not stop our authors, and for this we are incredibly grateful.

We are honored to have had the opportunity to work with renowned experts in presenting this issue, and we thank *Neurologic Clinics* for the invitation to guest edit. Without our mentors, past and present, we would not have had this opportunity, nor would we have been able to execute on it: thank you. We thank our patients and their families for their inspiration and our colleagues for their support. Finally, and most importantly, we thank our families: David, Isaac, Jacob, and Abigail Arslanian; and Elizabeth, Benjamin, and Grace Burns.

Joseph D. Burns, MD
Division of Neurology
Lahey Hospital and Medical Center
41 Mall Road
Burlington, MA 01805, USA

Anna M. Cervantes-Arslanian, MD
Boston University School of Medicine
72 East Concord Street, C3
Boston, MA 02118, USA

E-mail addresses:
joseph.d.burns@lahey.org (J.D. Burns)
anna.cervantes@bmc.org (A.M. Cervantes-Arslanian)

Acute Coma

Amra Sakusic, MD, PhD[a], Alejandro A. Rabinstein, MD[b],*

KEYWORDS

- Coma • Disorder of consciousness • Diagnosis • Treatment • Prognosis

KEY POINTS

- The term coma should be used to identify patients who cannot be aroused and cannot interact with the environment. Coma is an acute state that can evolve into prolonged disorder of consciousness, including unresponsive wakefulness, minimally conscious state, with different semiological features.
- Coma can be caused by structural brain injury or generalized brain dysfunction. Correct diagnosis of the cause of coma has enormous implications for treatment and prognosis.
- Evaluation of coma should be methodical. It is useful to keep a mental checklist to avoid missing important elements of differential diagnosis, examination, and testing.
- When evaluating a comatose patient, it is imperative to concentrate first on identifying diagnoses amenable to specific emergency treatments.
- Causes of coma can be treatable, nontreatable but reversible, or neither treatable nor reversible. After excluding diagnoses for which specific emergency treatment is available, it is always prudent to wait for reversibility before estimating a prognosis.

DEFINITION

Consciousness is the brain function that makes people who they are. It is composed of 2 domains: level and content. Level of consciousness refers to the degree of arousal, whereas content refers to the degree of awareness. Although there is no widely accepted formal definition of consciousness, its absence is better understood and is the topic of this review.

The deepest degree of impaired consciousness is known as coma. Comatose patients cannot be aroused and do not interact with the environment, even after painful stimulation.[1] A patient in coma is not alert and, consequently, is unaware.

Coma is not a disease, not even a syndrome. It is a state determined by the lack of certain major brain functions. It can also be considered as a condition reached through a final common pathway that many brain insults can follow when sufficiently severe. Coma can be caused by structural brain lesions, toxic exposures, metabolic

[a] Department of Neurology, Mayo Clinic, 4500 San Pablo Road South (Attention: Cannaday Building 3W CIM), Jacksonville, FL 32224, USA; [b] Department of Neurology, Mayo Clinic, 200 First Street Southwest, Rochester, MN 55905, USA
* Corresponding author.
E-mail address: rabinstein.alejandro@mayo.edu

Neurol Clin 39 (2021) 257–272
https://doi.org/10.1016/j.ncl.2021.01.001
0733-8619/21/© 2021 Elsevier Inc. All rights reserved.

disorders, inflammation, and seizures, to name just the main causes. Thus, saying a patient is comatose only indicates the manifestation of a critical brain dysfunction. The job of the clinician is to determine the cause of that brain dysfunction and whether it is reversible.

BASIC PATHOPHYSIOLOGIC CONSIDERATIONS

Although simplistic, the anatomic notion that coma results either from bilateral supra-tentorial or diencephalic brainstem dysfunction remains correct.[2] However, this cate-gorization is not exclusionary in practice. For instance, unilateral hemispheric lesions can cause contralateral hemispheric dysfunction and diencephalic-mesencephalic dysfunction through mass effect.

A classification based on causative mechanism is pragmatically more useful. Major categories include global anoxia-ischemia, cerebrovascular disease (ischemic or hemorrhagic), traumatic injury, seizures, infection, noninfectious inflammation, hydro-cephalus, neoplastic, metabolic and endocrine disorders, hypothermia, and various toxins. A detailed list of common causes of coma is presented in **Table 1**.

Another classification scheme has been proposed within the framework of the Curing Coma Campaign launched in 2019 by the Neurocritical Care Society.[3] This classification contemplates 4 categories (characterized as endotypes):

1. Disorder of consciousness (DOC) endotype without commensurate structural dam-age, a category that includes conditions that could be reversible with or without specific treatment (eg, seizures, drug overdose)
2. DOC endotype with structural or functional damage that is amenable to neurologic replacement or bypass therapy (eg, global anoxia or major stroke that could in the future be improved with stimulant drugs or brain-machine interfaces)
3. DOC endotype that is not amenable to pharmacologic or anatomic replacement or repair therapy (eg, end-stage infectious or degenerative process)
4. DOC mimics endotype, including conditions in which structural damage causes functional deficits that can be confused with coma (eg, severe abulia, locked-in syndrome)

This classification does not include another acutely treatable cause of DOC; namely, structural lesions amenable to emergency surgical therapy (eg, subdural or epidural hematoma with brain compression treatable with craniotomy and evacuation or acute internal carotid artery occlusion treatable with mechanical thrombectomy).

EMERGENCY EVALUATION AND MANAGEMENT

Every neurologist practicing in a hospital setting should have in-depth knowledge of coma. Not only neurologists but also emergency medicine physicians and hospitalists encounter comatose patients in their everyday clinical practice. Misunderstandings and misinformation related to diagnosis and management of comatose patients are common and may result in serious medical errors. Clinicians need to follow a method-ical and efficient approach to the evaluation of coma to prevent these errors.

In the emergency department, coma should be considered a medical emergency until proved otherwise. It often requires immediate action to prevent devastating com-plications. The first priority is to ensure the patient has a secure airway, adequate ventilation and oxygenation, and sufficient circulation. Once these vital functions have been stabilized, the clinician should obtain a detailed history of recent events and comorbidities, perform a focused but complete physical examination, and order investigations following a rational approach in order to uncover the cause of the

Table 1
Common causes of coma organized by mechanism

Structural Intracranial Disease	Diffuse Brain Dysfunction
Global anoxic-ischemic injury	Seizures
	Status epilepticus
	Postictal state
Cerebrovascular disease	Metabolic and endocrine disorder
Brainstem ischemia	Hypoglycemia
Massive hemispheric ischemia	Diabetic decompensation
Large areas of bilateral hemispheric ischemia	Hypercapnia
Bilateral thalamic ischemia	Hyponatremia
Poor-grade subarachnoid hemorrhage	Hypercalcemia
Large supratentorial intracerebral hemorrhage	Uremia
Large cerebellar hemorrhage	Hyperammonemia
Brainstem hemorrhage	Addison crisis
Deep venous sinus thrombosis	Myxedema
Extensive dural venous sinus thrombosis	Thiamine deficiency
Cerebral air embolism	
Trauma	Intoxications
Diffuse axonal injury	Carbon monoxide
Bilateral contusions	Cyanide
Extra-axial hemorrhage with mass effect	Opiate
Edema with intracranial hypertension	Alcohol and atypical alcohols
Cerebral fat embolism	Sedative-hypnotics
	Nonprescription sympathomimetics
	Serotonin syndrome
	Neuroleptic malignant syndrome
	Malignant catatonia
Tumor	Septic shock
Large supratentorial tumor with mass effect	
Cerebellar tumor with mass effect	
Brainstem tumor	
Infiltrative tumor (glioma, lymphoma)	
Pituitary apoplexy	
Acute hydrocephalus	Hypothermia
Infection	—
Fulminant bacterial meningitis	
Cerebral abscess with mass effect	
Epidural abscess with mass effect	
Viral encephalitis	
Advanced fungal meningoencephalitis	
Advanced tuberculous meningitis	
Posterior reversible encephalopathy syndrome	—
Fulminant demyelination	—
Inflammatory	
Osmotic	
Autoimmune encephalitis	—
Paraneoplastic	
Nonparaneoplastic	

coma. Although most therapeutic decisions depend on the cause of coma, some basic emergency interventions apply to all comatose patients.

Basic Tenets for the Emergency Management of Comatose Patients

The general principles of any medical emergency apply to the emergency management of coma. First, always think about ABC (airway, breathing, circulation):

- Airway and breathing
  - Assess the patient's ventilation and oxygenation
  - Supplement oxygen, if needed
  - Proceed with intubation and mechanical ventilation if:
    - Patient cannot protect the airway
    - Gas exchange is poor, with low oxygen saturation or hypercapnia
    - Breathing pattern is inefficient (note: Cheyne-Stokes breathing and central neurogenic hyperventilation do not always require mechanical ventilation)
    - There is a significant risk of aspiration

The concept that all comatose patients need to be immediately intubated is widespread, but unproved. Although it is true that most comatose patients require intubation because of 1 or more of the indications noted earlier, there are exceptions that generally involve coma causes expected to be short lived. For instance, a postictal patient who does not show compromise of airway patency, maintains a regular breathing pattern, and does not have major oxygen desaturation may be carefully observed without harm. Even if acidotic and hypercapnic initially, these patients typically clear their acidosis spontaneously and wake up after a variable length of time without complications, as long as recurrent seizures do not occur. Thus, the dictum that Glasgow Coma Scale (GCS) score less than 8 indicates the need for intubation should not be followed dogmatically. In contrast, noninvasive ventilation is not a safe option for comatose patients because of heightened risk of aspiration. If mechanical ventilation is deemed necessary for a comatose patient, tracheal intubation is indicated.

- Circulation
  - Obtain intravenous (IV) access
  - Ensure adequate blood pressure and sufficient organ perfusion
  - If hypotension is present (systolic blood pressure <90 mm Hg or mean arterial pressure <65 mm Hg), administer fluids
  - If the patient's blood pressure remains low after fluid resuscitation, consider giving vasopressors
  - Order 12-lead electrocardiogram and keep on continuous cardiac monitoring to exclude arrhythmias and corrected QT prolongation

Additional considerations that should be remembered when first evaluating any comatose patient include:

- If trauma is suspected, stabilize cervical spine.
- Give thiamine (100 mg IV) before dextrose (50% solution) to avoid Wernicke encephalopathy in malnourished patients.
- Give naloxone 0.4 to 2 mg IV if opioid overdose is deemed possible. Watch for delirium after rapid reversal of opioids caused by withdrawal.

Subsequent management steps should be guided by the results of the diagnostic work-up, which should always be geared toward identifying treatable neurologic and neurosurgical emergencies.

History Taking When Evaluating a Comatose Patient

Obtaining relevant historical details when evaluating a comatose patient can be challenging, especially if a companion is not available for interview and previous medical records are not accessible for review. However, it is crucial to maximize efforts to obtain relevant information on recent symptoms, previous illnesses, use of prescribed and nonprescription medications, and possible toxic exposures.

Often, most of the significant details are obtained from bystanders, work colleagues, a significant other, police officers, friends, or prehospital personnel. If necessary, phone calls should be made to reach out to witnesses even if they are already on the way to the hospital to prevent loss of valuable time. Indirect information should always be taken cautiously, but still can provide important clues to trim the differential diagnosis. Additional valuable sources of information are medical records, alert cards, bracelets, and pharmacy phone numbers that can be found in patients belongings. When possible, 1 team member should be assigned to seek out information while others stay at the bedside caring for the patient.

It is very important to establish whether the onset of coma was witnessed, when the patient was last known to be well, and the acuity of the presentation. It is crucial to determine whether the patient had respiratory or cardiac arrest at onset, and whether severe hypoxemia was noted on first evaluation.

Sudden onset of coma raises concern for stroke, seizure, or acute poisoning. A preceding headache points primarily to aneurysmal subarachnoid hemorrhage. Abnormal movements, urinary incontinence, and tongue bite signal a preceding seizure. A stuttering course may be the clue to diagnose basilar artery occlusion. In contrast, a gradual onset preceded by personality changes is more suspicious for an inflammatory process or a slowly expanding mass. If the onset was insidious or the patient had fluctuating decline, information regarding recent behavior at home and at work should be obtained.

While obtaining the history, clinicians should also focus on recent medications or changes in dosage of previously used medications, substance abuse, recent trauma, previous suicide attempts or suicidal ideation, other possible toxic exposures, and immunosuppression. When investigating comorbidities, it is important to pay attention to vascular risk factors and other conditions that require anticoagulation, renal or liver failure, epilepsy, brain tumor, and recent neurosurgery.

General Physical Examination

General inspection

The examination of a comatose patient should begin with a general visual inspection free of any stimulation. Simply by observing, the clinician can identify irregular breathing patterns, adventitious movements, asymmetry of movements, traumatic injuries (such as periorbital and retroauricular ecchymoses indicative of basilar skull fracture), and other signs that can be helpful in narrowing the differential diagnosis. Central neurogenic hyperventilation (ie, sustained tachypnea and hyperpnea) typically indicates bilateral thalamic lesions, whereas ataxic breathing (ie, irregular rate and irregular tidal volume) indicates pontine tegmentum lesions. Cheyne-Stokes breathing pattern (ie, oscillating periods of hyperventilation and hypoventilation) is more common but has less localizing value.

Vital signs and systemic features

Vital signs, fever, lateral tongue bite, skin changes, cardiac murmurs, signs of heart failure, and signs of portal hypertension can provide valuable information and help in establishing the correct diagnosis in a timely manner.

Fever should prompt consideration of central nervous system infection, but sepsis from other sources can also provoke coma. Fever can also be seen with several toxidromes, such as organophosphates, neuroleptic malignant syndrome, serotonin syndrome, or withdrawal of cerebral depressants.[4] Hypothermia and hyperthermia from heat stroke can cause coma. Presence of tachycardia or bradycardia can help in the differentiation of culprit toxins. Tachycardia can be seen with any cause of sympathetic activation. Bradycardia should raise concern for increased intracranial pressure and is especially prominent with acute hydrocephalus.

Detailed examination of the skin can be particularly informative. A purpuric rash can be a manifestation of thrombotic microangiopathy, bacterial meningitis (most notably by *Neisseria meningitidis*), rickettsial infection, disseminated intravascular coagulation, or vasculitis.[5] Needle puncture marks on the skin indicate IV drug abuse. Stigmata of liver failure, dark pigmentation in patients with Addison disease, cool and yellowish skin with myxedema, and extreme skin dryness with organophosphate intoxication are additional examples of the value of a careful dermatologic examination.

Neurologic Examination

The neurologic examination, despite its inherent limitations in comatose patients, is critically important to guide additional testing. It must be structured and efficient. The first step is to confirm that the patient is unresponsive to verbal or nonverbal commands and that arousal cannot be achieved with any form of auditory or painful stimulation. It is important to remember that lock-in patients may only be able to respond by blinking or vertical eye movements, which are often subtle and may be missed. Once it is established that the patient is comatose, the examination should be focused on assessing brainstem reflexes and motor responses to stimulation, and detecting signs of meningeal irritation and adventitious movements. Confounding factors, especially sedation and residual pharmacologic paralysis, must be taken into account when interpreting the findings of the neurologic examination. Hypothermia, hyperthermia, and hypotension can also act as confounders. Before reaching conclusions about the implications of neurologic findings, the examination should be repeated after these confounders are corrected or eliminated.

Examination of the eyes and brainstem

Careful observation of the eyes can be extremely helpful in comatose patients. First, the clinician should note their position. A slight divergence of the eyes is common in deeply sedated and comatose patients and it is often clinically insubstantial; however, a frankly disconjugate gaze (particularly vertical misalignment) may reflect a brainstem or cranial nerve lesion. Conjugate gaze deviation to one side can be seen with hemispheric lesions affecting the frontal lobe (gaze deviates to the side of the lesion) or with thalamic or pontine lesions (gaze deviates away from the side of the lesion). Downward gaze may signal hydrocephalus. Abnormal biphasic vertical eye excursions, of which the most common is ocular bobbing (with a fast initial phase downwards), can be seen with pontine damage but also in cases of global cerebral dysfunction; therefore, they have limited localization value.[6] Subtle nystagmoid jerks may be the only manifestation of status epilepticus. Periorbital myoclonus may be noticed after global anoxia.

Size, symmetry, and light reactivity should be gauged when examining the pupils. Very small pupils can be seen with pontine injury but also with opiate poisoning or CO_2 narcosis. Large reactive pupils are characteristic of hypersympathetic states, such as serotonin syndrome. Pupillary asymmetry in a comatose patient should always be considered a potential emergency unless it is known to be chronic. The typical unilateral large nonreactive pupil (so-called blown pupil) occurs from loss of parasympathetic innervation caused by compression of the brainstem or third cranial nerve and should raise immediate concern for uncal herniation when found in a comatose patient. Although characteristically ipsilateral to the side of the mass lesion, it can occasionally occur on the contralateral side.

Fundoscopy can provide additional useful information. Vitreous hemorrhage can be noted with aneurysmal subarachnoid hemorrhage. Papilledema is a fairly reliable indicator of increased intracranial pressure, but its absence does not exclude increased intracranial pressure because it may take time to develop and, in some patients, it may never occur.

Corneal reflexes should be optimally checked by touching the nasal aspect of the cornea because it may have greater innervation that the lateral part,[7] but what matters most is to ensure that the cornea and not the sclera is being stimulated. Sterile saline may initially be used for stimulation to reduce the risk of corneal damage; however, when no response (ie, blinking) is observed, it is advisable to recheck using a sterile cotton swab. Oculocephalic reflexes are tested by moving the head rapidly from side to side. A normal response in a comatose patient is a conjugate movement of the eyes away from the side of the head rotation (ie, so-called doll's eyes). This maneuver should only be conducted after the cervical spine has been cleared. Oculovestibular reflexes are elicited by irrigating the external auditory canal with ice water. A normal response in a comatose patient is a slow tonic deviation toward the irrigated ear. Gag and cough reflexes should also be tested by stimulating the pharynx and trachea, respectively.

Motor examination

A complete motor examination should include assessment of the muscle tone, spontaneous movements, and responses to pain. Any asymmetry should suggest the need to exclude a structural lesion. Motor response after central pain stimulation can be evaluated by pressing on temporomandibular joints or supraorbital notches. Central stimulation is necessary to determine whether the patient can localize pain. Peripheral pain stimulation is provoked by pressing on nailbeds. Clear response to central stimulation without response to stimulation of the extremities can be seen with cervical cord injury and in patients with critical illness neuromyopathy. Pain stimulation tests should be performed on all extremities and the best response should be recorded. A normal response to peripheral pain is to withdraw from the source of pain. Distinguishing flexion withdrawal from decorticate posturing may be challenging. Extensor (decerebrate) posturing is easier to recognize. However, it is important to realize that many patients with disinhibited motor responses have an initial extensor response that is followed by withdrawal; in such cases, the motor response should be consider withdrawal. Instead, true extensor posturing is sustained. A triple flexion response in the leg represents a spinal reflex. It can best be recognized by its stereotypical quality where any stimulation of the leg results in exactly and repeatedly the same response.

Myoclonus can be caused by metabolic abnormalities (renal or hepatic insufficiency, electrolyte disturbances), intoxication (opioid, lithium, serotonin agents, pesticides), anoxic-ischemic brain injury, or nonconvulsive status epilepticus.[8] Myoclonus can be differentiated from seizures by lack of rhythmicity. Any rhythmic movements, even if subtle, segmental, or solely visible after stimulation, should be considered highly suspicious for seizures.

Other aspects of the neurologic examination

Deep tendon reflexes, plantar responses, and presence of clonus should also be checked on every comatose patient. A unilateral Babinski sign may be the only sign of an underlying mass lesion. Clonus with preferential rigidity of the legs is characteristic of serotonin syndrome.[9]

The examination of a comatose patient is not complete without testing for signs of meningeal irritation. Although it is true that these signs lack high sensitivity and specificity,[10] they can be extremely helpful when unequivocally present.

Coma Scales: Value and Limitations

The 2 best-validated coma scales are the GCS[11] and the Full Outline of Unresponsiveness (FOUR) score.[12] These tools are helpful in facilitating everyday communication among health care providers and for the serial monitoring of patients' clinical evolution. However, they should not replace a more complete neurologic examination. The GCS is less useful in intubated patients because of the loss of ability to assess the verbal component. A modified version designed to overcome this shortcoming by resorting to certain assumptions has been proposed.[13] The GCS and FOUR score assess eye opening and motor responses, but the FOUR score also incorporates brainstem reflexes and respiratory pattern (**Fig. 1**).[12] Some studies have indicated that the FOUR score may outperform the GCS in predicting the prognosis of neurocritical patients evaluated in the emergency department[14] or the intensive care unit (ICU).[15]

DIAGNOSTIC TESTING

When ordering tests for the evaluation of coma, clinicians should be guided by some basic principles:

- First consider diagnoses that require emergency treatment
- Use the history and examination to steer the testing (ie, avoid a so-called gunshot approach)
- Excessive testing may lead to errors
- Sometimes it is necessary to be patient (ie, the diagnosis will declare itself over time)

The more tests are ordered, the higher the likelihood of finding abnormal results of unclear relevance, which can create a lot of confusion and result in inappropriate treatment. To avoid this, it is best to follow a methodical, stepwise approach directed by the information obtained through history and examination. However, it is crucial to think about the most common treatable causes of coma, particularly those for which emergency treatment (or lack thereof) will determine the prognosis (**Table 2**).

Routine emergency testing should include serum metabolic panel (preceded by point-of-care capillary glucose), complete blood count, serum lactic acid, serum ammonia, arterial blood gas, coagulation parameters, serum alcohol concentration, and urine drug screen. Febrile patients should have blood cultures. Noncontrast head computed tomography (CT) scan is often obtained in the emergency department, although the yield is low in patients without focal or lateralizing signs on neurologic examination and without history of trauma.[16,17]

Additional testing requires individualized decisions, and having a mental checklist may help avoid missing a relevant test (**Fig. 2**).[18,19] CT angiogram of the head to rule out basilar artery or intracranial carotid artery occlusion, lumbar puncture to exclude meningitis or encephalitis, and electroencephalogram to evaluate for status epilepticus need to be contemplated. MRI of the head (with gadolinium if possible) can be very informative for multiple diagnoses that are typically missed on CT scan, including global anoxic-ischemic injury,[20] posterior reversible encephalopathy syndrome,[21] herpes simplex virus-1 encephalitis,[22] cerebral fat embolism, fulminant demyelination, and some forms of autoimmune encephalitis (**Fig. 3**). When overdose is suspected, testing for serum concentration of specific prescription (eg, antiseizure)

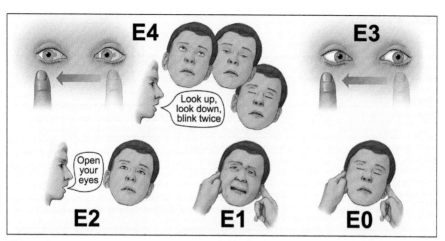

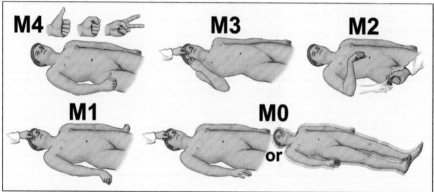

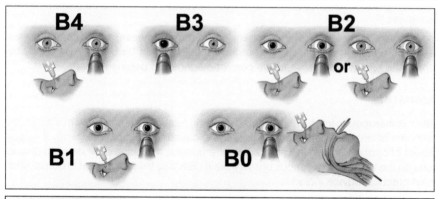

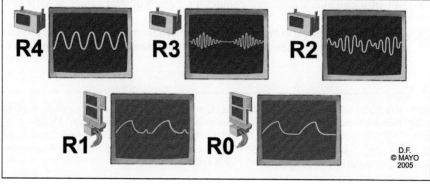

Table 2
Most frequent causes of emergently treatable acute coma

Diagnosis	Treatment
Hypoglycemia	Dextrose infusion (after thiamine)
Severe hyponatremia	Gradual serum sodium correction
CO_2 narcosis	Mechanical ventilation
CO intoxication	Hyperbaric oxygen
Opiate intoxication[a]	Naloxone
Intracranial hemorrhage	Surgical evacuation
Basilar artery occlusion	Reperfusion therapy (IV thrombolysis and/or mechanical thrombectomy)
Acute hydrocephalus	Ventriculostomy
Cerebral venous thrombosis	Anticoagulation
Status epilepticus	Antiseizure drugs
Fulminant bacterial meningitis	Antibacterial drugs with CNS penetration and dexamethasone
Herpes encephalitis	Acyclovir
Hypertensive encephalopathy	Gradual blood pressure reduction
Diabetic coma	Insulin
Uremic encephalopathy	Dialysis
Hyperammonemic encephalopathy	Lactulose, rifaximin
Sepsis	Antibiotics, fluids

Abbreviation: CNS, central nervous system

[a] Other less common intoxications with specific antidotes should also be considered when appropriate.[34]

or nonprescription (eg, acetaminophen) drugs may be necessary. Autoimmune encephalitis panels in serum and cerebrospinal fluid should be ordered prudently but can be the only way to arrive to the correct diagnosis in pertinent cases.[23]

TREATMENT

After the therapeutic interventions noted earlier in relation to emergency management, treatment of coma depends on the underlying cause.[24] A list of emergently treatable causes of coma is shown in **Table 2**. Other articles in this issue offer detailed discussions on the treatment of various primary brain diseases that may result in coma. Additional practical advice includes:

- If an intoxication is suspected, contact the poison control center or local toxicology specialist.
- When evaluating coma in the ICU, always remember to check the medication list and discontinue any medications that might be potential culprits or contributors

---

Fig. 1. The FOUR score. B, brainstem reflexes; E, eye response; M, motor response; R, respiration. Numbers indicate the score to be assigned for the response. (*From* Wijdicks EFM, Bamlet WR, Maramattom BV, Manno EM, McClelland RL: validation of a new Coma Scale: the FOUR score. Ann Neur, 2005:58:585-593; used with permission of Mayo Foundation for Medical Education and Research, all rights reserved.)

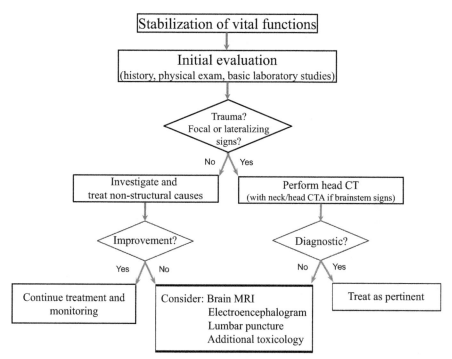

Fig. 2. Basic algorithm for the emergency evaluation of acute coma. Further details can be found on the text. CTA, CT angiogram.

to the pathogenesis of the coma (eg, sedatives, opiates, cefepime, serotonin-enhancing agents).[4,9,25]

- When the diagnosis remains uncertain and emergently treatable causes have been excluded, often it is best to wait (ie, when unsure what to do, better not to do anything).

- Supportive care is essential to optimize the chances of good recovery. Comatose patients are at risk of pneumonia, urinary infection, ileus, venous thromboembolism, gastroduodenal ulcers, cardiac arrhythmias, and medication toxicity. Prevention and early treatment of these and other complications demands close attention to detail. Sequential compression devices, deep venous prophylaxis with subcutaneous heparin or enoxaparin (if not contraindicated), stress ulcer prophylaxis, and a scheduled bowel regimen should be included in the routine management of any comatose patient.

The Curing Coma Campaign has been created to find new ways to treat comatose patients by refining the understanding of coma.[3] The initial priorities identified by the Scientific Advisory Council were defining coma endotypes with distinct recovery trajectories and possibilities for intervention, identifying novel biomarkers, and designing proof-of-concept clinical trials to promote recovery of consciousness.

PROGNOSIS

Prognosis is a major consideration in the care of comatose patients, and neurologists are sometimes consulted solely to estimate a prognosis after some time from the onset of the unresponsiveness. This delay is far from ideal. A neurologist should be

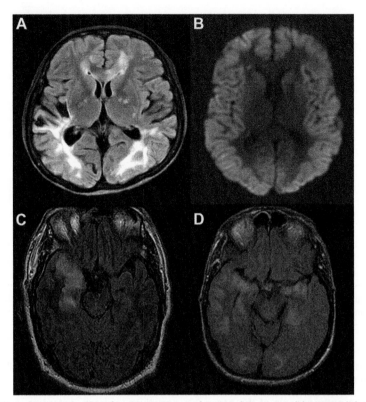

Fig. 3. Illustrative examples of various causes of coma documented by MRI. (*A*) Bilateral vasogenic edema predominantly affecting the occipital lobes in a patient with posterior reversible encephalopathy syndrome (fluid-attenuated inversion recovery [FLAIR] sequence). (*B*) Severe anoxic cortical injury after cardiac arrest (diffusion-weighted imaging sequence). (*C*) Inflammatory changes affecting the right temporal lobe in a patient with herpes simplex virus-1 encephalitis (FLAIR sequence). (*D*) Bilateral inflammatory changes predominantly affecting the limbic regions in a patient with paraneoplastic autoimmune encephalitis (FLAIR sequence). (Reproduced with permission from Rabinstein AA. Acute Coma. In: Rabinstein AA (editor). Neurological Emergencies: a practical approach. Switzerland: Springer Nature; 2020. p. 1-13.[19])

involved in the management of these patients from their first evaluation in the emergency department to assist in diagnosis and treatment. In general, prognosis should not be the first priority, although there are exceptions, such as patients with massive brainstem hemorrhages for whom aggressive treatment is likely to be futile. However, the guiding rule should be to avoid early therapeutic nihilism and to focus on diagnosis and emergency treatment first (**Fig. 4**).

Even more than for treatment, prognosis depends on the cause of coma. Discussions on prognosis for individual critical brain diseases are provided in other articles in this issue. Age, previous brain condition, degree of acute injury (severity, extent, and eloquence), and duration of coma are the basic determinants of prognosis, but many other factors need to be considered according to the primary diagnosis and other individual considerations.[26,27] Prognosis should always be expressed as estimation; gaps in prognostic ability exist for all major neurocritical diseases[28] and therefore

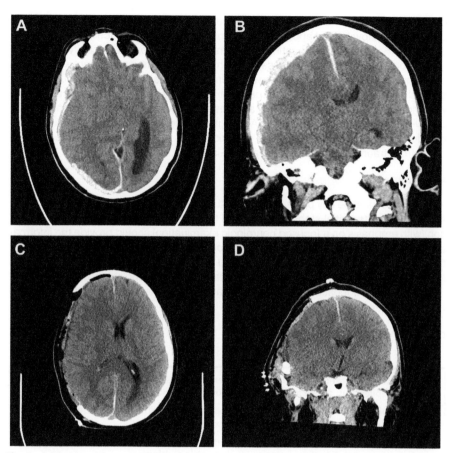

Fig. 4. A 32-year-old man without previous known medical problems was found unresponsive in his bed. His breathing was agonal and was intubated in the field. At the local emergency department he had bilaterally dilated, nonreactive pupils with extensor motor response on the left and no response on the right. Head CT scan (*A, B*) showed a massive right extra-axial hematoma with severe brain compression causing pronounced subfalcine and uncal herniation, and hydrocephalus from trapping of the contralateral ventricle. He was emergently transferred to our center while receiving 100 g of 20% mannitol en route. On arrival, he had regained pupillary reactivity on the left. He was immediately taken to the operating room where he underwent hematoma evacuation with right hemicraniectomy. During the operation, the neurosurgeons noted a pial arteriovenous malformation that was resected. Postoperative CT scan is shown in (*C*) and (*D*). The patient experienced a remarkably favorable evolution and 6 weeks later only had mild right III nerve palsy and very mild right hemiparesis (weakness ipsilateral to the side of the mass lesions can be explained by damage to the contralateral cerebral peduncle by the initial compression; this false localizing sign is known as the Kernohan-Woltman notch phenomenon).

it is impossible to be entirely conclusive. That estimation should then be put in the context of the patient's preferences and values in conversations with the family or other surrogates.

Our understanding of DOC is being enhanced by technology (functional MRI, PET, special electroencephalogram techniques) that is offering new venues to identify some evidence of covert consciousness in patients who appear comatose at the bedside.[29–31] How to best apply this new knowledge in daily practice remains a matter of debate.[32] When communicating with families, it is important to clarify that emergence from acute coma is a process in which some patients regain sleep-wake cycles but remain unaware (unresponsive wakefulness), others recover consciousness but only minimally and remain fully dependent (minimally conscious state), and those with more favorable evolution regain alertness and awareness with or without motor, behavioral, and cognitive deficits.[33] Although chances of recovery diminish with the duration of coma, improvement of consciousness is more likely after prolonged coma from trauma than from global anoxia-ischemia.[26]

SUMMARY

Neurologists must be key players on the multidisciplinary team caring for patients with acute coma. After initial stabilization of vital functions, history and physical examination (with emphasis on a focused neurologic examination) should provide the information to decide on subsequent testing. Conditions for which specific emergency treatment is possible should be considered first and therapeutic nihilism should be avoided. Estimating prognosis is an essential role of neurologists, but it is important not to rush to prognostication until it is clear that treatment or time cannot improve the condition of the patient.

CLINICS CARE POINTS

- After initial stabilization of vital functions, identify treatable neurologic emergencies, such as status epilepticus, stroke from large artery occlusion, and extra-axial hematoma.
- Always consider confounders (paralytics, sedatives, opiates, body temperature, metabolic disorders) when interpreting the neurologic examination.
- Keep a rational approach to testing by letting the history, general and neurologic examinations, and clinical evolution guide diagnostic decisions.
- When a treatable cause for the coma is not diagnosed, it is often best to just wait and follow the patient closely. Do not feel obliged to search for obscure diagnoses without effective treatment, do not embark on unsubstantiated empiric therapies, and do not rush prognostication.

FINANCIAL DISCLOSURE AND CONFLICTS OF INTEREST

The authors declare no pertinent financial conflicts of interest.

REFERENCES

1. Wijdicks EFM. Being comatose: why definition matters. Lancet Neurol 2012;11(8): 657–8.
2. Hocker S, Rabinstein AA. A clinical and investigative approach to the patient with diminished responsiveness. Neurol Clin 2011;29(4):739–47.
3. Provencio JJ, Hemphill JC, Claassen J, et al. The Curing Coma Campaign: framing initial scientific challenges-proceedings of the first curing coma campaign scientific advisory council meeting. Neurocrit Care 2020;33(1):1–12.
4. Cai A, Cai X. Toxin-induced acute delirium. Neurol Clin 2020;38(4):781–98.

5. Tsai J, Nagel MA, Gilden D. Skin rash in meningitis and meningoencephalitis. Neurology 2013;80(19):1808–11.
6. Mehler MF. The clinical spectrum of ocular bobbing and ocular dipping. J Neurol Neurosurg Psychiatry 1988;51(5):725–7.
7. Al-Aqaba MA, Fares U, Suleman H, et al. Architecture and distribution of human corneal nerves. Br J Ophthalmol 2010;94(6):784–9.
8. Levy A, Chen R. Myoclonus: pathophysiology and treatment options. Curr Treat Options Neurol 2016;18(5):21.
9. Pedavally S, Fugate JE, Rabinstein AA. Serotonin syndrome in the intensive care unit: clinical presentations and precipitating medications. Neurocrit Care 2014; 21(1):108–13.
10. Thomas KE, Hasbun R, Jekel J, et al. The diagnostic accuracy of Kernig's sign, Brudzinski's sign, and nuchal rigidity in adults with suspected meningitis. Clin Infect Dis 2002;35(1):46–52.
11. Teasdale G, Jennett B. Assessment of coma and impaired consciousness. A practical scale. Lancet 1974;2(7872):81–4.
12. Wijdicks EF, Bamlet WR, Maramattom BV, et al. Validation of a new coma scale: the FOUR score. Ann Neurol 2005;58(4):585–93.
13. Rutledge R, Lentz CW, Fakhry S, et al. Appropriate use of the Glasgow Coma Scale in intubated patients: a linear regression prediction of the Glasgow verbal score from the Glasgow eye and motor scores. J Trauma 1996;41(3):514–22.
14. Kevric J, Jelinek GA, Knott J, et al. Validation of the Full Outline of Unresponsiveness (FOUR) scale for conscious state in the emergency department: comparison against the Glasgow Coma Scale. Emerg Med J 2011;28(6):486–90.
15. Wijdicks EF, Kramer AA, Rohs T Jr, et al. Comparison of the Full Outline of UnResponsiveness score and the Glasgow Coma Scale in predicting mortality in critically ill patients*. Crit Care Med 2015;43(2):439–44.
16. Torres C, Zakhari N, Symons S, et al. Imaging the unconscious "found down" patient in the emergency department. Neuroimaging Clin N Am 2018;28(3):435–51.
17. Forsberg S, Hojer J, Ludwigs U, et al. Metabolic vs structural coma in the ED–an observational study. Am J Emerg Med 2012;30(9):1986–90.
18. Rabinstein AA. Coma and brain death. Continuum (Minneap Minn) 2018;24(6): 1708–31.
19. Rabinstein A. Acute coma. In: Rabinstein A, editor. Neurological emergencies: a practical approach. Lausanne, Switzerland: Springer Nature; 2020. p. 1–13.
20. Hirsch KG, Fischbein N, Mlynash M, et al. Prognostic value of diffusion-weighted MRI for post-cardiac arrest coma. Neurology 2020;94(16):e1684–92.
21. Fugate JE, Rabinstein AA. Posterior reversible encephalopathy syndrome: clinical and radiological manifestations, pathophysiology, and outstanding questions. Lancet Neurol 2015;14(9):914–25.
22. Singh TD, Fugate JE, Rabinstein AA. The spectrum of acute encephalitis: causes, management, and predictors of outcome. Neurology 2015;84(4):359–66.
23. Mittal MK, Rabinstein AA, Hocker SE, et al. Autoimmune encephalitis in the ICU: analysis of phenotypes, serologic findings, and outcomes. Neurocrit Care 2016; 24(2):240–50.
24. Hocker S, Rabinstein AA. Management of the patient with diminished responsiveness. Neurol Clin 2012;30(1):1–9, vii.
25. Singh TD, O'Horo JC, Day CN, et al. Cefepime is associated with acute encephalopathy in critically ill patients: a retrospective case-control study. Neurocrit Care 2020;33(3):695–700.

26. Kowalski RG, Buitrago MM, Duckworth J, et al. Neuroanatomical predictors of awakening in acutely comatose patients. Ann Neurol 2015;77(5):804–16.
27. Newman J, Blake K, Fennema J, et al. Incidence, predictors and outcomes of postoperative coma: an observational study of 858,606 patients. Eur J Anaesthesiol 2013;30(8):476–82.
28. Wartenberg KE, Hwang DY, Haeusler KG, et al. Gap analysis regarding prognostication in neurocritical care: a joint statement from the German Neurocritical Care Society and the Neurocritical Care Society. Neurocrit Care 2019;31(2):231–44.
29. Claassen J, Doyle K, Matory A, et al. Detection of brain activation in unresponsive patients with acute brain injury. N Engl J Med 2019;380(26):2497–505.
30. Kondziella D, Bender A, Diserens K, et al. European Academy of Neurology guideline on the diagnosis of coma and other disorders of consciousness. Eur J Neurol 2020;27(5):741–56.
31. Stender J, Gosseries O, Bruno M-A, et al. Diagnostic precision of PET imaging and functional MRI in disorders of consciousness: a clinical validation study. Lancet 2014;384(9942):514–22.
32. Peterson A, Owen AM, Karlawish J. Translating the discovery of covert consciousness into clinical practice. JAMA Neurol 2020;77(5):541–2.
33. Giacino JT, Katz DI, Schiff ND, et al. Practice guideline update recommendations summary: disorders of consciousness: report of the guideline development, dissemination, and implementation subcommittee of the American Academy of Neurology; the American Congress of Rehabilitation Medicine; and the National Institute on Disability, Independent Living, and Rehabilitation Research. Neurology 2018;91(10):450–60.
34. Edlow JA, Rabinstein A, Traub SJ, et al. Diagnosis of reversible causes of coma. Lancet 2014;384(9959):2064–76.

Neuromonitoring After Cardiac Arrest

Can Twenty-First Century Medicine Personalize Post Cardiac Arrest Care?

Rachel Beekman, MD[a],*, Carolina B. Maciel, MD, MSCR[b],
Ramani Balu, MD, PhD[c], David M. Greer, MD, MA[d],
Emily J. Gilmore, MD, MS[e]

KEYWORDS

- Neuromonitoring • Hypoxic-ischemic brain injury • Cardiac arrest
- Multimodal monitoring

KEY POINTS

- Invasive and noninvasive neuromonitoring provides insights into cerebral physiology, allowing an individualized approach to patient care.
- The degree of secondary brain injury, caused by an imbalance between cerebral metabolic demand and oxygen and glucose supply, is modifiable.
- Identification of secondary injury risk profiles, using neuromonitoring tools, may be key to evaluating therapeutic targets.
- Protocols for clinical implementation of noninvasive and invasive neuromonitoring and consensus for actionable values in the cardiac arrest population are warranted.
- Secondary injury after CA occurs due to an imbalance of cerebral metabolic demand and energy substrates
- Seizures, fever, and shivering are easily recognizable and treatable causes of increased cerebral metabolic demand

Continued

[a] Department of Neurology, Division of Neurocritical Care and Emergency Neurology, Yale University School of Medicine, P.O. Box 208018, 15 York Street, LLCI Building, 10th floor, New Haven, CT, 06520, USA; [b] Department of Neurology, UF Health Shands Hospital, University of Florida College of Medicine, PO Box 100236, Gainesville, FL 32610, USA; [c] Department of Neurology, Hospital of the University of Pennsylvania, 3400 Spruce Street, Philadelphia, PA 19104, USA; [d] Department of Neurology, Boston University School of Medicine, 75 Newton Street, Boston, MA 02118, USA; [e] Department of Neurology, Division of Neurocritical Care and Emergency Neurology, Yale University School of Medicine, 15 York Street, LLCI 810c, Box 208018, New Haven, CT 06510, USA
* Corresponding author. Department of Neurology, Division of Neurocritical Care and Emergency Neurology, Yale University School of Medicine, P.O. Box 208018, 15 York Street, LLCI Building, 10th floor, New Haven, CT, 06520
E-mail address: Rachel.Beekman@yale.edu

Neurol Clin 39 (2021) 273–292
https://doi.org/10.1016/j.ncl.2021.01.002
0733-8619/21/© 2021 Elsevier Inc. All rights reserved.

Continued

- Other factors that influence cerebral homeostasis, such as microcirculatory dysfunction, impaired autoregulation, and inflammation are not as easily recognized
- There is no "one-size-fits-all" approach for optimization of cerebral physiology after CA; neuromonitoring may assist in identifying individual and group level risk profiles for secondary injury

INTRODUCTION

Cardiac arrest (CA) is a major cause of morbidity and mortality globally; the incidence of out-of-hospital CA (OHCA) ranges from 24 to 186 per 100,000 person-years, and the incidence of in-hospital CA (IHCA) ranges from 1 to 5 per 1000 hospital admissions, depending on the region.[1–3] Sustained return of spontaneous circulation (ROSC) (>20 minutes) following cardiopulmonary resuscitation (CPR) occurs in 40% of patients with OHCA and 29% to 41% of patients with IHCA.[4,5] Of those successfully resuscitated, a mere 10.4% of patients with OHCA and 25.8% of patients with IHCA survive to hospital discharge.[6] Secondary brain injury, largely caused by an imbalance of cerebral metabolic demand and energy substrates,[7] contributes to poor neurologic outcome. Targeted temperature management (TTM) is the only therapy shown to modify secondary injury after CA and improve neurologic outcomes.[8–11] TTM and brain-centered resuscitation are the cornerstones of acute management in patients with CA (**Table 1**). Post-CA Syndrome (PCAS) is complex and heterogeneous; arrest-related factors (bystander CPR, etiology of arrest, rhythm), patient-related factors (degree of systemic inflammatory response syndrome, autoregulatory failure, risk for cerebral edema, and ongoing cerebral ischemia), and treatment-related factors (thrombolysis, hypothermia, extracorporeal cardiopulmonary resuscitation [ECMO]) influence the physiologic milieu. The use of neuromonitoring to evaluate individual cerebral physiology may provide new targets for secondary brain injury modulation. In this review, we outline the pathophysiology of secondary brain injury after CA, discuss the neuromonitoring tools used to identify those at risk for secondary injury, and explore potential future directions.

PATHOPHYSIOLOGY
Primary Injury

The brain uses 20% of the oxygen and 25% of the glucose produced by the human body.[12] Most cerebral energy demand is allocated to the maintenance and restoration of ion gradients, required for cell signaling and recycling of neurotransmitters.[12] During CA, oxygen and glucose delivery to neuronal tissue ceases, resulting in a shift to anaerobic metabolism, a rise in lactate, and sodium-potassium (Na/K) pump failure.[13] Spreading depolarizations (SDs), triggered by the failure of Na/K ATPases to maintain membrane polarity, result in a massive influx of cations into cells, a complete breakdown of transmembrane ionic gradients,[14] and osmotic movement of water into cells, causing neuronal swelling and distortion of the dendritic spines.[15] Neurons cannot fire action potentials due to sustained depolarization, causing electrical silence.[15] In the setting of prolonged ischemia, irreversible loss of Na/K ATPase function leads to terminal depolarization and cell death.[16] Restoration of blood flow alone is often insufficient to halt ongoing injury, as multiple pathophysiologic factors lead to a persistent imbalance between bioenergetics supply and demand.[7]

Table 1
Brain-centered goals for managing post cardiac arrest syndrome

Parameter	Goal
Temperature[a]	• 32–36°C for 24 h • Slow rewarming (0.1–0.25°C/h) • Fever avoidance, especially during the first 72 h • Aggressive treatment of shivering
Hemodynamics	Mean arterial pressure >65 mm Hg; consider individualized hemodynamic goals
Ventilation[b]	• O_2 Saturation >94% • Avoid Pao_2 <60 mm Hg or >300 mm Hg • $Paco_2$ 35–45 mm Hg
Glycemic control[c]	• Avoid hypoglycemia (glucose <72 mg/dL) • Avoid hyperglycemia

[a] The American Heart Association recommends (Class 1, level B) the use of targeted temperature management (TTM; 32°–36°C for at least 24 h after achieving target temperature) in adults who do not follow commands after return to spontaneous circulation, with any initial rhythm.[116] A post hoc analysis of 435 patients with cardiac arrest (CA) who received TTM between 32 to 36°C, suggests that patients with an initial lactate ≥12 mmol/L may benefit from 32 to 34°C more than 34 to 36°C.[117] A retrospective analysis of 1319 patients with CA treated with TTM between 32 to 36°C also found an association between illness severity (using Pittsburgh Cardiac Arrest Category) and outcome, suggesting that lower temperatures should be used in more severe post-CA syndrome.[118] A retrospective analysis of 628 patients with out-of-hospital CA with cardiac etiology found that initial core body temperature modified the effect of target temperature on outcomes; patients who presented with moderate hypothermia (defined by initial body temperature <35.5°C) had improved outcomes when treated with TTM <36°C.[119] Choice of target temperature depends on many factors, and significant variability exits between hospital systems.[120] There are few absolute contraindications to TTM other than premorbid terminal illness and intracerebral hemorrhage as the etiology of CA (rare in the United States); however, special circumstances that require an individualized risk benefit analysis include active bleeding, hemodynamic instability, pregnancy, and trauma.
[b] The partial pressure of oxygen (Pao_2) and carbon dioxide ($Paco_2$) have a U-shaped relationship with hospital mortality after CA[121]; avoiding hypoxia, hyperoxia, hypocapnia, and hypercapnia through optimization of ventilation and oxygenation are key to preventing secondary brain injury. Optimal targets are still the subject of ongoing work, but current guidelines recommend targeting an oxygen saturation of 92% to 98% and a $Paco_2$ goal of 35 to 45 mm Hg (Class 2b, Level B).[116]
[c] It is important to optimize glucose; however, optimal blood glucose range may differ in patients with diabetes and patients without diabetes.[122]

Secondary Injury

Microcirculatory dysfunction

The no-reflow phenomenon refers to suboptimal restoration of local tissue perfusion secondary to microcirculatory dysfunction after a period of ischemia. Mechanisms of no-reflow include endothelial injury causing localized swelling or endothelial blebs, leukocyte adhesion, mechanical compression from tissue edema, and activation of thrombotic cascades with micro-thromboses formation,[17] which may result in prolonged ischemic damage despite restoration of cardiac output.

Ischemia-reperfusion–induced microvascular dysfunction may be modifiable; exposure of post-capillary venules to nitric oxide (NO) attenuates leukocyte adherence to endothelial cells and decreases vascular leakage.[18] The use of heparin and recombinant tissue plasminogen activator (r-tPA) during CPR decreased no-reflow from 28% to 7% in a cat model of CA[19]; however, in human patients with OHCA, the use of thrombolysis (Tenecteplase) without adjunctive antithrombotic therapy during CPR has not translated into improved clinical outcomes (30-day survival, ROSC, or neurologic outcome).[20]

Seizures

Seizures are common after CA, occurring in 15% to 33% of patients post-CA treated with TTM,[21,22] with a resulting increase in the cerebral metabolic rate.[23,24] When arterial blood pressure, oxygenation, and glucose concentration are maintained, a rise in cerebral blood flow (CBF) is able to compensate for the increased cerebral metabolic rate and cerebral homeostasis is maintained.[23] Under conditions in which there is depletion of ATP and insufficient energy reserves, such as in hypoxic-ischemic brain injury (HIBI), seizures exacerbate brain injury.[25] In a piglet model of HIBI, MRI, electroencephalography (EEG), and histologic examination were used to identify the role of seizures in secondary brain injury; the presence of clinical and subclinical seizures was associated with lower cortical apparent diffusion coefficient on MRI (ADC, reflective of more severe HIBI), lower background amplitude on EEG, and greater histopathologic injury scores.[26]

Refractory status epilepticus (RSE), defined as clinical or nonconvulsive seizures lasting 30 minutes and unresponsive to benzodiazepines (first-line) and an adequately dosed parenteral second-line antiseizure drug (ASD), has been associated with poor prognosis after CA.[27,28] However, a recent prospective observational study evaluating outcome after RSE showed that using an aggressive treatment approach may improve outcomes in selected cases; patients with status myoclonus all had poor neurologic outcome.[28] Treatment of Electrographic Status Epilepticus after Cardiopulmonary Resuscitation (TELSTAR)[29] is a multicenter clinical trial with 2 parallel groups; patients who have electrographic status epilepticus are assigned to pharmacologic treatment aimed to suppress all epileptiform activity on EEG versus no treatment of electrographic status epilepticus.[29] Hopefully, this study will shed light on the impact of status epilepticus in CA, and whether aggressive treatment of electrographic status epilepticus impacts outcomes.

Fever/shivering

Fever is common within the first 48 hours after CA, occurring in up to 42% of patients, and is associated with increased mortality and worse neurologic outcomes (defined as cerebral performance category [CPC] 3–5).[30,31] TTM plays a critical role in fever avoidance; however, fever still occurs in up to 36% of patients during the post-TTM period, with a median onset of 36 hours after arrest.[30] Fever increases cerebral metabolic demand, and aggressive fever control may contribute to improved outcomes.[32] However, aggressive fever control may result in shivering, leading to significant energy expenditure and oxygen consumption,[33] which may decrease the efficacy of TTM. Management of shivering includes surface counter-warming, magnesium sulfate, buspirone, meperidine, sedation, and neuromuscular blockade.[34] In a multicenter study of 111 patients with OHCA, the use of early continuous neuromuscular blockade for 24 hours was associated with improved survival (78% vs 41%, $P = .005$) and lactic acid clearance at 24 hours (1.3 [0.9–2.0] vs 2.9 [1.5–5.5], $P < .001$) after CA.[35]

Impaired autoregulation

Under normal physiologic conditions, CBF remains constant across a range of mean arterial pressures (MAPs) to ensure that perfusion matches metabolic demands. Cerebral autoregulation involves a process of variable vasoconstriction and vasodilation to preserve CBF within an optimal range despite variations in MAP (**Fig. 1A**).[36] Impaired blood vessel reactivity, characteristic of autoregulatory failure, can cause either progression of ischemia or hyperemia, which may in turn contribute to cerebral edema.[37] Autoregulatory failure has been detected in 35% to 78% of patients post-CA,[38–40] and is associated with worse neurologic outcomes and lower likelihood of survival.[39,41]

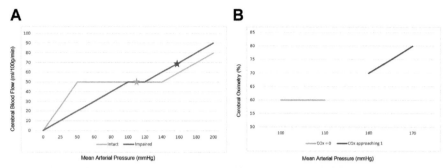

Fig. 1. Autoregulatory curve. (*A*) When autoregulation is intact (*blue line*), CBF remains constant across a wide range of MAPs. When autoregulation is impaired (*orange line* shows a right-shifted autoregulatory curve), CBF only remains constant in a narrow range of MAPs. (*B*) When autoregulation is intact (*green star* in *A*), COx is zero and rSO$_2$ remains constant despite a rise in MAP. When autoregulation fails (*red star* in *A*), COx approaches 1 because a rise in MAP is followed by a rise in rSO$_2$.

Cerebral autoregulation was assessed in 18 patients post-CA using transcranial Doppler (TCD) mean flow velocity (V$_{mean}$) in the middle cerebral artery as a proxy for CBF.[38] During a stepwise rise in MAP, achieved with titration of norepinephrine, 8 patients (44%) had absent cerebral autoregulation, 5 (28%) had a right-shifted lower limit of cerebral autoregulation, and 5 (28%) had normal cerebral autoregulation.[38] This suggests that autoregulatory failure after CA may have implications for the optimal MAP in a given individual to both achieve adequate cerebral perfusion and avoid hyperemia and subsequent cerebral edema.[38]

In the immediate post-resuscitation period, hypotension (MAP <60 or systolic blood pressure <100 mm Hg) is associated with worse neurologic outcomes and lower likelihood of survival.[42–44] Although some studies suggest improved neurologic outcomes with higher MAPs,[41,45,46] a large randomized trial of blood pressure augmentation after CA, the Neuroprotect post-CA trial,[47] showed no difference in neuroimaging evidence of HIBI (the primary outcome, determined by ADC on MRI). This trial randomized patients to an MAP of 65 mm Hg versus 85 to 100 mm Hg during the first 36 hours after CA.[47] The high MAP group had fewer adverse events, notably recurrent arrests, as well as higher cerebral oxygenation and a trend toward improved outcomes.[47] One of the limitations of this study was the broad application of MAP goals and failure to evaluate individualized perfusion targets.[47]

Inflammation

Activated endothelial cells and microglial cells, the resident macrophage of the brain, primed by ischemia and tissue injury, release reactive oxygen species, NO, and cytokines, initiating an inflammatory cascade similar to sepsis.[48] A sharp rise in inflammatory cytokines is seen as early as 3 hours after CA, and persists for several days.[49] The severity of this inflammatory response syndrome has implications for survival and neurologic outcomes. In a post hoc analysis of the Targeted Temperature Management trial,[10] levels of interleukin (IL)-6 correlated with severity of arrest (measured by doses of epinephrine required), time to ROSC, lactate levels at admission, and poor outcome.[50] In cerebral ischemia animal models, proinflammatory cytokines correlate with infarct volume.[51] The mechanism by which cytokines mediate brain, renal, and cardiovascular dysfunction in PCAS is not completely understood, and TTM, the only neuroprotective treatment after CA, has failed to demonstrate changes in inflammatory markers.[52] Tocilizumab, an IL-6 receptor antibody, is currently being evaluated for modulation of the systemic inflammatory response syndrome after CA (NCT03863015).

Cerebral edema

Derangements in ionic gradients, ensuing from cerebral ischemia, result in intracellular accumulation of sodium ions, cell swelling, loss of cytoskeletal integrity, and oncotic cell death.[53] After ROSC, reperfusion results in subsequent ionic and vasogenic edema due to loss of blood brain barrier integrity.[54] Cerebral edema, the pathologic accumulation of water within the intracellular and extracellular spaces of the brain, results in raised intracranial pressure (ICP),[55] and the subsequent decline in CBF and cerebral perfusion pressure (CPP) contribute to secondary ischemic injury.[56] Although therapeutics focused on mitigation of cerebral edema are emerging in stroke and traumatic brain injury (TBI), it is unknown if cerebral edema following CA provides a viable therapeutic target or marker of severe anoxic injury.[57]

What Is in Our Toolbox? How Can We Identify Pathophysiologic Mechanisms in Real Time?

Noninvasive neuromonitoring

Near-infrared spectroscopy. Near-infrared spectroscopy (NIRS) measures tissue absorbance of light, allowing for detection of changes in the concentration of oxygenated hemoglobin (**Fig. 2**).[58] This change in oxygenated hemoglobin allows for continuous noninvasive monitoring of cerebral oxygen saturation (rSO_2). In some studies, rSO_2 is used as a proxy for CBF. In a prospective, single-center study of 43 patients with OHCA, the main determinants of rSO_2 were MAP, partial pressure of oxygen (Pao_2), partial pressure of carbon dioxide ($Paco_2$), hematocrit, and temperature.[59] The Carbon dioxide, Oxygen and Mean Arterial pressure after Cardiac Arrest and REsuscitation (COMACARE) study was a randomized controlled trial comparing high MAP (80–100 mm Hg) versus normal-low MAP (65–75 mm Hg), moderate hyperoxia (150–188 mm Hg) versus normoxia (75–113 mm Hg), and low-normal (34–35 mm Hg) versus high-normal (43–45 mm Hg) $Paco_2$, which demonstrated significantly increased rSO_2 in the moderate hyperoxia and high-normal $Paco_2$ groups; however, no difference in rSO_2 was observed between MAP cohorts.[60,61] Although adjustment of ventilator settings to achieve brain-centered resuscitation may achieve increased rSO_2, the improvement in rSO_2 did not translate into clinical improvement; none of the prespecified clinical outcomes (neuron specific enolase, CPC 1–2 at 6 months, mortality at 3 months, hospital length of stay, and ventilator days) were achieved.[60]

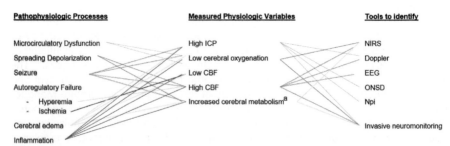

Fig. 2. Summary of pathophysiologic processes, measured physiologic variables, and tools to identify secondary brain injury in patients with CA. [a]Low glucose, high lactate, high lactate-pyruvate ratio, high glutamate, high glycerol.

The accuracy of rSO_2 as a surrogate of CBF depends on the ability to offload oxygen from hemoglobin in the microvasculature; this inability, called diffusion limitation, has been demonstrated as a pathophysiologic phenotype in HIBI.[62] In patients with diffusion limitation, the ratio of oxygenated to deoxygenated hemoglobin will be elevated, independent of CBF, limiting the accuracy of rSO_2 as a surrogate of CBF.[63] In fact, no relationship between brain tissue oxygen tension ($PbtO_2$) and rSO_2 was found in a small series of 10 patients with CA.[63,64] Furthermore, although HIBI reflects a global process, relative sparing of the frontal poles may result in falsely reassuring cerebral oximetry values; NIRS probes are placed on the forehead (where there is no hair) and only measure regional cerebral oxygenation.[65]

NIRS also can be used to detect autoregulatory failure after CA using the cerebral oximetry index (COx), a correlation coefficient derived from small changes in rSO_2 and MAP. When autoregulation is intact, rSO_2 remains constant despite changes in MAP, and thereby COx is zero or negative.[66] When COx approaches 1, this indicates a strong correlation between rSO_2 and MAP, interpreted as impaired autoregulation or MAP beyond the limits of autoregulation (**Fig. 1**B).[66,67] In a prospective study of 23 comatose patients with CA, COx was used to determine the association between impaired cerebrovascular autoregulation and outcomes after CA.[40] Seventy-eight percent of patients had impaired autoregulation, defined by COx greater than 0, between days 1 to 3 after CA, and autoregulatory failure was independently associated with mortality at 3 months (odds ratio [OR] 0.15, 95% confidence interval [0.01–0.50]).[40] A prospective observational study of 51 patients post-CA found that 35% had impaired autoregulation, identified by COx greater than 0 within the first 24 hours after CA, and patients with preexisting hypertension were especially vulnerable.[39] In this cohort, optimal MAP in those with disturbed autoregulation was at least 100 mm Hg, compared with 85 mm Hg in the preserved autoregulation group; furthermore, time spent below the individual optimal MAP goal was negatively associated with survival (OR 0.97 [0.96–0.99]).[39] An important caveat to these studies is that the validity of COx as a measure of autoregulation has not been definitively established. In a study evaluating cerebral autoregulation using pressure reactivity index (PRx) as the gold standard, COx failed to detect impairments in autoregulation, with a low area under the curve (AUC) of 0.488.[64]

Electroencephalogram. EEG monitoring after CA has increased dramatically over the past 15 years, but is still underused in centers where access is limited.[68] EEG detects nonconvulsive status epilepticus in approximately 12% to 32% of unconscious patients with CA undergoing TTM.[28,69–71] Intermittent EEG is more cost-effective than continuous EEG (cEEG); although cEEG has improved seizure detection in patients with CA[72] and results in modification of ASDs in critically ill patients with impaired consciousness,[73] this has not translated into clinical improvements, defined by CPC 1 to 2 and lower in-hospital mortality in patients with CA[72] or lower 6-month mortality in critically ill patients.[73] In an observational study of 759 comatose patients with CA, 414 patients (54.5%) developed epileptiform EEG activity and 26 (3.4%) developed potentially treatable seizures (defined as electrographic seizures and status epilepticus with continuous interictal background activity or periodic discharges >2.5 Hz with continuous background activity).[74] In this cohort, brief intermittent EEG provided comparable prognostic information to cEEG; however, it had lower sensitivity for detecting potentially treatable seizures.[74] To obtain 95% sensitivity for detection of potentially treatable seizures, patients with CA needed to be monitored for up to 53 hours.[74]

There are 3 main indications for cEEG monitoring in the intensive care unit: detection of nonconvulsive seizures or status epilepticus, prognostication, and diagnosis of ischemia.[75] EEG patterns, dichotomized into favorable (continuous) and unfavorable (isoelectric, low-voltage, or burst-suppression with identical bursts), after CA are highly predictive of neurologic outcomes[76–78]; however, the degree to which these patterns are intervenable remains unclear. Although status epilepticus may warrant aggressive treatment,[28] other malignant patterns such as burst-suppression and isoelectric background may reflect extensive anoxic injury.[77–80] The presence of epileptiform findings (defined as epileptiform transients [periodic discharges, spike wave discharges], seizures, or status epilepticus) on EEG within 72 hours after CA may be compatible with a favorable outcome.[81] A score of ≥ 2 using a novel prognostic score, NEC2RAS (No Epileptiform at 12–36 hours, Continuity $\geq 50\%$ at 12–36 hours, Reactivity at 2 timepoints [12–36 hours and 36–72 hours], normal background Amplitude at 36–72 hours, and Stimulus induced rhythmic, periodic, or ictal discharges at 36–72 hours), is 100% sensitive and 88% specific for predicting good outcome, defined as CPC 1 to 3.[81]

Quantitative EEG (qEEG) may be able to detect changes in EEG patterns that may not be identifiable with visual inspection of the raw EEG alone. qEEG is sensitive for detecting fluctuations in CBF, identified by a decrease in the alpha-delta ratio (ADR). A decline in ADR is a potential predictor of delayed cerebral ischemia in patients with subarachnoid hemorrhage (SAH)[82]; however, in a cohort of 10 comatose patients post-CA, ADRs in the first 72 hours after CA did not correlate with outcome.[83] Patients with poor outcome after CA, defined by lack of recovery of consciousness, had a graphical qEEG pattern with low or decreasing alpha and delta frequencies, as well as lower total power over 48 hours.[83] In a larger study of 138 comatose patients following CA, lower spectral power in the alpha and theta frequency ranges (5.2–13.2 Hz) within the first 24 hours after CA was highly specific for predicting unfavorable outcomes (CPC 3–5) at 3 months after CA.[84] However, EEG slowing that translates into worsening ADRs is a nonspecific finding, which could be a result of several different mechanisms and thus lacks specificity for ischemia. qEEG has the potential to identify early signs of secondary brain injury; however, further work is needed to advance our understanding of the utility of qEEG for ischemia monitoring, identification of epileptiform activity, and prognostication in the CA population.[85]

Transcranial Doppler. TCD sonography emits a high-frequency sound wave that resonates off moving red blood cells and is reflected back to the transducer, providing an estimate of the velocity of blood flow. TCDs can be performed at the bedside, but are highly operator-dependent and may be challenging to perform due to poor acoustic windows in up to 20% of patients.[86] Mean flow velocity (V_{mean}) can be used as a surrogate for CBF when the cross-sectional area of the blood vessel being measured remains constant; however, changes in blood vessel area, as seen in cerebral vasospasm, result in changes in V_{mean} that are independent of CBF.[87] Another physiologic variable assessed with TCDs is the pulsatility index (PI); calculated as the difference between systolic and diastolic flow velocities divided by the mean velocity, it reflects resistance in the vascular system.[88] PI has been evaluated as a proxy of ICP; Bellner and colleagues[89] found a strong correlation between PI and invasive ICP measurements; however, this has not been replicated.[90] TCDs only evaluate changes in arterial flow dynamics, and ICP may be affected by changes in arterial inflow, venous outflow, cerebral spinal fluid dynamics, and brain parenchymal volume[90]; therefore, PI only reflects ICP under select circumstances. Finally, TCD provides a static evaluation of CBF and ICP, which is constantly changing, and the trend over time may provide more valuable information regarding cerebral hemodynamics.[91]

In a cohort of 18 patients with OHCA treated with TTM, TCDs and measurements of cerebral oxygen extraction (CEO_2), obtained using retrograde jugular catheterization, were performed every 12 hours for 72 hours after CA to evaluate the cerebral supply-demand mismatch.[92] Shortly after CA admission, TCDs showed low V_{mean} (27.3 [21.5–33.6] cm/s) and high PI (1.6 [1.3–1.9]), which slowly normalized over 72 hours, whereas CEO_2 was normal at admission but decreased over 72 hours.[91] Furthermore, the decline in CEO_2 was almost fivefold higher in patients who did not survive to hospital discharge (25.8% [19.3–31.1] vs 5.7% [5.1–11.5], $P = .02$).[91] This suggests that CBF is low 12 hours after CA and improves over the subsequent 72 hours, whereas the cerebral metabolic rate decreases over 72 hours, likely influenced by hypothermia and HIBI,[91] creating a state of luxury perfusion.[93] The Early Transcranial Doppler Goal-Directed Therapy after Cardiac Arrest (GOODYEAR) study (NCT04000443) is currently using TCDs to evaluate the impact of MAP augmentation in response to cerebral hypoperfusion (defined as V_{mean} <30 cm/s, end-diastolic velocity <20 cm/s, and PI >1.4) during the first 12 hours after CA. This trial will provide important insights into early cerebral metabolism and blood flow after CA, as well as the use of TCDs to identify patients requiring interventions aimed at optimal CPP. Although cerebral autoregulatory curves can be assessed using TCDs,[38] this ideally requires continuous TCD measurements and the use of a probe helmet, which may not be feasible at most centers.

Optic nerve sheath diameter. The optic nerve complex contains the optic nerve sheath, the optic nerve, and subarachnoid space; increases in ICP are transmitted to the orbit, resulting in expansion of the optic nerve sheath diameter (ONSD).[94] Transorbital ultrasound is easily learned, low cost, and has high intraobserver agreement.[95,96] In 11 patients with CA with invasive ICP monitoring, ONSD ≥5.95 mm identified ICP ≥20 mm Hg with a sensitivity of 86%, specificity of 100%, and AUC 0.96 [95% CI limits 0.90–1.00].[97] In a prospective study of patients following CA, ONSD was assessed at 12, 24, and 48 hours after CA; ONSD ≥5.75 mm at 12 hours after CA predicted mortality with a sensitivity of 60% and specificity of 100%.[98] As a potential screening tool, ONSD may be helpful for detecting intracranial hypertension.

Neurologic pupil index. Automated pupillometry is a quantitative infrared system that tracks and analyzes the pupillary light response dynamics, and can provide objective data regarding pupil reactivity.[99] The neurologic pupil index (NPi) is an automated composite score of multiple variables, including minimum and maximum pupillary size, percentage constriction, latency, constriction velocity, maximum constriction velocity, and dilation velocity.[99] An NPi ≥3 indicates that pupil reactivity is within the normal distribution.[99] In a prospective study of patients with TBI, SAH, or intraparenchymal hemorrhage, the peak ICP in patients with an NPi less than 3 was higher than in patients with an NPi ≥3 (30.5 mm Hg vs 19.6 mm Hg, $P<.0014$).[99] In a cohort of 456 prospectively enrolled comatose patients with CA, an NPi ≤2 at any timepoint between day 1 and 3 after CA predicted unfavorable outcome, defined as CPC 3 to 5, with a sensitivity of 32% and specificity of 100%.[100] Automated pupillometry improved the prognostic value of standard manual pupillary light reflex testing, which was found to have a false positive rate of 10% on days 1 to 2 and 6% on day 3 post-CA.[100]

Invasive neuromonitoring
Invasive multimodal monitoring allows for direct, focal measurement of ICP, CBF, cerebrovascular autoregulation, partial pressure of brain tissue oxygen, cerebral metabolites (as measured by cerebral microdialysis), brain temperature, and electrocorticography.

Intracranial pressure. CPP is the net pressure gradient resulting in brain perfusion and is calculated as the MAP minus ICP. Direct measurement of ICP is accomplished most commonly through an external ventricular drain or an intraparenchymal monitor. In a study of 84 patients after CA monitored with an intracranial monitor, ICP greater than 25 mm Hg was present in 21.4% of patients on day 1 post-CA and 26.3% on day 2, and CPP less than 50 mm Hg was present in 39% of patients on day 1 and 55.9% on day 2.[101] Patients who survived to hospital discharge had lower ICP and higher CPP values.[101] In the setting of poor intracranial compliance, small changes in cerebral volume, due to development of cerebral edema, will lead to large changes in ICP. Continuous ICP monitoring allows for early identification of intracranial hypertension and strict control of CPP, despite a rise in ICP.[57]

The pressure reactivity index (PRx), a correlation coefficient between MAP and ICP, can be used to derive optimal MAP (MAP$_{OPT}$), the pressure needed to obtain adequate cerebral perfusion, without driving up ICP. In a prospective study of 10 patients with CA with invasive multimodal monitoring, PbtO$_2$ increased as the patients' MAP approached MAP$_{OPT}$; however, when MAP rose above MAP$_{OPT}$, this relationship did not persist.[102] This highlights the need for individualized blood pressure goals; raising MAP beyond the optimal goal for an individual patient may expose them to risks associated with vasopressor use, without clear physiologic benefit.[102]

Brain tissue oxygen tension. The most commonly used technology for measuring brain tissue oxygen tension (PbtO$_2$) is based on the Clark polarographic electrode; inside the probe, the cathode and anode are immersed in an electrolyte solution separated by a membrane, and measured current directly correlates with Pao$_2$.[103] A PbtO$_2$ less than 20 mm Hg represents compromised brain oxygenation; the Multidisciplinary Consensus Conference on Multimodality Monitoring in Neurocritical Care recommends interventions aimed at raising PbtO$_2$ above this threshold.[104]

In a swine model of CA, 10 swine were randomized to standard care (blinded to PbtO$_2$) versus titrated care in response to PbtO$_2$ values <20 mm Hg (100% fraction of inspired oxygen [Fio$_2$] for 10 minutes followed by increasing MAP by 20 mm Hg [if no rise in PbtO$_2$ >20 mm Hg with increased Fio$_2$] for 10 minutes).[105] Brain tissue hypoxia, defined as PbtO$_2$ less than 20 mm Hg, was common during standard care, occurring in 44% compared with only 2% in those with titrated care.[105] A rise in PbtO$_2$ was associated with higher ADR, suggesting that goal-directed therapy may mitigate secondary injury.[105]

Cerebral microdialysis. Cerebral microdialysis uses a fine double-lumen probe lined with a semipermeable dialysis membrane to determine the relative concentrations of lactate, pyruvate, glutamate, glucose, and glycerol in the brain. Monitoring of brain tissue biochemistry may allow for understanding of local ischemia, delivery and utilization of glucose, and excitotoxicity. The aim of using microdialysis is early identification of secondary injury to allow for implementation of neuroprotective strategies.[106] In a cohort of 10 patients post-CA, lactate:pyruvate ratio (LPR) did not differentiate outcome groups on day 1 post-CA (37 [30–40] versus 36 [26–52]; $P = .99$); however, patients with unfavorable outcome (defined as CPC 3–5 30 days after CA) had a progressive rise in LPR to values >40, which persisted between days 2 and 4 after CA, suggesting ongoing ischemia in patients with unfavorable outcomes.[107] In a small cohort of 4 patients post-CA treated with TTM, LPRs and glutamate levels were highest immediately after CA and during rewarming, suggesting that these 2 periods pose the greatest risk for secondary injury.[108]

Electrocorticography. Intracranial EEG has been used as part of invasive multimodal monitoring in SAH, TBI, and rarely CA, and uses a single electrode inserted into the brain parenchyma, also called a depth electrode.[109–111] Intracranial EEG can detect SDs and epileptiform activity not apparent on surface EEG,[110] and may be used in concert with other invasive monitors to detect physiologic consequences of epileptiform activity or seizures.[109–111]

There are several potential complications associated with invasive multimodal monitoring, including infection, technical failure, limitation of diagnostic testing (not compatible with MRI), and intracranial hemorrhage.[112] Given the risk profile and

Table 2
Summary of neuromonitoring tools

Neuromonitoring Tool	Physiology	Advantages	Disadvantages
NIRS	Cerebral oxygenation Cerebral autoregulation	Noninvasive Continuous monitoring Does not require skilled technician	Regional assessment Artifact may affect interpretation
EEG	Seizures/Status epilepticus Ischemia monitoring Cerebral metabolic state	Noninvasive Continuous monitoring Quantitative analysis provides an opportunity for machine learning	Requires skilled technician and interpretation Time-consuming
TCD	Relative cerebral blood flow Cerebral autoregulation	Noninvasive	Requires skilled technician and interpretation May be technically challenging
ONSD	Proxy of ICP	Noninvasive	Requires skilled technician May only provide supplemental information
NPi	Proxy of ICP	Noninvasive Easy to use	May only provide supplemental information
Intracranial ICP sensor	ICP CPP	Gold standard for measurement of ICP and CPP continuous	Invasive Complications can arise Regional assessment
PbtO$_2$	Cerebral oxygenation Cerebral autoregulation	Gold standard for measurement of cerebral oxygenation and autoregulation Allows for assessment of balance between oxygen delivery and demand Continuous	Invasive Complications can arise Regional assessment
Microdialysis	Cerebral metabolism	Allows for early detection of ischemia Allows for monitoring of cerebral metabolic state (energy failure, metabolic stress)	Focal measure Uncertain thresholds Invasive Complications can arise

Abbreviations: CPP, cerebral perfusion pressure; EEG, electroencephalography; ICP, intracranial pressure; NIRS, near-infrared spectroscopy; NPi, neurological pupil index; ONSD, optic nerve sheath diameter; PbtO$_2$, brain tissue oxygen tension, TCD, transcranial Doppler.

lack of high-grade evidence for use of invasive multimodal monitoring in patients with CA, invasive monitoring post-arrest is not currently commonly used except in specialized centers, and often only as part of a research study. **Table 2** has a summary of the available neuromonitoring tools, including the physiology assessed, advantages, and limitations of each tool.

FUTURE DIRECTIONS

There are no guidelines on how to integrate multimodal monitoring data in patients with CA to improve management. Appropriate patient selection is crucial. The ideal candidates for multimodal monitoring are patients for whom identification of cerebral metabolic distress will result in modification of treatment and prevention of secondary brain injury. Although multimodal monitoring may not improve outcomes in patients with severe HIBI, the data may be used to assist with neuroprognostication.

After a patient is selected for multimodal monitoring, physiologic variables must be interpreted in the context of patient-specific parameters, and no single data point should be used in isolation to make care decisions. For example, generalized periodic discharges may result in metabolic crisis for one patient, but may not be clinically relevant in another; in this case, markers of metabolic stress, such as $PbtO_2$, LPR, and ICP may be useful. Protocols for implementation of multimodal monitoring and consensus for actionable values are needed.

To develop protocols for invasive multimodal monitoring after CA, it is critical to determine if the data obtained from multimodal monitoring improves medical practice and patient outcomes. There are 4 important questions to be asked in a controlled clinical trial design:

1. Can physiologic changes putting the patient at risk for secondary neuronal injury be identified using multimodal monitoring?
2. Can progression to secondary injury be mitigated by changes in management in response to multimodal monitoring data?
3. In patients monitored with multimodal monitoring, can overall survival and neurologic outcomes be improved?
4. Is there a specific population of patients post-CA who might benefit from multimodal monitoring?

Similar to work in TBI,[113] a multicenter, parallel-group trial, with randomized assignment to multimodal monitoring versus standard care is a necessary first step to identify the utility of invasive multimodal monitoring in patients post-CA.

SUMMARY

There are many pathophysiologic mechanisms of secondary injury after global cerebral ischemia, and our current model of using a "one-size-fits-all" treatment approach is archaic. The Consensus Summary Statement of the International Multidisciplinary Consensus Conference on Multimodality Monitoring in Neurocritical Care[104] recommends ICP and CPP monitoring for those at risk of raised ICP, continuous bedside monitoring of autoregulation, brain tissue oxygen monitoring in patients at risk for cerebral ischemia, and cerebral microdialysis in patients at risk of cerebral ischemia, hypoxia, energy failure, and glucose deprivation.[104] Although these guidelines do not directly pertain to CA, PCAS may be the ideal population for multimodality monitoring given the relative homogeneity of brain injury and heterogeneity in systemic hemodynamics. The relatively homogeneous nature of brain injury in HIBI makes the location of parenchymal monitor placement less critical than in other acute brain injury phenotypes, such as in TBI, where probe location may not accurately reflect important changes remote from the probe location.[114]

Individualized monitoring may provide relevant data for identifying CA endotypes, key for appropriate patient selection into clinical trials. For example, hemodynamic augmentation may not improve brain hypoxia in patients with diffusion limitation.[115] Patients with an isoelectric EEG, with no evidence of improvement after 36 hours, may have a low likelihood of a positive outcome, regardless of the treatment. Broad enrollment of patients with CA in clinical trials may fail to identify therapeutic opportunities. Multimodal monitoring may also be beneficial for confirming mechanisms of new drug targets.

CONCLUSIONS

Invasive and noninvasive multimodal monitoring of patients post-CA increases our understanding of the pathophysiologic mechanisms underlying secondary brain injury, as well as the degree of variability between patients. It is the ideal time to leave clinical nihilism behind and reevaluate post-CA management in the era of multimodal monitoring. Identification of subgroups that have a reasonable likelihood of achieving a good outcome if not for withdrawal of life-sustaining therapy and those who will respond to physiologic augmentation or neuroprotective strategies will be key in designing future clinical trials.

CLINICS CARE POINTS

- Invasive and noninvasive neuromonitoring provides insights into cerebral physiology, allowing an individualized approach to patient care.

- The degree of secondary brain injury, caused by an imbalance between cerebral metabolic demand and oxygen and glucose supply, is modifiable.

- Identification of secondary injury risk profiles, using neuromonitoring tools, may be key to evaluating therapeutic targets.

- Protocols for clinical implementation of noninvasive and invasive neuromonitoring and consensus for actionable values in the CA population are warranted.

DISCLOSURE

All authors have nothing to disclose.

REFERENCES

1. Sandroni C, Nolan J, Cavallaro F, et al. In-hospital cardiac arrest: incidence, prognosis and possible measures to improve survival. Intensive Care Med 2007;33(2):237–45.
2. Nolan JP, Soar J, Smith GB, et al. Incidence and outcome of in-hospital cardiac arrest in the United Kingdom National Cardiac Arrest Audit. Resuscitation 2014; 85(8):987–92.
3. Berdowski J, Berg RA, Tijssen JG, et al. Global incidences of out-of-hospital cardiac arrest and survival rates: systematic review of 67 prospective studies. Resuscitation 2010;81(11):1479–87.
4. Soholm H, Hassager C, Lippert F, et al. Factors associated with successful resuscitation after out-of-hospital cardiac arrest and temporal trends in survival and comorbidity. Ann Emerg Med 2015;65(5):523–31.e2.

5. Skrifvars MB, Rosenberg PH, Finne P, et al. Evaluation of the in-hospital Utstein template in cardiopulmonary resuscitation in secondary hospitals. Resuscitation 2003;56(3):275–82.

6. Virani SS, Alonso A, Benjamin EJ, et al. Heart disease and stroke statistics-2020 update: a report from the American Heart Association. Circulation 2020;141(9): e139–596.

7. Sekhon MS, Ainslie PN, Griesdale DE. Clinical pathophysiology of hypoxic ischemic brain injury after cardiac arrest: a "two-hit" model. Crit Care 2017; 21(1):90.

8. Mild therapeutic hypothermia to improve the neurologic outcome after cardiac arrest. N Engl J Med 2002;346(8):549–56.

9. Bernard SA, Gray TW, Buist MD, et al. Treatment of comatose survivors of out-of-hospital cardiac arrest with induced hypothermia. N Engl J Med 2002;346(8): 557–63.

10. Nielsen N, Wetterslev J, Cronberg T, et al. Targeted temperature management at 33 degrees C versus 36 degrees C after cardiac arrest. N Engl J Med 2013; 369(23):2197–206.

11. Lascarrou JB, Merdji H, Le Gouge A, et al. Targeted temperature management for cardiac arrest with nonshockable rhythm. N Engl J Med 2019;381(24): 2327–37.

12. Belanger M, Allaman I, Magistretti PJ. Brain energy metabolism: focus on astrocyte-neuron metabolic cooperation. Cell Metab 2011;14(6):724–38.

13. Busl KM, Greer DM. Hypoxic-ischemic brain injury: pathophysiology, neuropathology and mechanisms. NeuroRehabilitation 2010;26(1):5–13.

14. Leao AA. Further observations on the spreading depression of activity in the cerebral cortex. J Neurophysiol 1947;10(6):409–14.

15. Dreier JP. The role of spreading depression, spreading depolarization and spreading ischemia in neurological disease. Nat Med 2011;17(4):439–47.

16. Krnjević K. Electrophysiology of cerebral ischemia. Neuropharmacology 2008; 55(3):319–33.

17. Reffelmann T, Kloner RA. The "no-reflow" phenomenon: basic science and clinical correlates. Heart 2002;87(2):162–8.

18. Kurose I, Wolf R, Grisham MB, et al. Modulation of ischemia/reperfusion-induced microvascular dysfunction by nitric oxide. Circ Res 1994;74(3):376–82.

19. Fischer M, Bottiger BW, Popov-Cenic S, et al. Thrombolysis using plasminogen activator and heparin reduces cerebral no-reflow after resuscitation from cardiac arrest: an experimental study in the cat. Intensive Care Med 1996;22(11): 1214–23.

20. Böttiger BW, Arntz HR, Chamberlain DA, et al. Thrombolysis during resuscitation for out-of-hospital cardiac arrest. N Engl J Med 2008;359(25):2651–62.

21. Lybeck A, Friberg H, Aneman A, et al. Prognostic significance of clinical seizures after cardiac arrest and target temperature management. Resuscitation 2017;114:146–51.

22. Knight WA, Hart KW, Adeoye OM, et al. The incidence of seizures in patients undergoing therapeutic hypothermia after resuscitation from cardiac arrest. Epilepsy Res 2013;106(3):396–402.

23. Meldrum BCA. Metabolic consequences of seizures. In: Siegel GJ, Agranoff BW, Albers RW, et al, editors. Basic neurochemistry: molecular, cellular and medical aspects. 6th edition. Philadelphia: Lippincott-Raven; 1999.

24. Wasterlain CG, Fujikawa DG, Penix L, et al. Pathophysiological mechanisms of brain damage from status epilepticus. Epilepsia 1993;34(Suppl 1):S37–53.

25. Yager JY, Armstrong EA, Miyashita H, et al. Prolonged neonatal seizures exacerbate hypoxic-ischemic brain damage: correlation with cerebral energy metabolism and excitatory amino acid release. Dev Neurosci 2002;24(5):367–81.

26. Björkman ST, Miller SM, Rose SE, et al. Seizures are associated with brain injury severity in a neonatal model of hypoxia-ischemia. Neuroscience 2010;166(1): 157–67.

27. Mayer SA, Claassen J, Lokin J, et al. Refractory status epilepticus: frequency, risk factors, and impact on outcome. Arch Neurol 2002;59(2):205–10.

28. Beretta S, Coppo A, Bianchi E, et al. Neurological outcome of postanoxic refractory status epilepticus after aggressive treatment. Epilepsy Behav 2019;101(Pt B):106374.

29. Ruijter BJ, van Putten MJ, Horn J, et al. Treatment of electroencephalographic status epilepticus after cardiopulmonary resuscitation (TELSTAR): study protocol for a randomized controlled trial. Trials 2014;15:433.

30. Gebhardt K, Guyette FX, Doshi AA, et al. Prevalence and effect of fever on outcome following resuscitation from cardiac arrest. Resuscitation 2013;84(8): 1062–7.

31. Bro-Jeppesen J, Hassager C, Wanscher M, et al. Post-hypothermia fever is associated with increased mortality after out-of-hospital cardiac arrest. Resuscitation 2013;84(12):1734–40.

32. Oddo M, Frangos S, Milby A, et al. Induced normothermia attenuates cerebral metabolic distress in patients with aneurysmal subarachnoid hemorrhage and refractory Fever. Stroke 2009;40(5):1913–6.

33. Badjatia N, Strongilis E, Gordon E, et al. Metabolic impact of shivering during therapeutic temperature modulation: the Bedside Shivering Assessment Scale. Stroke 2008;39(12):3242–7.

34. Jain A, Gray M, Slisz S, et al. Shivering treatments for targeted temperature management: a review. J Neurosci Nurs 2018;50(2):63–7.

35. Salciccioli JD, Cocchi MN, Rittenberger JC, et al. Continuous neuromuscular blockade is associated with decreased mortality in post-cardiac arrest patients. Resuscitation 2013;84(12):1728–33.

36. Pires PW, Dams Ramos CM, Matin N, et al. The effects of hypertension on the cerebral circulation. Am J Physiol Heart Circ Physiol 2013;304(12):H1598–614.

37. Jordan JD, Powers WJ. Cerebral autoregulation and acute ischemic stroke. Am J Hypertens 2012;25(9):946–50.

38. Sundgreen C, Larsen FS, Herzog TM, et al. Autoregulation of cerebral blood flow in patients resuscitated from cardiac arrest. Stroke 2001;32(1):128–32.

39. Ameloot K, Genbrugge C, Meex I, et al. An observational near-infrared spectroscopy study on cerebral autoregulation in post-cardiac arrest patients: time to drop 'one-size-fits-all' hemodynamic targets? Resuscitation 2015;90:121–6.

40. Pham P, Bindra J, Chuan A, et al. Are changes in cerebrovascular autoregulation following cardiac arrest associated with neurological outcome? Results of a pilot study. Resuscitation 2015;96:192–8.

41. Kilgannon JH, Roberts BW, Jones AE, et al. Arterial blood pressure and neurologic outcome after resuscitation from cardiac arrest*. Crit Care Med 2014; 42(9):2083–91.

42. Kilgannon JH, Roberts BW, Reihl LR, et al. Early arterial hypotension is common in the post-cardiac arrest syndrome and associated with increased in-hospital mortality. Resuscitation 2008;79(3):410–6.

43. Topjian AA, French B, Sutton RM, et al. Early postresuscitation hypotension is associated with increased mortality following pediatric cardiac arrest. Crit Care Med 2014;42(6):1518–23.

44. Kaji AH, Hanif AM, Thomas JL, et al. Out-of-hospital cardiac arrest: early in-hospital hypotension versus out-of-hospital factors in predicting in-hospital mortality among those surviving to hospital admission. Resuscitation 2011;82(10): 1314–7.

45. Bhate TD, McDonald B, Sekhon MS, et al. Association between blood pressure and outcomes in patients after cardiac arrest: a systematic review. Resuscitation 2015;97:1–6.

46. Roberts BW, Kilgannon JH, Hunter BR, et al. Association between elevated mean arterial blood pressure and neurologic outcome after resuscitation from cardiac arrest: results from a multicenter prospective cohort study. Crit Care Med 2019;47(1):93–100.

47. Ameloot K, De Deyne C, Eertmans W, et al. Early goal-directed haemodynamic optimization of cerebral oxygenation in comatose survivors after cardiac arrest: the Neuroprotect post-cardiac arrest trial. Eur Heart J 2019;40(22):1804–14.

48. Xiang Y, Zhao H, Wang J, et al. Inflammatory mechanisms involved in brain injury following cardiac arrest and cardiopulmonary resuscitation. Biomed Rep 2016;5(1):11–7.

49. Adrie C, Laurent I, Monchi M, et al. Postresuscitation disease after cardiac arrest: a sepsis-like syndrome? Curr Opin Crit Care 2004;10(3):208–12.

50. Bro-Jeppesen J, Kjaergaard J, Wanscher M, et al. Systemic inflammatory response and potential prognostic implications after out-of-hospital cardiac arrest: a substudy of the target temperature management trial. Crit Care Med 2015;43(6):1223–32.

51. Pantoni L, Sarti C, Inzitari D. Cytokines and cell adhesion molecules in cerebral ischemia: experimental bases and therapeutic perspectives. Arterioscler Thromb Vasc Biol 1998;18(4):503–13.

52. Jou C, Shah R, Figueroa A, et al. The role of inflammatory cytokines in cardiac arrest. J Intensive Care Med 2020;35(3):219–24.

53. Kahle KT, Simard JM, Staley KJ, et al. Molecular mechanisms of ischemic cerebral edema: role of electroneutral ion transport. Physiology (Bethesda) 2009;24: 257–65.

54. Stokum JA, Gerzanich V, Simard JM. Molecular pathophysiology of cerebral edema. J Cereb Blood Flow Metab 2016;36(3):513–38.

55. Wilson MH. Monro-Kellie 2.0: the dynamic vascular and venous pathophysiological components of intracranial pressure. J Cereb Blood Flow Metab 2016;36(8): 1338–50.

56. Rodríguez-Boto G, Rivero-Garvía M, Gutiérrez-González R, et al. Basic concepts about brain pathophysiology and intracranial pressure monitoring. Neurologia 2015;30(1):16–22.

57. Hayman EG, Patel AP, Kimberly WT, et al. Cerebral edema after cardiopulmonary resuscitation: a therapeutic target following cardiac arrest? Neurocrit Care 2018;28(3):276–87.

58. Villringer A, Planck J, Hock C, et al. Near infrared spectroscopy (NIRS): a new tool to study hemodynamic changes during activation of brain function in human adults. Neurosci Lett 1993;154(1–2):101–4.

59. Bouglé A, Daviaud F, Bougouin W, et al. Determinants and significance of cerebral oximetry after cardiac arrest: a prospective cohort study. Resuscitation 2016;99:1–6.

60. Jakkula P, Reinikainen M, Hastbacka J, et al. Targeting two different levels of both arterial carbon dioxide and arterial oxygen after cardiac arrest and resuscitation: a randomised pilot trial. Intensive Care Med 2018;44(12):2112–21.

61. Jakkula P, Pettilä V, Skrifvars MB, et al. Targeting low-normal or high-normal mean arterial pressure after cardiac arrest and resuscitation: a randomised pilot trial. Intensive Care Med 2018;44(12):2091–101.

62. Sekhon MS, Ainslie PN, Menon DK, et al. Brain hypoxia secondary to diffusion limitation in hypoxic ischemic brain injury postcardiac arrest. Crit Care Med 2020;48(3):378–84.

63. Hoiland RL, Griesdale DE, Sekhon MS. Assessing autoregulation using near infrared spectroscopy: more questions than answers. Resuscitation 2020;156: 280–1.

64. Hoiland RL, Sekhon MS, Cardim D, et al. Lack of agreement between optimal mean arterial pressure determination using pressure reactivity index versus cerebral oximetry index in hypoxic ischemic brain injury after cardiac arrest. Resuscitation 2020;152:184–91.

65. Tosh W, Patteril M. Cerebral oximetry. BJA Educ 2016;16(12):417–21.

66. Steppan J, Hogue CW Jr. Cerebral and tissue oximetry. Best Pract Res Clin Anaesthesiol 2014;28(4):429–39.

67. Moerman A, De Hert S. Recent advances in cerebral oximetry. Assessment of cerebral autoregulation with near-infrared spectroscopy: myth or reality? F1000Res 2017;6:1615.

68. Rush B, Ashkanani M, Romano K, et al. Utilization of electroencephalogram post cardiac arrest in the United States: a nationwide retrospective cohort analysis. Resuscitation 2017;110:141–5.

69. Rittenberger JC, Popescu A, Brenner RP, et al. Frequency and timing of nonconvulsive status epilepticus in comatose post-cardiac arrest subjects treated with hypothermia. Neurocrit Care 2012;16(1):114–22.

70. Dragancea I, Backman S, Westhall E, et al. Outcome following postanoxic status epilepticus in patients with targeted temperature management after cardiac arrest. Epilepsy Behav 2015;49:173–7.

71. Amorim E, van der Stoel M, Nagaraj SB, et al. Quantitative EEG reactivity and machine learning for prognostication in hypoxic-ischemic brain injury. Clin Neurophysiol 2019;130(10):1908–16.

72. Crepeau AZ, Fugate JE, Mandrekar J, et al. Value analysis of continuous EEG in patients during therapeutic hypothermia after cardiac arrest. Resuscitation 2014;85(6):785–9.

73. Rossetti AO, Schindler K, Sutter R, et al. Continuous vs routine electroencephalogram in critically ill adults with altered consciousness and no recent seizure: a multicenter randomized clinical trial. JAMA Neurol 2020;77(10):1–8.

74. Elmer J, Coppler PJ, Solanki P, et al. Sensitivity of continuous electroencephalography to detect ictal activity after cardiac arrest. JAMA Netw Open 2020; 3(4):e203751.

75. Caricato A, Melchionda I, Antonelli M. Continuous electroencephalography monitoring in adults in the intensive care unit. Crit Care 2018;22(1):75.

76. Sondag L, Ruijter BJ, Tjepkema-Cloostermans MC, et al. Early EEG for outcome prediction of postanoxic coma: prospective cohort study with cost-minimization analysis. Crit Care 2017;21(1):111.

77. Hofmeijer J, Beernink TM, Bosch FH, et al. Early EEG contributes to multimodal outcome prediction of postanoxic coma. Neurology 2015;85(2):137–43.

78. Sivaraju A, Gilmore EJ, Wira CR, et al. Prognostication of post-cardiac arrest coma: early clinical and electroencephalographic predictors of outcome. Intensive Care Med 2015;41(7):1264–72.

79. Ruijter BJ, Tjepkema-Cloostermans MC, Tromp SC, et al. Early electroencephalography for outcome prediction of postanoxic coma: a prospective cohort study. Ann Neurol 2019;86(2):203–14.

80. Scarpino M, Lolli F, Lanzo G, et al. Neurophysiology and neuroimaging accurately predict poor neurological outcome within 24 hours after cardiac arrest: the ProNeCA prospective multicentre prognostication study. Resuscitation 2019;143:115–23.

81. Barbella G, Lee JW, Alvarez V, et al. Prediction of regaining consciousness despite an early epileptiform EEG after cardiac arrest. Neurology 2020;94(16): e1675–83.

82. Yu Z, Wen D, Zheng J, et al. Predictive accuracy of alpha-delta ratio on quantitative electroencephalography for delayed cerebral ischemia in patients with aneurysmal subarachnoid hemorrhage: meta-analysis. World Neurosurg 2019; 126:e510–6.

83. Wiley SL, Razavi B, Krishnamohan P, et al. Quantitative EEG metrics differ between outcome groups and change over the first 72 h in comatose cardiac arrest patients. Neurocrit Care 2018;28(1):51–9.

84. Kustermann T, Nguepnjo Nguissi NA, Pfeiffer C, et al. Electroencephalography-based power spectra allow coma outcome prediction within 24 h of cardiac arrest. Resuscitation 2019;142:162–7.

85. Elmer J, Rittenberger JC. Quantitative EEG after cardiac arrest: new insights from an old technology. Resuscitation 2019;142:184–5.

86. Sarkar S, Ghosh S, Ghosh SK, et al. Role of transcranial Doppler ultrasonography in stroke. Postgrad Med J 2007;83(985):683–9.

87. Blanco P, Abdo-Cuza A. Transcranial Doppler ultrasound in neurocritical care. J Ultrasound 2018;21(1):1–16.

88. de Riva N, Budohoski KP, Smielewski P, et al. Transcranial Doppler pulsatility index: what it is and what it isn't. Neurocrit Care 2012;17(1):58–66.

89. Bellner J, Romner B, Reinstrup P, et al. Transcranial Doppler sonography pulsatility index (PI) reflects intracranial pressure (ICP). Surg Neurol 2004;62(1):45–51 [discussion: 51].

90. Cardim D, Robba C, Bohdanowicz M, et al. Non-invasive monitoring of intracranial pressure using transcranial doppler ultrasonography: is it possible? Neurocrit Care 2016;25(3):473–91.

91. Lau VI, Arntfield RT. Point-of-care transcranial Doppler by intensivists. Crit Ultrasound J 2017;9(1):21.

92. Lemiale V, Huet O, Vigue B, et al. Changes in cerebral blood flow and oxygen extraction during post-resuscitation syndrome. Resuscitation 2008;76(1):17–24.

93. Lassen NA. The luxury perfusion syndrome. Scand J Clin Lab Invest Suppl 1968;102:X. A.

94. Soldatos T, Chatzimichail K, Papathanasiou M, et al. Optic nerve sonography: a new window for the non-invasive evaluation of intracranial pressure in brain injury. Emerg Med J 2009;26(9):630–4.

95. Bauerle J, Lochner P, Kaps M, et al. Intra- and interobsever reliability of sonographic assessment of the optic nerve sheath diameter in healthy adults. J Neuroimaging 2012;22(1):42–5.

96. Ballantyne SA, O'Neill G, Hamilton R, et al. Observer variation in the sonographic measurement of optic nerve sheath diameter in normal adults. Eur J Ultrasound 2002;15(3):145–9.

97. Cardim D, Griesdale DE, Ainslie PN, et al. A comparison of non-invasive versus invasive measures of intracranial pressure in hypoxic ischaemic brain injury after cardiac arrest. Resuscitation 2019;137:221–8.

98. Ertl M, Weber S, Hammel G, et al. Transorbital sonography for early prognostication of hypoxic-ischemic encephalopathy after cardiac arrest. J Neuroimaging 2018;28(5):542–8.

99. Chen JW, Gombart ZJ, Rogers S, et al. Pupillary reactivity as an early indicator of increased intracranial pressure: the introduction of the Neurological Pupil index. Surg Neurol Int 2011;2:82.

100. Oddo M, Sandroni C, Citerio G, et al. Quantitative versus standard pupillary light reflex for early prognostication in comatose cardiac arrest patients: an international prospective multicenter double-blinded study. Intensive Care Med 2018; 44(12):2102–11.

101. Gueugniaud PY, Garcia-Darennes F, Gaussorgues P, et al. Prognostic significance of early intracranial and cerebral perfusion pressures in post-cardiac arrest anoxic coma. Intensive Care Med 1991;17(7):392–8.

102. Sekhon MS, Gooderham P, Menon DK, et al. The burden of brain hypoxia and optimal mean arterial pressure in patients with hypoxic ischemic brain injury after cardiac arrest. Crit Care Med 2019;47(7):960–9.

103. Stewart C, Haitsma I, Zador Z, et al. The new Licox combined brain tissue oxygen and brain temperature monitor: assessment of in vitro accuracy and clinical experience in severe traumatic brain injury. Neurosurgery 2008;63(6):1159–64 [discussion: 1164–5].

104. Le Roux P, Menon DK, Citerio G, et al. Consensus summary statement of the International Multidisciplinary Consensus Conference on Multimodality Monitoring in Neurocritical Care: a statement for healthcare professionals from the Neurocritical Care Society and the European Society of Intensive Care Medicine. Neurocrit Care 2014;21(Suppl 2):S1–26.

105. Elmer J, Flickinger KL, Anderson MW, et al. Effect of neuromonitor-guided titrated care on brain tissue hypoxia after opioid overdose cardiac arrest. Resuscitation 2018;129:121–6.

106. Tisdall MM, Smith M. Cerebral microdialysis: research technique or clinical tool. Br J Anaesth 2006;97(1):18–25.

107. Hifumi T, Kawakita K, Yoda T, et al. Association of brain metabolites with blood lactate and glucose levels with respect to neurological outcomes after out-of-hospital cardiac arrest: a preliminary microdialysis study. Resuscitation 2017; 110:26–31.

108. Nordmark J, Rubertsson S, Mortberg E, et al. Intracerebral monitoring in comatose patients treated with hypothermia after a cardiac arrest. Acta Anaesthesiol Scand 2009;53(3):289–98.

109. Witsch J, Frey HP, Schmidt JM, et al. Electroencephalographic periodic discharges and frequency-dependent brain tissue hypoxia in acute brain injury. JAMA Neurol 2017;74(3):301–9.

110. Vespa P, Tubi M, Claassen J, et al. Metabolic crisis occurs with seizures and periodic discharges after brain trauma. Ann Neurol 2016;79(4):579–90.

111. Ko SB, Ortega-Gutierrez S, Choi HA, et al. Status epilepticus-induced hyperemia and brain tissue hypoxia after cardiac arrest. Arch Neurol 2011;68(10): 1323–6.

112. Bailey RL, Quattrone F, Curtin C, et al. The safety of multimodality monitoring using a triple-lumen bolt in severe acute brain injury. World Neurosurg 2019;130: e62–7.

113. Chesnut RM, Temkin N, Carney N, et al. A trial of intracranial-pressure monitoring in traumatic brain injury. N Engl J Med 2012;367(26):2471–81.

114. Ponce LL, Pillai S, Cruz J, et al. Position of probe determines prognostic information of brain tissue PO2 in severe traumatic brain injury. Neurosurgery 2012;70(6):1492–502 [discussion: 1502–3].

115. Hoiland RL, Robba C, Menon DK, et al. Differential pathophysiologic phenotypes of hypoxic ischemic brain injury: considerations for post-cardiac arrest trials. Intensive Care Med 2020;46(10):1969–71.

116. Panchal AR, Bartos JA, Cabañas JG, et al. Part 3: adult basic and advanced life support: 2020 American Heart Association Guidelines for Cardiopulmonary Resuscitation and Emergency Cardiovascular Care. Circulation 2020; 142(16_suppl_2):S366–468.

117. Okazaki T, Hifumi T, Kawakita K, et al. Targeted temperature management guided by the severity of hyperlactatemia for out-of-hospital cardiac arrest patients: a post hoc analysis of a nationwide, multicenter prospective registry. Ann Intensive Care 2019;9(1):127.

118. Callaway CW, Coppler PJ, Faro J, et al. Association of initial illness severity and outcomes after cardiac arrest with targeted temperature management at 36 °C or 33 °C. JAMA Netw Open 2020;3(7):e208215.

119. Kim JH, Park JH, Shin SD, et al. Effects of moderate hypothermia versus normothermia on survival outcomes according to the initial body temperature in out-of-hospital cardiac patients: a nationwide observational study. Resuscitation 2020; 151:157–65.

120. Deye N, Vincent F, Michel P, et al. Changes in cardiac arrest patients' temperature management after the 2013 "TTM" trial: results from an international survey. Ann Intensive Care 2016;6(1):4.

121. McKenzie N, Williams TA, Tohira H, et al. A systematic review and meta-analysis of the association between arterial carbon dioxide tension and outcomes after cardiac arrest. Resuscitation 2017;111:116–26.

122. Wang CH, Chang WT, Huang CH, et al. Associations between intra-arrest blood glucose level and outcomes of adult in-hospital cardiac arrest: a 10-year retrospective cohort study. Resuscitation 2020;146:103–10.

Brain Herniation and Intracranial Hypertension

Aleksey Tadevosyan, MD[a],*, Joshua Kornbluth, MD[b]

KEYWORDS

- Cerebral herniation • Herniation syndromes • Intracranial pressure
- Intracranial hypertension • Dialysis disequilibrium syndrome
- Hepatic encephalopathy

KEY POINTS

- Cerebral herniation is a devastating event, with high rates of morbidity and mortality, and may manifest with symptoms, such as increased nausea, somnolence, and agitation.
- Intracranial hypertension and cerebral herniation are not synonymous. Although most events of herniation do occur in the setting of intracranial hypertension, patients with spontaneous intracranial hypotension and sinking skin flap syndrome may have cerebral herniation with low or normal intracranial pressure.
- Treatment of intracranial hypertension involves conservative measures, such as head of bed elevation and midline maintenance of neck position to improve intracranial venous drainage, augmentation of mean arterial pressure to maintain appropriate cerebral perfusion pressure, and higher-tiered therapies, such as hyperosmolar therapy, sedation and pentobarbital coma, temporary paralysis, hypothermia, and surgical decompression.
- Critically ill patients with sepsis and multiorgan failure (liver failure or acute kidney injury) and intracranial pathology are at higher risk of developing cerebral edema, intracranial hypertension, and herniation. Care should be taken with seemingly innocuous therapies, such as dialysis, because volume shifts may cause or exacerbate cerebral edema.

INTRODUCTION

Intracranial pressure (ICP) is defined as the pressure measured within the intracranial vault. This is a dynamic pressure consisting of a systolic, diastolic, and derived mean pressure and may fluctuate physiologically. Normal ICP (measured as the mean) typically is 10 cm H_2O to 20 cm H_2O, or 7 mm Hg to 14 mm Hg. ICP is governed by the relationship between volumes of brain tissue, cerebrospinal fluid (CSF), and intracranial blood in the arterial and venous compartments. Expansion of any 1 of these results

[a] Department of Neurology, Tufts University School of Medicine, Beth Israel Lahey Hospital and Medical Center, 41 Mall Road, Burlington, MA 01805, USA; [b] Department of Neurology, Tufts University School of Medicine, Tufts Medical Center, 800 Washington Street, Box#314, Boston, MA 02111, USA
* Corresponding author.
E-mail address: aleksey.tadevosyan@lahey.org

Neurol Clin 39 (2021) 293–318
https://doi.org/10.1016/j.ncl.2021.02.005
0733-8619/21/© 2021 Elsevier Inc. All rights reserved.
neurologic.theclinics.com

in compensatory decrease in 1 or more of the other, resulting in limited changes in ICP. Furthermore, the cranium is considered nonexpansile after closure of the fontanelles and, therefore, once these compensatory mechanisms are exhausted, an increase in volume causes a pathologic increase in ICP (**Fig. 1**). This classically is referred to as the Monro-Kellie doctrine, although recent data suggest that in vivo, the doctrine might not be completely accurate.[1]

ICP is an important determinant of cerebral perfusion pressure (CPP). Based on the Monro-Kellie doctrine, it can be extrapolated that mean CPP = mean arterial pressure − mean ICP.[2] In the uninjured brain with intact cerebral autoregulation, cerebral blood flow (CBF) remains relatively constant within a wide range of CPP (approximately 50–150 mm Hg), although this exact range may vary between individual patients, where patients who are chronically hypertensive have the CBF/CPP curve shifted to the right (**Fig. 2**).[3] These patients may be more susceptible to cerebral ischemia in setting of systemic hypotension (such as during septic shock). Autoregulation is maintained largely via cerebral arteriolar reactivity, whereby, with preserved autoregulation, with an increase in CPP. there is progressive vessel constriction maintaining an unchanged CBF.[4] As CPP increases past the point of maximal autoregulation, there is passive vasodilation leading to increased blood flow and progressive hyperemia (see **Fig. 2**).[4] In patients with severe brain injury with complete loss of autoregulation, an increase in systemic blood pressure, and therefore CPP, inadvertently may increase CBF. This leads to increased cerebral blood volume in a brain with an already elevated ICP, causing a further worsening of intracranial hypertension (see **Fig. 2**).

The individual patient characteristics, trends, and dynamics of ICP generally are more important to patient management than isolated values, but mean ICP exceeding

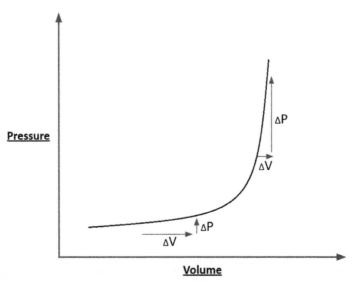

Fig. 1. Cerebral compliance—pressure versus volume curve. In a compliant brain, relatively larger changes in volume cause a small increase in ICP. As the various compartments of the brain become full (mass lesion, edema or hemorrhage in the brain parenchyma, venous congestion from cerebral sinus thrombosis, and hydrocephalus), however, even with the slightest change in volume, there may be a large change in pressure. If untreated, this may lead to intracranial hypertension and herniation. ΔV = Change in Volume, ΔP = Change in Pressure.

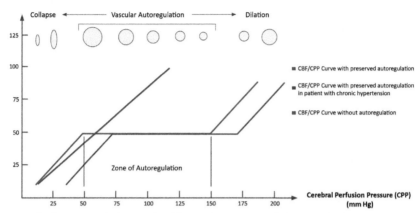

Fig. 2. Cerebral autoregulation. In healthy patients, as CPP is increased, the CBF remains largely stable within the zone of autoregulation, where arteriolar muscle reactivity leads to vasoconstriction in the face of increasing pressure. Under low pressures where vascular tone is low, increase in pressure causes an increase in flow. Above the zone of autoregulation, further increase in pressure leads to passive vessel dilation, hyperemia, and ischemia, leading to hypertensive encephalopathy. In patients who are chronically hypertensive, the zone of autoregulation is shifted to the right as a protective measure against systemic hypertension. These patients may be more susceptible to cerebral ischemia with systemic hypotension (such as in shock). In patients with severe brain injury, autoregulation may be lost; thereby, increase in perfusion pressure leads directly to increased CBF, increased intravascular volume, and worsening of an already existing ICP crisis.

20 mm Hg to 25 mm Hg is defined as intracranial hypertension and generally is treated aggressively.[5,6] Intracranial hypertension may reduce CPP based on these principles and lead to cerebral hypoperfusion and ischemia. Guidelines suggest a CPP greater than 60 is a useful lower threshold of cerebral perfusion to maximize outcomes in brain-injured patients.[7] In addition to analysis of mean ICP, analysis of ICP waveform when monitored may provide useful information about intracranial compliance and may help guide care.[8] An assessment of the degree of change in ICP to phasic changes in the respiratory cycle or to provocative maneuvers, such as jugular vein occlusion, also may give an examiner information about intracranial compliance.

CLINICAL AND RADIOGRAPHIC SIGNS OF ELEVATED INTRACRANIAL PRESSURE AND BRAIN HERNIATION

For purposes of this review, acute intracranial hypertension and herniation are focused on. More chronic causes of intracranial hypertension (eg, idiopathic intracranial hypertension) and herniation (eg, slow-growing brain tumors) may cause significant changes in anatomy and physiology separate from the acute changes discussed in this article.

Intracranial hypertension may occur relatively uniformly in the cranium due to diffuse injury, for example, anoxic brain injury or subarachnoid hemorrhage, or may occur in 1 or more brain compartments and cause a differential of pressure across intracranial structures. This may lead to cerebral herniation, defined as a shift of brain tissue through a naturally occurring opening in another tissue, which is a life-threatening emergency and is associated with poor outcomes in a variety of neurologic disorders.[9] Cerebral herniation may occur as a result of intracranial mass lesions, either focal or diffuse, or of disorders of CSF circulation, and the clinical consequences are due to the cause of herniation, the tissue that herniates, the degree of derangement of adjacent brain, and the time course at which herniation proceeds and is reversed. Cerebral herniation is the common final pathway for many different diseases and may happen along with an increase in ICP.

Initial signs of intracranial hypertension are somewhat nonspecific and include headache, nausea, vomiting, increased somnolence and obtundation, and, at times, worsening agitation. In the inpatient setting especially, it is difficult to ascertain whether a patient's worsening mental status is due to rising ICP or myriad other causes, such as worsening infection, uremia, hyperammonemia, polypharmacy, hypercarbia, and other acute central nervous system events, including seizure and acute stroke. Although in most instances uncontrolled and rising ICP leads to herniation, there are cases where herniation occurs in the setting of normal or even low ICP as well.[10] Therefore, intracranial hypertension and cerebral herniation are not synonymous. In the appropriate clinical context, brain herniation should be in the differential in patients having an acute change in mental status. One of the most concerning features of brain herniation is further injury to the brain microvasculature, and at times larger vessels, which in turn can cause further tissue ischemia, increasing cytotoxic edema and hemorrhage and worsening herniation. There are multiple anatomic patterns of cerebral herniation, and, although most forms of herniation share certain clinical features, such as acute change in mental status, they also may present with unique and nuanced clinical manifestations, as discussed later and summarized in **Table 1**.

Subfalcine Herniation

Subfalcine herniation consists of midline shift of the medial structures of the brain, primarily movement of the ipsilateral cingulate gyrus underneath the falx cerebri (also called cingulate herniation), caused by mass effect in the ipsilateral cerebral hemisphere (**Fig. 3**A).[11] Degree of herniation is quantified by measuring the midline shift of the septum pellucidum at the level of foramen of Monro.[12] Clinically, patients demonstrate findings consistent with medial frontal lobe dysfunction, including abulia, emergence of frontal release signs, and loss of initiative.[13] In severe cases, subfalcine herniation can cause unilateral or bilateral compression of the anterior cerebral arteries, pericallosal artery leading to unilateral or rarely bilateral leg weakness, and acute urinary retention.[14–16]

Descending Transtentorial Herniation

Descending transtentorial herniation (DTH) occurs when there is downward herniation of brain matter past the tentorium cerebelli and can occur in 2 separate patterns: lateral DTH and central DTH.[11,12,17] Lateral DTH occurs with the displacement of the parahippocampal gyrus past the edge of the tentorium (**Fig. 3**B).[18,19] Most commonly, this involves the herniation of the most medial part of the anterior temporal lobe (uncus) causing compression of the midbrain and the contralateral cerebral peduncle against the tentorial edge.[12] Ipsilateral midbrain injury at this level manifests with worsening of mental status and ipsilateral cranial third nerve palsy, resulting in a dilated and unresponsive pupil. The ipsilateral posterior cerebellar artery (PCA) also can be compressed with infarctions in the occipital lobe and medial temporal lobe. Compression of the contralateral cerebral peduncle containing the uncrossed descending corticospinal and corticobulbar pathways results in weakness ipsilateral

Table 1
Review of herniation syndromes[11,12]

Type of Herniation	Displaced Structures	Clinical Manifestation
DTH • Anterior lateral • Posterior lateral • Central	Anterior temporal lobe/uncus Posterior parahippocampal gyrus Midbrain and diencephalon	Ipsilateral CN3 palsy, ipsilateral weakness, PCA territory infarction, Parinaud syndrome PCA/SCA infarction, coma, various cranial nerve injuries (pontine Duret hemorrhages)
Ascending cerebellar transtentorial herniation	Midbrain and median cerebellar structures	Pinpoint pupils, coma, bradycardia, ventricular arrhythmia, respiratory arrest
Tonsillar herniation	Cerebellar tonsils, medulla, and pons	PICA infarcts, obtundation, respiratory arrest, hemodynamic instability
Transalar herniation • Descending • Ascending	Inferior frontal gyrus Anterior temporal horn	Ipsilateral MCA stroke Ipsilateral MCA/ACA stroke
Subfalcine herniation	Cingulate gyrus	Ipsilateral or bilateral leg weakness, frontal lobe syndromes, acute urinary retention, somnolence
Transcalvarial herniation	Area of brain herniating through craniectomy, with compression of brain along edges of bony defect	Symptoms may be determined by area of brain adjacent to defect

Abbreviations: ACA, anterior cerebral artery; CN3, cranial nerve 3; PICA, posterior inferior cerebellar artery.

to the culprit supratentorial mass lesion (known as the false localizing sign) with a
newly upgoing toe an early finding.[20]

Increased mass effect in the posterior temporal lobe and occipital lobe can cause
herniation of the posterior component of the parahippocampal gyrus, resulting in
the effacement of the lateral quadrigeminal plate cistern as well as displacement
and torsion of the brainstem.[11,19] The unique clinical manifestation of this type of herniation often is Parinaud syndrome, followed by coma if pressure is not relieved.[11,12,21]

Central herniation occurs when bihemispheric supratentorial mass effect results in a
downward herniation of the thalamus and midbrain through tentorial incisura and the
medulla through the foramen magnum.[11] Radiographic findings occur in the rostral to
caudal direction with the effacement of the perimesencephalic cisterns, inferior
displacement of the quadrigeminal plate, and the basilar artery resulting in Duret hemorrhages.[22,23] This is followed by acute obstructive hydrocephalus with increased
downward pressure as well as infarction of the vascular territories supplied by the
PCAs, resulting in increased cytotoxic edema and further compression on the brainstem
as herniation continues. Clinically, patients develop agitation, followed by obtundation,
with bilaterally poorly reactive and at times fixed midposition pupils, and then decorticate followed by decerebrate posturing, Cushing triad, and coma, and death.[12,24]

Tonsillar Herniation

Cerebellar tonsillar herniation can occur in isolation in the setting of increased mass
effect in the posterior fossa or as a result of supratentorial pressure, in which case

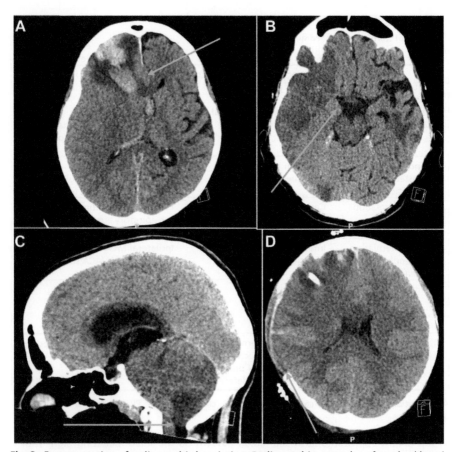

Fig. 3. Representation of radiographic herniation. Radiographic examples of cerebral herniation. All are CT images without contrast. (*A*) Subfalcine herniation after intracerebral hemorrhage. Arrow points to cingulate gyrus under the falx. (*B*) Uncal herniation after large right MCA stroke. Arrow points to uncus causing displacement of the midbrain. (*C*) Transforaminal tonsillar herniation after cerebellar stroke. Arrow points to cerebellar tonsil below the level of the foramen magnum. (*D*) Transcalvarial herniation after DC for treatment of severe TBI. Arrow points to the area of the brain compressed against bony defect and herniation.

tonsillar herniation accompanies downward transtentorial herniation (**Fig. 3**C).[11,12] Acute tonsillar herniation (not to be confused with chronic or congenital tonsillar herniation, as seen in Chiari malformations) occurs when 1 or both of the cerebellar tonsils herniate caudally through the foramen magnum. As with other types of herniation, tonsillar herniation also can cause obstructive hydrocephalus with the effacement of the fourth ventricle. Compression of the medulla causes decreased mental status, hemodynamic instability, and respiratory arrest.[25] The posterior inferior cerebellar arteries can be compressed, leading to cerebellar infarcts.[11,17]

Ascending Cerebellar Transtentorial Herniation

Ascending cerebellar transtentorial herniation also occurs in the setting of increased mass effect in the posterior fossa. Pressure within the medial structures of the cerebellum may push the cerebellar vermis and cerebellar hemispheres superiorly through the tentorial incisura.[26] In some instances, rapid decompression of a supratentorial mass or evacuation of hemorrhage may lead to this type of herniation.[17] This also can occur in patients with sinking skin flap syndrome who had undergone surgical decompression for large SDH, severe traumatic brain injury (TBI), or acute stroke and are postcranioplasty. Cranioplasty, especially with placement of a negative pressure subgaleal drain, is thought to induce a negative pressure environment supratentorially, thereby pulling the posterior fossa anteriorly and cranially.[9,27] As with other types of herniation with pontomedullary compression, initial clinical symptoms include obtundation, hemodynamic and respiratory instability, severe bradycardia, life-threatening arrhythmias, and pinpoint pupils.[28,29] There is evolution of pupillary size from severely miotic to midposition fixed as herniation progresses with upward movement of the midbrain.[26] As with DTH, vascular compromise can occur with impingement of unilateral or bilateral superior cerebellar artery (SCA) or PCA.[26,30] Importantly, patients with ATH usually do not have elevated ICP; therefore, clinicians should not ignore the signs of herniation even with normal ICP if a monitor is present.

Transalar Herniation

Descending herniation occurs from mass effect in the frontal lobe whereby the inferior frontal gyrus is displaced posteriorly and caudally with respect to the sphenoid wing.[11] Ascending herniation occurs with the displacement of the anterior temporal lobe anteriorly in the cranial direction over the sphenoid ridge.[11] The middle cerebral artery (MCA) and supraclinoid internal carotid artery are displaced and compressed against anterior clinoid process, resulting in ipsilateral anterior circulation stroke.[11,12,17]

Extracranial Herniation

Extracranial herniation describes protrusion of brain matter through a cranial defect that was caused by trauma or surgery (**Fig. 3**D). As herniation progresses, brain tissue may compress against the edges of the skull, causing both venous and arterial infarction. Clinical findings depend on the area of brain tissue that is herniating.

SPONTANEOUS INTRACRANIAL HYPOTENSION AND HERNIATION

Although most instances of brain herniation occur in patients with elevated ICP, it also has been described in patients with intracranial hypotension. Spontaneous intracranial hypotension (SIH) usually occurs in the setting of a spinal CSF leak.[31,32] Targeted or blind epidural blood patch (EBP) is the mainstay of therapy. The most common clinical manifestation is acute-onset orthostatic headache.[33,34] Brain imaging often shows smooth diffuse dural enhancement on magnetic resonance imaging (MRI), whereas in other conditions with dural enhancement, such as carcinomatous, granulomatous, or bacterial meningitis, dural involvement is nodular, localized, and patchy.[35,36] In severe cases, patients rapidly can develop stupor followed by coma.[37] On imaging, such clinical deterioration coincides with caudal displacement of the brainstem, termed, brain sagging, resulting in downward displacement of the thalamus onto the posterior fossa, compression of the pons and midbrain against the clivus, impingement of cerebral peduncles, and effacement of the basal cisterns, leading to obstructive hydrocephalus.[38–40] Subdural hemorrhage (SD) and hygromas can be present and usually are bilateral; however, unilateral collections occur as well.[41–43] A diagnosis of SIH may be missed or delayed in patients presenting with SD, especially if MRI, demonstrating the typical features of SIH, is not completed. In lieu of this, it is important to recognize the possibility of SIH, not hypertension, as the cause of neurologic decline in patients admitted with nontraumatic SD. Some patients with bilateral subdurals and intracranial hypotension may have bilateral midposition hypoactive and at times nonreactive pupils with preserved consciousness. Without treating the underlying etiology responsible for SIH, surgical decompression of SD while leading to temporary improvement in clinical status leads to recurrent subdural collection formation usually within hours of procedure and worsening caudal herniation because the brain now exposed is to atmospheric pressure.[42,43] On the other hand, when EBP is performed prior to SDH evacuation and the leak is treated, patients rapidly may develop intracranial hypertension because the mass effect from SDH remains. Henceforth, clinicals should monitor patients with intracranial mass lesions who undergo EBP carefully.

In this condition, low ICP not always may be present; it is estimated that approximately 30% to 50% of patients with SIH have normal and sometimes even elevated ICP.[44,45] This makes accurate estimation of ICP in patients with SIH challenging, especially those with SD with midline shift and herniation from the subdural itself. Trendelenburg positioning has been used as a diagnostic and therapeutic tool in patients with SIH and SD.[46] Failure to improve neurologically after Trendelenburg positioning may imply presence of intracranial hypertension from mass effect and may necessitate evacuation of subdural fluid collections if the patient is in extremis, followed by treatment of SIH.[47]

MEDICAL TREATMENT OF INTRACRANIAL HYPERTENSION

Management of intracranial hypertension is one of the main tenets of neurocritical care. Elevated ICP from a distinct pathology if left untreated can cause further secondary neurology injury, with subsequent further increase in ICP leading to a difficult to control feedback loop. Management can be divided into tiers, ranging from the fundamental neuroprotective measures of tier 0 to tier 3 therapies, such as hypothermia and high-dose barbiturate coma, used in selected groups of patients (**Table 2**). The ICP monitoring and treatment modalities presented in this section largely are from the TBI literature; given the quality and depth of the clinical studies, however, they can in part be generalizable to other conditions causing intracranial hypertension (**Table 3**).

Hyperosmolar Therapy

Hyperosmolar therapy long has been a mainstay in treating acutely elevated ICP, with the most frequently used formulations being 20% mannitol boluses and hypertonic saline (HTS), 2%, 3% 7.5%, or 23.4%, in the United States. Although recognizing the utility in decreasing ICP, given the paucity of high-quality studies, the most recent guidelines from the Brain Trauma Foundation do not explicitly recommend the use of hyperosmolar therapy in patients suffering from intracranial hypertension with

Table 2	
Tiers of therapy for intracranial pressure control	
Tiers	**Treatments**
Tier 0	HOB >30°, head/neck midline (facilitates venous drainage), euglycemia, eucapnia, euthermia, Spo_2 >94%, avoidance of hyponatremia and hypotonic fluids, ICP <22 mm Hg, CPP goal >60 mm Hg
Tier 1	Hyperosmolar therapy, EVD placement for CSF diversion
Tier 2	Temporary hyperventilation, increased sedation, neuromuscular blockade
Tier 3	Barbiturates to achieve burst suppression, hypothermia, decompression

Table 3
General overview of conditions causing intracranial hypertension

Primary Causes of Acute Intracranial Hypertension	Main Treatments (in Addition to Tier 1 Therapies)
TBI	Hyperosmolar therapy, decompression, burst suppression, hypothermia
Acute ischemic and hemorrhagic stroke	Hyperosmolar therapy, decompression
Acute hydrocephalus	EVD placement
Subarachnoid hemorrhage	Hyperosmolar therapy, vasospasm management, EVD
Brain tumor	Dexamethasone or alternative, decompression
Cardiac arrest	Therapeutic hypothermia/targeted temperature management
Acute liver failure	Hyperosmolar therapy, RRT (aggressive ammonia treatment)
Meningitis/encephalitis/abscess	Hyperosmolar therapy, antimicrobials, corticosteroids

TBI.[48] Many of the studies investigating the use of mannitol and HTS in decreasing ICP have been small retrospective studies and case series as well as meta-analyses pooling a heterogenous group of patients (TBI, stroke, and intracranial hemorrhage).[49–53] In 2008, a small prospective trial by Francony and colleagues[54] compared the effects of single infusion of equiosmolar doses of 20% mannitol and 7.45% of HTS on ICP. Each arm had 10 patients and of 20 patients 17 were TBI patients and 3 with acute ischemic stroke. After a prolonged infusion of approximately 20 minutes, both treatment modalities seemed to have an equivalent decrease in ICP (by 37%–41%) with sustained effect of approximately 120 minutes (with continued decrease in ICP by 23%–32%).[54] In a 2015 study by Mangat and colleagues,[55] the New York State database of the Brain Trauma Foundation TBI-trac was analyzed retrospectively for patients admitted with severe TBI with Glasgow Coma Scale score (GCS) less than 8, who had received either mannitol or HTS. There were 35 patients who received HTS and 477 who received mannitol, and, after matching of baseline characteristics, 25 patients from each group were reviewed. There were no statistically significant differences in mortality at 2 weeks of therapy. In a follow-up study with the same database, use of HTS was associated with a reduction in total number and percentage of days with high ICP and low CPP.[56]

In 4 recent meta-analyses, there were no significant differences in mortality or favorable neurologic outcome between HTS and mannitol, although improved control of intracranial hypertension with HTS.[57–60] In the recent Seattle International Severe Traumatic Brain Injury Consensus Conference (SIBCC) expert panel recommendations, sodium and osmolarity thresholds of 155 mEq/L and 320 mEq/L, respectively, are recommended, above which administration of further hyperosmolar therapy likely is futile.[61] In the authors' institution, alternating boluses of 3% HTS, 250 mL to 500 mL, and mannitol, 0.5 g/kg to 1 g/kg, are used.

Corticosteroids

Steroids most often are used in patients with vasogenic and not cytotoxic cerebral edema in an acute setting.[62,63] Conditions in which vasogenic edema predominates include brain tumors; demyelinating conditions, such as multiple sclerosis and acute disseminated encephalomyelitis; and cerebral abscesses. The utility of corticosteroids in treatment of cytotoxic edema, such as in ischemic stroke, intracranial hemorrhage, and TBI, has been studied; however, there is no clear evidence of clinical benefit. In a meta-analysis by Wintzer and colleagues[64] that included 7 randomized controlled trials (RCTs) where dexamethasone was studied in patients with spontaneous intracerebral hemorrhage, there was no improvement in risk of death or morbidity, and there was a nonsignificant trend toward increased risk of complications (hyperglycemia, psychiatric symptoms, hypokalemia, and gastrointestinal bleeding). In a prospective observational diffusion tensor imaging MRI study, dexamethasone administration in TBI patients was associated with significant decrease in degree of pericontusional edema, although there were no changes in clinical outcome.[65]

Sedation and Analgesia

Sedation and analgesia are important and universally utilized treatments in managing patients with intracranial hypertension.[66] The most common agents used in the neurological intensive care units in the United States for this purpose include fentanyl, propofol, and midazolam, and, if burst suppression is deemed necessary, barbiturates.[67,68] It is thought that sedation decreases cerebral metabolic rate and oxygen consumption, leading to decreasing blood flow and blood volume and thereby lower ICP.[66,69–71] Sedation and analgesia also blunt the response to pain from trauma and discomfort of the endotracheal tube, thereby minimizing episodes of hypertension, which, in patients with impaired autoregulation, may lead to ICP spikes.[68] The most common and concerning side effect of sedation is decreased cardiac output and hypotension, which, if not anticipated, can have an adverse impact on CPP by decreasing the mean arterial pressure.[66,68] Other well-known common side effects include bradycardia with dexmedetomidine use, ileus and possible bowel obstruction with opiate use (especially in conjunction with paralytics for ICP control), refractory hypokalemia with pentobarbital coma followed by rebound hyperkalemia, and propofol infusion syndrome with propofol use, especially with doses higher than 4 mg/kg/h to 5 mg/kg/h.[72–76] Propofol and midazolam are thought to be equivalent in their role in ICP reduction.[77] Addition of propofol to morphine improved outcomes compared with morphine alone in a small RCT.[78]

Despite the pervasive notion that ketamine may raise ICP, there has been renewed interest in its use for sedation given hemodynamically inert properties and perceived decreased propensity in causing delirium compared with opiates and benzodiazepines.[68,79] According to 3 review articles of available literature, ketamine use was not associated with significantly increased ICP.[80–82] Most studies reviewed were small prospective cohort and retrospective studies, and only 6 were focused on patients with elevated ICP. In these 6 studies, however, no deleterious effect of ketamine on ICP was noted.[83–88] In a newly published review, Gregers and colleagues[89] concluded that although no studies have clearly shown that ketamine is harmful in patients with elevated ICP, the quality of data available does not allow for a strong recommendation of use of ketamine in patients with intracranial hypertension.

For hemodynamically stable patients with suprarefractory intracranial hypertension not responsive to tier 1 and tier 2 interventions to control ICP, barbiturates have been used to achieve electroencephalogram burst suppression for ICP control. In a multicenter prospective RCT from the 1980s by Eisenberg and colleagues,[90] patients with severe TBI (GCS 4–7 with reactive pupils) and elevated ICP for specified duration (with different ICP targets for patients who had a craniectomy) were randomized into a conventional therapy arm (control) and treatment arm (pentobarbital loading dose, followed by continuous infusion after). Conventional therapy included head of bed (HOB) elevation, hyperventilation, morphine, paralytics, mannitol therapy, and ventriculostomy. Some patients also had undergone craniectomy. Most patients in the control arm eventually crossed over and received pentobarbital as well. Patients who received pentobarbital were observed to have a significant decrease in ICP, had an improved mortality outcome at 1 month, and neurologic outcome at 6 months (death and vegetative state).[90] In a prospective observational study from Europe, outcomes of patients with severe TBI who received barbiturates at 2 doses (high-dose group receiving >2 g/24 h for 3 consecutive days or until death, n = 71; and low-dose group, n = 140) were compared with those who received conventional therapy only (n = 961).[91] After adjusting for age, GCS score, and Injury Severity Score, no statistically significant differences were observed in mortality at hospital discharge and at 6 months.[91] In a recent Cochrane review, use of barbiturates was associated with decreased ICP, but this did not translate to improvement in mortality or neurologic morbidity.[92] The most recent BTF guidelines recommend use of high dose barbiturate for suprarefractory intracranial hypertension in hemodynamically stable patients.[48]

Hypothermia

Hypothermia after cardiac arrest has been known to improve mortality and neurologic outcomes in patients with cardiac arrest.[93,94] It is less clear whether hypothermia also improves outcomes in patients who have intracranial injury from other pathologic processes, with TBI remaining the most feverishly studied pathology. It has been theorized that hypothermia conveys its beneficial effects via multiple mechanisms, including reduction of mitochondrial dysfunction and free radical formation, blunting of reperfusion injury, preservation of blood-brain barrier with a resultant decrease in vasogenic edema, and antithrombotic effects leading to decreased cerebral vascular microthrombosis.[95–97] It is unclear in which patient population hypothermia should be instituted, including its timing and duration. A few small, earlier trials have shown that hypothermia may improve mortality and neurologic outcomes in patients with severe TBI.[98–101] In a meta-analysis of 20 RCTs between 1993 and 2011 comparing therapeutic hypothermia (<36°C) versus normothermia that included 1885 adult patients with severe TBI, hypothermia was associated with significant reduction in poor neurologic outcome and mortality, albeit the investigators themselves state of inherent bias and low quality of some of the included trials.[102] In recent years, there have been few large, RCTs that evaluated both prophylactic and therapeutic use of hypothermia in patients with severe TBI. In a multicenter RCT (National Acute Brain Injury Study: Hypothermia II [NABIS: H II]), patients with severe TBI were randomized to normothermia and hypothermia groups where cooling was administered to 33°C for 48 hours within 4 hours to 5 hours of randomization.[103] This study did not show a difference in death or severe disability within 6 months of follow-up. In a subgroup analysis of patients who received surgical evacuation of hematoma with bone flap off to relieve pressure, however, those who underwent concurrent hypothermia did statistically better than the control group.[103] Similar conclusions were reached in a previous small RCT, where patients with severe TBI who had undergone unilateral craniectomy on admission were found to have favorable neurologic outcome at 12 months after admission after undergoing moderate hypothermia (33°C–35°C) for approximately 4 days after surgery.[104] In the larger Eurotherm3235 RCT, patients with severe TBI who had undergone hypothermia (32°C–35°C) for 48 hours as rescue therapy and replacement for hyperosmolar therapy (followed by hyperosmolar therapy if needed) did not have improved neurologic outcomes at 6 months and had a statistically significant increase in unfavorable outcome and all-cause mortality.[105] Similarly, in the most recent trial (Prophylactic

Hypothermia Trial to Lessen Traumatic Brain Injury-Randomized Clinical Trial), in which patients with severe TBI were prophylactically cooled to 33°C for 72 hours on initial contact (including out-of-hospital cooling to 35°C and re-evaluation on arrival to emergency room), compared with standard therapy, there were no differences in neurologic outcome or death at 6 months.[106] One weakness of these studies is that higher-tiered therapies perhaps were instituted more aggressively than necessary thereby diluting the effect of the intervention being studied. Another caveat is that maintenance of normocapnia during hypothermia may induce a hypocarbic state and, therefore, chronically decreased cerebral perfusion in patients undergoing hypothermia as because-corrected $Paco_2$ is lower than measured.[107,108] The Targeted Therapeutic Mild Hypercapnia After Resuscitated Cardiac Arrest: A Phase III Multi-Centre Randomised Controlled Trial (TAME Cardiac Arrest Trial) currently is investigating this concept.

SURGICAL TREATMENT OF INTRACRANIAL HYPERTENSION

The decision for any surgical treatment of high ICP and/or cerebral herniation must be based on the likelihood of benefit to the patient's outcome. Surgical treatment of intracranial hypertension and herniation usually is targeted at the site of the most mass effect from the acute injury. Surgical treatment targeted at augmenting CSF drainage through ventriculostomy catheter placement remains the primary surgical intervention in diffuse brain injuries. Intracranial hypertension and herniation due to acute hydrocephalus is best treated with extraventricular drain (EVD) placement and is preferred over the use of a lumbar drain due to the risk of transforaminal herniation. EVD placement with continuous CSF drainage currently is supported by the guidelines for ischemic cerebellar stroke,[109] spontaneous ICH,[110] and TBI.[48]

Surgical Resection of Mass Lesion

Surgical resection of lesions causing mass effect may immediately lower ICP and reduce herniation, although not always associated with a prompt and significant improvement in patient condition. Expedient surgical intervention has shown the most benefit for extra-axial hematomas and for cerebellar ICH greater than 3 cm in diameter or with hydrocephalus and/or brainstem compression.[110] The STITCH II trial included 601 patients with spontaneous lobar ICH without IVH and showed a nonstatistically significant but nevertheless clinically relevant benefit for spontaneous superficial ICH.[111] Surgical evacuation may still be considered as a life-saving measure for select patients.

Decompressive Craniectomy in Traumatic Brain Injury

Decompressive craniectomy (DC) involves creating a large unilateral or bilateral bone window(s), with or without durotomy, to allow for a larger compartment for a swollen brain and negating the Monro-Kellie doctrine. The DECRA trial showed that early (within 72 h of injury) bifrontotemporoparietal DC decreased ICP but was not associated with a better outcome than the control arm.[112] The follow-up, the RESCUEicp trial, allowed for unilateral or bilateral DC and resulted in a lower mortality for patients randomized to receive surgery though with higher rates of vegetative state and severe disability compared with medical care.[113] An important distinction is that in the RESCUEicp trial, surgical decompression was reserved as a last resort therapy after other higher-tiered medical interventions were exhausted (excluding barbiturate coma).

Hemicraniectomy in Large Hemispheric Stroke

DC also has been considered for treatment if elevated ICP and herniation after large hemispheric stroke. A meta-analysis of 3 RCTs, DECIMAL, HAMLET, and Destiny, looking at DC for large hemispheric stroke showed that early (<48 h after onset) DC significantly improved survival (78% DC vs. 29% control) and resulted in varying levels of the severity of disability measured at 1 year.[114] A more recent review and meta-analysis reached the same conclusion.[115] Decision making regarding DC in large hemispheric stroke must be made with the understanding the DC may be life-saving and should be predicated on the degree of infarction and patient-specific characteristics and preferences. It must be stressed, however, that across these trials approximately 50% of surviving patients under 60 years old and approximately 80% above 60 years old survived with severe functional disability (modified Rankin scale score 4–5) at 12 months' follow-up.

SPECIAL CONSIDERATIONS
Hepatic Encephalopathy and Intracranial Hypertension

Hepatic encephalopathy (HE) refers to a wide spectrum of neuropsychiatric symptoms in the setting of acute or chronic liver dysfunction and is classified via the following 4 factors: underlying disease, severity of manifestation, time course, and existence of precipitating factors (**Table 4**).[116,117] Conditions causing HE include drugs, toxins,

Table 4
Characteristics of hepatic encephalopathy[116,117]

Classification	Subclassification	Features
Underlying disease process	Type A	Acute liver failure
	Type B	Portosystemic bypass
	Type C	Cirrhosis
Severity of symptoms	Minimal	Subtle clues identified on neuropsychiatric testing
	Grade I	Trivial lack of awareness
	Grade II	Euphoria or anxiety
	Grade III	Shortened attention span with impairment of addition or subtraction
	Grade IV	Altered sleep rhythm
		Lethargy or apathy
		Disorientation for time
		Obvious personality change, with inappropriate behavior
		Dyspraxia
		Asterixis
		Somnolence to semistupor but responsive to stimuli
		Confused with gross disorientation
		Bizarre behavior
		Coma
Time course	Episodic	Episodes of self-limited HE during lifetime
	Recurrent	Multiple events of HE occurring at <6 mo
	Persistent	Symptoms always present with varying severity
Precipitating factors	None	Infections, electrolyte and metabolic disturbance, gastrointestinal bleeding
	Precipitated	

and infections leading to acute liver failure, decompensated chronic cirrhosis, and certain inborn errors of metabolism.[118–121] Cytotoxic and vasogenic edema is a hallmark of HE and is in part mediated by hyperammonemia. A detailed discussion of the complex and incompletely understood pathophysiology of ammonia-induced cerebral edema is outside the scope of this article, but in short it includes a complex interplay between direct cerebral neurotoxicity of ammonia and other cytokines and impaired cerebral perfusion as a result of a sepsis-like physiology with high output cardiac failure, low systemic resistance, and hypotension from seepage of proinflammatory mediators from the splanchnic circulation into the systemic circulation.[122–124] Ammonia metabolism primarily occurs in the liver, where it is converted to urea. It also occurs in the skeletal muscle tissues and the brain, where ammonia is metabolized into glutamine.[121] The kidneys play an important role in excretion of ammonia: in healthy patients, approximately 20% of daily ammonia clearance occurs via renal excretion.[121,125,126] Therefore, critically ill patients with liver dysfunction and acute kidney injury (often caused by the liver dysfunction itself) are at higher risk of developing hyperammonemia.

Although it is thought that abnormal ammonia levels in the serum do not always correlate with neurologic symptoms, it has been demonstrated that high levels (>200 µmol/L) seem to be associated with increased risk of cerebral edema, intracranial hypertension, and herniation.[127–129] Treatment of hyperammonemia primarily involves increased gut excretion, with lactulose and rifaximin being mainstays of therapy, whereas decreasing protein intake. Renal replacement therapy (RRT) is another important treatment of elevated ICP in patients with hyperammonemia.[130,131] Timing and duration of RRT remain understudied, but it is argued that early initiation may lead to better outcomes.[132,133] In a prospective clinical trial, Slack and colleagues[134] showed an average 22% median decrease in serum ammonia levels within 24 hours of continuous RRT and directly correlated with filtration rate. Methods of RRT are important to consider as well. Although it would be quicker to perform intermittent hemodialysis (HD), there is some evidence that continuous RRT might be a safer option given the graded removal of ammonia and less risk of rebound cerebral edema.[135,136] Current guidelines from the European Association for the Study of the Liver recommend continuous forms of RRT over intermittent HD in patients with hyperammonemia.[137]

As in patients with primary neurologic injury (TBI or acute stroke), there is evidence that hyperosmolar therapy can decrease ICP in patients with acute liver failure, and sodium level of at least 145 mmol/L is recommended.[120,131,138] In the authors' institution, hyperosmolar therapy usually is instituted after serial head CT scans show progressive edema in conjunction with worsening clinical status and rising ammonia levels. Many patients with hyperammonemia concurrently are hyponatremic; thus, care should be taken to not raise the sodium level too rapidly given concerns of osmotic demyelination syndrome. Therapeutic hypothermia has been used in patients with acute liver failure with intracranial hypertension with variable success.[139,140] In a prospective study by Jalan and colleagues,[141] 14 patients with intracranial hypertension and acute liver failure were cooled to 32°C to 33°C as a bridge to liver transplantation after failing standard medical therapy. Prior to cooling, the mean ICP was 36.5 mm Hg and CPP of 40.1 mm Hg, and at 4 hours the mean ICP decreased to 16.3 mm Hg and CPP increased to 66.4 mm Hg. These changes persisted for at least the next 24 hours. Of the 14 patients, 1 patient died of brain herniation, and the rest underwent liver transplantation within a median of 32 hours of cooling with complete neurologic recovery. In a prospective nonblinded RCT by Bernal and colleagues,[142] 46 patients with acute liver failure and intracranial hypertension were randomized into a

33°C (moderate hypothermia [MH]) and 36°C (control) groups for 72 hours. No statistically significant differences were noted in hospital mortality (41%–46%) or rate of complications. In the MH group, however, none of the patients who received transplantation died whereas in the control group 33% of the patients (4/12) undergoing transplantation passed away. Other treatments of hyperammonemia with variable success include medications and ammonia scavenging agents, such as high dose L-carnitine, hydroxocobalamin, biotin, arginine, L-ornithine phenylacetate, and sodium benzoate.[143–146]

Dialysis Disequilibrium Syndrome

HD is a frequently used procedure for RRT in patients with end-stage renal disease (ESRD). The primary aim of RRT is to mimic the function of the kidneys by removing the excess body water, urea, and other generated toxic solutes by ultrafiltration. Removal of solutes via HD may cause intracerebral volume shifts. Increased brain volume after HD has been described in both animal and human studies.[147,148] Clinical manifestations of rapid removal of volume and solute via HD has been termed, *dialysis disequilibrium syndrome (DDS)*, and can present with benign symptoms, such as headache, nausea, and dizziness, to severe signs, such as stupor and coma.[149] Presentation usually is within 24 hours of dialysis and often during the procedure itself.[150,151] It is postulated that in patients with ESRD there is an increase in cerebral intraparenchymal urea and other hyperosmolar solutes (idiogenic osmoles) to maintain brain-blood osmolar steady state in response to increased overall serum osmolarity.[147,151,152] During HD, as volume and solutes are rapidly removed, the osmolarity in brain tissue is thought to exceed that of plasma, causing influx of water into the brain leading to cerebral edema.[150,153,154] In a second hypothesis, correction of acidosis after HD results in elevation of serum bicarbonate and carbon dioxide, which after diffusion into brain tissue causes in situ acidosis after conversion into carbonic acid, further augmenting formation of osmolar solutes.[150,155–157] In a study by Walters and colleagues,[148] the average increase in brain volume after HD was approximately 3% of total brain volume.

Although in most patients these shifts may cause some mild symptoms during dialysis, in critically ill patients with brain injury and elevated ICP, even the slightest increase in volume may induce cerebral herniation.[158] In a small case series by Kumar and colleagues,[159] 1 patient with acute IPH and 1 patient with bilateral acute SDH while undergoing HD for baseline ESRD developed clinical signs of herniation. Head CT imaging in both patients showed effacement of basal cisterns and worsened edema without change in size of hemorrhage. Although most commonly occurring in patients with an already compromised blood-brain barrier, elevated ICP, and reduced intracranial compliance, DDS with herniation also has been described in critically ill patients with sepsis undergoing HD for acute renal failure without known intracranial pathology.[160,161] Other conditions associated with DDS include severe metabolic acidosis, especially in the contexts of extremes of age,[162,163] new dialysis, having missed multiple dialysis sessions,[164,165] carcinomatous and bacterial meningitis,[166] hydrocephalus,[167] and hypertensive emergency[149,168] (**Box 1**). There also are case reports of patients developing leukoencephalopathy and osmotic demyelination instead of generalized edema and herniation.[169–171]

In place of intermittent high-volume HD, continuous venovenous HD (CVVHD) with lower rate of filtration has been proposed as a safer alternative.[150,160] Even with CVVHD, however, there have been 2 cases of DDS during dialysis.[172] Clinicians should be mindful that patients who have been receiving hyperosmolar therapy and now are hypernatremic may have an acute drop in sodium levels if the default bath

---

Box 1
Risk factors associated with development of dialysis disequilibrium syndrome

Primary intracranial processes with elevated ICP (ischemic and hemorrhagic stroke, TBI, SD, subarachnoid hemorrhage)

Conditions causing cerebral edema (acute demyelinating conditions, encephalitis, hypertensive emergency, hyperammonemia)

Conditions leading to breakdown of blood-brain barrier (neoplastic, inflammatory and infectious meningitis, sepsis, Thrombotic thrombocytopenic purpura–hemolytic uremic syndrome, disseminated intravascular coagulation)

Hyperosmolar state (hyperglycemic nonketotic coma, uremia, hypernatremia)

Severe metabolic acidosis

Missed dialysis days or new to dialysis

Extremes of age

---

composition is used where sodium concentration usually is 135 mEq/L to 140 mEq/L. At the authors' institution, 3% saline infusion frequently is continued simultaneously with CVVHD to dampen the serum sodium fall. Especially in patients with intracranial injury undergoing any form of RRT, clinicians should rapidly recognize signs of clinical decompensation and act to relieve cerebral edema and ICP.

FUTURE DIRECTIONS

Improved methods of rapid identification and prediction of those at highest risk of developing intracranial hypertension and herniation as well as patients most likely to benefit from aggressive treatments are needed. Potential tools for making these determinations may include a combination of the neurologic examination, radiographic imaging, assessments of cerebral ischemia and tissue stress, ICP, regional CBF, cerebrovascular reactivity, electrophysiology, and others. This approach to assessment is termed multimodal monitoring.[173] Currently, evidence remains weak for robust recommendation of certain aspects of multimodal monitoring (mainly surgical placement of intracranial monitors), given its invasive nature, resource utilization, cost, and generalizability. In addition, noninvasive technologies, such as automated pupillometry,[174] optic nerve sheath diameter detection with ultrasound,[175] near-infrared spectroscopy,[176] cranial accelerometry, and electroencephalogram spectrum analysis,[177] among others, all are showing promise to screen for cerebral herniation, measure ICP, and trend response to therapy without need for invasive surgical procedures.

DISCLOSURE

The authors have nothing to disclose.

REFERENCES

1. Mascarenhas S, Vilela GHF, Carlotti C, et al. The new ICP minimally invasive method shows that the Monro-Kellie doctrine is not valid. Acta Neurochir Suppl 2012;114:117–20.

2. Miller JD, Stanek A, Langfitt TW. Concepts of cerebral perfusion pressure and vascular compression during intracranial hypertension. Prog Brain Res 1972;411–32. https://doi.org/10.1016/S0079-6123(08)60102-8.
3. Steiner L a, Czosnyka M, Piechnik SK, et al. Continuous monitoring of cerebrovascular pressure reactivity allows determination of optimal cerebral perfusion pressure in patients with traumatic brain injury. Crit Care Med 2002;30(4):733–8.
4. Partington T, Farmery A. Intracranial pressure and cerebral blood flow. Anaesthesia & Intensive Care Medicine 2014;15(4):189–94.
5. Freeman WD. Management of intracranial pressure. Continuum (Minneap Minn) 2015;21(5 Neurocritical Care):1299–323.
6. Naidech AM. Diagnosis and management of spontaneous intracerebral hemorrhage. Continuum (Minneap Minn) 2015;21(5 Neurocritical Care):1288–98.
7. Marehbian J, Muehlschlegel S, Edlow BL, et al. Medical management of the severe traumatic brain injury patient. Neurocrit Care 2017;27(3):430–46.
8. Czosnyka M. Monitoring and interpretation of intracranial pressure. J Neurol Neurosurg Psychiatry 2004;75(6):813–21.
9. Kalanuria A a, Geocadin RG, Püttgen H a. Brain code and coma recovery: aggressive management of cerebral herniation. Semin Neurol 2013;33(2):133–41.
10. Woo PYM, Lo WHY, Wong HT, et al. The "negative" impact of a subgaleal drain: post-cranioplasty negative pressure subgaleal drain-induced ascending transtentorial herniation. Asian J Neurosurg 2019;14(1):256–61.
11. Gilardi BR, López JIM, Villegas ACH, et al. Types of cerebral herniation and their imaging features. Radiographics 2019;39(6):1598–610.
12. Johnson PL, Eckard DA, Chason DP, et al. Imaging of acquired cerebral herniations. Neuroimaging Clin N Am 2002;12:217–28.
13. Paradiso S, Chemerinski E, Yazici KM, et al. Frontal lobe syndrome reassessed: comparison of patients with lateral or medial frontal brain damage. J Neurol Neurosurg Psychiatry 1999;67(5):664–7.
14. Kang SY, Kim JS. Anterior cerebral artery infarction: stroke mechanism and clinical-imaging study in 100 patients. Neurology 2008;70(24 Pt 2):2386–93.
15. Byard RW. Patterns of cerebral and cerebellar herniation. Forensic Sci Med Pathol 2013;9(2):260–4.
16. Herath HM, Matthias AT, Kulatunga A. Acute on chronic bilateral subdural hematoma presenting with acute complete flaccid paraplegia and urinary retention mimicking an acute spinal cord injury: a case report. BMC Res Notes 2017;10(1):627.
17. Laine FJ, Shedden AI, Dunn MM, et al. Acquired intracranial herniations: MR imaging findings. AJR Am J Roentgenol 1995;165:967–73.
18. Inao S, Kuchiwaki H, Kuchiwaki H, et al. Magnetic resonance imaging assessment of brainstem distortion associated with a supratentorial mass. J Neurol Neurosurg Psychiatry 1993;56(3):280–5.
19. Stovring J. Descending tentorial herniation: findings on computed tomography. Neuroradiology 1977;14(3):101–5.
20. Zhang CH, DeSouza RM, Kho JS, et al. Kernohan-Woltman notch phenomenon: a review article. Br J Neurosurg 2017;31(2):159–66.
21. Lyons AR, Olson SL. Parinaud syndrome as an unusual presentation of intracranial hypotension. Surg Neurol Int 2020;11:98.
22. Parizel PM, Makkat S, Jorens PG, et al. Brainstem hemorrhage in descending transtentorial herniation (Duret hemorrhage). Intensive Care Med 2002;28(1):85–8.

23. Ishizaka S, Shimizu T, Ryu N. Dramatic recovery after severe descending trans-tentorial herniation-induced Duret haemorrhage: a case report and review of literature. Brain Inj 2014;28:374–7.

24. Reich JB, Sierra J, Camp W, et al. Magnetic resonance imaging measurements and clinical changes accompanying transtentorial and foramen magnum brain herniation. Ann Neurol 1993;33:159–70.

25. Ishikawa M, Kikuchi H, Fujisawa I, et al. Tonsillar herniation on magnetic resonance imaging. Neurosurgery 1988;22(1 Pt 1):77–81.

26. Cuneo RA, Caronna JJ, Pitts L, et al. Upward transtentorial herniation: seven cases and a literature review. Arch Neurol 1979;36:618–23.

27. Karamchandani K, Chouhan RS, Bithal PK, et al. Severe bradycardia and hypo-tension after connecting negative pressure to the subgaleal drain during craniotomy closure. Br J Anaesth 2006;96:608–10.

28. Yamaura A, Makino H. Neurological deficits in the presence of the sinking skin flap following decompressive craniectomy. Neurol Med Chir (Tokyo) 1977;17:43–53.

29. Annan M, De Toffol B, Hommet C, et al. Sinking skin flap syndrome (or syndrome of the trephined): a review. Br J Neurosurg 2015;29:314–8.

30. Honeybul S. Sudden death following cranioplasty: a complication of decompressive craniectomy for head injury. Br J Neurosurg 2011;25:343–5.

31. Chung SJ, Kim JS, Lee MC. Syndrome of cerebrospinal fluid hypovolemia: clinical and imaging fea-tures and outcome. Neurology 2000;55:1321–7.

32. Schievink WI, Maya MM, Jean-Pierre S, et al. A classification system of spontaneous spinal CSF leaks. Neurology 2016;87:673–9.

33. Leep-Hunderfund AN, Mokri B. Second-half-of-the-day headache as a manifestation of spontaneous CSF leak. J Neurol 2012;259(2):306–10.

34. Mea E, Chiapparini L, Savoiardo M, et al. Headache attributed to spontaneous intracranial hypotension. Neurol Sci 2008;29(Suppl 1):S164–5.

35. Pannullo SC, Reich JB, Krol G, et al. MRI changes in intracranial hypotension. Neurology 1993;43:919–26.

36. Kranz PG, Gray L, Amrhein TJ. Spontaneous intracranial hypotension: 10 myths and misperceptions. Headache 2018;58:948–59.

37. Schievink WI, Maya MM, Moser FG, et al. A serious complication of spontaneous intracranial hypotension. Neurology 2018;90(19):e1638–45.

38. Shah LM, McLean LA, Heilbrun ME, et al. Intracranial hypotension: improved MRI detection with diagnostic intracranial angles. AJR Am J Roentgenol 2013;200:400–7.

39. Kranz PG, Gray L, Malinzak MD, et al. Spontaneous intracranial hypotension: pathogenesis, diagnosis, and treatment. Neuroimaging Clin N Am 2019;29:581–94.

40. Aghaei Lasboo A, Hurley MC, Walker MT, et al. Emergent image-guided treatment of a large CSF leak to reverse "in-extremis" signs of intracranial hypotension. AJNR Am J Neuroradiol 2008;29:1627–9.

41. Takahashi K, Mima T, Akiba Y. Chronic subdural hematoma associated with spontaneous intracranial hypotension: therapeutic strategies and outcomes of 55 cases. Neurol Med Chir (Tokyo) 2016;56:69–76.

42. Osada Y, Shibahara I, Nakagawa A, et al. Unilateral chronic subdural hematoma due to spontaneous intracranial hypotension: a report of four cases. Br J Neurosurg 2020;34(6):632–7.

43. Ferrante E, Rubino F, Beretta F, et al. Treatment and outcome of subdural hematoma in patients with spontaneous intracranial hypotension: a report of 35 cases. Acta Neurol Belg 2018;118(1):61–70.

44. Kranz PG, Tanpitukpongse TP, Choudhury KR, et al. How common is normal cerebrospinal fluid pressure in spontaneous intracranial hypotension? Cephalalgia 2016;36:1209–17.

45. Luetmer PH, Schwartz KM, Eckel LJ, et al. When should I do dynamic CT myelography? Predicting fast spinal CSF leaks in patients with spontaneous intracranial hypotension. AJNR Am J Neuroradiol 2012;33:690–4.

46. Dhillon AK, Rabinstein AA, Wijdicks EF. Coma from worsening spontaneous intracranial hypotension after subdural hematoma evacuation. Neurocrit Care 2010;12(3):390–4.

47. Loya JJ, Mindea SA, Yu H, et al. Intracranial hypotension producing reversible coma: a systematic review, including three new cases. J Neurosurg 2012;117: 615–28.

48. Carney N, Totten AM, O'Reilly C, et al. Guidelines for the management of severe traumatic brain injury. Fourth Edition. Neurosurgery 2017;80(1):6–15.

49. Horn P, Münch E, Vajkoczy P, et al. Hypertonic saline solution for control of elevated intracranial pressure in patients with exhausted response to mannitol and barbiturates. Neurol Res 1999;21:758–64.

50. Kerwin AJ, Schinco MA, Tepas JJ 3rd, et al. The use of 23.4% hypertonic saline for the management of elevated intracranial pressure in patients with severe traumatic brain injury: a pilot study. J Trauma 2009;67(2):277–82.

51. Ware ML, Nemani VM, Meeker M, et al. Effects of 23.4% sodium chloride solution in reducing intracranial pressure in patients with traumatic brain injury: a preliminary study. Neurosurgery 2005;57:727–36.

52. Battison C, Andrews PJ, Graham C, et al. Randomized, controlled trial on the effect of a 20% mannitol solution and a 7.5% saline/6% dextran solution on increased intracranial pres-sure after brain injury. Crit Care Med 2005;33: 196–202.

53. Rockswold GL, Solid CA, Paredes-Andrade E, et al. Hypertonic saline and its effect on intracranial pressure, cerebral perfusion pressure, and brain tissue oxygen. Neurosurgery 2009;65:1035–42.

54. Francony G, Fauvage B, Falcon D, et al. Equimolar doses of mannitol and hypertonic saline in the treatment of increased intracranial pressure. Crit Care Med 2008;36:795–800.

55. Mangat HS, Chiu Y-L, Gerber LM, et al. Hypertonic saline reduces cumulative and daily intracranial pressure burdens after severe traumatic brain injury. J Neurosurg 2015;122:202–10.

56. Mangat HS, Wu X, Gerber LM, et al. Hypertonic saline is superior to mannitol for the combined effect on intracranial pressure and cerebral perfusion pressure burdens in patients with severe traumatic brain injury. Neurosurgery 2020;86: 221–30.

57. Gu J, Huang H, Huang Y, et al. Hypertonic saline or mannitol for treating elevated intracranial pressure in traumatic brain injury: a meta-analysis of randomized controlled trials. Neurosurg Rev 2019;42:499–509.

58. Chen H, Song Z, Dennis JA. Hypertonic saline versus other intracranial pressure-lowering agents for people with acute traumatic brain injury. Cochrane Database Syst Rev 2019;12:CD010904.

59. Shi J, Tan L, Ye J, et al. Hypertonic saline and mannitol in patients with traumatic brain injury: a systematic and meta-analysis. Medicine (Baltimore) 2020;99(35). https://doi.org/10.1097/MD.0000000000021655.

60. Miyoshia Y, Kondo Y, Suzuki H, et al. Effects of hypertonic saline versus mannitol in patients with traumatic brain injury in prehospital, emergency department, and intensive care unit settings: a systematic review and meta-analysis. J Intensive Care 2020;12(8):61.

61. Hawryluk GWJ, Aguilera S, Buki A, et al. A management algorithm for patients with intracranial pressure monitoring: the seattle international severe traumatic brain injury consensus conference (SIBICC). Intensive Care Med 2019;45:1783–94.

62. Schroeder T, Bittrich P, Noebel C, et al. Efficiency of dexamethasone for treatment of vasogenic edema in brain metastasis patients: a radiographic approach. Front Oncol 2019;30(9):695.

63. Dietrich J, Rao K, Pastorino S, et al. Corticosteroids in brain cancer patients: benefits and pitfalls. Expert Rev Clin Pharmacol 2011;4(2):233–42.

64. Wintzer S, Heckmann JG, Huttner HB, et al. Dexamethasone in patients with spontaneous intracerebral hemorrhage: an updated meta-analysis. Cerebrovasc Dis 2020;49(5):495–502.

65. Moll A, Lara M, Pomar J, et al. Effects of dexamethasone in traumatic brain injury patients with pericontusional vasogenic edema: a prospective-observational DTI-MRI study. Medicine (Baltimore) 2020;99(43). https://doi.org/10.1097/MD.0000000000022879.

66. Roberts DJ, Hall RI, Kramer AH, et al. Sedation for critically ill adults with severe traumatic brain injury: a systematic review of randomized controlled trials. Crit Care Med 2011;39(12):2743–51.

67. Vincent JL, Berré J. Primer on medical management of severe brain injury. Crit Care Med 2005;33(6):1392–9.

68. Oddo M, Crippa IA, Mehta S, et al. Optimizing sedation in patients with acute brain injury. Crit Care 2016;20(1):128.

69. Bilotta F, Gelb AW, Stazi E, et al. Pharmacological perioperative brain neuroprotection: a qualitative review of randomized clinical trials. Br J Anaesth 2013;110(Suppl 1):i113–20.

70. Adembri C, Venturi L, Pellegrini-Giampietro DE. Neuroprotective effects of propofol in acute cerebral injury. CNS Drug Rev 2007;13(3):333–51.

71. Albanèse J, Viviand X, Potie F, et al. Sufentanil, fentanyl, and alfentanil in head trauma patients: a study on cerebral hemodynamics. Crit Care Med 1999;27(2):407–11.

72. Urwin SC, Menon DK. Comparative tolerability of sedative agents in head-injured adults. Drug Saf 2004;27(2):107–33.

73. Mijzen EJ, Jacobs B, Aslan A, et al. Propofol infusion syndrome heralded by ECG changes. Neurocrit Care 2012;17(2):260–4.

74. Kang TM. Propofol infusion syndrome in critically ill patients. Ann Pharmacother 2002;36(9):1453–6.

75. Awad M, Bonitz J, Pratt A. Pentobarbital induced hypokalemia: a worrying sequela. Int J Surg Case Rep 2020;71:323–6.

76. Otterspoor LC, Kalkman CJ, Cremer OL. Update on the propofol infusion syndrome in ICU management of patients with head injury. Curr Opin Anaesthesiol 2008;21(5):544–51.

77. Ghori KA, Harmon DC, Elashaal A, et al. Effect of midazolam versus propofol sedation on markers of neurological injury and outcome after isolated severe head injury: a pilot study. Crit Care Resusc 2007;9(2):166–71.
78. Kelly DF, Goodale DB, Williams J, et al. Propofol in the treatment of moderate and severe head injury: a randomized, prospective double-blinded pilot trial. J Neurosurg 1999;90(6):1042–52.
79. White PF, Way WL, Trevor AJ. Ketamine–its pharmacology and therapeutic uses. Anesthesiology 1982;56(2):119–36.
80. Himmelseher S, Durieux ME. Revising a dogma: ketamine for patients with neurological injury? Anesth Analg 2005;101(2):524–34, table of contents.
81. Zeiler FA, Teitelbaum J, West M, et al. The ketamine effect on intracranial pressure in nontraumatic neurological illness. J Crit Care 2014;29(6):1096–106.
82. Cohen L, Athaide V, Wickham ME, et al. The effect of ketamine on intracranial and cerebral perfusion pressure and health outcomes: a systematic review. Ann Emerg Med 2015;65(1):43–51.e2.
83. Bourgoin A, Albanèse J, Wereszczynski N, et al. Safety of sedation with ketamine in severe head injury patients: comparison with sufentanil. Crit Care Med 2003;31(3):711–7.
84. Albanèse J, Arnaud S, Rey M, et al. Ketamine decreases intracranial pressure and electroencephalographic activity in traumatic brain injury patients during propofol sedation. Anesthesiology 1997;87(6):1328–34.
85. Kolenda H, Gremmelt A, Rading S, et al. Ketamine for analgosedative therapy in intensive care treatment of head-injured patients. Acta Neurochir (Wien) 1996; 138(10):1193–9. Erratum in: Acta Neurochir (Wien) 1997;139(12):1193.
86. Mayberg TS, Lam AM, Matta BF, et al. Ketamine does not increase cerebral blood flow velocity or intracranial pressure during isoflurane/nitrous oxide anesthesia in patients undergoing craniotomy. Anesth Analg 1995;81(1):84–9.
87. Bourgoin A, Albanèse J, Léone M, et al. Effects of sufentanil or ketamine administered in target-controlled infusion on the cerebral hemodynamics of severely brain-injured patients. Crit Care Med 2005;33(5):1109–13.
88. Schmittner MD, Vajkoczy SL, Horn P, et al. Effects of fentanyl and S(+)-ketamine on cerebral hemodynamics, gastrointestinal motility, and need of vasopressors in patients with intracranial pathologies: a pilot study. J Neurosurg Anesthesiol 2007;19(4):257–62.
89. Gregers MCT, Mikkelsen S, Lindvig KP, et al. Ketamine as an anesthetic for patients with acute brain injury: a systematic review. Neurocrit Care 2020;33(1): 273–82.
90. Eisenberg HM, Frankowski RF, Contant CF, et al. High-dose barbiturate control of elevated intracranial pressure in patients with severe head injury. J Neurosurg 1988;69(1):15–23.
91. Majdan M, Mauritz W, Wilbacher I, et al. Barbiturates use and its effects in patients with severe traumatic brain injury in five European countries. J Neurotrauma 2013;30(1):23–9.
92. Roberts I, Sydenham E. Barbiturates for acute traumatic brain injury. Cochrane Database Syst Rev 2012;12(12):CD000033.
93. Nielsen N, Wetterslev J, Cronberg T, et al, TTM Trial Investigators. Targeted temperature management at 33°C versus 36°C after cardiac arrest. N Engl J Med 2013;369(23):2197–206.
94. Chandrasekaran PN, Dezfulian C, Polderman KH. What is the right temperature to cool post-cardiac arrest patients? Crit Care 2015;19:406.

95. Sinclair HL, Andrews PJ. Bench-to-bedside review: hypothermia in traumatic brain injury. Crit Care 2010;14(1):204.

96. Tokutomi T, Morimoto K, Miyagi T, et al. Optimal temperature for the management of severe traumatic brain injury: effect of hypothermia on intracranial pressure, systemic and intracranial hemodynamics, and metabolism. Neurosurgery 2007;61(1 Suppl):256–65.

97. Polderman KH. Application of therapeutic hypothermia in the ICU: opportunities and pitfalls of a promising treatment modality. Part 1: indications and evidence. Intensive Care Med 2004;30(4):556–75.

98. Jiang J, Yu M, Zhu C. Effect of long-term mild hypothermia therapy in patients with severe traumatic brain injury: 1-year follow-up review of 87 cases. J Neurosurg 2000;93(4):546–9.

99. Jiang JY, Xu W, Li WP, et al. Effect of long-term mild hypothermia or short-term mild hypothermia on outcome of patients with severe traumatic brain injury. J Cereb Blood Flow Metab 2006;26(6):771–6.

100. Liu WG, Qiu WS, Zhang Y, et al. Effects of selective brain cooling in patients with severe traumatic brain injury: a preliminary study. J Int Med Res 2006;34(1): 58–64.

101. Zhi D, Zhang S, Lin X. Study on therapeutic mechanism and clinical effect of mild hypothermia in patients with severe head injury. Surg Neurol 2003;59(5): 381–5.

102. Crossley S, Reid J, McLatchie R, et al. A systematic review of therapeutic hypothermia for adult patients following traumatic brain injury. Crit Care 2014; 18(2):R75.

103. Clifton GL, Valadka A, Zygun D, et al. Very early hypothermia induction in patients with severe brain injury (the national acute brain injury study: hypothermia II): a randomised trial. Lancet Neurol 2011;10(2):131–9.

104. Qiu W, Zhang Y, Sheng H, et al. Effects of therapeutic mild hypothermia on patients with severe traumatic brain injury after craniotomy. J Crit Care 2007;22(3): 229–35.

105. Andrews PJ, Sinclair HL, Rodriguez A, et al, Eurotherm3235 Trial Collaborators. Hypothermia for intracranial hypertension after traumatic brain injury. N Engl J Med 2015;373(25):2403–12.

106. Cooper DJ, Nichol AD, Bailey M, et al. POLAR trial investigators and the ANZICS Clinical trials group. effect of early sustained prophylactic hypothermia on neurologic outcomes among patients with severe traumatic brain injury: the POLAR randomized clinical trial. JAMA 2018;320(21):2211–20.

107. Docherty A, Emelifeonwu J, Andrews PJD. Hypothermia after traumatic brain injury. JAMA 2018;320(21):2204–6.

108. Alston TA. Blood gases and pH during hypothermia: the "-stats. Int Anesthesiol Clin 2004;42(4):73–80.

109. Powers WJ, Rabinstein AA, Ackerson T, et al. 2018 Guidelines for the early management of patients with acute ischemic stroke: a guideline for healthcare professionals from the American heart association/American stroke association. Stroke 2018;49. https://doi.org/10.1161/STR.0000000000000158.

110. Hemphill JC, Greenberg SM, Anderson CS, et al. Guidelines for the management of spontaneous intracerebral hemorrhage: a guideline for healthcare professionals from the American heart association/American stroke association. Stroke 2015;46(7):2032–60.

111. Mendelow AD, Gregson BA, Rowan EN, et al. Early surgery versus initial conservative treatment in patients with spontaneous supratentorial lobar intracerebral haematomas (STICH II): A randomised trial. Lancet 2013;382(9890):397–408.

112. Cooper DJ, Rosenfeld JV, Murray L, et al. Decompressive craniectomy in diffuse traumatic brain injury. N Engl J Med 2011;364(16):1493–502.

113. Hutchinson PJ, Kolias AG, Timofeev IS, et al. Trial of decompressive craniectomy for traumatic intracranial hypertension. N Engl J Med 2016;375(12): 1119–30.

114. Vahedi K, Hofmeijer J, Juettler E, et al. Early decompressive surgery in malignant infarction of the middle cerebral artery: a pooled analysis of three randomised controlled trials. Lancet Neurol 2007;6(3):215–22.

115. Alexander P, Heels-Ansdell D, Siemieniuk R, et al. Hemicraniectomy versus medical treatment with large MCA infarct: a review and meta-analysis. BMJ Open 2016;6(11):e014390.

116. American Association for the Study of Liver Diseases. European association for the study of the liver. hepatic encephalopathy in chronic liver disease: 2014 practice guideline by the European association for the study of the liver and the American association for the study of liver diseases. J Hepatol 2014; 61(3):642–59.

117. Ferenci P, Lockwood A, Mullen K, et al. Hepatic encephalopathy–definition, nomenclature, diagnosis, and quantification: final report of the working party at the 11th World Congresses of Gastroenterology, Vienna, 1998. Hepatology 2002;35(3):716–21.

118. Auron A, Brophy PD. Hyperammonemia in review: pathophysiology, diagnosis, and treatment. Pediatr Nephrol 2012;27(2):207–22.

119. Wakim-Fleming J. Hepatic encephalopathy: suspect it early in patients with cirrhosis. Cleve Clin J Med 2011;78(9):597–605.

120. Canalese J, Gimson AE, Davis C, et al. Controlled trial of dexamethasone and mannitol for the cerebral oedema of fulminant hepatic failure. Gut 1982;23(7): 625–9.

121. Walker V. Ammonia metabolism and hyperammonemic disorders. Adv Clin Chem 2014;67:73–150.

122. Trewby PN, Williams R. Pathophysiology of hypotension in patients with fulminant hepatic failure. Gut 1977;18(12):1021–6.

123. Larsen FS, Ejlersen E, Hansen BA, et al. Functional loss of cerebral blood flow autoregulation in patients with fulminant hepatic failure. J Hepatol 1995;23(2): 212–7.

124. Bémeur C, Butterworth RF. Liver-brain proinflammatory signalling in acute liver failure: role in the pathogenesis of hepatic encephalopathy and brain edema. Metab Brain Dis 2013;28(2):145–50.

125. Weiner ID, Verlander JW. Renal ammonia metabolism and transport. Compr Physiol 2013;3(1):201–20.

126. Wright G, Noiret L, Olde Damink SW, et al. Interorgan ammonia metabolism in liver failure: the basis of current and future therapies. Liver Int 2011;31(2): 163–75.

127. Clemmesen JO, Larsen FS, Kondrup J, et al. Cerebral herniation in patients with acute liver failure is correlated with arterial ammonia concentration. Hepatology 1999;29(3):648–53.

128. Ozanne B, Nelson J, Cousineau J, et al. Threshold for toxicity from hyperammonemia in critically ill children. J Hepatol 2012;56(1):123–8.

129. Ong JP, Aggarwal A, Krieger D, et al. Correlation between ammonia levels and the severity of hepatic encephalopathy. Am J Med 2003;114(3):188–93.

130. Gupta S, Fenves AZ, Hootkins R. The Role of RRT in Hyperammonemic Patients. Clin J Am Soc Nephrol 2016;11(10):1872–8.

131. Warrillow SJ, Bellomo R. Preventing cerebral oedema in acute liver failure: the case for quadruple-H therapy. Anaesth Intensive Care 2014;42(1):78–88.

132. Bernal W, Wendon J. Acute liver failure. N Engl J Med 2013;369(26):2525–34.

133. Bernal W, Lee WM, Wendon J, et al. Acute liver failure: a curable disease by 2024? J Hepatol 2015;62(1 Suppl):S112–20.

134. Slack AJ, Auzinger G, Willars C, et al. Ammonia clearance with haemofiltration in adults with liver disease. Liver Int 2014;34(1):42–8.

135. Davenport A, Will EJ, Davison AM. Early changes in intracranial pressure during haemofiltration treatment in patients with grade 4 hepatic encephalopathy and acute oliguric renal failure. Nephrol Dial Transplant 1990;5(3):192–8.

136. Bernal W, Hyyrylainen A, Gera A, et al. Lessons from look-back in acute liver failure? A single centre experience of 3300 patients. J Hepatol 2013;59(1):74–80.

137. Clinical practice guidelines panel, Wendon J, Panel members, Cordoba J, Dhawan A, Larsen FS, Manns M, Samuel D, Simpson KJ, Yaron I, EASL Governing Board representative, Bernardi M. EASL clinical practical guidelines on the management of acute (fulminant) liver failure. J Hepatol 2017;66(5):1047–81.

138. Murphy N, Auzinger G, Bernel W, et al. The effect of hypertonic sodium chloride on intracranial pressure in patients with acute liver failure. Hepatology 2004; 39(2):464–70.

139. Jacob S, Khan A, Jacobs ER, et al. Prolonged hypothermia as a bridge to recovery for cerebral edema and intracranial hypertension associated with fulminant hepatic failure. Neurocrit Care 2009;11(2):242–6.

140. Karvellas CJ, Todd Stravitz R, Battenhouse H, et al. US acute liver failure study group. Therapeutic hypothermia in acute liver failure: a multicenter retrospective cohort analysis. Liver Transpl 2015;21(1):4–12.

141. Jalan R, Olde Damink SW, Deutz NE, et al. Moderate hypothermia in patients with acute liver failure and uncontrolled intracranial hypertension. Gastroenterology 2004;127(5):1338–46.

142. Bernal W, Murphy N, Brown S, et al. A multicentre randomized controlled trial of moderate hypothermia to prevent intracranial hypertension in acute liver failure. J Hepatol 2016;65(2):273–9.

143. Sakpal SV, Reedstrom H, Ness C, et al. High-dose hydroxocobalamin in end-stage liver disease and liver transplantation. Drugs Ther Perspect 2019;35(9): 442–6.

144. Malaguarnera M, Pistone G, Elvira R, et al. Effects of L-carnitine in patients with hepatic encephalopathy. World J Gastroenterol 2005;11(45):7197–202.

145. Misel ML, Gish RG, Patton H, et al. Sodium benzoate for treatment of hepatic encephalopathy. Gastroenterol Hepatol (N Y) 2013;9(4):219–27.

146. De Las Heras J, Aldámiz-Echevarría L, Martínez-Chantar ML, et al. An update on the use of benzoate, phenylacetate and phenylbutyrate ammonia scavengers for interrogating and modifying liver nitrogen metabolism and its implications in urea cycle disorders and liver disease. Expert Opin Drug Metab Toxicol 2017;13(4):439–48.

147. Arieff AI, Massry SG, Barrientos A, et al. Brain water and electrolyte metabolism in uremia: effects of slow and rapid hemodialysis. Kidney Int 1973;4(3):177–87.

148. Walters RJ, Fox NC, Crum WR, et al. Haemodialysis and cerebral oedema. Nephron 2001;87(2):143–7.

149. Patel N, Dalal P, Panesar M. Dialysis disequilibrium syndrome: a narrative review. Semin Dial 2008;21(5):493–8.
150. Mistry K. Dialysis disequilibrium syndrome prevention and management. Int J Nephrol Renovasc Dis 2019;12:69–77.
151. Kennedy AC, Linton AL, Eaton JC. Urea levels in cerebrospinal fluid after haemodialysis. Lancet 1962;1(7226):410–1.
152. Silver SM, Sterns RH, Halperin ML. Brain swelling after dialysis: old urea or new osmoles? Am J Kidney Dis 1996;28(1):1–13.
153. Krane NK. Intracranial pressure measurement in a patient undergoing hemodialysis and peritoneal dialysis. Am J Kidney Dis 1989;13(4):336–9.
154. Chen CL, Lai PH, Chou KJ, et al. A preliminary report of brain edema in patients with uremia at first hemodialysis: evaluation by diffusion-weighted MR imaging. AJNR Am J Neuroradiol 2007;28(1):68–71.
155. Sabatini S, Kurtzman NA. Bicarbonate therapy in severe metabolic acidosis. J Am Soc Nephrol 2009;20(4):692–5.
156. Arieff AI. Dialysis disequilibrium syndrome: current concepts on pathogenesis and prevention. Kidney Int 1994;45(3):629–35.
157. rachtman H, Futterweit S, Tonidandel W, et al. The role of organic osmolytes in the cerebral cell volume regulatory response to acute and chronic renal failure. J Am Soc Nephrol 1993;3(12):1913–9.
158. Lund A, Damholt MB, Strange DG, et al. Increased intracranial pressure during hemodialysis in a patient with anoxic brain injury. Case Rep Crit Care 2017; 2017:5378928.
159. Kumar A, Cage A, Dhar R. Dialysis-induced worsening of cerebral edema in intracranial hemorrhage: a case series and clinical perspective. Neurocrit Care 2015;22(2):283–7.
160. Bagshaw SM, Peets AD, Hameed M, et al. Dialysis disequilibrium syndrome: brain death following hemodialysis for metabolic acidosis and acute renal failure–a case report. BMC Nephrol 2004;5:9.
161. Osgood M, Compton R, Carandang R, et al. Rapid unexpected brain herniation in association with renal replacement therapy in acute brain injury: caution in the neurocritical care unit. Neurocrit Care 2015;22(2):176–83.
162. Doorenbos CJ, Bosma RJ, Lamberts PJ. Use of urea containing dialysate to avoid disequilibrium syndrome, enabling intensive dialysis treatment of a diabetic patient with renal failure and severe metformin induced lactic acidosis. Nephrol Dial Transplant 2001;16(6):1303–4.
163. Mah DY, Yia HJ, Cheong WS. Dialysis disequilibrium syndrome: a preventable fatal acute complication. Med J Malaysia 2016;71(2):91–2.
164. Dalia T, Tuffaha AM. Dialysis disequilibrium syndrome leading to sudden brain death in a chronic hemodialysis patient. Hemodial Int 2018;22(3):E39–44.
165. Adapa S, Konala VM, Aeddula NR, et al. Dialysis disequilibrium syndrome: rare serious complication of hemodialysis and effective management. Cureus 2019; 11(6):e5000.
166. Tsuchida Y, Takata T, Ikarashi T, et al. Dialysis disequilibrium syndrome induced by neoplastic meningitis in a patient receiving maintenance hemodialysis. BMC Nephrol 2013;14:255.
167. Flannery T, Shoakazemi A, McLaughlin B, et al. Dialysis disequilibrium syndrome: a consideration in patients with hydrocephalus. J Neurosurg Pediatr 2008;2(2):143–5.
168. Zepeda-Orozco D, Quigley R. Dialysis disequilibrium syndrome. Pediatr Nephrol 2012;27(12):2205–11.

169. Tarhan NC, Agildere AM, Benli US, et al. Osmotic demyelination syndrome in end-stage renal disease after recent hemodialysis: MRI of the brain. AJR Am J Roentgenol 2004;182(3):809–16.

170. Chang CH, Hsu KT, Lee CH, et al. Leukoencephalopathy associated with dialysis disequilibrium syndrome. Ren Fail 2007;29(5):631–4.

171. Aydin OF, Uner C, Senbil N, et al. Central pontine and extrapontine myelinolysis owing to disequilibrium syndrome. J Child Neurol 2003;18(4):292–6.

172. Tuchman S, Khademian ZP, Mistry K. Dialysis disequilibrium syndrome occurring during continuous renal replacement therapy. Clin Kidney J 2013;6(5): 526–9.

173. Le Roux P, Menon DK, Citerio G, et al. Consensus summary statement of the international multidisciplinary consensus conference on multimodality monitoring in neurocritical care: a statement for healthcare professionals from the neurocritical care society and the european society of intensive C. Neurocrit Care 2014; 21:S1–26. Suppl 2(S2).

174. Jahns FP, Miroz JP, Messerer M, et al. Quantitative pupillometry for the monitoring of intracranial hypertension in patients with severe traumatic brain injury. Crit Care 2019;23(1):155.

175. Kim SE, Hong EP, Kim HC, et al. Ultrasonographic optic nerve sheath diameter to detect increased intracranial pressure in adults: a meta-analysis. Acta Radiol 2019;60(2):221–9.

176. Fantini S, Sassaroli A, Tgavalekos KT, et al. Cerebral blood flow and autoregulation: current measurement techniques and prospects for noninvasive optical methods. Neurophotonics 2016;3(3):031411.

177. Chen H, Wang J, Mao S, et al. A new method of intracranial pressure monitoring by EEG power spectrum analysis. Can J Neurol Sci 2012;39(4):483–7.

Anesthesia Considerations in Neurological Emergencies

Anil Ramineni, MD[a], Erik A. Roberts, BS[b], Molly Vora, BS[b],
Sohail K. Mahboobi, MD[c,d], Ala Nozari, MD, PhD[b,e],*

KEYWORDS

- Neurologic emergencies • Anesthetic pharmacology • Airway management
- Endotracheal intubation • Ventilation • Sedation

KEY POINTS

- General anesthesia is often required in neurologic emergencies for airway control and to aid with management.
- Several general anesthetics can be neuroprotective and decrease cerebral metabolism.
- Hypotension during anesthesia induction is associated with cerebral ischemia and poor outcome.
- Rapid sequence intubation is generally preferred for anesthesia induction in neurologic emergencies, although awake fiberoptic intubation may be needed in cases of acute cervical spinal cord injury.
- Ventilation should be adjusted to maintain eucapnia and optimize cerebral perfusion.

INTRODUCTION

Upper airway obstruction and respiratory failure are common complications of neurologic emergencies. General anesthesia may be required in these patients for endotracheal intubation and to enable mechanical ventilation. Moreover, patients with neurologic emergencies and confusional states may be unable to tolerate important diagnostic and therapeutic interventions, requiring pharmacologic control of their agitation, anxiety, or delirium. General anesthesia is frequently needed to enable emergent procedures, such as endovascular treatment of ischemic strokes or craniotomies, and also may be needed to induce burst suppression in patients with status

[a] Department of Neurology, Lahey Hospital and Medical Center, 41 Mall Road, Burlington, MA 01805, USA; [b] Boston University School of Medicine, 72 East Concord Street, Boston, MA 02118, USA; [c] Department of Anesthesiology, Lahey Hospital and Medical Center, 41 Mall Road, Burlington, MA 01805, USA; [d] Tufts University School of Medicine, 136 Harrison Avenue, Boston, MA 02111, USA; [e] Department of Anesthesiology, Boston Medical Center, 750 Albany Street, Power Plant 2R, Boston, MA 02118, USA
* Corresponding author. Department of Anesthesiology, Boston Medical Center, 750 Albany Street, Boston, MA 02118.
E-mail address: Ala.Nozari@bmc.org

Neurol Clin 39 (2021) 319–332
https://doi.org/10.1016/j.ncl.2021.01.007
0733-8619/21/© 2021 Elsevier Inc. All rights reserved.

neurologic.theclinics.com

epilepticus or as treatment for reducing intracranial hypertension. Importantly, many patients with neurologic emergencies require sedation in the emergency department and intensive care unit (ICU), and it is therefore prudent to recognize the physiologic effects, pharmacologic properties, and common side effects of these agents. In this article, we address anesthetic and airway management considerations that are important and often unique to patients with neurologic emergencies.

AIRWAY MANAGEMENT

Neurologic emergencies often lead to airway complications or respiratory failure necessitating ventilatory support. Airway management, intubation, ventilation, and choice of sedatives directly influence cerebral perfusion and physiology.[1] Noninvasive positive pressure ventilation may be considered in patients with low risk of aspiration, but this requires very careful patient selection and monitoring. Most patients with neurologic emergencies will require intubation to secure the airway.

Indications for intubation include difficulty with oxygenation or ventilation and anticipated cardiopulmonary decline. In neurologic emergencies, of particular concern is a failure of airway protection (related to depressed level of consciousness and/or oropharyngeal incoordination), neuromuscular respiratory fatigue, and/or anticipated neurologic decline.[1] Despite its historical use, the absence of gag reflex is not a reliable indicator of airway protection in patients with neurologic emergencies, especially because up to 25% of healthy individuals lack the reflex.[2] Airway protection is dependent on multiple variables, including strength of cough reflex, quantity and quality of secretions, and ability to swallow.[3] A Glasgow Coma Scale score ≤8 is also suggestive of lost protective airway reflexes, and intubation has been shown to be associated with lower mortality in those patients.[4] Whenever possible, urgent management of airway should coincide with a focused neurologic examination.

Initial evaluation should include assessment for difficulty in bag-mask ventilation and intubation. Helpful mnemonics include "MOANS" (**Box 1**) for difficulty of bag-mask ventilation and "LEMON" (**Box 2**) to predict difficult endotracheal intubations.

ANESTHETIC INDUCTION

To minimize risks of hemodynamic instability, exacerbation of neurologic injury, respiratory complications, and aspiration of gastric contents, rapid sequence intubation (RSI) is the method of choice, as described in the Emergency Neurologic Life Support (ENLS) algorithm.[1] The sympathetic response associated with laryngoscopy is of particular concern in patients with neurologic emergencies, as the associated hypertension may be deleterious. Although data are limited, pharmacologic pretreatment with a timely bolus of intravenous lidocaine has been reported to mitigate this

---

Box 1
MOANS mnemonic for difficulty in bag-mask ventilation

Mask seal (facial hair, facial anatomy, secretions, ability to apply pressure to face)

Obesity, upper airway obstruction

Age >55, results in loss of tissue elasticity

No teeth

Stiff lungs, or c-Spine precautions

> **Box 2**
> **LEMON mnemonic for difficulty in intubation**
>
> Look externally (eg, jaw abnormalities, teeth, beards, tongue, large incisors)
>
> Evaluate 3-3-2 (number of fingers for interincisor, hyoid-mental, hyoid-thyroid distance)
>
> Mallampati
>
> Obstruction, obesity (eg, head and neck cancer, burn injury, Ludwig angina, hematoma)
>
> Neck mobility (spine precautions, elderly, arthritis)

hemodynamic response and its intracranial pressure (ICP) effect,[5] with a recommended dose of 1.5 mg/kg administered 60 to 90 seconds before laryngoscopy.[5–7] Pretreatment with a short-acting opioid also may be considered, for example, fentanyl at a dose of 2 to 3 μg/kg over 30 to 60 seconds before laryngoscopy.[1] However, this should be avoided in patients with significant hemodynamic instability, or those reliant on sympathetic tone, because of the risk of hypotension.[8]

Attention to hemodynamics with anticipation of peri-intubation hypotension is important, and it is prudent to have vasopressors at the bedside and ideally connected through an intravenous line. A mean arterial pressure (MAP) of 80 to 110 mm Hg should be maintained or a cerebral perfusion pressure (CPP) greater than 60 mm Hg if the ICP is known.[9] According to the ENLS guidelines, induction may be performed with etomidate (0.3 mg/kg) or ketamine (2 mg/kg).[1] However, propofol (1 to 2 mg/kg) is still commonly used for anesthesia induction in these patients. However, for many patients with neurological emergencies lower induction doses may be required to minimize the hemodynamic side effects. Paralysis is typically achieved with either succinylcholine or rocuronium. Sedation and analgesia should be readily available at the bedside to be continued following induction. Noxious stimuli such as tracheal suctioning should be minimized, as these could potentially elevate ICP.

VENTILATION

In patients who are intubated, mechanical ventilation must be carefully adjusted to maintain physiologic homeostasis, as $Paco_2$ is a potent acute mediator of cerebral vascular tone and cerebral blood flow. Hyperventilation should in general be avoided given the associated risk of cerebral vasoconstriction and decreased cerebral blood flow (CBF).[10,11] In patients with critical ICP and impending herniation, hyperventilation may be transiently used pending other therapeutic measures.[12] It is, however, important to consider the risks associated with excessive vasoconstriction and critical CBF reduction that is caused by hyperventilation. A brief course, less than 2 hours, of hyperventilation to a $Paco_2$ of 30 to 35 mm Hg may be considered, while definitive treatment is provided. Hyperventilation is not safe or effective for longer periods of time due to cerebrospinal fluid buffering among other mechanisms.[13,14] In patients with central neurogenic hyperventilation who are at high risk for exacerbation of brain injury by ischemia, targeted therapies to suppress the respiratory drive may be considered (e.g., intravenous opioids, benzodiazepines, or even general anesthetics), in addition to therapies aimed at treating the underlying pathophysiology.[15] Hypoventilation also can be harmful, particularly in patients with intracranial hypertension, by causing deleterious cerebral vasodilation. Likewise, in the setting of metabolic acidosis, suppression of compensatory respiratory drive with sedation or neuromuscular blockade can worsen the metabolic derangement.[1]

Although hypoxia is widely known to cause brain injury, hyperoxia (Pao_2 >300 mm Hg) also can lead to reperfusion injury due to reactive oxygen species, ultimately leading to worse outcomes in patients with traumatic brain injury (TBI) and global hypoxic-ischemic injury after cardiac arrest.[16,17] Following successful intubation, oxygen should thus be weaned to the lowest fraction of inspired oxygen (Fio_2) that will maintain an O_2 saturation of greater than 94%.

Moderate positive end-expiratory pressure (PEEP) (<12 cmH2O) has not been shown to significantly affect the ICP or CPP in patients with acute ischemic stroke, and likely this can be generalized to most patients with acute neurologic injury.[18] High levels of PEEP can potentially worsen intracranial hypertension through its effect on intrathoracic and venous pressures.[19] Caution should be exercised depending on the clinical scenario, understanding that impaired oxygenation or ventilation as a result of inadequate PEEP also can be detrimental. ICP monitoring is advisable for patients who are at risk for elevated ICP in whom a high level of PEEP is needed to ensure adequate oxygenation.

ANESTHESIA AND SEDATION

Sedation and analgesia may be necessary in intubated patients with neurologic emergencies for endotracheal tube tolerance, ventilator synchronization, and minimization of ICP. The objective is to use the lowest dose of sedative/analgesic that maintains comfort and ventilator synchrony, avoiding oversedation and preserving the ability to clinically assess a patient's neurologic status. Due to its effectiveness and relatively short duration of action, propofol is a favored agent in neurologic ICUs. Dexmedetomidine, a centrally acting alpha$_2$-adrenoceptor agonist, is also commonly used and well tolerated by most patients. Caution should be exercised, as dexmedetomidine may cause bradycardia and hypotension in both a dose-dependent and idiosyncratic fashion, especially of concern with bolus dosing.[20,21] Also, weaning should be performed carefully, taking into consideration its long context-sensitive half time, although some patients also may exhibit dexmedetomidine withdrawal characterized by tachycardia, hypertension and agitation. Benzodiazepines are not ideal sedatives for these patients due to a more prolonged effect and an association with delirium and cognitive dysfunction, although their anticonvulsant properties are important for patients with seizures. This is particularly important, as delirium is common among patients with neurologic emergencies, with a reported association with neurologic deficits.[22] Therefore, if used outside of management of seizures, benzodiazepines are best administered as single boluses rather than continuous infusions.

Structured and individualized sedation strategies such as targeted sedation and delirium scores, daily sedation interruption or minimization, linked spontaneous awakening and breathing trials, and early mobilization of the ICU patients can reduce the risk of excessive or prolonged sedation and have been associated with improvements in patient outcomes.[23] These important measures must, nevertheless, be tailored to the individual needs and capabilities of the neurologically injured patient. For instance, spontaneous breathing trials are not ideal in patients with elevated ICP or active seizures, and early mobilization may prove harmful early after a stroke.

An emerging trend for ICU sedation is the use of inhaled anesthetics for ICU sedation, although more studies are needed to further explore the safety of long-term use of inhaled agents.[24]

PHARMACOLOGY OF COMMON ANESTHETIC AND SEDATIVE AGENTS

It is important to be aware of the physiologic effects (**Table 1**), pharmacologic properties (**Table 2**), and side effects of anesthetic agents and sedatives.

Table 1
Anesthetic cerebral metabolic and physiologic effects

Medication	CMR	CBF	CBV	ICP
Barbiturates	−	−	−	−
Benzodiazepines	−	−	−	− or n.c.
Etomidate	−	−	−	−
Propofol	−	−	−	−
Ketamine	+ or n.c.	+	+	+
Dexmedetomidine	− or n.c.	−	−	n.c.
Opioids	n.c.	n.c.	− or n.c.	n.c.
Lidocaine	−	−	−	−
Sevoflurane	−	+	+	+
Isoflurane	−	+	+	+
Desflurane	−	+	+	+

Increase (+), decrease (−), and no change (n.c.).
Abbreviations: CBF, cerebral blood flow; CBV, cerebral blood volume; CMR, cerebral metabolic rate; CSF, cerebrospinal fluid; ICP, intracranial pressure.

Propofol is commonly used for induction, including in critically ill patients. It is thought to act by increasing the duration of the gamma-aminobutyric acid (GABA-A)–activated opening of chloride channels, resulting in cell membrane hyperpolarization.[25] However, propofol should be used cautiously in neurologic emergencies, as it can cause vasodilation and negative inotropic effects leading to a significant reduction in systemic blood pressure, particularly in older patients and those with cardiomyopathy. This effect is most pronounced after bolus doses. Its use is best considered in patients with severe hypertension.[9] It has anticonvulsant effects and is commonly used in the management of patients with refractory status epilepticus.[26] Prolonged treatment with high doses of propofol is associated with a risk of developing propofol infusion syndrome (PRIS), which can lead to cardiac failure, rhabdomyolysis and kidney failure, and metabolic acidosis. Early recognition of these clinical signs (the opening shot is generally an unexplained lactic acidosis) and discontinuation of propofol infusion when PRIS is suspected are crucial to reducing risk of serious complications and death.

Because of its favorable hemodynamic effects, *etomidate* remains a popular anesthetic induction agent for emergent cases, including neurologic emergencies. It is a carboxylated imidazole derivative that enhances the function of neural GABA-A receptors.[27] Some providers use etomidate sparingly due to concern about causing adrenal insufficiency, particularly in septic patients, although this remains controversial and is generally not a major concern in patients with neurologic emergencies.[28–30]

Ketamine is a useful secondary agent to consider for induction in neurologic emergencies. It is a highly lipid-soluble phencyclidine derivate with strong analgesic properties, acting via inhibition of the N-methyl-D-aspartate (NMDA) receptor complex. Ketamine can produce a transient increase in systemic blood pressure and cardiac output through sympathetic stimulation, but is also reported to have direct myocardial depressant properties, which may lead to hypotension. Ketamine is a potent bronchodilator that can be used in patients with asthma or bronchospasm. Historically, ketamine was avoided in neurologic emergencies due to concerns about increasing ICP and cerebral metabolism. However it is increasingly being considered in this setting

Table 2
Context-sensitive half time (CSHT) of various anesthetic medications

Medications	Elimination Half Time (min)	CSHT (min)		
		3-h Infusion	4-h Infusion	8-h Infusion
Fentanyl	462	>100	180	285
Sufentanil	577	26	28	38
Alfentanil	111	51	59	50
Remifentanil	48	<5	<10	<10
Morphine	120	25	30	80
Midazolam	173	50	61	70
Propofol	280	15	20	31
Thiopental	420–1000	120	135	178–200
Etomidate	174–318	6	10	15
Ketamine	150	20	25	35
Dexmedetomidine	180	75	75	75
Diazepam	1200–3000	Massive accumulation		

because of its advantageous hemodynamic profile as well as emerging evidence of neuroprotective effects of NMDA antagonists.[6,31,32] Ketamine is also an anticonvulsant and is recommended as an alternative agent for refractory status epilepticus.[26,33]

Alternative induction agents include benzodiazepines and opioids, although these are rarely used alone. Benzodiazepines act by enhancing activity at the GABA-A receptor complex. Although cardiac output is not affected, a modest decrease in peripheral vascular resistance can lead to systemic hypotension, particularly in the hypovolemic patient. Respiratory depression is not significant, but occurs when larger doses are administered, particularly in combination with opioids. Benzodiazepines have strong anticonvulsant properties and are considered first-line in the treatment of status epilepticus.[26] The onset of intermediate-acting agents (eg, lorazepam) can take minutes at lower doses, so care must be taken to avoid stacking doses and causing oversedation.

Opioids bind to opioid receptors and have relatively modest cardiovascular side effects. In patients with neurologic emergencies, in whom there is significant hyperactivity of the sympathetic nervous system due to brain injury, respiratory distress, or both, however, the sympatholytic effect of opiates can lead to significant drops in blood pressure. When large doses of opioid agonists are administered, this may result in stiff-chest syndrome or skeletal muscle rigidity ("wooden chest syndrome") that can make mask ventilation difficult. This is particularly a concern with fentanyl administered at doses greater than 10 μg/kg, although it may rarely occur with other opioids and at lower doses.[34–36]

Barbiturates such as thiopental and methohexital were the primary anesthesia induction agents before the introduction of propofol. Barbiturates act primarily by prolonging and potentiating the action of GABA on GABA-A receptors, although their diverse clinical activities are also attributed to a blockade of the α-amino-3-hydroxy-5-methyl-4-isoxazolepropionic acid (AMPA)/kainate glutamate receptors and inhibition of glutamate release.[37] Although recovery after a single bolus is rapid, their long context-sensitive half time results in markedly prolonged recovery if administered as repeated boluses or a continuous infusion (see **Table 2**). Similar to propofol, barbiturates can produce a decrease in systemic blood pressure through peripheral vasodilation, and to a lesser extent negative inotropic effects. While rarely used for induction in modern medicine, these may be considered in the setting of alcohol withdrawal or for refractory status epilepticus due to their anticonvulsant properties.[7] Pentobarbital may be used to induce coma in the setting of refractory intracranial hypertension. An electroencephalogram (EEG) should be used to monitor for adequate burst suppression (2–5 bursts/min). Notably, possible adverse effects include hypotension, ileus, and propylene glycol toxicity manifesting with acute renal dysfunction, lactic acidosis, and arrhythmias.[38,39]

Neuromuscular blocking agents (NMBA) may be required to produce skeletal muscle relaxation to facilitate tracheal intubation of patients with neurologic emergencies. For neuromuscular blockade, the 2 rapid-acting agents (succinylcholine or rocuronium) are favored, as they provide optimal intubation conditions without the need for prolonged mask ventilation. In patients with neurologic emergencies that affect the neuromuscular transmission, for example, those with myasthenic crisis, there are additional considerations (see *Acute Neuromuscular Respiratory Failure* section).

Succinylcholine, a depolarizing NMBA, should be avoided in patients more than 24 to 72 hours from acute denervating injury (eg, stroke, spinal cord injury) and in patients with chronic denervating disease (eg, amyotrophic lateral sclerosis, multiple sclerosis) due to a higher risk of severe hyperkalemia.[9] There is a theoretic concern of causing or worsening elevated ICP with succinylcholine.[40] Retrospective data suggest an association between use of succinylcholine and mortality in patients with severe TBI in the emergency department requiring RSI.[41] However, alternative data suggest the effect is likely nonexistent or minimal.[42]

Rocuronium, a non-depolarizing NMBA, is a reasonable alternative in most patients with neurologic emergencies. It should be noted, however, that because of its long duration of action with sustained paralysis, rocuronium is not always ideal for induction of neuromuscular blockade. The clinical duration of RSI doses of rocuronium can exceed 60 minutes, so reversal with sugammadex may be required.[9]

ELEVATED INTRACRANIAL PRESSURE AND/OR CEREBRAL HERNIATION

Intracranial hypertension and acute cerebral herniation are potentially catastrophic neurologic emergencies that require immediate recognition and treatment to prevent irreversible brain injury and death. Although caution should be undertaken with ABCs in any medical emergency, particular attention to their intricacies and heightened awareness of hemodynamics become paramount in this clinical scenario.

In the setting of elevated ICP and/or cerebral herniation, when possible, it is preferable to pursue intubation on an urgent semi-elective basis rather than emergently.[9] This requires anticipating decline and having a low threshold to secure the airway via intubation. If feasible, a conversation should occur between providers and patients/family to clarify wishes regarding intubation and resuscitation.

Before and surrounding the time of intubation, it is important to be diligent in bedside interventions for elevated ICP/herniation. This begins with maintaining head of bed elevation, to a minimum of 30° but ideally as high as is practical. In addition, it is important to ensure that the head and neck is kept midline and that nothing is tight around the neck to facilitate cerebral venous drainage. When the head is lowered for intubation, this should be done at the latest possible moment, and it should be elevated as soon as safely possible following intubation. Only iso-osmotic or hyperosmotic fluids should be used as intravenous solutions. Hyperosmolar therapy with mannitol or hypertonic saline should be considered before, or simultaneously with, intubation.[9] With regard to the intubation, RSI should be pursued whenever possible. Given the theoretical risk of increasing the ICP, succinylcholine may not always be the ideal NMBA in these cases.

ACUTE NEUROMUSCULAR RESPIRATORY FAILURE

Patients presenting with acute neuromuscular respiratory failure require a different evaluation process as compared with standard acute respiratory failure. In addition to constantly assessing the airway and potential need for ventilation, it is important to consider general, subjective, and objective features that more subtly indicate the need for intubation. Also, it is safest to err on the side of caution when encountering acute neuromuscular respiratory failure with a low threshold for ICU monitoring, as the condition may deteriorate quickly.[9] Noninvasive positive pressure ventilation (NIPPV) may be considered on a case-by-case basis, although must be pursued quite cautiously, as handling of secretions may limit bilevel positive airway pressure and continuous positive airway pressure utilization. In general, although NIPPV may be useful in select patients with potentially rapidly treatable conditions like myasthenic crisis, it is not appropriate for patients with neuromuscular respiratory failure due to typically more protracted conditions like Guillain-Barré syndrome. High-flow nasal cannula may provide a false sense of reassurance with regard to oxygenation while allowing hypoventilation-related hypercapnia to worsen.

Unfortunately, no single measure is perfect to predict need for intubation. Important considerations include the patient's sensation of dyspnea, poor handling of secretions, worsening use of accessory muscles, or abdominal paradoxic breathing (**Table 3**). Although objective measures such as negative inspiratory force and forced vital capacity may be considered, these can be misleading and limited by patient's ability to form a mouth seal. Hypoxemia and hypercapnia are often late findings and foretell respiratory collapse.

In patients with acute neuromuscular respiratory failure, bulbar and skeletal weakness increases the risk of aspiration, which makes RSI preferable. An important consideration is the appropriate use of paralytics in this setting. In general, succinylcholine should be avoided if there is evidence of underlying progressive neuromuscular disease such as Guillain-Barré syndrome, chronic neuromuscular weakness, or prolonged immobilization, as it may precipitate acute hyperkalemia.[9] Due to the reduction in available acetylcholine receptors in myasthenia gravis (MG), succinylcholine may be ineffective to achieve paralysis unless a higher dose is used ($\sim$2.5 times the standard dose).[9] Conversely, patients with MG may be extraordinarily sensitive to non-depolarizing NMBA and it is recommended to use half the dose (rocuronium 0.5–0.6 mg/kg) and to consider reversal with sugammadex, or to avoid NMBAs altogether.[9]

Given many conditions that precipitate acute neuromuscular respiratory failure may be associated with dysautonomia, it is prudent to prepare atropine/glycopyrrolate, fluids, and vasopressors before intubation if there is evidence of autonomic instability. It is important to avoid medications that may precipitate myasthenia, and exercise caution with the use of anticholinesterases, which may increase secretions and/or precipitate cholinergic crisis.[9]

ACUTE ISCHEMIC STROKE

Acute ischemic stroke is a time-sensitive neurologic emergency that may require treatment via intravenous thrombolysis or mechanical thrombectomy (MT). Optimal

Table 3
Findings in acute neuromuscular respiratory failure to consider intubation

General	Subjective	Objective
• Increasing generalized muscle weakness • Dysphagia • Dysphonia • Dyspnea on exertion and at rest	• Rapid shallow breathing • Tachycardia • Weak cough • Interrupted or staccato speech (gasping for air) • Use of accessory muscles for breathing • Abdominal paradoxic breathing • Orthopnea • Weakness of trapezius and neck muscles (inability to lift head) • Inability to perform single breath count of 1–20 • Cough after swallowing	• Decreased level of consciousness • Hypoxemia • Vital capacity <1 L or 20 mL/kg, or 50% decrease in 1 d • Maximum inspiratory pressure > −30 cm H_2O • Maximum expiratory pressure <40 cm H_2O • Nocturnal desaturation • Hypercarbia

management requires diligent attention to hemodynamics as well as optimization of procedural anesthesia in the event MT is required.

Initial retrospective studies showed worse outcomes with general anesthesia (GA) as compared with conscious sedation or monitored anesthesia care (MAC)[43,44]; however, more recent prospective trials show equivalent or improved outcomes with both GA and MAC.[45–47] Ultimately the appropriate choice of anesthesia should be individualized to patient and provider. Consider MAC if GA is thought to carry a high risk of hemodynamic instability or consequential delay in intervention. If the patient is unable to cooperate, or when airway control and ventilation may be compromised, GA may be a better choice. Patients requiring conversion to GA during endovascular therapy have worse outcomes, and so it may be prudent to select GA if there is uncertainty.[48]

Before clot retrieval in patients with stroke due to large-vessel occlusion, perfusion of salvageable ischemic brain tissue (the penumbra) is dependent on tenuous collateral blood flow. As such, preservation of blood pressure in this setting is crucial. An arterial line for invasive blood pressure monitoring is useful but should not delay the procedure. The femoral arterial sheath side-port can be transduced in most cases. Blood pressure reduction before recanalization is associated with larger infarct volumes and worse functional outcomes for patients affected by large-vessel intracranial occlusion stroke.[49] Studies have shown that a 10% blood pressure drop from baseline, for more than 10 minutes, during MT is strongly associated with worse neurologic outcomes.[50] For patients undergoing MT under GA, single MAP drops below 60 mm Hg are independently related to unfavorable 3-month outcome.[51] Therefore, every effort should be made to anticipate and prevent hypotensive episodes, especially below this threshold. It may be reasonable to err on the side of modest hypertension rather than hypotension before recanalization, accounting for other factors, such as tissue plasminogen activator administration.

Following recanalization, stringent attention to blood pressure remains paramount. However, at this time, the focus should surround aggressive control of hypertension to reduce the risk of reperfusion injury. Higher blood pressure within the first 24 hours after successful MT is associated with a higher likelihood of symptomatic ICH, mortality, and requiring hemicraniectomy.[52] Although it is likely prudent for blood pressure to be reduced below 160 mm Hg,[53] it is possible that even further antihypertensive control below 140 mm Hg[54] or lower may be appropriate for some patients.[55,56] Further investigation is likely required to better elucidate optimal blood pressure control following MT, and there are ongoing randomized clinical trials.[57]

ACUTE CERVICAL SPINAL CORD INJURY

Patients with traumatic spinal cord injury (SCI) involving the cervical spine are at very high risk for respiratory failure due to a combination of factors including trauma-related airway edema, loss of diaphragmatic innervation (C3, C4, and C5) with failure to ventilate, and loss of chest and abdominal wall strength. All patients with a complete cervical traumatic SCI should be considered for early, elective intubation and mechanical ventilation.[9] Patients with incomplete or lower injuries will have variability in their ability to maintain adequate oxygenation and ventilation. Considerations in these patients include shortness of breath, vital capacity less than 10 mL/kg, or decreasing vital capacity. Also, the appearance of "quad breathing," when the abdomen goes out sharply with inspiration, suggests the need for intubation. When in doubt, it is better to intubate a patient with a cervical traumatic SCI electively rather than wait until it needs to be done emergently.[1]

Generally, patients with cervical traumatic SCI who require intubation should be intubated using a fiberoptic approach by an experienced provider.[9,58] Video- or direct laryngoscopy are reasonable alternatives in emergent scenarios, or if fiberoptic equipment is not available.[59] Cervical stabilization is paramount regardless of the method of intubation chosen. Aspiration precaution should always be taken and RSI considered, although depolarizing NMBAs may need to be avoided (see above). When choosing an induction regimen, caution should be undertaken, as these patients frequently have loss of vasomotor tone caused by the SCI, so sympatholytic medications may result in new or exacerbated hypotension and bradycardia. Caution should be undertaken to evaluate for concomitant injuries that may impact intubation and mechanical ventilation, such as pulmonary contusions, pneumothorax, and rib fractures. Noninvasive ventilation may not be ideal as the inability to cough and clear secretions increases aspiration risk.[9]

Patients with traumatic SCI above T6 often develop neurogenic shock, which is a form of distributive shock characterized by hypotension and bradycardia. Patients may be hypotensive with warm, dry skin due to loss of sympathetic tone. In patients with traumatic injury, other potential sources of hypotension, such as hemorrhage, must be carefully evaluated. In managing hypotension, it is generally accepted to target a MAP of 85 to 90 mm Hg for the first 7 days, although strong evidence supporting this tactic is lacking.[9] This begins with adequate volume resuscitation with intravenous fluids and if necessary colloids and blood transfusions. Thereafter, if there is persistent hypotension, pursue addition of second-line therapy with vasopressors and inotropes. Norepinephrine is preferred, given its alpha and beta activity to treat both hypotension and bradycardia.[9] Phenylephrine is often used due to ease of administration and titration; however, caution should be exercised, as this does not address bradycardia and may worsen it through reflexive mechanisms.[9] Corticosteroids are commonly avoided in traumatic SCI, as data have shown increased risk of complications without neurologic benefit.[60]

SUMMARY

Neurologic emergencies often require GA and mechanical ventilation. It is important to understand the unique airway management, ventilation strategies, and anesthetic considerations in this setting because these choices can affect cerebral physiology and subsequently patient outcomes. RSI is generally preferred for intubation, and ventilation should be adjusted to maintain eucapnia and optimize cerebral perfusion. Knowledge of specific anesthesiological considerations for the scenarios of elevated ICP, neuromuscular respiratory failure, acute ischemic stroke, and acute cervical SCI is paramount to minimize secondary neurologic injury.

CLINICS CARE POINTS

- Patients with neurologic emergencies are at a greater risk of aspiration; RSI may be preferable.
- In patients with elevated ICP, hyperosmolar therapy with mannitol or hypertonic saline should be considered before intubation.
- Hypotension on anesthesia induction for patients with ischemic stroke is associated with worse outcome and should be avoided.
- Patients with cervical traumatic SCI should be intubated with manual inline stabilization or using an awake fiberoptic approach by an experienced provider.

DISCLOSURE

The authors have nothing to disclose.

REFERENCES

1. Rajajee V, Riggs B, Seder DB. Emergency neurological life support: airway, ventilation, and sedation. Neurocrit Care 2017;27(S1):4–28.
2. Davies AE, Stone SP, Kidd D, et al. Pharyngeal sensation and gag reflex in healthy subjects. The Lancet 1995;345(8948):487–8.
3. Walls RM, Hockberger RM, Gausche-Hill M. Rosen's emergency medicine: concepts and clinical practice. 9th Edition. Philadelphia, PA: Elsevier; 2018.
4. Winchell RJ, Hoyt DB. Endotracheal intubation in the field improves survival in patients with severe head injury. Trauma Research and Education Foundation of San Diego. Arch Surg 1997;132(6):592–7.
5. Zeiler FA, Sader N, Kazina CJ. The impact of intravenous lidocaine on ICP in neurological illness: a systematic review. Crit Care Res Pract 2015;2015:485802.
6. Bucher J, Koyfman A. Intubation of the neurologically injured patient. J Emerg Med 2015;49(6):920–7.
7. Bilotta F, Branca G, Lam A, et al. Endotracheal lidocaine in preventing endotracheal suctioning-induced changes in cerebral hemodynamics in patients with severe head trauma. Neurocrit Care 2008;8(2):241–6.
8. Roppolo LP, Walters K. Airway management in neurological emergencies. Neurocrit Care 2004;1(4):405–14.
9. Venkatasubramanian C, Lopez GA, O'Phelan KH, et al. Emergency neurological life support: fourth edition, updates in the approach to early management of a neurological emergency. Neurocrit Care 2020;32(2):636–40.
10. Dumont TM, Visioni AJ, Rughani AI, et al. Inappropriate prehospital ventilation in severe traumatic brain injury increases in-hospital mortality. J Neurotrauma 2010;27(7):1233–41.
11. Rangel-Castilla L, Lara LR, Gopinath S, et al. Cerebral hemodynamic effects of acute hyperoxia and hyperventilation after severe traumatic brain injury. J Neurotrauma 2010;27(10):1853–63.

12. Qureshi AI, Geocadin RG, Suarez JI, et al. Long-term outcome after medical reversal of transtentorial herniation in patients with supratentorial mass lesions. Crit Care Med 2000;28(5):1556–64.
13. Stocchetti N, Maas AIR, Chieregato A, et al. Hyperventilation in head injury: a review. Chest 2005;127(5):1812–27.
14. Zhang Z, Guo Q, Wang E. Hyperventilation in neurological patients: from physiology to outcome evidence. Curr Opin Anaesthesiology 2019;32(5):568–73.
15. Pantelyat A, Galetta SL, Pruitt A. Central neurogenic hyperventilation: a sign of CNS lymphoma. Neurol Clin Pract 2014;4(6):474–7.
16. Brücken A, Kaab AB, Kottmann K, et al. Reducing the duration of 100% oxygen ventilation in the early reperfusion period after cardiopulmonary resuscitation decreases striatal brain damage. Resuscitation 2010;81(12):1698–703.
17. Yamamoto R, Yoshizawa J. Oxygen administration in patients recovering from cardiac arrest: a narrative review. J Intensive Care 2020;8:60.
18. Georgiadis D, Schwarz S, Baumgartner RW, et al. Influence of positive end-expiratory pressure on intracranial pressure and cerebral perfusion pressure in patients with acute stroke. Stroke 2001;32(9):2088–92.
19. Huseby JS, Pavlin EG, Butler J. Effect of positive end-expiratory pressure on intracranial pressure in dogs. J Appl Physiol Respir Environ Exerc Physiol 1978;44(1):25–7.
20. Smuszkiewicz P, Wiczling P, Ber J, et al. Pharmacokinetics of dexmedetomidine during analgosedation in ICU patients. J Pharmacokinet Pharmacodyn 2018; 45(2):277–84.
21. Weerink MAS, Struys MMRF, Hannivoort LN, et al. Clinical pharmacokinetics and pharmacodynamics of dexmedetomidine. Clin Pharmacokinet 2017;56(8): 893–913.
22. von Hofen-Hohloch J, Awissus C, Fischer MM, et al. Delirium screening in neurocritical care and stroke unit patients: a pilot study on the influence of neurological deficits on CAM-ICU and ICDSC outcome. Neurocrit Care 2020;33(3):708–17.
23. Sessler CN, Wilhelm W. Analgesia and sedation in the intensive care unit: an overview of the issues. Crit Care 2008;12(Suppl 3):S1.
24. Herzog-Niescery J, Seipp HM, Weber TP, et al. Inhaled anesthetic agent sedation in the ICU and trace gas concentrations: a review. J Clin Monit Comput 2018; 32(4):667–75.
25. Trapani G, Altomare C, Liso G, et al. Propofol in anesthesia. Mechanism of action, structure-activity relationships, and drug delivery. Curr Med Chem 2000;7(2): 249–71.
26. Brophy GM, Bell R, Claassen J, et al. Guidelines for the evaluation and management of status epilepticus. Neurocrit Care 2012;17(1):3–23.
27. Pejo E, Cotten JF, Kelly EW, et al. In vivo and in vitro pharmacological studies of methoxycarbonyl-carboetomidate. Anesth Analg 2012;115(2):297–304.
28. Albert SG, Ariyan S, Rather A. The effect of etomidate on adrenal function in critical illness: a systematic review. Intensive Care Med 2011;37(6):901–10.
29. Chan CM, Mitchell AL, Shorr AF. Etomidate is associated with mortality and adrenal insufficiency in sepsis: a meta-analysis*. Crit Care Med 2012;40(11):2945–53.
30. Gu WJ, Wang F, Tang L, et al. Single-dose etomidate does not increase mortality in patients with sepsis: a systematic review and meta-analysis of randomized controlled trials and observational studies. Chest 2015;147(2):335–46.
31. Gregers MCT, Mikkelsen S, Lindvig KP, et al. Ketamine as an anesthetic for patients with acute brain injury: a systematic review. Neurocrit Care 2020;33(1): 273–82.

32. Bell JD. In vogue: ketamine for neuroprotection in acute neurologic injury. Anesth Analgesia 2017;124(4):1237–43.
33. Pribish A, Wood N, Kalava A. A review of nonanesthetic uses of ketamine. Anesthesiol Res Pract 2020;2020:5798285.
34. Neidhart P, Burgener MC, Schwieger I, et al. Chest wall rigidity during fentanyl- and midazolam-fentanyl induction: ventilatory and haemodynamic effects. Acta Anaesthesiol Scand 1989;33(1):1–5.
35. Çoruh B, Tonelli MR, Park DR. Fentanyl-induced chest wall rigidity. Chest 2013; 143(4):1145–6.
36. Torralva R, Janowsky A. Noradrenergic mechanisms in fentanyl-mediated rapid death explain failure of naloxone in the opioid crisis. J Pharmacol Exp Ther 2019;371(2):453–75.
37. Löscher W, Rogawski MA. How theories evolved concerning the mechanism of action of barbiturates. Epilepsia 2012;53(Suppl 8):12–25.
38. Bernstein JE, Ghanchi H, Kashyap S, et al. Pentobarbital coma with therapeutic hypothermia for treatment of refractory intracranial hypertension in traumatic brain injury patients: a single institution experience. Cureus 2020;12(9):e10591.
39. Chen HI, Malhotra NR, Oddo M, et al. Barbiturate infusion for intractable intracranial hypertension and its effect on brain oxygenation. Neurosurgery 2008;63(5): 880–6 [discussion: 886–7].
40. Cottrell JE. Succinylcholine and intracranial pressure. Anesthesiology 2018; 129(6):1159–62.
41. Patanwala AE, Erstad BL, Roe DJ, et al. Succinylcholine is associated with increased mortality when used for rapid sequence intubation of severely brain injured patients in the emergency department. Pharmacotherapy 2016;36(1): 57–63.
42. Kovarik WD, Mayberg TS, Lam AM, et al. Succinylcholine does not change intracranial pressure, cerebral blood flow velocity, or the electroencephalogram in patients with neurologic injury. Anesth Analg 1994;78(3):469–73.
43. Löwhagen Hendén P, Rentzos A, Karlsson JE, et al. General anesthesia versus conscious sedation for endovascular treatment of acute ischemic stroke: the anstroke trial (anesthesia during stroke). Stroke 2017;48(6):1601–7.
44. Schönenberger S, Uhlmann L, Hacke W, et al. Effect of conscious sedation vs general anesthesia on early neurological improvement among patients with ischemic stroke undergoing endovascular thrombectomy: a randomized clinical trial. JAMA 2016;316(19):1986–96.
45. Cappellari M, Pracucci G, Forlivesi S, et al. General anesthesia versus conscious sedation and local anesthesia during thrombectomy for acute ischemic stroke. Stroke 2020;51(7):2036–44.
46. Wan TF, Xu R, Zhao ZA, et al. Outcomes of general anesthesia versus conscious sedation for Stroke undergoing endovascular treatment: a meta-analysis. BMC Anesthesiol 2019;19(1):69.
47. Zhang Y, Jia L, Fang F, et al. General anesthesia versus conscious sedation for intracranial mechanical thrombectomy: a systematic review and meta-analysis of randomized clinical trials. J Am Heart Assoc 2019;8(12):e011754.
48. Simonsen CZ, Schönenberger S, Hendén PL, et al. Patients requiring conversion to general anesthesia during endovascular therapy have worse outcomes: a post hoc analysis of data from the saga collaboration. AJNR Am J Neuroradiol 2020; 41(12):2298–302.

49. Petersen NH, Ortega-Gutierrez S, Wang A, et al. Decreases in blood pressure during thrombectomy are associated with larger infarct volumes and worse functional outcome. Stroke 2019;50(7):1797–804.
50. Valent A, Sajadhoussen A, Maier B, et al. A 10% blood pressure drop from baseline during mechanical thrombectomy for stroke is strongly associated with worse neurological outcomes. J Neurointerv Surg 2020;12(4):363–9.
51. Fandler-Höfler S, Heschl S, Argüelles-Delgado P, et al. Single mean arterial blood pressure drops during stroke thrombectomy under general anaesthesia are associated with poor outcome. J Neurol 2020;267(5):1331–9.
52. Anadani M, Orabi MY, Alawieh A, et al. Blood pressure and outcome after mechanical thrombectomy with successful revascularization. Stroke 2019;50(9): 2448–54.
53. Matusevicius M, Cooray C, Bottai M, et al. Blood pressure after endovascular thrombectomy: modeling for outcomes based on recanalization status. Stroke 2020;51(2):519–25.
54. Cernik D, Sanak D, Divisova P, et al. Impact of blood pressure levels within first 24 hours after mechanical thrombectomy on clinical outcome in acute ischemic stroke patients. J Neurointerv Surg 2019;11(8):735–9.
55. Chang JY, Han MK. Postthrombectomy systolic blood pressure and clinical outcome among patients with successful recanalization. Eur Neurol 2019; 81(5–6):216–22.
56. Anadani M, Orabi Y, Alawieh A, et al. Blood pressure and outcome post mechanical thrombectomy. J Clin Neurosci 2019;62:94–9.
57. Mazighi M, Labreuche J, Richard S, et al. Blood Pressure Target in Acute Stroke to Reduce HemorrhaGe After Endovascular Therapy: The Randomized BP TARGET Study Protocol. Front Neurol 2020;11:480.
58. Dutta K, Sriganesh K, Chakrabarti D, et al. Cervical spine movement during awake orotracheal intubation with fiberoptic scope and mcgrath laryngoscope in patients undergoing surgery for cervical spine instability: a randomized control trial. J Neurosurg Anesthesiol 2020;32(3):249–55.
59. Robitaille A, Williams SR, Tremblay MH, et al. Cervical spine motion during tracheal intubation with manual in-line stabilization: direct laryngoscopy versus GlideScope laryngoscopy. Anesth Analg 2008;106(3):935–41, table of contents.
60. Sultan I, Lamba N, Liew A, et al. The safety and efficacy of steroid treatment for acute spinal cord injury: a systematic review and meta-analysis. Heliyon 2020; 6(2):e03414.

Neuromuscular Respiratory Failure

Tarun D. Singh, MBBS, Eelco F.M. Wijdicks, MD, PhD*

KEYWORDS

- Neuromuscular weakness • Myasthenia • GBS • ALS

KEY POINTS

- Normal ventilation depends on the ability to maintain adequate tidal volume and respiratory rate with the diaphragm, manage secretions with oropharyngeal muscles, and clear secretions with the abdominal muscles.
- The diagnosis of neuromuscular weakness is primarily clinical.
- Appropriate triage is essential, particularly in patients with bulbar or severe appendicular weakness.
- The prognosis of patients with neuromuscular weakness depends on cause, appropriate therapy, and meticulous intensive care unit care.

INTRODUCTION

The incidence of neuromuscular disorders (NMDs) ranges from 0.05 to 9 per 100,000/y and the prevalence is between 1 and 10 per 100,000 population.[1] However, they are the primary causes of ICU admission in less than 0.5% of all cases and usually consist of a new diagnosis or a complication of a preexisting disorder.[2] The earliest well-documented cases describing the critical care management of patients with NMDs date back to the 1950s when the National Hospital of Neurology and Neurosurgery in London, United Kingdom, started admitting patients with poliomyelitis, myasthenia gravis (MG), and tetanus,[3] thus starting early critical care neurology. Knowledge of neuromuscular respiratory failure is largely based on years of clinical practice, because clinical studies are hampered by low prevalence of these diseases.

Respiratory mechanics can become impaired in an acutely evolving NMD, leading to aspiration or hypercarbia. These patients can present with early signs of respiratory failure, including tachycardia, tachypnea, increased sweating, and use of accessory muscles, or more obvious findings such as dysphonia, pooling secretions, and hypoxemia. This article discusses the most common neuromuscular conditions that require ICU management, including Guillain-Barré syndrome (GBS), MG, critical illness neuromyopathy (CINM), and amyotrophic lateral sclerosis (ALS). A neuromuscular diagnosis

Division of Critical Care Neurology, Mayo Clinic, 200 First Street South West, Rochester, MN 55905, USA
* Corresponding author.
E-mail address: wijde@mayo.edu

Neurol Clin 39 (2021) 333–353
https://doi.org/10.1016/j.ncl.2021.01.010
0733-8619/21/© 2021 Elsevier Inc. All rights reserved.

can be established with a careful history, examination, laboratory tests, electrodiagnostic and (occasionally) histopathologic evaluation. Determination of neuromuscular respiratory failure is far more difficult and is sometimes arbitrary, particularly when judging severity and need for ventilator support.

CENTRAL COMPONENT OF MECHANICAL RESPIRATORY FAILURE

The medulla oblongata is the location of the central respiratory breathing generator with feedback from chemoreceptors and mechanoreceptors. The ventral respiratory group contains the inspiratory and expiratory neurons, which control the upper airway muscles of inspiration, and the spinal respiratory neurons innervating the intercostal and abdominal muscles. Inhibitory neurons within the pre-Bötzinger complex generate central apneas, including the Ondine curse (central hypoventilation from loss of automaticity of breathing). The nucleus ambiguus innervates the dilator muscles of the soft palate, pharynx, and larynx. Central respiratory chemoreceptors present in the serotonergic raphe neurons in the pons, medulla, and retrotrapezoid nucleus respond to hypercarbia and are relatively immune to acute injury and metabolic insults.

An acquired form of Ondine curse has been described with acute stroke, infections, multiple sclerosis, and some brainstem tumors. Furthermore, acute spinal cord lesions rostral to C3 to C5 levels of the cervical spinal cord can cause complete paralysis of the muscles of inhalation and exhalation, resulting in immediate dependence on mechanical ventilation. Lesions below this level do not affect the diaphragm but may affect the abdominal and intercostal muscles, resulting in reduced expiratory effort.

PERIPHERAL COMPONENT OF MECHANICAL RESPIRATORY FAILURE

There are 4 groups of muscles that are primarily involved in ventilation and respiration. The bulbar muscles are responsible for maintaining the airways open and clearing secretions. The most important inspiratory muscle is the diaphragm, which is responsible for two-thirds of ventilatory effort at rest. It is composed of similar proportions of slow and fast twitch muscle fibers with rich blood supply, making it resistant to fatigue. When the work of breathing is increased, the accessory inspiratory muscles, which include the external intercostal, scalene, and sternocleidomastoid muscles, take over more responsibility. Normal expiration predominantly occurs by passive recoil of the thoracic cage with internal intercostal (thoracic segments 1–12) and abdominal wall muscles (thoracic segments 7–12) helping with forced expiration. More importantly, the abdominal muscles assist in coughing, and weakness in these muscles results in failure to clear secretions.

PATIENT WITH AN ACUTE NEUROMUSCULAR EMERGENCY
History

The evaluation of a patient with suspected acute neuromuscular failure begins with a thorough history, with the true initial diagnostic consideration being whether the problem is of a new onset or whether is an acute exacerbation of an underlying chronic condition. Patients and their families should be asked about developmental history; recent infections, surgeries, and vaccinations; changes in medications; and new/old symptoms. The timing of onset of new symptoms, pattern of muscular weakness, and the pace of progression are crucial for evaluating the need for respiratory support. The most common symptom of neuromuscular respiratory failure is dyspnea that worsens when lying flat (orthopnea). Ascending weakness and hyporeflexia or areflexia are characteristic of GBS, but predominantly bulbar presentation may also occur in Miller Fisher syndrome. Acute inflammatory demyelinating polyneuropathy (AIDP) is often preceded by a viral illness. Some forms of viral acute flaccid paralysis are associated with systemic prodromal symptoms, including fever, malaise, nausea/vomiting, abdominal cramps, diarrhea, rash, lymphadenopathy, and headaches. Tetanus should be suspected in individuals who are unvaccinated with recent wound injuries or drug abuse. Foodborne botulism may result from inadequately sterilized canned products or honey consumption in infants. Rarely, botulism occurs in patients receiving botulinum toxin for therapeutic and cosmetic purposes. Botulism is characterized by rapidly descending paralysis where bulbar muscles are affected first, and may be associated with signs and symptoms of autonomic disturbance such as urinary retention and ileus. Patients with chronic symptoms also complain of nonrefreshing sleep, morning headaches, somnolence, and fatigue.

Physical Examination

The onset of symptoms, pattern of muscle weakness, and acuity of progression are crucial in predicting the need for mechanical ventilation. On inspection, the patient appears tired, has an unpleasant feeling of not catching enough air, and may struggle to breathe. The failure of respiratory mechanics leads to restlessness, tachycardia (>100 beats/min), tachypnea (>20 breaths/min), staccato speech (failure to string more than a few words together in a sentence), gurgling mucus, dysphagia, and dysphonia. The use of accessory muscles, including sternocleidomastoid and scalene muscles, is prominent. The most important sign is the presence of a paradoxic breathing pattern caused by thoracoabdominal dyssynchrony. Normally the abdomen and chest expand and contract in a synchronized manner. During inspiration, downward movement of the diaphragm displaces the abdominal contents down and out as the rib margins are lifted and moved out, raising both the chest and abdomen. In patients with neuromuscular respiratory failure, the movements are not coordinated because of the diaphragmatic failure and create a rocking-horse effect leading to hypoventilation and failure of alveoli deployment, leading to oxygen shunting and hypoxia. The degree of dyssynchrony depends on the severity of the respiratory muscle weakness and is highly suggestive of the need for ventricular assistance. This need can be confirmed by having the patient lay down and laying one hand on the chest and another one on the abdomen and asking the patient to take a deep breath. Furthermore, the neck flexion strength should also be tested because weakness here indicates diaphragmatic weakness. Vital capacity (VC) can be evaluated by asking the patient to count from 1 to 20 in a single breath, with inability to count to 20 being an indication of respiratory compromise. The breathing pattern of acute cervical spinal cord injury usually includes small tidal volumes, tachypnea, but no change in minute ventilation. Patients with chronic disorders such as motor neuron disease (MND)/ALS or Duchenne muscular dystrophy may lapse into respiratory failure with few of these signs and symptoms. The examination should be completed by full assessment of the bulbar, facial, and appendicular muscle weakness, including testing for sustained upgaze and fatigability. Areflexia, dysautonomia, and flaccid tone might suggest a neurogenic disorder, whereas preserved reflexes are more likely in acute myopathy and disorders of the neuromuscular junction. The various signs and symptoms that are suggestive of neuromuscular respiratory failure are listed in **Table 1**.

Diagnostic Evaluation of Neuromuscular Respiratory Failure

The differential diagnosis of acute neuromuscular respiratory failure and localization are shown in **Fig. 1** and **Table 2**. All patients with unclear history should be evaluated

Table 1
Factors associated with neuromuscular respiratory failure

Signs	Symptoms	Diagnostic Studies
Paradoxic respiration	Dyspnea without exertion	Breath count <20
Severe bulbar weakness	Cough after swallowing	Hypercapnia
Decreased consciousness	Diaphoresis	Vital Capacity<20 mL/kg
Accessory muscle use	Tachypnea	or <1 Liter
Rapid clinical decline	Shallow breathing	Maximum inspiratory
Staccato speech	Difficulty handling secretions	pressure >30 cm H_2O
Orthopnea	Restlessness	Maximum expiratory
Weak/absent cough	Morning headaches (chronic)	pressure <40 cm H_2O
Neck flexion weakness	Excessive daytime sleepiness	Progressive decline in spirometry
Severe dysautonomia		values over time
		Normal $Paco_2$ in tachypnea
		Decrease in Pao_2 without
		desaturation
		Atelectasis on chest radiograph
		Diaphragm paralysis on
		ultrasonography

for reversible underlying causes of respiratory failure. Patients with signs of impending failure should be admitted to the ICU for close monitoring. Chest radiograph should be done to exclude underlying pulmonary issues such as pneumonia. Bedside pulmonary function tests provide the most vital information to monitor worsening respiratory failure and need for mechanical ventilation.

Forced VC (FVC), maximum inspiratory pressure (MIP)/negative inspiratory force, and maximum expiratory pressure (MEP) are the most common spirometry measures used to evaluate respiratory function. An FVC of less than 20 mL/kg or a 30% decline or more over 24 hours, MIP of less than −30 cm H_2O, and an MEP of less than 40 cm H_2O are indicators of impending respiratory failure (also known as the 20/30/40 rule).[4] Furthermore a decrease in FVC exceeding 20% from upright to supine also suggests diaphragmatic weakness. The trend of these measurements rather than an abnormal value is most important ,and all effort should be made to measure these in the same body position every time. It is crucial to ensure that the patient provides maximal effort, has a good seal around the spirometer (masks can be used in patients with bulbar weakness), and multiple efforts, choosing the best of 3 attempts, should be used for reliability.

Measurement of the sniff nasal inspiratory pressures in patients with GBS has suggested better correlation with worsening weakness than spirometry, because these patients have circumventing leaks from facial diplegia. The sniff nasal inspiratory pressure test is performed by wedging a bung into 1 nostril, through which a thin catheter connected to a pressure transducer has been passed (completely obstructs flow through that nostril). The patient is instructed to sniff as strongly as possible through the contralateral unobstructed nostril. The pressure measured in the obstructed nostril is an indicator of inspiratory muscle strength. Nasal sniff pressures should be preferred in chronic conditions where the mouth seal is impaired, as in patients with bulbar weakness. Although important to detect hypoxemia, pulse oximetry does not identify abnormalities of CO_2. Overnight pulse oximetry can suggest nocturnal hypoventilation as a sign of respiratory muscle weakness.

Because the primary pattern of respiratory failure in patients with NMDs is restrictive, patients develop atelectasis at the lung bases, causing blood shunting leading

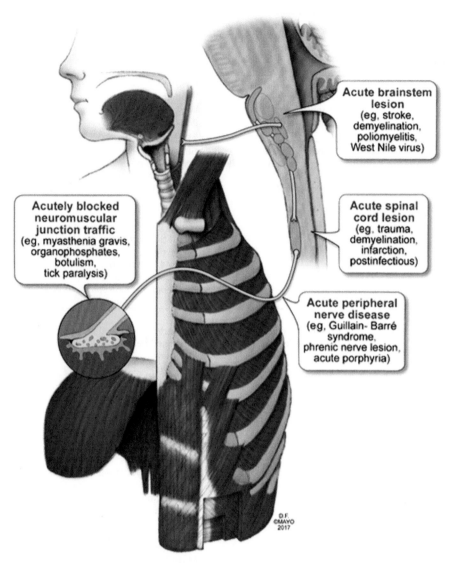

Fig. 1. The muscles involved in inspiration; the diaphragm and its peripheral innervation; the main causes of acute respiratory failure.

to mild hypoxia. As patients become more fatigued, they develop alveolar hypoventilation, as shown by normal Pco_2 and slightly low levels of Pao_2 on arterial blood gases (ABGs). In the later stages of the respiratory failure with worsening weakness, alveoli start to collapse and tidal volumes get progressively smaller, eventually leading to hypercapnia,[5] causing a mixed hypoxemic-hypercapnic respiratory failure. Thus the arterial Pco_2 increases to greater than normal when the diaphragm becomes adynamic and a normal arterial Pco_2 in a tachypneic patient may signal impending fatigue and respiratory failure.

Neurophysiologic testing for neuromuscular disease includes electromyography (EMG) and nerve conduction studies (NCSs), including repetitive nerve stimulation

Table 2
Differential diagnosis of acute neuromuscular failure by localization within the peripheral nervous system

Localization	Clinical Examination	Diseases
Anterior horn cell	Proximal and distal weakness No sensory loss Increased reflexes in ALS	MND Polio and postpolio syndrome West Nile virus Paraneoplastic MND Kennedy disease
Peripheral nerve	Weakness dependent on the nerve/nerves involved Sensory loss Decreased reflexes	GBS Polyneuropathies Acute onset of chronic inflammatory demyelinating polyneuropathy Toxins Trauma Critical illness polyneuropathy Vasculitic neuropathy Porphyria Amyloid neuropathy Malignant infiltration Paraneoplastic neuropathy Phrenic nerve injury
Neuromuscular junction	Generalized weakness No sensory loss Normal reflexes	MG Lambert-Eaton myasthenic syndrome Prolonged neuromuscular blockade Botulism Organophosphorus poisoning Tick paralysis Snake bite Hypermagnesemia
Muscle	Proximal weakness No sensory loss Normal reflexes	Critical illness myopathy Rhabdomyolysis Polymyositis Periodic paralysis Metabolic myopathies (hyperkalemia, hypokalemia, hypernatremia, hypophosphatemia, hyperthyroidism) Inflammatory myopathies Toxins Mitochondrial myopathy Acid maltase deficiency Muscular dystrophy

and phrenic nerve stimulation. The phrenic nerve can be easily stimulated underneath the posterior border of the sternocleidomastoid, and needle diaphragm EMG can be performed by needle entry at the sixth or seventh intercostal space. Some recent studies have also used fluoroscopy and ultrasonography to show the absence of diaphragmatic excursion during voluntary sniffing.[6] These tests can also be used to assess potential functional diaphragm recovery.[7]

Other tests to consider in the evaluation of neuromuscular respiratory failure include creatinine kinase, chemistry panel, antibodies for MG and Lambert-Eaton myasthenic syndrome (LEMS), antiganglioside antibodies, lumbar puncture, and biopsy of nerve/muscle for severe cases. Dynamic MRI for accessing diaphragm function with a short acquisition times of less than 30 minutes will potentially be useful in future.[8–10]

Respiratory Support

Any respiratory distress signal requires intensive care admission. Oxygen administration should be used cautiously to achieve saturation between 90% and 95%, but prolonged oxygen administration can lead to CO_2 retention in patients with neuromuscular respiratory failures resulting in hypercapnic coma or respiratory arrest.[11]

Noninvasive ventilation with bilevel positive airway pressure (BiPAP) is a very good option for patients with respiratory failure caused by MG, ALS presenting acutely, and chronic muscular disorders, because it provides positive airway pressure during inspiration and expiration with oxygen flow and hence helps to improve oxygenation and ventilation.[12] BiPAP has shown considerable benefit in patients with MG exacerbations with respiratory failure.[13] However, it is unreliable in patients with GBS, in whom diaphragmatic failure is often too severe to be treated with pressure support alone and should not be continued if these patients continue to use accessory muscles despite being on BiPAP. Typical settings for BiPAP are an inspiratory positive airway pressure of 10 cm H_2O (range 5–25 cm H_2O) and an expiratory positive airway pressure of 5 cm H_2O (range 0–30 cm H_2O) with a backup rate of 12 to 16 breaths/min. BiPAP could also be considered as a rescue therapy in postextubation patients who are showing increased work of breathing and possible need for reintubation but who maintain adequate ability to manage secretions.[14] Limitations of BiPAP include discomfort from the close-fitting mask, failure to rest and sleep, leaks, and gastric distention. BiPAP should not be used in patients with inability to clear secretions because of aspiration risk. It is also not successful in patients with profound cholinergic symptoms. Clinical evaluation of the patient's comfort is the best judge of using BiPAP. High-flow nasal cannula has been considered as an alternative to BiPAP in mild respiratory weakness because it provides up to 70 L/min and an fraction of inspired oxygen (Fio_2) of 100% via large-bore binasal prongs, but it must be used judiciously to avoid hypercarbia and these patients should be monitored closely.[15] Other diseases that can benefit from BiPAP are progressive NMDs such as ALS and muscular dystrophies when an acute illness causes a sudden decompensation in the patient's respiratory function.[16,17]

Mechanical support is often short term in MG and prolonged in GBS.[18] Several clinical decisions dictate the timing of intubation. Clear clinical signs, including patient distress, inability to clear secretions, weak cough, tachypnea, hemodynamic instability, abnormal ABGs suggesting hypoxia, or early hypercapnia, favor immediate intubation. Patients who present with more subtle signs such as restlessness, anxiety, accessory respiratory muscles use, nasal flaring, mouth opening, and increased oxygen demand despite correcting hypoxemia could be preemptively intubated rather than guided by pulmonary function tests. Patients who present with worsening pulmonary function tests and progressive symptoms are a practical dilemma, and many factors might play into the decision regarding intubation and mechanical support. The patient's diagnosis and the natural course of the disease, oropharyngeal weakness, dysphonia, worsening pulmonary function tests with a continuous decline of VC reaching 10 to 15 mL/kg, and the 20/30/40 rule in GBS may guide practitioners.

As the symptoms improve for the intubated patients, spontaneous breathing trials are recommended and it is preferred to monitor them for at least 24 hours on pressure support before extubation. The process can be initiated once VC reaches 10 to 15 mL/kg and spontaneous tidal volumes of 7 mL/kg are attained. In GBS, maximal inspiratory mouth pressures exceeding −50 cm H_2O and VC improvement by 4 mL/kg from preintubation to preextubation were associated with successful extubation, but measurement of pulmonary function tests depends on patient effort and is difficult while still intubated, and these volitional measurements should not be seen as a definitive threshold. No single value is a predictor of extubation success.[4] In MG, one important priority is to achieve satisfactory treatment of the myasthenic symptoms. Age more than 50 years, low peak FVC values in the first week, and increased bicarbonate level at baseline are predictive factors of longer time on mechanical intubation.[19]

GUILLAIN-BARRÉ SYNDROME AND RELATED DISORDERS

The term GBS is applied to a group of acute radiculoneuropathies, including AIDP, Miller Fisher syndrome, acute motor axonal neuropathy (AMAN), and acute motor and sensory axonal neuropathy. It is an acute immune polyradiculoneuropathy characterized by ascending flaccid weakness with areflexia and can lead to neuromuscular respiratory failure. In Europe and North America, GBS incidence is between 0.8 and 1.9 per 100,000 people with a slight male predominance,[20] and the incidence increases with age up to 2.7 per 100,000 people per year in patients older than 80 years.[21] GBS is responsible for more than 6000 hospital admissions per year in the United States.[22] Miller Fisher syndrome comprises up to 5% of the GBS cases in Western Europe, with higher rates in Japan and Taiwan.[23]

GBS often occurs with antecedent infection by *Campylobacter jejuni*, Cytomegalovirus, Epstein-Barr virus, influenza A, *Haemophilus influenzae*, *Mycoplasma*, or Zika virus among others. Pathogenesis of GBS is thought to be secondary to an autoimmune response caused by a preceding infection that cross reacts with peripheral nerve components, causing the immune system to attack the peripheral nerves and spinal roots.

Clinical Presentation

Patients usually present with rapidly worsening weakness that typically begins 10 to 14 days after a viral illness, usually an upper respiratory or diarrheal illness. The first symptoms are often lumbar pain with a tight feeling around the torso and distal leg paresthesias, followed by symmetric progressive weakness (often called ascending, but weakness often involves both arms and legs). Symptoms usually reach their nadir by 2 weeks but can worsen up to 4 weeks after symptom onset. Bulbar involvement is present in approximately 50% of patients and bilateral facial weakness predominates, followed by oropharyngeal weakness and ophthalmoparesis.[24] Patients with Miller Fisher variant present with primary involvement of oculomotor muscles and ataxia. Miller Fisher variant often becomes more generalized with oropharyngeal and extremity weakness.

Dysautonomia is a major feature of severe GBS and can lead to cardiac arrhythmias, hemodynamic instability, gastroparesis, paralytic ileus, and urinary retention. Neuropathic pain is present in up to 70% of patients and may be disabling and refractory. It is usually radiculopathic and is accompanied by severe allodynia. Respiratory failure occurs in approximately 25% of patients with classic GBS.[5] The most severely affected patients with GBS can develop a locked-in state. This state occurs mostly in the axonal variants, with rapid progression of symptoms in a matter of days.

Diagnosis

The diagnosis of GBS is primarily clinical and can be supported by cerebrospinal fluid (CSF) abnormalities and electrophysiologic findings. Imaging has a limited role and is used to exclude structural lesions. The clinical criteria are progressive ascending paresis, usually symmetric with hyporeflexia or areflexia. The most prominent abnormalities are seen typically about 2 weeks into the course of the disease.[25] In the demyelinating form of GBS, electrodiagnostic findings include increased F-wave latency (earliest sign), prolonged distal motor latency, decrease in compound muscle action potential (CMAP), conduction block, and temporal dispersion with normal sensory nerve potentials.[26] In axonal forms, NCSs show decreased motor or sensory amplitudes, based on the nerve involvement. EMG shows decreased recruitment, fibrillations, positive sharp waves, and polyphasic motor unit action potentials.[26] Fibrillations are more prominent between 6 and 10 weeks and polyphasic motor unit action potentials between 9 and 15 weeks after symptoms onset. Albuminocytologic dissociation (increased CSF protein levels without pleocytosis) is the characteristic abnormality in the CSF. CSF protein level can be normal within the early course of the disease (24–48 hours), but is expected to increase later in the course of disease. Blood tests have a minimal role in the diagnosis. The most relevant is the presence of antiganglioside antibodies, most notably GM1a, GM1b, GD1a, GalNac-GD1a in AMAN related to *C. jejuni* infection and GQ1b in Miller Fisher syndrome.

Management

The priority in patients with suspected GBS is to determine the best level of monitoring that the patient will require. It is extremely important to recognize the signs of early respiratory failure as discussed in **Table 1**, and the presence of severe progressive weakness, bulbar muscle involvement, signs of diaphragmatic insufficiency, and dysautonomia indicate ICU admission. Noninvasive ventilation is not a good option and these patients should be intubated because the muscle involvement will take weeks to improve.

Clinical trials have established the use of either intravenous immunoglobulin (IVIg) or plasma exchange (PLEX) as standard treatment.[27,28] It is imperative to initiate therapy as early as possible, because the beneficial effects of IVIg and PLEX have been shown when they are administered within 2 weeks of the onset of symptoms. The choice of agent should be based on the experience of the hospital facility and treating physicians. In patients who fail the first course of IVIg, a second course might be beneficial. Combining IVIg and PLEX does not provide any additional benefit.[29] Corticosteroids alone are not beneficial, whereas the combination of IVIg and high-dose methylprednisolone could have some short-term benefits compared with IVIg alone, but their use is not recommended because of the side effect profile of high-dose steroids.[30] The comparison of IVIg and PLEX is shown in **Table 3**.

Various systemic complications can occur during the course of the disease. These complications and their recommended treatments are listed in **Table 4**.

Long-Term Outcome

The outcome and prognosis of GBS depends on the clinical phenotype. Factors associated with poor outcome include age greater than 60 years, rapid progression to severe weakness (7 days or less), need for ventilator support, mean distal CMAP amplitude of less than 20%, and a preceding diarrheal illness.[31,32] Approximately 20% of patients with GBS are not able to walk without assistance at 6 months, and most patients continue to experience fatigue and pain.[33] The mortality varies between 2.4% and 6.4% and can be as high as 15% to 30% in mechanically ventilated patients.[34]

MYASTHENIA GRAVIS IN THE INTENSIVE CARE UNIT

MG is the most common autoimmune disorder of the neuromuscular junction (NMJ) and is caused by antibodies against the postsynaptic acetylcholine receptors

Table 3
Comparison of immunoglobulin with plasma exchange

	Immunoglobulin	PLEX
Dose	2 g/kg divided into 5 doses of 0.4 g/kg or 2 doses of 1 g/kg	5 treatments performed on alternate days with removal of ~3 L
Symptoms	Chest pain Infusion reaction: headache, shivering, myalgia	Hypotension
Practical considerations	May need to check IgA levels before treatment	Hemodialysis catheter needed
Advantages	Shorter course, widely available	Lower cost, faster response in MG
Disadvantages	Higher cost and occasional shortages (in United States)	Central access needed, needs access to specialized equipment
Procedure-related complications	Hyperviscosity (risk of arterial and venous thrombosis) Aseptic meningitis Anaphylaxis (if IgA deficient) Acute kidney injury TRALI)	Venous catheter-related infection, pneumothorax, local hematoma Mild coagulopathy Hypocalcemia TRALI
Contraindications	Congenital IgA deficiency, CHF, hypercoagulable state	Sepsis

Abbreviations: CHF, congestive heart failure; Ig, immunoglobulin; TRALI, transfusion-related acute lung injury.

(AChR) or muscle-specific tyrosine kinase (MuSK) affecting NMJ transmission. The incidence of MG varies from 0.25 to 2 per 1 million people, with prevalence of 40 to 180 per 1 million people worldwide with 10% in the pediatric population.[35,36] MG has a bimodal distribution with early-onset disease seen more commonly in women in the second and third decades of life and late onset in men during the sixth to eighth decades of life.[37] About 85% of the antibodies are directed against AChR and 40% of patients who are AChR seronegative have MuSK.[36] Lipoprotein-related protein 4 (LRP4) autoantibodies were identified in 2011 and are positive in 9% of patients who are negative for both AChR and MuSk antibodies.[38]

Myasthenic crisis is defined by the presence of respiratory failure and occurs in 10% to 60% of patients with MG, and about one-fifth of patients have at least 1 crisis during their disease course.[39]

Clinical Presentation

Fatigable muscle weakness is the hallmark of the disease. The typical examination features include ptosis, diplopia caused by ocular motility deficits that cannot be localized to specific cranial nerves, jaw or tongue weakness, neck flexion/extension weakness, and dysarthric speech. The muscle weakness is asymmetric and fluctuates during the day. Head drop and bulbar weakness are more common with MuSK antibodies.[40] Nearly 50% to 80% of patients who initially present with ocular symptoms develop systemic MG within 2 years of initial presentation.[41] About 20% of patients have a crisis within the first year of diagnosis, which is usually triggered by a precipitating factor such an infection, illness, surgery, pregnancy, emotional stress, or exposure to medications such as aminoglycosides. Medications that have been implicated in precipitating myasthenic crisis are shown in **Table 5**. Poor respiratory capacity can

Table 4
Possible complications associated with Guillain-Barré syndrome and suggested treatments

System	Complications	Prevention/Treatment
Neurologic/ psychiatric	Neuropathic pain Depression Anxiety Insomnia Delirium	Pain medications with antidepressant actions: gabapentin/pregabalin, SNRI, TCAs Avoid opioids (can worsen ileus) Sleep aids Delirium precautions, including avoiding sedative drugs (eg, benzodiazepines)
Cardiac	Labile blood pressure Cardiac arrhythmias Tachycardia/bradycardia Atrioventricular blocks Asystole	Continuous cardiac monitoring Avoid β-blockers Atropine at bedside Low-dose short-acting drugs preferred (eg, nicardipine, clevidipine, hydralazine) Fluids for hypotensive episodes Low-dose vasopressors Avoidance of vagal maneuvers
Pulmonary	Respiratory failure Aspiration Pneumonia Ventilator-associated complications Mucous plugging Need for tracheostomy Pulmonary embolism	Avoid succinylcholine for induction for intubation Elective intubation, avoid rapid sequence intubation Aggressive pulmonary hygiene Daily bedside spirometry Adequate mobilization when possible DVT prophylaxis
Gastrointestinal	Adynamic ileus Gastroparesis Need for nasogastric tube/PEG tube Stress ulcers	Aggressive bowel regimens including use of daily suppositories Avoid metoclopramide and neostigmine if dysautonomia Minimize opioids Stress ulcer prophylaxis
Genitourinary	Urinary retention Urinary incontinence	Intermittent or continuous catheterization
Endocrinology	Syndrome of inappropriate secretion of antidiuretic hormone (hyponatremia)	Fluid restriction Hypertonic saline
Musculoskeletal	Pressure ulcers DVT Critical illness neuropathy/ myopathy	DVT prophylaxis Mobilization Early involvement of PMR/PT/ OT

Abbreviations: DVT, deep vein thrombosis; OT, occupational therapy; PEG, percutaneous endoscopic gastrostomy; PMR, physical medicine and rehabilitation; PT, physical therapy, SNRI, serotonin-norepinephrine reuptake inhibitor; TCAs, tricyclic antidepressants.

Table 5 Medications that may exacerbate myasthenia gravis	
Anesthetic agents: Isoflurane Halothane Lidocaine Bupivacaine	Neuromuscular blockers: Depolarizing: succinylcholine Nondepolarizing: vecuronium, rocuronium
Cardiac medications: β-Blockers Calcium channel blockers Verapamil	Ophthalmologic medications: Timolol
Antibiotics: Tetracyclines Macrolides Fluoroquinolones Aminoglycosides Nitrofurantoin	Anticonvulsant medications: Carbamazepine Phenytoin Phenobarbital Ethosuximide Gabapentin
Psychiatric drugs: Lithium Haloperidol Chlorpromazine Phenothiazine Amitriptyline	Miscellaneous: Magnesium Interleukin Pembrolizumab Glucocorticoids

be assessed by asking the patient to count from 1 to 20 in a single breath, with each number equating to ~100 mL of FVC. Pain or sensory deficits are uncommon in MG and neither bladder/bowel dysfunction nor autonomic involvement occurs.

Cholinergic crisis can also result in respiratory failure mimicking a myasthenic crisis. These patients usually present with signs of cholinergic toxicity, including increased salivation, bronchial secretions, miosis, sweating, bradycardia, diarrhea, and fasciculations. MG with MuSk can have an increased sensitivity to cholinergic effects.[42]

Diagnosis

The diagnosis of MG can be made by combination of history, typical physical examination that shows the presence of NMJ failure, electrophysiologic studies, or serologic testing. The bedside testing used for diagnosis includes the edrophonium test and the ice-pack test. These tests have high sensitivity but have fallen out of favor because of low specificity and high interpreter variability.

The edrophonium test begins with administration of 2 mg intravenously followed by 2 mg every 60 seconds up to a total of 10 mg. A positive test is characterized by rapid improvement of symptoms and has a sensitivity of 80% to 90%. Testing should be avoided in elderly patients, cardiac abnormalities, or with bronchospasm, and should only be performed in the inpatient setting with atropine available at the bedside because the patients can develop cholinergic side effects. The ice-pack test is only useful in patients with ptosis and is performed by placing an ice pack on the ptotic eye for 2 minutes. Immediate improvement in ptosis constitutes a positive test.

Single-fiber EMG is the gold standard of diagnosis of MG and shows increased jitter. Slow (2–3 Hz) repetitive nerve stimulation has a sensitivity of 80% in patients with generalized MG, but less than 50% in those with only ocular symptoms.[43] A decrement of more than 10% in CMAP amplitude is seen and is more pronounced between the first and second stimuli. In the ICU, these tests are only necessary to establish a new diagnosis or if the diagnosis is in question.

Chest computed tomography should be obtained in a new diagnosis of MG to exclude thymoma. Serologic testing for AChR-binding antibodies should be performed. Additional antibody testing includes antistriational antibodies, MuSk, and LRP4 antibodies.

Management

Myasthenic crisis consists of respiratory failure and hence these patients should be assessed for clinical signs of respiratory distress, oxygen desaturation, and hypercapnia. Patients with bulbar weakness and respiratory distress should be evaluated for prompt initiation of mechanical ventilation. Immediate BiPAP support has been found to decrease the need for intubation and decrease the length of stay in the ICU.[44] However, endotracheal intubation is seldom avoided in patients with increasing $Paco_2$ values. Elective intubation should be considered in patients with significant bulbar weakness, severe hypercapnia, profound hypoxia, and those with contraindication to BiPAP. Weaning from invasive ventilation can be challenging, and extubation failure occurs in 25% of patients.[45] Ventilator weaning directly to BiPAP may increase the chances of successful extubation.

Immunotherapy with IVIg or PLEX should be administered as soon as possible. Both interventions are well tolerated and equally effective, but combination therapy does not add benefit.[46,47] There is minimal evidence suggesting IVIg may be safer in elderly patients and those with complex medical comorbidities.[48] Concomitant steroid administration is the standard of care, and prednisone 1 mg/kg ideal body weight is most commonly used. Patients receiving high-dose steroids can experience worsening of weakness; hence, patients on noninvasive ventilation should be monitored carefully. The beneficial effects of steroids usually manifest after 2 to 6 weeks. Early BiPAP with administration of PLEX or IVIg has been shown to successfully treat some patients with myasthenic crisis with lower rates of pulmonary complications.

Cholinesterase inhibitors, including pyridostigmine and neostigmine, provide symptomatic treatment, and dosage depends on the severity of symptoms. These medications should be transiently discontinued after intubation to reduce secretions but should never be stopped in patients with noninvasive ventilation.

Steroid-sparing agents such as azathioprine (total dose of 2–3 mg/kg) in combination with steroids have been shown to shorten time to remission and reduce relapses compared with steroids alone.[49] The dose of azathioprine can be decreased by 25% with addition of allopurinol, which reduces its metabolism and hence decreases the toxicity.[50] Other second-line agents to consider include methotrexate, cyclosporine, cyclophosphamide, mycophenolate mofetil, and tacrolimus. Rituximab is an alternative monotherapy in refractory MG, especially in patients with MuSK antibodies. Thymectomy has shown an increased rate of remission in patients with generalized and severe MG but is not recommended for patients who are positive for MuSK antibodies.[51]

Long-Term Outcome

The mortality from MG has improved greatly in the second half of the twentieth century, decreasing from 30% to less than 5%.[39] This improvement is likely attributable in part to better understanding of the disease, as well as advancements in critical care, including ventilatory support.

AMYOTROPHIC LATERAL SCLEROSIS

ALS is a progressive, incurable neurodegenerative disease that affects both upper and lower motor neurons (LMNs). It is the most common MND, with an incidence of about

2 in 100,000 and the average age of onset in the seventh decade.[52] In the United States, the cumulative lifetime risk is 1 in 400 and death occurs because of respiratory paralysis within 3 to 5 years.[52,53]

Clinical Presentation

The hallmark of ALS is progressive asymmetric weakness with both upper motor neuron (spasticity, hyperreflexia) and LMN (flaccid weakness, fasciculations, and diminished reflexes) signs. ALS is broadly classified as limb-onset ALS, which comprises nearly 80% of cases, and bulbar onset, which is characterized by early dysarthria and dysphagia. A small minority of patients present with isolated respiratory symptoms.

Diagnosis

The diagnosis of ALS is primarily based on history and examination. Laboratory work-up and imaging are obtained to exclude other potential causes. The differential diagnosis of MND is shown in **Table 6**. NCSs support the diagnosis by demonstrating

Table 6
Mimickers of amyotrophic lateral sclerosis in the intensive care unit with the disease characteristics

Diagnosis	Motor Neuron Involvement	Characteristics
Kennedy disease	Lower	Gynecomastia Peripheral neuropathy Perioral fasciculations X-linked
Spinal muscular atrophy 4	Lower	Onset>30 y Axial>limb weakness
Multifocal motor neuropathy	Lower in bibrachial pattern	Arm and hand weakness Increased anti-GM1 antibodies Response with IVIg
Cervical radiculomyelopathy	Upper and lower, upper, lower	Sensory loss Focal reflex loss
Primary lateral sclerosis	Upper	Slow progression
MG	None	Diplopia, ptosis Fluctuating weakness
Infectious myelitis (West Nile virus, poliovirus, coxsackie B virus)	Lower	History of exposure Subacute presentation
AIDP and variants	Lower	Ascending sensorimotor symptoms Diffuse hyporeflexia
Lymphoma	Lower	Cranial neuropathies Lumbar polyradiculopathy
Paraneoplastic (ANNA-1, ANNA-2)	Upper, lower, or both	Subacute onset Encephalitis Type B symptoms
Myopathy (inclusion body myositis, acid maltase deficiency, necrotizing autoimmune myopathy)	None	Proximal>distal weakness Increased creatine kinase level

Abbreviations: ANNA, antineuronal nuclear antibodies.

intact sensory studies and motor conduction velocities in the presence of decreased CMAP amplitudes. Fibrillation potential and reduced recruitment of the motor units on needle EMG with tall long-motor units further support the diagnosis.

Management

There are 2 medications that are approved for the treatment of ALS. Riluzole given at a dosage of 50 mg/d has been shown to increase the survival by 2 to 3 months.[54] The second medication, edaravone (Radicava), was approved in 2017 and is associated with a slower decline over 6 months.[55] Although these medications can modestly increase survival, the mainstay of management of ALS is symptomatic treatment. **Table 7** summarizes the pharmacologic and nonpharmacologic approach to symptom management.

The most common cause of death from ALS is respiratory failure. FVC is the most commonly used parameter to assess respiratory function, but it is not a very sensitive test. An FVC cutoff of 75% of predicted is suggested for monitoring of respiratory function and ventilatory assistance.[56] Sniff nasal pressure has shown greater predictive power than FVC because it detected hypercapnia with a sensitivity of 90% and specificity of 87%.[57] A mean oxygen saturation (Sao_2) of less than 93%, nocturnal desaturation of less than 90%, as well as an apnea-hypopnea index greater than 5 in polysomnography are also associated with poor outcome.[58]

Both invasive and noninvasive ventilatory support play significant roles in the treatment of respiratory failure in ALS. Noninvasive ventilation, typically BiPAP, has been shown to improve the median survival by 205 days and to improve quality of life in patients with ALS with severe bulbar dysfunction.[59] In patients who do not tolerate noninvasive ventilation, invasive ventilation via tracheostomy should be offered as an alternative. Tracheostomy not only prolongs the survival (10.4 vs 0.8 months) but also offers a comparable quality of life with noninvasive ventilation for patients with ALS.[60] Once the tracheostomy is in place, the most common cause of mortality is acute respiratory tract infection.[61] Diaphragmatic pacing has not been shown to be an effective procedure for ALS because it was associated with decreased survival and increased adverse events.[62]

Patients with ALS often have trouble with handling oral secretions because of bulbar weakness. These problems are further exacerbated by sialorrhea and difficulty coughing

Table 7		
Approach to symptom management of amyotrophic lateral sclerosis		
Symptom	**Pharmacologic Treatment**	**Nonpharmacologic Treatment**
Spasticity	Baclofen, tizanidine, botulinum toxin injections	Stretching exercises, early involvement with PT/OT
Cramps	Levetiracetam, quinine, mexiletine	Stretching, adequate hydration
Sialorrhea	Scopolamine patch, amitriptyline, atropine, glycopyrrolate, salivary gland botulinum injections	Oral care
Constipation	Laxatives, fiber supplements	Hydration, exercise
Pseudobulbar affect	Dextromethorphan/quinidine, SSRIs	Education

Abbreviation: SSRIs, selective serotonin reuptake inhibitors.

because of the weak expiratory muscles. Medical management includes anticholinergic bronchodilators, beta-receptor agonists, mucolytics such as guaifenesin, procedures including botulinum toxin injections, and radiotherapy to the salivary glands. Mechanical insufflation-exsufflation with an inflated cuff aids in clearing secretions by increasing the peak cough expiratory flows, especially in patients with bulbar weakness.[63,64] High-frequency chest wall oscillation is also helpful in decreasing the symptom of breathlessness.[65]

Dysphagia from bulbar weakness increases the patient's risk of aspiration. Gastrostomy feeding tube placement is vital in providing feeds and an alternative route for medication administration. Placement is recommended before the FVC decreases to less than 50% of the predicted value.[66] Placement of a percutaneous endoscopic gastrostomy, radiologically inserted gastrostomy, and peroral gastrostomy are all considered equally safe in patients with ALS.[67]

CRITICAL ILLNESS NEUROMYOPATHY

Critically ill patients in the ICU can develop severe weakness of the respiratory and limb muscles from axonal polyneuropathy or myopathy or both. Critical illness polyneuropathy (CIP) is a length-dependent sensorimotor axonal polyneuropathy, whereas critical illness myopathy (CIM) is a preferential loss of myosin filaments, reduced ATPase activity, and muscle inexcitability secondary to sodium channelopathy.[68] Despite substantial improvement in the mortality of patients with sepsis and critical illness over the last decade, up to 70% of patients have residual disability, largely caused by critical illness neuromyopathy (CINM). Risk factors for CINM include immobility, severe sepsis, multiorgan failure, ventilation for more than 72 hours, systemic inflammatory response syndrome without sepsis, high-dose glucocorticoids, and prolonged use of neuromuscular blocking agents.

Clinical Features

CINM mostly presents as a flaccid quadriparesis with failure to wean from mechanical ventilation, although the pattern of clinical signs/symptoms depends on the proportion of CIP and CIM. The differentiating clinical features and laboratory findings are shown in **Table 7**.

Diagnosis

Although CINM is a clinical diagnosis, electrophysiologic studies and muscle biopsy can help distinguish between CIP and CIM. CIP shows reduced amplitude of CMAP and sensory nerve action potential with normal or mildly reduced conduction velocities, meanwhile CIM shows myopathic motor unit potentials with abnormal spontaneous activity (fibrillation potentials and positive sharp waves). Prolongation of CMAP is the earliest sign of CIM.[69] In undifferentiated cases, nerve/muscle biopsies can help further differentiate between CIP and CIM, as shown in **Table 8**.

Management

Many strategies have been proposed for the management of CIP and CIM, but no specific regimen has emerged as a definitive treatment strategy. These interventions include minimizing sedation, spontaneous breathing trials, and early rehabilitation. In patients who cannot be mobilized, active and passive cycle ergometry and muscle stimulation have shown some promise for improving disability. Intensive insulin

Table 8
Features of critical illness myopathy and polyneuropathy

	Critical Illness Myopathy	CIP
Presentation	Typically exposed to NM blocking agents or corticosteroids in setting of critical illness	Critically ill (sepsis and multiorgan failure)
Physical examination	Flaccid symmetric atrophy and weakness of limbs and neck flexors Proximal>distal Cranial nerves spared Normal sensation Reflexes reduced, but may be preserved Respiratory muscle weakness	Flaccid symmetric atrophy and weakness of limbs Distal>proximal Lower>upper limbs Cranial nerves spared Reduced sensation Reflexes reduced or absent Respiratory muscle weakness
Laboratory investigations	Creatine kinase level may be increased	Creatine kinase level normal
EMG	Low motor amplitudes (<80% of lower limit of normal) Preserved sensory response Myopathic motor unit potentials Normal repetitive nerve stimulation	Reduced or absent motor potentials Reduced or absent sensory Neurogenic motor unit potentials Active denervation Normal repetitive nerve stimulation
Biopsy	Myosin filament loss Muscle necrosis	Axonal neuropathy Muscle denervation

therapy has been validated as a method for preventing CINM by 2 randomized controlled trials.[70,71]

Long-Term Outcome

CINM is independently associated with higher short-term and long-term mortality, with greater physical disability and poorer quality of life in survivors. Elderly patients and patients with CIP have less favorable outcomes, although patients who are younger and with less severe disease have better recovery.

SUMMARY

Acute neuromuscular respiratory failure can represent a diagnostic challenge for neurologists, but prompt identification of cause and signs of impending respiratory failure and appropriate triage of these patients are essential to improve prognosis. Improvements in the ICU management of these diseases have clearly improved the mortality in the last decade, but there still remain major gaps in knowledge. Determining the optimal timing of intubation and weaning off the ventilator remain challenging. Newer bedside techniques such as bedside diaphragmatic ultrasonography may more clearly visualize diaphragmatic function and may guide clinical decisions. Preemptive treatment with antibiotics with the first signs of tracheobronchitis may reduce time on the ventilator, but such an aggressive approach requires careful study. Ventilator-associated infections require far more attention in patients with acute neuromuscular respiratory failure. There are unexplored aspects of understanding failing respiratory mechanics and how best to assess and manage this condition in acute neurology, which is undoubtedly a reflection of the rarity of the disorders described, which precludes large clinical trials.

There needs to be better development of diagnostic tests measuring respiratory control and breathing instability, to identify the causes of neuromuscular weakness in which the diagnosis could not be made despite extensive work-up and to shift the focus of research outcomes from mortality to short-term and long-term functional outcome, because these patients usually have a poor functional prognosis.

DISCLOSURES

The authors have nothing to disclose.

REFERENCES

1. Deenen JC, Horlings CG, Verschuuren JJ, et al. The epidemiology of neuromuscular disorders: a comprehensive overview of the literature. J Neuromuscul Dis 2015;2(1):73–85.
2. Damian MS, Ben-Shlomo Y, Howard R, et al. The effect of secular trends and specialist neurocritical care on mortality for patients with intracerebral haemorrhage, myasthenia gravis and Guillain-Barré syndrome admitted to critical care : an analysis of the intensive care national audit & research centre (ICNARC) national United Kingdom database. Intensive Care Med 2013;39(8):1405–12.
3. Wijdicks EF. The history of neurocritical care. Handb Clin Neurol 2017;140:3–14.
4. Lawn ND, Fletcher DD, Henderson RD, et al. Anticipating mechanical ventilation in Guillain-Barré syndrome. Arch Neurol 2001;58(6):893–8.
5. Rabinstein AA, Wijdicks EF. Warning signs of imminent respiratory failure in neurological patients. Semin Neurol 2003;23(1):97–104.
6. Sarwal A, Walker FO, Cartwright MS. Neuromuscular ultrasound for evaluation of the diaphragm. Muscle Nerve 2013;47(3):319–29.
7. Summerhill EM, El-Sameed YA, Glidden TJ, et al. Monitoring recovery from diaphragm paralysis with ultrasound. Chest 2008;133(3):737–43.
8. Mogalle K, Perez-Rovira A, Ciet P, et al. Quantification of diaphragm mechanics in pompe disease using dynamic 3D MRI. PLoS One 2016;11(7):e0158912.
9. Wens SC, Ciet P, Perez-Rovira A, et al. Lung MRI and impairment of diaphragmatic function in Pompe disease. BMC Pulm Med 2015;15:54.
10. Wens SC, Ciet P, Perez-Rovira A, et al. Cine-MRI as a new tool to evaluate diaphragmatic dysfunction in pompe disease. J Neuromuscul Dis 2015;2(s1):S57.
11. O'Driscoll BR, Howard LS, Davison AG. BTS guideline for emergency oxygen use in adult patients. Thorax 2008;63(Suppl 6):vi1–68.
12. Nava S, Hill N. Non-invasive ventilation in acute respiratory failure. Lancet 2009; 374(9685):250–9.
13. Rabinstein A, Wijdicks EF. BiPAP in acute respiratory failure due to myasthenic crisis may prevent intubation. Neurology 2002;59(10):1647–9.
14. Bach JR, Gonçalves MR, Hamdani I, et al. Extubation of patients with neuromuscular weakness: a new management paradigm. Chest 2010;137(5):1033–9.
15. Frat JP, Thille AW, Mercat A, et al. High-flow oxygen through nasal cannula in acute hypoxemic respiratory failure. N Engl J Med 2015;372(23):2185–96.
16. Radunovic A, Annane D, Rafiq MK, et al. Mechanical ventilation for amyotrophic lateral sclerosis/motor neuron disease. Cochrane Database Syst Rev 2013;(3): CD004427.
17. Villanova M, Brancalion B, Mehta AD. Duchenne muscular dystrophy: life prolongation by noninvasive ventilatory support. Am J Phys Med Rehabil 2014;93(7): 595–9.

18. Lawn ND, Wijdicks EF. Tracheostomy in Guillain-Barré syndrome. Muscle Nerve 1999;22(8):1058–62.
19. Thomas CE, Mayer SA, Gungor Y, et al. Myasthenic crisis: clinical features, mortality, complications, and risk factors for prolonged intubation. Neurology 1997; 48(5):1253–60.
20. Sejvar JJ, Baughman AL, Wise M, et al. Population incidence of Guillain-Barré syndrome: a systematic review and meta-analysis. Neuroepidemiology 2011; 36(2):123–33.
21. Willison HJ, Jacobs BC, van Doorn PA. Guillain-Barré syndrome. Lancet 2016; 388(10045):717–27.
22. Frenzen PD. Hospital admissions for Guillain-Barré syndrome in the United States, 1993-2004. Neuroepidemiology 2007;29(1–2):83–8.
23. Lyu RK, Tang LM, Cheng SY, et al. Guillain-Barré syndrome in Taiwan: a clinical study of 167 patients. J Neurol Neurosurg Psychiatry 1997;63(4):494–500.
24. Fokke C, van den Berg B, Drenthen J, et al. Diagnosis of Guillain-Barré syndrome and validation of Brighton criteria. Brain 2014;137(Pt 1):33–43.
25. Hadden RD, Cornblath DR, Hughes RA, et al. Electrophysiological classification of Guillain-Barré syndrome: clinical associations and outcome. Plasma Exchange/Sandoglobulin Guillain-Barré syndrome trial group. Ann Neurol 1998; 44(5):780–8.
26. Vucic S, Cairns KD, Black KR, et al. Neurophysiologic findings in early acute inflammatory demyelinating polyradiculoneuropathy. Clin Neurophysiol 2004; 115(10):2329–35.
27. Hughes RA, Raphaël JC, Swan AV, et al. Intravenous immunoglobulin for Guillain-Barré syndrome. Cochrane Database Syst Rev 2014;(1):CD002063.
28. Raphael JC, Chevret S, Hughes RA, et al. Plasma exchange for Guillain-Barré syndrome. Cochrane Database Syst Rev 2012;(7):CD001798.
29. Randomised trial of plasma exchange, intravenous immunoglobulin, and combined treatments in Guillain-Barré syndrome. Plasma exchange/sandoglobulin guillain-barré syndrome trial group. Lancet 1997;349(9047):225–30.
30. van Koningsveld R, Schmitz PI, Meché FG, et al. Effect of methylprednisolone when added to standard treatment with intravenous immunoglobulin for Guillain-Barré syndrome: randomised trial. Lancet 2004;363(9404):192–6.
31. Rajabally YA, Uncini A. Outcome and its predictors in Guillain-Barre syndrome. J Neurol Neurosurg Psychiatry 2012;83(7):711–8.
32. Walgaard C, Lingsma HF, Ruts L, et al. Early recognition of poor prognosis in Guillain-Barre syndrome. Neurology 2011;76(11):968–75.
33. Drenthen J, Jacobs BC, Maathuis EM, et al. Residual fatigue in Guillain-Barre syndrome is related to axonal loss. Neurology 2013;81(21):1827–31.
34. Wijdicks EF, Klein CJ. Guillain-Barré Syndrome. Mayo Clin Proc 2017;92(3): 467–79.
35. Carr AS, Cardwell CR, McCarron PO, et al. A systematic review of population based epidemiological studies in Myasthenia Gravis. BMC Neurol 2010;10:46.
36. Statland JM, Ciafaloni E. Myasthenia gravis: five new things. Neurol Clin Pract 2013;3(2):126–33.
37. Boldingh MI, Maniaol AH, Brunborg C, et al. Increased risk for clinical onset of myasthenia gravis during the postpartum period. Neurology 2016;87(20): 2139–45.
38. Zhang B, Tzartos JS, Belimezi M, et al. Autoantibodies to lipoprotein-related protein 4 in patients with double-seronegative myasthenia gravis. Arch Neurol 2012; 69(4):445–51.

39. Alshekhlee A, Miles JD, Katirji B, et al. Incidence and mortality rates of myasthenia gravis and myasthenic crisis in US hospitals. Neurology 2009;72(18): 1548–54.

40. Rivner MH, Pasnoor M, Dimachkie MM, et al. Muscle-specific tyrosine kinase and myasthenia gravis owing to other antibodies. Neurol Clin 2018;36(2):293–310.

41. Grob D, Brunner N, Namba T, et al. Lifetime course of myasthenia gravis. Muscle Nerve 2008;37(2):141–9.

42. Koneczny I, Herbst R. Myasthenia gravis: pathogenic effects of autoantibodies on neuromuscular architecture. Cells 2019;8(7).

43. Witoonpanich R, Dejthevaporn C, Sriphrapradang A, et al. Electrophysiological and immunological study in myasthenia gravis: diagnostic sensitivity and correlation. Clin Neurophysiol 2011;122(9):1873–7.

44. Seneviratne J, Mandrekar J, Wijdicks EF, et al. Noninvasive ventilation in myasthenic crisis. Arch Neurol 2008;65(1):54–8.

45. Seneviratne J, Mandrekar J, Wijdicks EF, et al. Predictors of extubation failure in myasthenic crisis. Arch Neurol 2008;65(7):929–33.

46. Barth D, Nabavi Nouri M, Ng E, et al. Comparison of IVIg and PLEX in patients with myasthenia gravis. Neurology 2011;76(23):2017–23.

47. Gajdos P, Chevret S, Toyka K. Intravenous immunoglobulin for myasthenia gravis. Cochrane Database Syst Rev 2012;12(2):CD002277.

48. Mandawat A, Kaminski HJ, Cutter G, et al. Comparative analysis of therapeutic options used for myasthenia gravis. Ann Neurol 2010;68(6):797–805.

49. Palace J, Newsom-Davis J, Lecky B. A randomized double-blind trial of prednisolone alone or with azathioprine in myasthenia gravis. Myasthenia gravis study group. Neurology 1998;50(6):1778–83.

50. Sparrow MP. Use of allopurinol to optimize thiopurine immunomodulator efficacy in inflammatory bowel disease. Gastroenterol Hepatol (N Y) 2008;4(7):505–11.

51. El-Salem K, Yassin A, Al-Hayk K, et al. Treatment of MuSK-Associated Myasthenia Gravis. Curr Treat Options Neurol 2014;16(4):283.

52. Chio A, Logroscino G, Traynor BJ, et al. Global epidemiology of amyotrophic lateral sclerosis: a systematic review of the published literature. Neuroepidemiology 2013;41(2):118–30.

53. Forsgren L, Almay BG, Holmgren G, et al. Epidemiology of motor neuron disease in northern Sweden. Acta Neurol Scand 1983;68(1):20–9.

54. Fang T, Al Khleifat A, Meurgey JH, et al. Stage at which riluzole treatment prolongs survival in patients with amyotrophic lateral sclerosis: a retrospective analysis of data from a dose-ranging study. Lancet Neurol 2018;17(5):416–22.

55. Writing G, Edaravone ALSSG. Safety and efficacy of edaravone in well defined patients with amyotrophic lateral sclerosis: a randomised, double-blind, placebo-controlled trial. Lancet Neurol 2017;16(7):505–12.

56. Radunovic A, Mitsumoto H, Leigh PN. Clinical care of patients with amyotrophic lateral sclerosis. Lancet Neurol 2007;6(10):913–25.

57. Miller RG, Jackson CE, Kasarskis EJ, et al. Practice parameter update: the care of the patient with amyotrophic lateral sclerosis: drug, nutritional, and respiratory therapies (an evidence-based review): report of the quality Standards Subcommittee of the American Academy of Neurology. Neurology 2009;73(15):1218–26.

58. Jackson CE, Rosenfeld J, Moore DH, et al. A preliminary evaluation of a prospective study of pulmonary function studies and symptoms of hypoventilation in ALS/MND patients. J Neurol Sci 2001;191(1–2):75–8.

59. Bourke SC, Tomlinson M, Williams TL, et al. Effects of non-invasive ventilation on survival and quality of life in patients with amyotrophic lateral sclerosis: a randomised controlled trial. Lancet Neurol 2006;5(2):140–7.
60. Sancho J, Servera E, Díaz JL, et al. Home tracheotomy mechanical ventilation in patients with amyotrophic lateral sclerosis: causes, complications and 1-year survival. Thorax 2011;66(11):948–52.
61. Chio A, Calvo A, Ghiglione P, et al. Tracheostomy in amyotrophic lateral sclerosis: a 10-year population-based study in Italy. J Neurol Neurosurg Psychiatry 2010; 81(10):1141–3.
62. Diep B, Wang A, Kun S, et al. Diaphragm pacing without tracheostomy in congenital central hypoventilation syndrome patients. Respiration 2015;89(6): 534–8.
63. Sancho J, Servera E, Díaz J, et al. Efficacy of mechanical insufflation-exsufflation in medically stable patients with amyotrophic lateral sclerosis. Chest 2004;125(4): 1400–5.
64. Sancho J, Servera E, Vergara P, et al. Mechanical insufflation-exsufflation vs. tracheal suctioning via tracheostomy tubes for patients with amyotrophic lateral sclerosis: a pilot study. Am J Phys Med Rehabil 2003;82(10):750–3.
65. Lange DJ, Lechtzin N, Davey C, et al. High-frequency chest wall oscillation in ALS: an exploratory randomized, controlled trial. Neurology 2006;67(6):991–7.
66. Czell D, Bauer M, Binek J, et al. Outcomes of percutaneous endoscopic gastrostomy tube insertion in respiratory impaired amyotrophic lateral sclerosis patients under noninvasive ventilation. Respir Care 2013;58(5):838–44.
67. ProGas Study G. Gastrostomy in patients with amyotrophic lateral sclerosis (ProGas): a prospective cohort study. Lancet Neurol 2015;14(7):702–9.
68. Zhou C, Wu L, Ni F, et al. Critical illness polyneuropathy and myopathy: a systematic review. Neural Regen Res 2014;9(1):101–10.
69. Goodman BP, Harper CM, Boon AJ. Prolonged compound muscle action potential duration in critical illness myopathy. Muscle Nerve 2009;40(6):1040–2.
70. Hermans G, Wilmer A, Meersseman W, et al. Impact of intensive insulin therapy on neuromuscular complications and ventilator dependency in the medical intensive care unit. Am J Respir Crit Care Med 2007;175(5):480–9.
71. Van den Berghe G, Schoonheydt K, Becx P, et al. Insulin therapy protects the central and peripheral nervous system of intensive care patients. Neurology 2005;64(8):1348–53.

Headache Emergencies

David Kopel, MD[a], Crandall Peeler, MD[b], Shuhan Zhu, MD[a,*]

KEYWORDS

- Thunderclap headache • Subarachnoid hemorrhage • Elevated intracranial pressure
- Intracranial hypotension • Venous sinus thrombosis
- Reversible cerebral vasoconstriction syndrome • Giant cell arteritis • Papilledema

KEY POINTS

- The majority of patients who seek care for headache have primary headache; a small subset have secondary causes associated with high morbidity and mortality.
- A systematic history assessing for "red flag" features along with a careful neurologic examination is required to appropriately diagnose secondary causes.
- Secondary causes include subarachnoid hemorrhage, reversible cerebral vasoconstriction syndrome, elevated intracranial pressure, hydrocephalus, cerebral venous sinus thrombosis, arterial dissection, central nervous system infection, and inflammatory vasculitis.
- Patients who are pregnant, immunocompromised, elderly, or have known malignancy have higher risks of secondary disorders therefore.
- Clinicians should have a different threshold to obtain additional diagnostic evaluations in high-risk patients.

INTRODUCTION

Nontraumatic headache is responsible for approximately 2% of all emergency department (ED) visits.[1] With roughly 145 million total ED visits per year,[2] this means an average of nearly 8000 patients visit an ED for headache each day. Although the majority of nontraumatic headaches are benign, a small fraction (about 3%)[3] are due to underlying causes associated with significant morbidity and mortality.

The most common cause of ED visits for nontraumatic headache is migraine headaches, which, despite their severity and significant impact on quality of life, are not in and of themselves dangerous. Yet migraine is important because the symptoms of migraine headaches overlap with those caused by far more dangerous secondary conditions such as aneurysmal subarachnoid hemorrhage (SAH), reversible cerebral

State on conflict of interest: The authors listed have no relevant conflicts of interest related to information and topics reviewed within this article.
[a] Department of Neurology, 725 Albany Street, Suite 7B, Boston, MA 02118, USA;
[b] Department of Ophthalmology and Neurology, 85 East Concord Street 8th Floor, Boston, MA 02118, USA
* Corresponding author.
E-mail address: shuhan.zhu@bmc.org

vasoconstriction syndrome (RCVS), elevated intracranial pressure (ICP), hydrocephalus, cerebral venous sinus thrombosis (CVST), arterial dissection, central nervous system (CNS) infection, and inflammatory vasculitis, which can carry high morbidity and mortality if not appropriately diagnosed and treated. Additionally, because primary headaches are very common, they often coexist with secondary causes.

The keystone of evaluation begins with thorough history taking. Without a guiding history, the physical examination, imaging, and other studies that are obtained may be inappropriate for the diagnosis at hand and can lead to false reassurance with normal results. This review provides clinicians with the knowledge needed to appropriately and confidently distinguish patients with headache emergencies from the more common yet superficially similar patients with benign causes of headache.

THE ROLE OF HISTORY AND NEUROLOGIC EXAMINATION

Owing to significant overlap in symptoms of benign and dangerous causes of headache, and the fact that most patients with headache ultimately have primary causes, clinicians must use a systematic approach each time to avoid misdiagnosis in the patients with dangerous secondary causes. Because the causes of secondary headaches range from intracranial bleeding to altered ICP to CNS inflammatory disease, clinicians must first be guided by history to obtain the appropriate diagnostic studies.

Various mnemonics have been developed to assist the clinician in efficiently obtaining a headache history aimed at identifying dangerous secondary etiologies. When consistently used, the SNOOP4 mnemonic[4] can be quite effective at this task. Each component of the mnemonic represents a red flag that, when present, can signify the presence of a dangerous secondary cause. Diagnoses such as SAH, RCVS, elevated ICP, hydrocephalus, CVST, arterial dissection, CNS infection, and inflammatory vasculitis would all trigger multiple red flags using this mnemonic.

This review discusses the clinical application of key red flags and how to evaluate for their possible causes. We focus on thunderclap headache, positional headache, patients with abnormal physical examinations, and special very high-risk patient populations because we believe these are the most important to an efficient emergency headache evaluation. We also recommend that the reader review the original publication by Dr Dodick for additional guidance on the use of SNOOP4. For the readers' reference, we have summarized the SNOOP4 mnemonic in **Table 1**.

A prospective, observational study with 90 patients[5] from Thailand using SNOOP4 for detection of serious causes of secondary headaches showed a high negative predictive value (96.4%) but a low positive predictive value (25.9%) for serious causes such as intracerebral hemorrhage, infarction, CNS infection, or neoplasm. The low positive predictive value is likely a reflection of the fact that only a small percentage of all patients with nontraumatic headaches have a dangerous underlying cause. Patients who do not have any of the SNOOP4 red flags are unlikely to have a dangerous secondary cause; patients who do have a red flag require additional evaluation or consideration to further delineate whether a dangerous secondary cause may be present.

Although clinical guides can be very helpful, it is also important to keep in mind that no single guideline or mnemonic can capture all the clinical variations of a particular condition or provide all relevant evaluations and possible causes. In particular, patients who are pregnant, immunocompromised, elderly, or have known malignancy have higher risks of secondary disorders. Therefore, clinicians should have a higher a priori clinical suspicion for a dangerous secondary headache etiology and a different threshold to obtain additional diagnostic evaluations in such patients.

Table 1
SNOOP4 mnemonic (Dodick 2010)

	Symptoms to Assess for	Secondary Causes to Consider:
Systemic symptoms	Fever, chills, night sweats, myalgias, weight loss, malignancy history, immunocompromised state	Vasculitis, CNS infection, metastatic malignancy
Neurologic symptoms	Unilateral weakness, diplopia, gait changes, speech changes, personality/behavior changes	CNS neoplasm, inflammatory lesion, infection or vascular disease
Sudden Onset ("thunderclap")	Sudden severe pain	SAH, RCVS, venous thrombosis, arterial dissection
Onset after age 50	New headaches later in life	CNS neoplasm, vasculitis, inflammatory disease, infection
Pattern change/ progressive	Worsening of previous headache patterns	Base on review of other SNOOP4 symptoms
Valsalva Precipitation	Headache triggered with straining or coughing	CSF flow obstruction, elevated intracranial pressure
Postural aggravation	Worse with lying down	Elevated intracranial pressure
Papilledema	Transient visual obscurations, double vision, visual field loss	Elevated intracranial pressure, hydrocephalus, CSF flow obstruction

Adapted from Dodick DW. Pearls: headache. *Semin Neurol.* 2010;30(1):74-81.

The role of the neurologic examination is often emphasized in the evaluation of headache and other neurologic problems, but it should be noted that a detailed examination without an appropriate history for context is rarely helpful. The examination should be guided and informed by the history, and the findings should be interpreted in the context of the history. The history can help clinicians to hone in on the most important examination components to perform and appreciate subtle findings that may be missed otherwise. In addition to the general neurologic examination, physicians should also perform a fundoscopic examination to assess for papilledema. In some patients with an elevated ICP, this may be the only abnormal examination finding.

In cases for which there are no red flags and the history is consistent with a primary headache disorder, a careful neurologic examination should still be performed with the goal of demonstrating normal findings and, thus, supporting the diagnosis made based on history. Neurologic abnormalities that are unexplained should alert the clinician to further review the patient's history and/or reassess in the context of the patient's history and presentation.

THUNDERCLAP HEADACHE

The most well-known worrisome headache pattern is the thunderclap headache, typically associated with aneurysmal SAH. Given the high degree of morbidity and mortality associated with SAH, the emphasis is appropriately placed on its rapid and accurate diagnosis. However, it is important to highlight several more subtle components of the headache history that may guide management in cases of thunderclap headache, as well as to highlight some other possible causes that should not be missed.

Subarachnoid Hemorrhage

The majority of patients presenting with SAH in a recent study reported that their headache reached peak intensity within 1 second of onset, a so-called apoplectic headache.[6] Eighty percent of patients with a SAH stated that their headache had peaked in intensity within 1 minute. In contrast, of patients presenting with headaches unrelated to SAH, 10% and 17% reported peak intensity within 1 second and 1 minute, respectively. Other clinical features in this study that were significantly associated with SAH as a headache etiology included occipital location, a stabbing quality, and the presence of meningismus.

A clinical decision rule known as the Ottawa SAH (OSAH) rule has been proposed in a study of more than 1000 patients with an acute headache and externally validated in several subsequent studies of hundreds of patients.[7–9] The aim of this rule is to stratify patients with nontraumatic headache peaking within 1 hour (without impaired consciousness, focal deficits, or historical features such as past aneurysmal bleeding placing them at high risk) as high or low risk for aneurysmal SAH. According to the OSAH rule, one should look for the following features: age greater than 40 years, neck pain, neck stiffness, limitations in neck flexion, apoplectic headache onset, headache onset during exertion, or loss of consciousness at any point. The absence of all these features had a sensitivity and negative predictive value of essentially 100% to rule out SAH.[7–9] Although the OSAH rule has been validated for other types of intracerebral bleeding,[9] the absence of these features should not reassure a provider against other dangerous causes of headache.

We recommend the use of the OSAH rule to rule out SAH in patients presenting with acute onset headache who have none of the red flags. For those who do have one of these concerning features, further history taking and examination are required before deciding on imaging. This practice is in line with the American College of Emergency Physicians' guidelines, which state that the OSAH rule should be used to rule out SAH, but owing to low specificity, should not be used to rule in this disorder.[10] A computed tomography (CT) scan of the brain is nearly 100% sensitive and specific for SAH if done within 6 hours of headache onset. However, sensitivity decreases to 93% by 24 hours and continues to decrease after that.[11] The sensitivity of lumbar puncture (LP) to look for xanthochromia is poor in the first 2 hours or so after headache onset and peaks at about 12 hours from headache onset.[12] Thus, we recommend LP for all patients under investigation for SAH with a negative head CT scan more than 6 hours after symptom onset. When the head CT scan is negative within the first 6 hours, other diagnoses should be considered.

Reversible Cerebral Vasoconstriction Syndrome

RCVS should be considered in all patients presenting with thunderclap headache, especially if the headache is recurrent. The headache onset can be very rapid, as in SAH, but the headaches tend to be shorter, lasting 1 to 3 hours[13] and often include a moderate headache between recurrent exacerbations, as opposed to the headache of SAH, which often persists for days or weeks in our clinical experience. Traditionally, the headache of RCVS is posterior and bilateral at onset, then becomes holocranial, although significant variations exist.[14] It can be triggered by exertion or a Valsalva maneuver. About one-half of the time, there is a history of exposure to vasoactive compounds (some are listed in **Table 2**) or the patient is recently post partum.[14] There may be focal neurologic deficits or seizures. Women are at greater risk and are less likely to have a clear vasoactive trigger identified than men.[13]

Table 2
Vasoactive compounds associated with RCVS

Drug Categories	Examples of Offending Drugs
Drugs of abuse	Cannabis, cocaine, amphetamines, LSD
Antidepressants	Selective serotonin reuptake inhibitors and selective norepinephrine reuptake inhibitors like fluoxetine, paroxetine, duloxetine and venlafaxine
Alpha sympathomimetics	Enteral or nasal decongestants like ephedrine and pseudoephedrine, norepinephrine
Triptans	Sumatriptan, rizatriptan, frovatriptan
Ergot alkaloid derivatives	Methergine, bromocriptine, lisuride
Others	Intravenous immunoglobulin, interferon, nicotine patches, ginseng, binge drinking, phenytoin

RCVS can cause ischemic and hemorrhagic stroke and is associated with sulcal SAH at the convexity. Brain edema and posterior white matter changes resembling the posterior reversible encephalopathy syndrome (PRES) can occur and these 2 disorders may have related pathophysiology.[13] In a retrospective case series, although 55% of patients had normal imaging at the time of presentation, 39% developed infarcts, 34% had convexity SAH, 20% had lobar hemorrhage, and 38% had brain edema on reimaging later in the disease course.[15] Conventional angiography is the best test to look for the characteristic segmental narrowing and dilatation of multiple vessels.[13]

CT angiography and MR angiography have about 70% of the sensitivity of conventional angiography,[14] and reimaging is key because it is thought that vasoconstriction begins with small distal vessels that may not be seen on angiography and progresses proximally with maximum MCA branch vasoconstriction seen about 16 days after clinical onset.[13] On diagnosis, vasoactive medications are stopped, patients are advised to avoid exertion, and they are often treated with nimodipine, the early administration of which significantly improves headaches.[13] It is not yet clear whether treatment with nimodipine helps to prevent the neurologic complications of RCVS.

Cerebral Venous Sinus Thrombosis

CVST is traditionally associated with subacutely progressive headache, but can present with a thunderclap headache in a minority of cases. Risk factors for CVST include an underlying hypercoagulable state, head injury, exogenous estrogens through contraceptive pills, and pregnancy.[16]

Occlusion of the cortical and deep veins disrupts normal blood flow, leading to venous infarct and/or hemorrhage, which can cause focal neurologic deficits or alteration in mental status in about one-half of the cases.[16] Occlusion of the sinuses impairs cerebral spinal fluid (CSF) outflow leading to an increased ICP, headache, and papilledema. Hemorrhages or infarcts that do not respect expected arterial vascular territories raise concern for a venous stroke. When there is intracranial hemorrhage, substantial early perihematomal edema can suggest a venous source; studies have shown that decreased venous drainage is associated with an increase in edema around a parenchymal bleed.[17] Although a thrombus may appear hyperintense on T1- and T2-weighted MRI, dedicated MR venography or CT venography is often helpful in making the diagnosis. Diagnostic angiography is rarely necessary, but can be useful in subtle cases. CVST should be treated with anticoagulation, even if there is intracerebral hemorrhage present, because studies have indicated that such treatment helps to prevent death and dependency.[18] Anticoagulation arrests the growth of the thrombus and helps to prevent pulmonary embolism.[16] The role of endovascular treatment is uncertain, and the current practice is to reserve it for refractory cases that would otherwise have a poor prognosis.

Arterial Dissection

Another diagnosis to consider in patients presenting with rapid onset headache, especially after trauma or exertion, is arterial dissection of the cervical portions of the carotid and/or vertebral arteries. Less commonly, dissection of large intracranial arteries can also cause sudden headache.[19] Although there are clear cases with head or neck trauma followed by neck pain, headaches, and focal neurologic deficits, most cases are more subtle.

Carotid dissection usually causes a unilateral headache. When it is unilateral, the sidedness of the headache is almost always ipsilateral to the location of the dissection.[20] Carotid dissection can present without any pain or with isolated headache and orbital or facial pain; however, in most cases there are some neurologic manifestations such as transient ischemic attacks or strokes, ipsilateral Horner syndrome, transient monocular vision loss, pulsatile tinnitus (corresponding to carotid bruit on examination), and dysgeusia.[20]

Vertebral dissection usually presents with unilateral or bilateral posterior headache, but the pain can be more diffuse. Migraineurs are less likely to confuse this headache for a typical migraine compared with that of carotid dissection.[20] Neurologic findings can be transient or permanent and symptoms are variable depending on the location of the ischemia or infarct. These symptoms can include complete or partial Wallenberg syndrome, visual field deficits, cranial neuropathies, and area postrema syndrome, among others.[20]

Conventional or noninvasive (CT angiography, MR angiography) angiography can be used to diagnose a dissection. In centers with radiologists who are experienced in its interpretation, MR vessel wall imaging is a technique that may detect small, subadventitial dissections with greater sensitivity than traditional imaging modalities by demonstrating thrombus in the false lumen.[21] **Fig. 1** shows carotid dissection with thrombus seen on vessel wall imaging (T1 fat saturation).There is controversy regarding the use of anticoagulation or antiplatelet therapy for treatment and a recent randomized clinical trial did not find a significant difference between the 2 in stroke prevention.[22] In our experience, anticoagulation is usually reserved for cases with intraluminal thrombus, where one can definitively rule out intracranial extension of the dissection.

POSITIONAL HEADACHE

Headaches with a strong positional component should raise clinicians' suspicion for altered ICP, which may be due to serious underlying causes. Classically, patients with increased ICP report more and/or worsening headaches (which may be accompanied by nausea) on first waking in the morning, with the Valsalva maneuver, or with lying down, which improve or resolve with sitting or standing. Patients with decreased ICP owing to CSF leak typically report the opposite, with headaches that improve or resolve with reclining and the onset of headaches with sitting or standing, although some patients with intracranial hypotension have paradoxic worsening while supine.

Assessing a patient's headache symptomatology for high or low pressure features can be challenging, because many primary headache disorders can have a positional

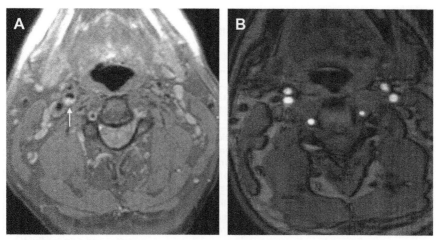

Fig. 1. MR vessel wall imaging. Vessel wall imaging (*A*) with a T1 fat-saturation sequence demonstrates hyperintense crescent of intramural hematoma (*arrow*) within the dissection, which is not visualized on usual time of flight vascular imaging (*B*).

component. A diagnostic feature of migraine is "aggravation by or causing avoidance of routine physical activity (eg, walking or climbing stairs)"[23]; in these cases, the migraine pain is worsened by stimulus in general, which includes physical activity (as well as other forms of stimulus such as noise and/or light). Additionally, morning-predominant headaches may also be seen in other settings, such as obstructive sleep apnea and migraine, because approximately 25% of migraineurs report headaches starting overnight.[24]

Elevated Intracranial Pressure

Although both high and low ICP can result in headaches, the causes of elevated ICP are more likely to be associated with significant morbidity and mortality than the causes of decreased ICP.

Some conditions associated with elevated ICP, such as mass lesions, CNS infections, or hydrocephalus (which can be due to many different etiologies) carry a risk for coma and death if left untreated. Others, such as idiopathic intracranial hypertension (IIH), are not acutely life threatening but can be associated with significant morbidity, such as permanent loss of vision. In cases of suspected high ICP, initial brain imaging with a CT scan can offer rapid information on whether acutely dangerous conditions such as hydrocephalus, mass lesions, diffuse edema, or CVST may be present. The absence of overt hydrocephalus on an initial CT scan does not always exclude an elevated ICP, because hydrocephalus is a relative finding that is subject to the baseline degree of brain and CSF volume; mild hydrocephalus may be difficult to diagnose on imaging, particularly in patients who are elderly or have a preexisting brain injury with encephalomalacia. A comparison with prior imaging is critical if it is available.

A clear understanding of the patient's medical background and risk factors can be very helpful because the pretest probability of a potential ICP disorder is highly dependent on such information. **Table 3** reviews the major groups of disorders that can lead to elevated ICP with additional considerations and risk factors to assess for in each patient.

Table 3
Major groups of disorders leading to altered ICP

	Immediate Causes	Secondary Evaluations/ Considerations
Elevated ICP		
Obstructive hydrocephalus	Mass-occupying lesion(s) owing to tumor or infectious lesion	Assess patients for systemic cancer diagnoses and immunosuppressed status
Nonobstructive hydrocephalus	Inadequate CSF resorption by arachnoid granulations owing to inflammation, hemorrhage in subarachnoid space or obstruction in dural venous sinuses	Assess for systemic inflammatory disorders, immunosuppression or hypercoagulable state
Diffuse edema	CNS infection, hypoxic injury, metabolic derangement (hyponatremia, hyperammonemia)	Assess for risk factors for CNS infection, immunosuppressed status and risks for fluid/ electrolyte imbalances
Normal imaging	Idiopathic increased ICP (IIH)	Assess for risk factors based on age, gender, body mass and medication exposures
Decreased ICP		
Iatrogenic	Dural defect from medical procedure or overshunting	Assess for epidural procedures, ENT surgeries, spinal surgeries and evaluate for overshunting
Traumatic	Dural defect owing to traumatic head injury	Assess for recent head injury in previous days to weeks
Spontaneous	Dural defect owing to tear from perineural nerve root cyst tear or calcified disc leading to dural puncture	Assess for underlying connective tissue disorders that may predispose to spontaneous dural defects

A fundoscopic examination for papilledema is required when evaluating patients for possible elevation of ICP. The presence of papilledema can help to confirm the diagnosis of an elevated ICP. The severity of papilledema is measured by the Frisen grade (**Fig. 2**), with higher grades reflecting effects of higher ICP. In patients with papilledema (of any Frisen grade) accompanied by features such as altered mental status or thunderclap headache, an emergent evaluation must be conducted because these findings are worrisome for SAH, CVST, rapid expansion of a mass lesion, or a severe CNS infection.

It must also be noted that the absence of papilledema does not exclude the presence of an elevated ICP, particularly in cases of an acutely elevated ICP, because the finding of papilledema itself can take several days to develop. In acute cases, when papilledema may not be a reliable feature, the absence of spontaneous retinal venous pulsations (SVP) may be a more sensitive marker for an elevated ICP.[25,26] In healthy individuals, SVPs are seen as rhythmic pulsations in the diameter of the retinal veins as they cross the optic disc and are the result of the interplay between the pulse pressure in the intraocular space and the CSF. SVPs are detectable in approximately 90% of healthy individuals and cease to be present when ICP is greater than 19 mm H_2O[26]; they may be absent in some healthy individuals owing to anatomic variations

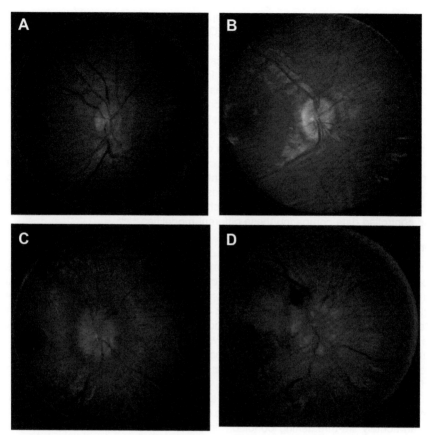

Fig. 2. Frisen grading of papilledema. Frisen grading of papilledema. (*A*) Grade 1 shows nasal blurring of the disc margin with sparing of the temporal edge. (*B*) Grade 2 shows circumferential disc blurring. (*C*) Grade 3 papilledema leading to partial obscuration of major vessels as they pass over the disc margin. (*D*) Grade 4 papilledema leading to obscuration of major vessel centrally over the disc.

within the optic disc and vasculature.[26] The presence of SVPs (along with absence of papilledema) can be helpful clues to the patient's ICP; however, the absence of SVP must be interpreted within the clinical context because this can be a normal finding.

The use of ultrasound examination to measure the optic nerve sheath diameter has been studied as a noninvasive method to assess for elevated ICP in patients with IIH[24] and severe brain injury.[27] Although these studies showed an association between a larger optic nerve sheath diameter and increased ICP, this technique is not yet routinely applied in clinical practice owing the lack of consensus on an acceptable optic nerve sheath diameter cut-off value, perhaps in part because of baseline variations in optic nerve sheath anatomy across normal patient populations.[28]

In cases of elevated ICP owing to obstructive hydrocephalus or supratentorial masses where an LP is contraindicated, ventricular shunting may be performed to divert CSF and prevent coma and/or vision loss. Surgical or medical treatment of the underlying lesion(s) varies depending on the nature of the lesion.

In patients with IIH, those with severe papilledema (Frisen grade 3 or 4) are at higher risk for vision loss from irreversible optic nerve injury and warrant urgent treatment. An

LP should be performed urgently, and the opening pressure should be measured with the patient in the lateral decubitus position. CSF drainage during the LP can be temporarily therapeutic by decreasing the CSF pressure. In cases when an LP cannot be obtained urgently either owing to a contraindication (such as anticoagulation) or technical limitation, intravenous methylprednisolone in conjunction with acetazolamide[29] may provide a temporizing measure to decrease the risk of vision loss. The long-term use of steroids for IIH, however, is not recommended owing to other risks of chronic steroid exposure. After acute ICP control, patients should be initiated on treatments to maintain ICP reduction with agents such as acetazolamide or topiramate[30] in addition to long-term treatments of weight loss and dietary management. In patients who are refractory to these treatments, surgical procedures such as optic nerve fenestration, venous sinus stenting, or ventricular shunting may be required to prevent vision loss. The selection of the procedure depends on the procedural availabilities and procedurals risks based on individual patient characteristics owing to a lack of randomized controlled data comparing these different modalities.[31,32]

Decreased Intracranial Pressure

Decreased ICP can occur spontaneously (more commonly in at-risk patients such as those with connective tissue disorders), owing to trauma, or owing to iatrogenic causes such as postprocedural complications from an LP, epidural injection, surgeries (skull base, ENT, or spinal) or CSF shunt overdrainage. The pathognomonic, and oftentimes only, feature is orthostatic headache owing to decreased buoyancy of the brain leading to traction on pain-sensitive structures, such as the dura and vasculature when patients are upright. The orthostatic headache is often accompanied by neck pain, nausea, and dizziness or vertigo; patients may also report muffled hearing or tinnitus with orthostatic stress.

The neurologic examination and imaging are typically normal, which can make this a very difficult diagnosis, particularly in cases of spontaneous leaks. Although generally not an acutely life-threatening condition, in some cases of rapid leaks, a severely decreased ICP lead to disorders of consciousness or coma from brain sag with compression of the brainstem.[33–35] This diagnosis should be considered in patients who do not otherwise have an explanation for coma or cranial nerve palsies. Special care should be used during the examination of vision and eye movements as associated cranial nerve palsies frequently include the sixth, fourth, or third nerves and can be subtle.

Imaging may show supportive features, although normal findings do not entirely exonerate this diagnosis owing to the positioning of the patient during imaging (supine) and lack of imaging sensitivity by any 1 criteria alone. The changes seen on imaging are related to the physical effects of brain sag and compensatory vascular changes.[36,37] With brain sag, imaging may show ventricular collapse, decreased mamillopontine distance, decreased prepontine cisterns, posterior fossa crowding or secondary Chiari malformation, subdural hematoma, and/or hygroma may be seen if bridging vein tear occurs. Compensatory increases in blood flow to the intracranial space may result in an enlargement of the venous sinuses, engorgement of the pituitary vasculature, and pachymeningeal enhancement on MRI. A classification system published by Dobrocky and associates[38] in JAMA Neurology in 2019 stratifies imaging findings into 3 major criteria scored as 2 points each (pachymeningeal enhancement, engorgement of venous sinuses, effacement of suprasellar cistern) and 3 minor criteria scored at 1 point each (subdural fluid collection, effacement of the prepontine cisterns and reduced mamillopontine distance) showed that a high score of 5 or higher was associated with a very high probability of CSF leak (78.6%

sensitivity and 98.3% specificity) and should be referred quickly for epidural blood patch. In patients with a low score of 2 or less, the probability of CSF leak is very low (92.9% sensitivity and 93.3% specificity) additional noninvasive imaging with MRI of the spine to assess for epidural CSF collections should be performed before consideration for invasive diagnostic procedures.

In patients who are suspected to have spontaneous CSF leaks, an empiric spinal epidural blood patch[39] can be performed because most spontaneous leaks occur in the spinal column (thoracic being most common). In patients who are refractory to the initial patch, MR imaging of the whole spinal column (with sagittal and axial T2 sequences for better visualization of possible epidural spinal fluid collections) can be performed to attempt to identify the site of the leak to guide additional targeted treatment. For patients with persistent leaks despite empiric blood patching, CT scan or radioisotope myelography may be obtained to assess for the source of leak. Rapid leaks are more difficult to detect on CT myelopathy owing to the rapid equilibration of contrast between the intradural and extradural CSF spaces; in these cases, the use of digital subtraction myelography may be required.[40,41]

In iatrogenic cases, when the dural puncture is small as in subarachnoid block, LP, or epidural injection and there are no indwelling devices, the majority of patients will recover with conservative care after several days (rarely, an epidural blood patch is necessary). Patients with orthostatic headaches who have had larger surgical access should have investigation to determine the site of the leak to assess the risk for CNS infection or need for surgical revision.

HEADACHE WITH ABNORMAL EXAMINATION

Patients with headache accompanied by symptoms such as persistent fever, hemiplegia, or diplopia generally undergo further diagnostic testing, but probing for more subtle abnormalities with an eye toward potentially devastating causes is essential in evaluating and triaging patients with a headache. It is worth noting that migraine can be associated with hemiparesis, brainstem aura, hemianesthesia, visual field abnormalities, and other neurologic symptoms. However, when such findings are present, migraine is a diagnosis of exclusion and should only be made with confidence in patients diagnosed with migraines associated with those features consistently in the past. A high index of suspicion should be maintained to avoid the morbidity associated with intracranial pathology.

Although intracerebral hemorrhage is known to cause headache, ischemic stroke can also cause headache in about 14% of cases.[42] Ischemia is more likely to cause headache when it involves the cerebellum, is not lacunar, and when the patient is female, young, and has a history of migraine.[43] This finding highlights the importance of a thorough cerebellar examination screening for appendicular dysmetria, dysdiadochokinesia, truncal ataxia, and gait abnormalities in all patients presenting with headache associated with dizziness or nausea, even if there is a history of migraine (particularly considering that patients suffering from migraine with aura are at a greater risk of stroke).[44] Cerebellar strokes are frequently misdiagnosed and pitfalls in the initial history and examination have been shown to be a major cause of these errors.[45]

Altered mentation, presenting as new onset confusion, lethargy, or behavioral alterations, is not commonly associated with primary headache and should always raise suspicion for secondary headache owing to an intracranial process such as CNS infection or increased ICP. Patients suspected to have meningitis should undergo a CT of the brain before an LP if they have papilledema, focal deficits, a Glasgow

Coma Scale score of less than 10, new-onset seizures, or if they are immunocompromised.[46] Empiric treatment should be initiated with haste to cover *Streptococcus pneumoniae* and *Neisseria meningitidis* in all patients and *Listeria monocytogenes* in neonates, pregnant women, the elderly, and the immunocompromised.[46] Coverage for herpes simplex meningoencephalitis should be considered when the patient has seizures, altered consciousness, or language/behavioral disturbances.[46] In herpes simplex virus meningoencephalitis, imaging may show abnormalities of the temporal lobes (MRI is most sensitive and can show diffusion restriction early in the course of illness) and the initial CSF tests may show lymphocytic pleocytosis, increased red blood cells, and a positive polymerase chain reaction test for herpes simplex virus (even if treatment with acyclovir has been initiated).[46]

SPECIAL POPULATIONS

In addition to headaches that raise red flags owing to their semiology or associated examination abnormalities, any new headache in patients with certain demographic risk factors should cause concern. Although primary headache disorders can occur in patients who are pregnant, immunocompromised, elderly, or have a known malignancy, special care should be taken in these groups before ascribing a benign diagnosis to new headaches.

Pregnant Patients

About 87% of women with migraines report improvement in their headaches in the third trimester, 83% in the second trimester, and 47% in the first trimester.[47] Notably, this trend may not apply to patients who have migraine with aura or chronic migraine. Accordingly, new or changing headaches (including longer headache duration) during pregnancy or the postpartum period is unusual and should always be a cause for concern because several secondary headaches are more likely during this time.

Patients with migraines are at increased risk for eclampsia, and other headache etiologies to consider in a pregnant or postpartum patient with new headache include CVST, RCVS, PRES, intracranial hypotension, and pneumocephalus (especially after dural puncture for epidural anesthesia), SAH, arterial dissection, pituitary apoplexy, and ischemic stroke.

Hypertension may raise concern for preeclampsia, but should also prompt evaluation for overlapping vasculopathies including PRES or RCVS leading to ischemic or hemorrhagic stroke. A thunderclap pattern may raise concern for SAH, but can also be due to RCVS, arterial dissection, CVST, or pituitary apoplexy. Papilledema suggests increased ICP and, although IIH is possible, CVST and space-occupying lesions need to be ruled out. This point is especially true when a headache is brought about by a Valsalva maneuver during delivery (which should also prompt investigation for arterial dissection and aneurysmal SAH).

Bitemporal hemianopia suggests pituitary apoplexy, but this diagnosis can present with less classical visual field alterations[48] that may include vision loss in 1 eye more than the other owing to asymmetric optic nerve and chiasm compression.[49] There is usually a sudden headache that can be associated with nausea, vomiting, ophthalmoplegia, and severe endocrine dysfunction, such as hemodynamic instability and diabetes insipidus.[50] Vision alterations or loss in a pregnant patient with headache can also suggest preeclampsia, PRES, or CVST. MRI is typically recommended over a CT scan in pregnant patients to limit fetal radiation exposure and, depending on the headache semiology and associated examination findings, there should be a low threshold for arterial and venous imaging as well.[51]

Immunosuppressed Patients

Patients at risk for an infectious etiology of acute headache include those with cranial trauma, recent neurosurgery, endocarditis, chronic and/or recent ear infection, sinusitis, and those who are immunocompromised such as patients with human immunodeficiency virus infection, cancer, or who are on immunosuppressive medications. Etiologies to consider include viral, bacterial, parasitic, and fungal infections of the meninges and brain parenchyma, as well as space-occupying lesions, such as subdural empyema, brain abscess, and granulomas, which can cause an increased ICP. A chronic headache in immunosuppressed patients can be owing to meningeal or parenchymal infection with slow-growing pathogens including fungi like *Cryptococcus* and mycobacteria like tuberculosis. Cryptococcal infection is often associated with a dramatically elevated ICP and papilledema. CSF studies are critical after ruling out obstructive hydrocephalus in immunocompromised patients with acute or chronic headache.

Patients with Underlying Malignancies

Patients with known malignancy who present with headache should undergo appropriate studies to assess for intracranial metastasis (particularly in those with sites of primary malignancy that have a tendency to metastasize to the brain or meninges such as breast, lung, kidney, and melanoma). Other crucial diagnoses to consider in patients with cancer with acute headache include CVST, ischemic stroke owing to hypercoagulable state, and infection owing to immunosuppression from the malignancy or its treatment. Brain metastases or primary brain cancer can cause headache owing to meningeal irritation without significantly increasing ICP. In these cases, there may not be features such as papilledema or headache intensity that is worse in the morning. In cases of known malignancy presenting with new headache and normal imaging, CSF cytology should be done to evaluate for leptomeningeal metastasis.[48] Patients who have received cerebral radiation therapy may develop stroke-like migraine attacks after radiation therapy syndrome years later, characterized by unilateral migraine headache with stroke-like symptoms and signs and imaging showing dramatic contrast enhancement in the affected hemisphere.[52]

Older Patients

Patients presenting with new or changing headaches after the age of 50 should be evaluated for vascular and oncologic etiologies. In addition to an increased risk of stroke, there is risk in these patients for arteritis, most notably giant cell arteritis. Giant cell arteritis classically presents with constant unilateral or bilateral temporal headache refractory to analgesia, scalp tenderness, jaw claudication, transient vision loss, and/or systemic symptoms such as fever, weight loss, and myalgias.[53] Its incidence increases with advancing age.[53] A feared complication is vision loss owing to arteritic ischemic optic neuropathy or central retinal artery occlusion. Physical examination may demonstrate temporal artery tenderness, an absence of temporal artery pulse, or a prominent, enlarged temporal artery, although it should be noted that absence of these findings does not exonerate giant cell arteritis, because early examination is often normal. The finding of prominent, enlarged temporal artery is the most specific[54] and occurs more commonly when the patient is presenting with a nonheadache chief complaint (65% of the time vs 20% in those presenting with headache).[55] The erythrocyte sedimentation rate and C-reactive protein should be checked and although neither is specific, the C-reactive protein is more sensitive (95%–98% vs 77%–86%).[56] Color-coded duplex ultrasound examination can show stenoses and occlusions as well as hypoechoic wall thickening that indicates sites of inflammation, which may be good candidates for biopsy.[53] Providers should not delay therapy while awaiting biopsy because it can still be diagnostic up to 14 days after the initiation of treatment.[53] To prevent vision loss, steroids should be started early if giant cell arteritis is considered. Patients often need prolonged steroid therapy to avoid recurrence; agents that can decrease the necessary steroid maintenance dose include methotrexate, azathioprine, and tocilizumab.[53,57]

SUMMARY

Consistent and systematic application of an appropriate history and neurologic examination in patients with headache can help clinicians to appropriately diagnose dangerous secondary conditions for optimal clinical outcomes. Owing to the overlapping symptoms of primary and secondary causes of headache, a systematic approach is required when obtaining history to identify patients with dangerous secondary causes. The SNOOP4 mnemonic provides a rapid and systematic approach to obtaining history, which can guide triage, examination, and additional clinical studies. Physical examination, particularly with attention to mental status and funduscopic findings, can offer additional clues to the presence of secondary causes. The history and examination should be used to guide appropriate imaging and laboratory studies and interpretations of their results.

SAH carries very high morbidity and mortality if not diagnosed appropriately and rapidly. Other secondary causes with significant risks if not diagnosed in timely fashion include RCVS, elevated ICP, CVST, arterial dissection, CNS infection and inflammatory vasculitis. In addition to the history, physical examination, and laboratory studies, the patient's medical background can offer key clues when evaluating for these possible disorders. Patients who are pregnant are at an increased risk for CVST, and patients who are older and immunocompromised are at greater risk for CNS infection and inflammatory vasculitis. Patients with underlying cancer and new headaches should be evaluated for cerebral metastasis and vascular etiologies arising from a hypercoagulable state.

KEY CLINICAL POINTS

- The majority of patients who seek care for headache have primary headache, but a small subset have secondary causes associated with high morbidity and mortality.
- A systematic history assessing for red flag features along with a careful neurologic examination is required to appropriately diagnose secondary causes such as SAH, RCVS, elevated ICP, hydrocephalus, CVST, arterial dissection, CNS infection, and inflammatory vasculitis.
- Patients who are pregnant, immunocompromised, elderly, or have known malignancy have higher risks of secondary disorders therefore, clinicians should have a different threshold to obtain additional diagnostic evaluations in these patients.

CLINICS CARE POINTS

- Headaches with thunderclap onset always require close evaluation for dangerous underlying etiologies such as SAH, RCVS, and elevated ICP that, if left untreated, are associated with a high degree of morbidity and mortality.

- A CT scan of the brain is nearly 100% sensitive and specific for SAH if performed within 6 hours of headache onset. However, sensitivity decreases to 93% by 24 hours and continues to decrease after that; therefore, an LP is recommended for patients who are suspected of having SAH, especially if it has been more than 6 hours since the onset of the headache.

- Altered mentation, presenting as new onset confusion, lethargy, or behavioral alterations, is not commonly associated with primary headache and should always raise suspicion for secondary headache owing to an intracranial process such as CNS infection or an increased ICP.

- Headaches with a strong positional component should raise clinicians' suspicion for altered ICP, which may be due to serious underlying causes. Although both high and low ICP can result in headaches, the causes of elevated ICP are more likely to be associated with significant morbidity and mortality than the causes of decreased ICP. A fundoscopic examination for papilledema is required when evaluating patients for possible elevation of the ICP.

- Although generally not an acutely life-threatening condition, in some cases of rapid leaks, a severely decreased ICP leads to disorders of consciousness or coma from brain sag with compression of the brainstem. This diagnosis should be considered in patients who do not otherwise have an explanation for coma or cranial nerve palsies.

REFERENCES

1. Goldstein JN, Camargo CA Jr, Pelletier AJ, et al. Headache in United States emergency departments: demographics, work-up and frequency of pathological diagnoses. Cephalalgia 2006;26(6):684–90.
2. Centers for Disease Control and Prevention. National Hospital Ambulatory Medical Care Survey: 2017 Emergency Department Summary Tables. 2017. Available at: https://www.cdc.gov/nchs/data/nhamcs/web_tables/2017_ed_web_tables-508.pdf. Accessed August 17, 2020.
3. Chu KH, Howell TE, Keijzers G, et al. Acute headache presentations to the emergency department: a statewide cross-sectional study. Acad Emerg Med 2017; 24(1):53–62.
4. Dodick DW. Pearls: headache. Semin Neurol 2010;30(1):74–81.
5. Wongtanasarasin W, Wittayachamnankul B. Clinical availability of SNOOP4 in acute non-traumatic headache patients admitted to the emergency department. Hong Kong Journal of Emergency Medicine 2020. 102490792092868.
6. Mac Grory B, Vu L, Cutting S, et al. Distinguishing characteristics of headache in nontraumatic subarachnoid hemorrhage. Headache 2018;58(3):364–70.
7. Bellolio MF, Hess EP, Gilani WI, et al. External validation of the Ottawa subarachnoid hemorrhage clinical decision rule in patients with acute headache. Am J Emerg Med 2015;33(2):244–9.
8. Perry JJ, Stiell IG, Sivilotti ML, et al. High risk clinical characteristics for subarachnoid haemorrhage in patients with acute headache: prospective cohort study. BMJ 2010;341:c5204.
9. Wu WT, Pan HY, Wu KH, et al. The Ottawa subarachnoid hemorrhage clinical decision rule for classifying emergency department headache patients. Am J Emerg Med 2020;38(2):198–202.
10. American College of Emergency Physicians Clinical Policies Subcommittee (Writing Committee) on Acute Headache. Clinical policy: critical issues in the evaluation and management of adult patients presenting to the emergency department with acute headache: approved by the ACEP board of directors

June 26, 2019 Clinical Policy Endorsed by the Emergency Nurses Association (July 31, 2019). Ann Emerg Med 2019;74(4):e41–74.

11. Dubosh NM, Bellolio MF, Rabinstein AA, et al. Sensitivity of early brain computed tomography to exclude aneurysmal subarachnoid hemorrhage: a systematic review and meta-analysis. Stroke 2016;47(3):750–5.

12. Edlow JA, Wyer PC. Evidence-based emergency medicine/clinical question. How good is a negative cranial computed tomographic scan result in excluding subarachnoid hemorrhage? Ann Emerg Med 2000;36(5):507–16.

13. Ducros A. Reversible cerebral vasoconstriction syndrome. Lancet Neurol 2012; 11(10):906–17.

14. Ducros A, Boukobza M, Porcher R, et al. The clinical and radiological spectrum of reversible cerebral vasoconstriction syndrome. A prospective series of 67 patients. Brain 2007;130(Pt 12):3091–101.

15. Singhal AB, Hajj-Ali RA, Topcuoglu MA, et al. Reversible cerebral vasoconstriction syndromes: analysis of 139 cases. Arch Neurol 2011;68(8):1005–12.

16. Stam J. Thrombosis of the cerebral veins and sinuses. N Engl J Med 2005; 352(17):1791–8.

17. Chen L, Xu M, Yan S, et al. Insufficient cerebral venous drainage predicts early edema in acute intracerebral hemorrhage. Neurology 2019;93(15):e1463–73.

18. Coutinho JM, de Bruijn SF, deVeber G, et al. Anticoagulation for cerebral venous sinus thrombosis. Stroke 2012;43(4):e41–2.

19. Debette S, Compter A, Labeyrie M-A, et al. Epidemiology, pathophysiology, diagnosis, and management of intracranial artery dissection. Lancet Neurol 2015; 14(6):640–54.

20. Silbert PL, Mokri B, Schievink WI. Headache and neck pain in spontaneous internal carotid and vertebral artery dissections. Neurology 1995;45(8):1517–22.

21. Alexander MD, Yuan C, Rutman A, et al. High-resolution intracranial vessel wall imaging: imaging beyond the lumen. J Neurol Neurosurg Psychiatry 2016; 87(6):589–97.

22. Markus HS, Levi C, King A, et al, Cervical Artery Dissection in Stroke Study I. Antiplatelet therapy vs anticoagulation therapy in cervical artery dissection: the Cervical Artery Dissection in Stroke Study (CADISS) randomized clinical trial final results. JAMA Neurol 2019;76(6):657–64.

23. Olesen J. International classification of headache disorders. Lancet Neurol 2018; 17(5):396–7.

24. de Tommaso M, Delussi M. Circadian rhythms of migraine attacks in episodic and chronic patients: a cross sectional study in a headache center population. BMC Neurol 2018;18(1):94.

25. Jacks AS, Miller NR. Spontaneous retinal venous pulsation: aetiology and significance. J Neurol Neurosurg Psychiatry 2003;74(1):7–9.

26. Levin BE. The clinical significance of spontaneous pulsations of the retinal vein. Arch Neurol 1978;35(1):37–40.

27. Geeraerts T, Merceron S, Benhamou D, et al. Non-invasive assessment of intracranial pressure using ocular sonography in neurocritical care patients. Intensive Care Med 2008;34(11):2062–7.

28. Kishk NA, Ebraheim AM, Ashour AS, et al. Optic nerve sonographic examination to predict raised intracranial pressure in idiopathic intracranial hypertension: the cut-off points. Neuroradiol J 2018;31(5):490–5.

29. Liu GT, Glaser JS, Schatz NJ. High-dose methylprednisolone and acetazolamide for visual loss in pseudotumor cerebri. Am J Ophthalmol 1994;118(1):88–96.

30. Scotton WJ, Botfield HF, Westgate CS, et al. Topiramate is more effective than acetazolamide at lowering intracranial pressure. Cephalalgia 2019;39(2):209–18.
31. Fonseca PL, Rigamonti D, Miller NR, et al. Visual outcomes of surgical intervention for pseudotumour cerebri: optic nerve sheath fenestration versus cerebrospinal fluid diversion. Br J Ophthalmol 2014;98(10):1360–3.
32. Lai LT, Danesh-Meyer HV, Kaye AH. Visual outcomes and headache following interventions for idiopathic intracranial hypertension. J Clin Neurosci 2014;21(10): 1670–8.
33. Lyons AR, Olson SL. Parinaud syndrome as an unusual presentation of intracranial hypotension. Surg Neurol Int 2020;11:98.
34. Pleasure SJ, Abosch A, Friedman J, et al. Spontaneous intracranial hypotension resulting in stupor caused by diencephalic compression. Neurology 1998;50(6): 1854–7.
35. Schievink WI, Maya MM, Moser FG, et al. Coma: a serious complication of spontaneous intracranial hypotension. Neurology 2018;90(19):e1638–45.
36. Mokri B. Spontaneous CSF leaks: low CSF volume syndromes. Neurol Clin 2014; 32(2):397–422.
37. Schievink WI. Spontaneous spinal cerebrospinal fluid leaks and intracranial hypotension. JAMA 2006;295(19):2286–96.
38. Dobrocky T, Grunder L, Breiding PS, et al. Assessing spinal cerebrospinal fluid leaks in spontaneous intracranial hypotension with a scoring system based on brain magnetic resonance imaging findings. JAMA Neurol 2019;76(5):580–7.
39. Sencakova D, Mokri B, McClelland RL. The efficacy of epidural blood patch in spontaneous CSF leaks. Neurology 2001;57(10):1921–3.
40. Hoxworth JM, Trentman TL, Kotsenas AL, et al. The role of digital subtraction myelography in the diagnosis and localization of spontaneous spinal CSF leaks. AJR Am J Roentgenol 2012;199(3):649–53.
41. Kim DK, Brinjikji W, Morris PP, et al. Lateral decubitus digital subtraction myelography: tips, tricks, and pitfalls. AJNR Am J Neuroradiol 2020;41(1):21–8.
42. Harriott AM, Karakaya F, Ayata C. Headache after ischemic stroke: a systematic review and meta-analysis. Neurology 2020;94(1):e75–86.
43. Tentschert S, Wimmer R, Greisenegger S, et al. Headache at stroke onset in 2196 patients with ischemic stroke or transient ischemic attack. Stroke 2005; 36(2):e1–3.
44. Merikangas KR, Fenton BT, Cheng SH, et al. Association between migraine and stroke in a large-scale epidemiological study of the United States. Arch Neurol 1997;54(4):362–8.
45. Savitz SI, Caplan LR, Edlow JA. Pitfalls in the diagnosis of cerebellar infarction. Acad Emerg Med 2007;14(1):63–8.
46. Richie MB, Josephson SA. A practical approach to meningitis and encephalitis. Semin Neurol 2015;35(6):611–20.
47. Sances G, Granella F, Nappi RE, et al. Course of migraine during pregnancy and postpartum: a prospective study. Cephalalgia 2003;23(3):197–205.
48. Chou DE. Secondary headache syndromes. Continuum (Minneap Minn) 2018; 24(4, Headache):1179–91.
49. Abbott J, Kirkby GR. Acute visual loss and pituitary apoplexy after surgery. BMJ 2004;329(7459):218–9.
50. Ranabir S, Baruah MP. Pituitary apoplexy. Indian J Endocrinol Metab 2011; 15(Suppl 3):S188–96.
51. Robbins MS. Headache in pregnancy. Continuum (Minneap Minn) 2018;24(4, Headache):1092–107.

52. Black DF, Bartleson JD, Bell ML, et al. SMART: stroke-like migraine attacks after radiation therapy. Cephalalgia 2006;26(9):1137–42.
53. Ness T, Bley TA, Schmidt WA, et al. The diagnosis and treatment of giant cell arteritis. Dtsch Arztebl Int 2013;110(21):376–85 [quiz: 386].
54. Smetana GW, Shmerling RH. Does this patient have temporal arteritis? JAMA 2002;287(1):92–101.
55. Gonzalez-Gay MA, Barros S, Lopez-Diaz MJ, et al. Giant cell arteritis: disease patterns of clinical presentation in a series of 240 patients. Medicine (Baltimore) 2005;84(5):269–76.
56. Gonzalez-Gay MA, Lopez-Diaz MJ, Barros S, et al. Giant cell arteritis: laboratory tests at the time of diagnosis in a series of 240 patients. Medicine (Baltimore) 2005;84(5):277–90.
57. Stone JH, Tuckwell K, Dimonaco S, et al. Trial of tocilizumab in giant-cell arteritis. N Engl J Med 2017;377(4):317–28.

Acute Dizziness, Vertigo, and Unsteadiness

Barbara Voetsch, MD, PhD[a,b,*], Siddharth Sehgal, MD[a,b]

KEYWORDS

- Dizziness • Vertigo • Vestibular syndrome • Vertebrobasilar stroke
- Posterior circulation stroke • Benign paroxysmal positional vertigo
- Vestibular neuritis • HINTS examination

KEY POINTS

- Dizziness and vertigo are common chief complaints in the emergency department and have a broad differential diagnosis. Vertigo is a symptom, not a diagnosis.
- Relying on the character of dizziness is associated with a greater risk of misdiagnosis. The history should instead be focused on timing and triggers of vestibular symptoms.
- Stroke is the most concerning condition presenting with dizziness, and its prompt recognition is critical for timely treatment.
- The HINTS (head impulse, nystagmus, test of skew) examination is the most important bedside clinical test to differentiate peripheral from central vertigo, but it is diagnostic only when the patient is symptomatic.
- Head computed tomography should not be used to rule out stroke. Brain MRI is the diagnostic test of choice in appropriately selected patients.

INTRODUCTION

Dizziness, vertigo, and disequilibrium are among the most common chief complaints in patients referred for neurologic evaluation or presenting to the emergency department (ED). These symptoms account for 3.3% to 4% of ED visits annually in the United States.[1,2] This corresponds to almost 4.5 million emergent visits, and recent studies indicate that this number is steadily increasing.[2] However, the term dizziness encompasses a wide range of symptoms with variable clinical significance. Although most conditions are benign and self-limited, such as semicircular canal dysfunction or orthostatic hypotension, in a subset of patients they may signal the presence of a potentially life-threatening neurologic event, including vertebrobasilar ischemia or brainstem hemorrhage. Serious causes of dizziness may also be medical in origin, such as cardiac arrhythmias and electrolyte derangements, which poses a challenging problem for treating

[a] Department of Neurology, Lahey Hospital and Medical Center, 41 Mall Road, Burlington, MA 1805, USA; [b] Tufts University School of Medicine, Burlington, MA, USA
* Corresponding author. Department of Neurology, Lahey Hospital and Medical Center, 41 Mall Road, Burlington, MA 1805.
E-mail address: Barbara.Voetsch@lahey.org

Neurol Clin 39 (2021) 373–389
https://doi.org/10.1016/j.ncl.2021.01.008
0733-8619/21/© 2021 Elsevier Inc. All rights reserved.

clinicians or consultant neurologists: identifying the small number of patients with an ominous condition among a large number of patients with less concerning causes of dizziness and vertigo. In addition, because of the paucity of reliable clinical criteria, there is a high rate of misdiagnosis for acutely dizzy patients in the ED.[3] A cross-sectional study of almost 9500 ED patients with dizziness showed that about one-fourth are given a symptom diagnosis only, highlighting the difficulty of determining a specific underlying cause.[1] In an international survey of emergency physicians, development of clinical decision rules for acute vertigo was identified as one of the topmost priorities.[4]

NEUROANATOMY

Three different systems participate in the regulation of balance and equilibrium: the vestibular, the proprioceptive, and the visual systems. The vestibular system includes the vestibular apparatus in the inner ear (labyrinth), the vestibular portion of the eighth cranial nerve (the vestibulocochlear nerve), and the vestibular nuclei in the brainstem with their central connections.

The labyrinth is located within the petrous portion of the temporal bone and consists of the utricle, saccule, and 3 semicircular canals, which lie in orthogonal planes to each other.[5] These structures are filled with endolymph and contain neuroepithelial hair cells, which serve as exquisitely motion-sensitive kinetic receptors and transmit impulses indicating position and movement of the head to the brainstem, via the vestibular (Scarpa) ganglion situated in the internal auditory meatus. The utricle and saccule contain small calcified crystals called otoliths, which stimulate the hair cells when activated by movement, gravity, or inertia to transmit linear acceleration, whereas the semicircular canals are sensitive to angular acceleration.

The central fibers originating from the bipolar cells of the vestibular ganglion form the vestibular nerve, which joins the cochlear nerve and traverses the cerebellopontine angle alongside the facial nerve to enter the brainstem at the level of the pontomedullary junction. These fibers then terminate in the vestibular nuclear complex (composed of the superior, lateral, medial, and inferior or descending vestibular nuclei, as shown in **Fig. 1**) located on each side of the floor of the fourth ventricle and rostral medulla, where they relay with secondary neurons.

The vestibular nuclei play a critical role in the adjustment of posture, muscle tone, and eye position in response to tilt and acceleration of the head in space. This adjustment occurs through projections to the contralateral vestibular nuclei, extraocular nuclei, cerebellum, and spinal cord.[5] These main connections are:

- The lateral and medial vestibular nuclei give rise to the lateral and medial vestibulospinal tracts, respectively (see **Fig. 1**). The lateral vestibulospinal tract descends ipsilaterally throughout the length of the spinal cord and connects to motor neurons to maintain extensor tone and balance. The medial vestibulospinal tract extends only to the cervical and upper thoracic level, playing an important role in controlling neck and head position.
- Fibers arising primarily from the medial vestibular nucleus, with contributions from all other vestibular nuclei, ascend in the heavily myelinated medial longitudinal fasciculus to the oculomotor, trochlear, and abducens nuclei. This pathway mediates the vestibulo-ocular reflex (VOR), described in more detail later.
- Some fibers from the vestibular nerve bypass the vestibular nuclei and connect directly to the flocculonodular lobe of the cerebellum, also called the vestibulocerebellum or archicerebellum. The flocculonodular lobe and cerebellar vermis also receive impulses from the vestibular nuclei, with which it has several reciprocal connections.

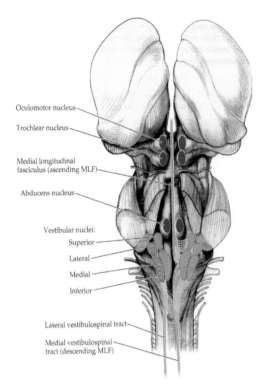

Oculomotor nucleus

Trochlear nucleus

Medial longitudinal
fasciculus (ascending MLF)

Abducens nucleus

Vestibular nuclei:

Superior

Lateral

Medial

Inferior

Lateral vestibulospinal tract

Medial vestibulospinal
tract (descending MLF)

Fig. 1. The vestibular nuclei and their connections. (*From* Blumenfeld H. Brainstem I: Surface Anatomy and Cranial Nerves. In: Neuroanatomy through Clinical Cases, 2nd ed. Sunderland: Sinauer Associates; 2010. p. 524.)

- An ascending pathway through the ventral posterior thalamus to the cortex provides an awareness of head position that is integrated with visual and tactile spatial information in the parietal association cortex.
- In addition, the vestibular nuclei receive reciprocal connections from the cerebellum, reticular formation, spinal cord, and contralateral vestibular nuclei.

Taken together, impulses arising in the receptors of the labyrinth form the afferent limb of the reflex arcs that serve to coordinate the extraocular, nuchal, and body muscles to ensure that balance and tone are preserved with every position and movement of the head. The VOR is an important example of these reflex arcs. The semicircular canals provide a head velocity signal, which is transmitted through the vestibular division of the eighth cranial nerve to the vestibular nuclei. The vestibular nuclei on both sides then integrate with the oculomotor nuclei and generate an equal and opposite eye velocity signal to keep the eyes in place while the head moves. This ability allows objects of interest to be kept in visual focus while the head moves; for example, while walking or driving. The brainstem connections involved in the VOR are shown in **Fig. 1.**

CAUSE

A lesion affecting the vestibular pathways at any point from the labyrinth to the vestibular nuclei or its central connections can result in symptoms of vertigo, dizziness, and imbalance. A commonly used classification divides the broad range of possible causes into 3 main categories: peripheral, central, and systemic. The characteristics of the dizziness and examination findings associated with each of these conditions can vary greatly, as further discussed later.

Peripheral causes result from dysfunction of the vestibular end organs in the labyrinth or of the vestibular portion of the eighth cranial nerve. This dysfunction includes peripheral vestibulopathy such as vestibular neuritis or labyrinthitis, benign paroxysmal positional vertigo (BPPV), Menière disease, and vestibular schwannoma, although vestibular schwannoma, if large enough, can affect additional surrounding posterior fossa structures. Less common causes include semicircular canal dehiscence syndrome and herpes zoster oticus. In addition, ototoxicity from drugs such as aminoglycosides, notably gentamicin, are considered in this group.

Central causes result from lesions or dysfunction of the vestibular nuclei within the brainstem and their central connections, and are less common than either peripheral or systemic causes. Typically, additional complaints or neurologic signs on examination are present, but their absence should not exclude the possibility of a central cause. Central vertigo most commonly occurs as a result of posterior circulation ischemia affecting the central vestibular structures in the brainstem and cerebellum in elderly patients and those with vascular risk factors. Brainstem or cerebellar hemorrhage can have a similar presentation and occurs more commonly in patients with hypertension and diabetes. In younger patients, acute demyelination in the setting of multiple sclerosis is on the differential diagnosis. Other less common causes include posterior fossa brain tumors, central nervous system infection, and trauma. In the absence of structural lesions, vestibular migraines must be considered in patients with episodic vestibular symptoms and headache.

In addition, approximately 50% of dizzy patients presenting to the ED have a widespread range of underlying systemic causes, such as toxic, metabolic, infectious, and cardiovascular conditions, including arrhythmias.[1] These causes include cardiovascular conditions such as hypotension and cardiac arrhythmias, systemic infections, medications (eg, toxicity caused by common anticonvulsants such as phenytoin, phenobarbital, and carbamazepine), anemia, and metabolic and endocrine disorders. Rarely, dizziness can be a primary manifestation of carbon monoxide poisoning. Associated symptoms (eg, gastrointestinal bleeding, fever) or context (eg, new antihypertensive medications) often suggest these diagnoses.

In contrast with the outpatient setting, where only a minority of cases is attributed to dangerous causes such as cerebrovascular accident (6%) or cardiac arrhythmia (1%), small studies have estimated that, in the ED, up to 30% of patients with dizziness have a serious disorder, including 15% with stroke, transient ischemic attack (TIA), cardiac arrhythmia, acute infection, or anemia.[1]

In addition, the patients presenting to the ED with these symptoms are typically older, with 25% to 30% being more than 65 years of age, which has led to a general trend toward more neuroimaging studies and higher costs of care in this patient population.[2]

DIAGNOSTIC APPROACH

Diagnosis of the underlying disease requires that the complaint of dizziness be analyzed carefully. The first step is to take a detailed and accurate history, which guides the physical examination and provides a clinical framework for the differential diagnosis and subsequent diagnostic work-up.

Clinical History

Dizziness is a vague term used by patients to describe a variety of different abnormal sensory experiences. These experiences can include a feeling of rotation or movement, as well as swaying, faintness, lightheadedness, or unsteadiness. Episodes of blurry vision, confusion, disorientation, or even brief seizures can be described by patients as dizzy spells. In the past, there has been an emphasis on categorizing dizziness into true vertigo and nonvertiginous symptoms. Vertigo is defined as a subjective illusion of motion, classically with a rotatory component. It is the predominant symptom that arises from an acute asymmetry or dysfunction of the vestibular system and can be attributed to central or peripheral causes, as discussed earlier.[6] Importantly, vertigo is a symptom, not a diagnosis. Some patients perceive this as self-motion, whereas others describe movement of the environment.

Recent studies have shown this method of focusing on the character of dizziness to be notoriously unreliable and associated with a high rate of misdiagnosis.[7] Patients are often unable to give an accurate and consistent description of symptoms, and, in addition to common words such as spinning, lightheadedness, or unsteadiness, may use vague terms such as woozy, foggy, or confused.[8] In the past few years, a different approach to emergency evaluation of dizziness has therefore been proposed, which focuses on the timing and triggers of symptoms.[9] Timing refers to the onset, duration, and evolution of the dizziness, whereas triggers refer to movements, actions, or situations that provoke the onset of dizziness. Using these criteria results in a few possible patterns of symptoms that, when combined with a targeted neurologic examination focused on signs of brainstem and cerebellar dysfunction, can then be used to narrow down the differential diagnostic considerations and determine the need for further investigations.[9,10] Of note, the term vestibular in this context refers to vestibular symptoms (vertigo, dizziness, unsteadiness) rather than signifying a vestibular cause. These symptom subtypes are listed later and are summarized in **Table 1**.

- Episodic vestibular syndrome (EVS): intermittent episodes that arise either spontaneously and last from minutes or hours up to several days or are triggered by head movement, change in body position, or other specific situation. EVS typically lasts from seconds to less than a minute and, in the absence of the specific trigger, patients are symptom free. The most common conditions causing

Table 1
Main benign and high-risk causes of episodic and acute vestibular syndromes

Syndrome Type	High-Risk Causes	Benign Causes
Spontaneous episodic vestibular syndrome	• TIA • Cardiac arrhythmia • Hypoglycemia	• Vestibular migraine • Menière disease • Panic attack
Triggered episodic vestibular syndrome	• Bow-hunter syndrome • Midline cerebellar stroke (CPPV)	• BPPV • Semicircular canal dehiscence syndrome • Orthostatic hypotension
Acute vestibular syndrome	• Stroke • Brainstem or cerebellar hemorrhage • Tumor • Demyelinating lesion • CO poisoning	• Vestibular neuritis • Viral labyrinthitis • Ramsay Hunt syndrome • Medications

Abbreviation: CPPV, central paroxysmal positional vertigo.

triggered EVS include BPPV and orthostatic hypotension, whereas vestibular migraines and TIAs account for most spontaneous EVS.

- Acute vestibular syndrome (AVS): sudden onset of persistent dizziness lasting days to weeks. Although symptoms can worsen with head or body movement, these patients remain symptomatic even in the absence of movement or other specific triggers. The differential diagnosis includes primarily vestibular neuritis/labyrinthitis and posterior circulation stroke. Most AVS is spontaneous but it can be triggered by antecedent exposure to trauma or toxic causes.
- Chronic vestibular syndrome: prolonged dizziness that lasts for weeks, months, or even longer, caused by conditions that are beyond the scope of this review.

The terms dizziness and vertigo are used interchangeably in the remainder of this article given their limited diagnostic utility without the associated duration and trigger characteristics.

Spontaneous episodic vestibular syndromes

Spontaneous episodic vestibular spells typically last for minutes to a few hours, less commonly for days.[11] In addition to dizziness, patients generally also experience nausea and vomiting, gait unsteadiness, and nystagmus causing vision disturbance. Spontaneous vestibular symptoms do not have an obvious trigger. Although patients may report worsening with head movement or body position changes, the symptoms are still present in the absence of those factors. Because these patients may be asymptomatic at the time of initial medical evaluation with a normal physical and neurologic examination, and their symptoms cannot be provoked in the absence of a known trigger, the diagnostic evaluation hinges on a detailed history and the clinical context.

Vestibular migraine is the most common reported cause of EVS, with a prevalence of about 1% in the general population.[12] It is characterized by episodic vestibular symptoms in patients who generally have an established history of migraines with or without aura, but the dizziness and the headache do not necessarily occur simultaneously.[13] Photophobia, phonophobia, motion intolerance, and decreased hearing can occur. Neurologic examination is normal apart from possible nystagmus during an attack. Because migraine is a central process, the nystagmus can be of central type (direction changing, vertical, or torsional, as further discussed later). The diagnostic criteria for vestibular migraine are listed in **Box 1**. Because these criteria require

---

Box 1
Diagnostic criteria for vestibular migraine according to the International Classification of Headache Disorders[14]

- A current or past history of migraine (with or without aura)
- At least 5 episodes fulfilling the following 2 criteria:
  - Vestibular symptoms of moderate or severe intensity, lasting between 5 minutes and 72 hours
  - At least 50% of episodes are associated with at least 1 of the following 3 migrainous criteria:
    - Headache with at least 2 of the following characteristics (unilateral, pulsating, moderate or severe intensity, aggravation by routine physical activity)
    - Photophobia and phonophobia
    - Visual aura
- Symptoms not better accounted for by another diagnosis

at least 5 episodes with vestibular symptoms, this diagnosis cannot be established after a single event.[14]

Other benign causes of spontaneous EVSs include Menière disease, anxiety attacks, and vasovagal syncope. Menière disease is characterized by recurrent episodes of vertigo or dizziness lasting between 20 minutes and 12 hours, tinnitus or aural fullness, and audiometrically documented low-frequency to midfrequency hearing loss, which is presumed to be secondary to endolymphatic hydrops.[15] The course of Menière disease is variable, but about two-thirds of patients tend to experience vertigo attacks in clusters. Because the condition extends over years, it is much less commonly seen in the ED. Panic attacks can present with episodic dizziness in the absence of the classic hyperventilation and occasionally without an obvious antecedent provocation. Symptoms usually begin rapidly and can last for several minutes, typically peaking at about 10 minutes.[16]

TIA in the vertebrobasilar circulation is the most important serious cause for spontaneous EVS. Although often additional posterior circulation findings such as dysarthria, diplopia, gait unsteadiness, and nausea or vomiting can be present, isolated dizziness does not exclude the possibility of a TIA. In a recent study of transient brainstem symptoms preceding posterior circulation stroke, 8.4% of patients had episodes of isolated dizziness leading up to the event, mostly in the previous 48 hours.[17] In all cases, the vertigo was of sudden onset and unprovoked.

Vertebral artery dissection should be considered in young patients with acute dizziness and severe headache, especially if associated with sudden neck pain without photophobia or phonophobia. In older patients with traditional vascular risk factors, vertebral artery or basilar artery stenosis often present with recurrent TIAs before leading to a stroke. Among patients with basilar artery occlusive disease in the New England Medical Center Posterior Circulation Registry, two-thirds of patients initially had TIAs, of whom almost 60% progressed to stroke.[18]

Although less common, paroxysmal cardiac rhythm disorders and hypoglycemia are other dangerous conditions that need to be considered. Cardiac arrhythmia is an important diagnostic consideration for presentations with episodes of exertion-induced dizziness or syncope. Interestingly, the dizziness caused by cardiac arrhythmias can be described by patients as vertigo,[19] which is another reason for not relying on the character of dizziness during the diagnostic process.

Triggered episodic vestibular syndromes

Triggered EVS is characterized by brief episodes of vertigo or dizziness that are precipitated by specific factors such as head movement or body position changes. Patients have associated nausea, vomiting, and gait unsteadiness but are asymptomatic in between spells in the absence of the provocative trigger.

The most common cause of triggered EVS is BPPV, which is the prototypical triggered episodic vestibular syndrome and accounts for about 10% of all dizziness presentations in the ED. Prevalence increases with age, with peak onset between 50 and 60 years of age.[20] BPPV can be idiopathic, secondary to whiplash or head trauma, which can be mild, or a residual effect of several vestibular disorders. It is caused by calcium debris from the utricular sac that migrates into the semicircular canals and leads to inappropriate movement of the endolymph with head acceleration, leading to a perceived sensation of spinning.[20] Because of its anatomic-dependent position, the posterior semicircular canal is the most common site of canalithiasis and accounts for about four-fifths of cases of BPPV. Common triggers include head movement and body position changes, bending the head forward or backward, and rolling over in bed, which precipitates brief attacks of severe dizziness or vertigo lasting for seconds to minutes. Hearing loss and tinnitus are typically absent. Between episodes, patients are symptom free, but bouts can recur for weeks or even months if not treated. Although the condition is benign, the symptoms of BPPV can be uncomfortable and dramatic, explaining the common ED presentation. Observing nystagmus during a provoking maneuver solidifies the diagnosis of BPPV in patients with a typical history (discussed later in relation to physical examination).

Orthostatic hypotension causes EVS, which is triggered by getting up from a seated or supine position. This condition is generally benign and is caused by hypovolemia, but it can be a presenting symptom of serious conditions such as internal hemorrhage, myocardial infarction, or severe metabolic derangement.[21] Dizziness from orthostatic hypotension is not triggered by rolling over in bed or lying down, which can help in the differential diagnosis with BPPV.

Semicircular canal dehiscence syndrome is an uncommon condition in which thinning of the bone overlying the superior semicircular canal allows pressure to be transmitted to the inner ear.[22] This pressure leads to episodes of dizziness, hyperacusis, and nausea triggered by an increase in pressure such as coughing, sneezing, or Valsalva maneuver. Episodes can also be triggered by loud sound (Tullio phenomenon) and there may be cochlear hypersensitivity and pulsatile tinnitus. These patients should be referred to an otorhinolaryngologist. The diagnosis is established with high-resolution computed tomography (CT) of the temporal bone and, in some patients, surgical repair is required.

It is rare for cerebrovascular disorders to present with classic triggered episodes, with few exceptions, which are discussed next. However, it is important to stress that isolated dizziness as well as triggered episodes or intermittent worsening of episodes associated with specific circumstances, although uncommon manifestations of a cerebrovascular event, should not rule out this possibility and constitute a potential pitfall in these patients.

Acute vestibular syndromes

Patients with acute spontaneous vestibular syndromes present with persistent dizziness or vertigo, at times severe, and often associated with nausea, vomiting, and persistent postural instability. Symptoms last for several days, with a gradual course of improvement over the subsequent weeks. Unlike the episodic cases, these patients are symptomatic at the time of their initial clinical evaluation, and a careful physical and neurologic examination can provide helpful information to establish a diagnosis.[23] These patients have symptoms at rest that typically worsen with head movement, an important and frequently misinterpreted clinical feature when differentiating these conditions from triggered episodic syndromes, in which patients are asymptomatic at rest.[24]

Vestibular neuritis is the classic AVS. It is a self-limiting condition thought to be secondary to herpes simplex viral infections or idiopathic.[25] Viral labyrinthitis presents in a similar manner with an additional component of hearing impairment. The most concerning differential diagnosis of AVS is posterior circulation stroke, which, in most cases, is ischemic, but hemorrhagic strokes can also occur. Ischemic stroke in the cerebellum or brainstem accounts for up to 10% of AVSs, with some estimates being even higher, depending on the age group.[23] Distinguishing stroke from vestibular neuritis or labyrinthitis is critical to ensure that treatment is initiated promptly and the underlying stroke mechanism is evaluated. The characteristics of cerebrovascular disorders presenting with dizziness are discussed further later.

Trauma or chemical intoxication can also present with acute persistent vestibular symptoms. The antecedent history of exposure or trauma is usually evident but may not be obvious in some circumstances when a reliable history cannot be obtained because of coexisting mental status alteration. For patients experiencing dizziness after an acute blunt head trauma, it is important to think about a traumatic vertebral artery dissection and posterior skull fracture as concomitant causes for the vestibular symptoms. Medications known to cause vestibular dysfunction include anticonvulsants[26] and aminoglycosides. Rarely, carbon monoxide poisoning can present with isolated dizziness with other nonspecific symptoms.[27]

Cerebrovascular disorders presenting with dizziness

Although posterior circulation ischemia remains the most serious and potentially life-threatening neurologic problem in dizzy patients, most have substantially less concerning conditions, posing a particularly vexing diagnostic challenge for emergency physicians and neurologists. TIA and ischemic stroke should be on the differential diagnosis for any patient with spontaneous vestibular syndrome, acute or episodic. Dizziness and vertigo are the presenting symptoms in almost half of patients with posterior circulation ischemic events.[18] Given the proximity of several brainstem nuclei, and ascending and descending tracts, there are typically several associated neurologic signs and symptoms. Although discussing individual ischemic brainstem and cerebellar syndromes is not within the scope of this review, it is worth noting the most common associated findings. In the more than 400 patients reviewed in the New England Medical Center Posterior Circulation Registry,[18] the most frequent presenting signs other than dizziness were unilateral limb weakness, gait or unilateral limb ataxia, dysarthria, and headache. Nystagmus was present in about one-quarter of patients and slightly more had nausea and vomiting. Horner syndrome is a common sign in lateral medullary syndrome (Wallenberg syndrome). Even with underlying basilar artery occlusive disease, the most severe form of posterior circulation ischemia, more than 50% of patients reported dizziness or vertigo as a chief symptom. Although isolated vertigo is less common, it does not exclude a posterior circulation event. Similarly, unilateral hearing loss typically indicates a peripheral event; however, acute stroke in the anterior inferior cerebellar artery distribution should be considered when a patient presents with acute vertigo accompanied by unilateral hearing loss.[28]

Diagnosis of ischemic stroke in the posterior circulation can be less obvious than an anterior circulation stroke. The National Institutes of Health Stroke Scale (NIHSS) is skewed toward anterior circulation symptoms and therefore tends to underestimate the severity of vertebrobasilar infarcts. The NIHSS score can be zero, as in the case of vermian cerebellar infarcts, for example.[29] In a meta-analysis including more than 15,000 patients with acute stroke, approximately 9% were misdiagnosed at the initial clinical encounter, with about 15% of these patients presenting with isolated dizziness/vertigo as their chief complaint.[30] A large review of ED visits and hospital discharges identified dizziness to be the most important factor correlating with a missed stroke diagnosis.[31] As a result, patients with posterior circulation stroke are significantly more likely to receive a wrong or delayed diagnosis at the initial medical evaluation compared with those presenting with a carotid distribution ischemic event. A study analyzing time from symptom onset to diagnosis in patients presenting with basilar artery occlusion found that both in the prehospital phase and in the emergency room there were highly significant delays in diagnosis compared with patients presenting with left middle cerebral artery occlusion.[32] This finding is even more true among younger patients, who have fewer vascular risk factors and are thought to be at a lower risk of stroke. Patients with posterior circulation stroke more frequently have transient neurologic symptoms in the days to weeks leading up to a vertebrobasilar stroke, compared with anterior circulation infarcts.[17] However, patients do not always seek immediate medical attention for these nonspecific symptoms and, when they do, they are often not recognized as a sign of a major impending cerebrovascular event. These errors are missed opportunities to provide acute stroke treatments and initiate secondary prevention measures.

Typically, the vestibular symptoms associated with acute infarcts of the posterior circulation are spontaneous, of sudden onset, and continuous, but in rare instances patients with well-defined triggered episodes may harbor a cerebrovascular cause, such as patients with midline cerebellar infarcts.[33] Another rare cause of vertebrobasilar ischemia presenting with episodic symptoms is bow-hunter syndrome, which is triggered by head and neck movement.[34] Patients develop external compression or even occlusion of the vertebral artery against the atlantoaxial or subaxial level during head and neck turning to one side. In general, the symptoms develop while the patient is standing, which helps differentiate this condition from BPPV. Barring these rare exceptions, patients with classic triggered episodic vestibular symptoms do not have an underlying cerebrovascular cause for their symptoms.

Physical Examination

As in all neurologic conditions, the physical examination of a dizzy patient begins with a general assessment. Important initial elements include the vital signs, including orthostatics and general appearance. Skin pallor or cyanosis may be a sign of severe anemia or hypoxia. Cardiac examination may indicate an arrhythmia (eg, prolonged supraventricular tachycardia causing hypotension) or atrial fibrillation and valvular heart disease as potential embolic sources for embolic stroke. The presence of a neck bruit suggests underlying carotid or vertebral artery stenosis. In addition, a skin rash around the external ear and vesicles in the auditory canal, especially with concomitant ipsilateral facial palsy, should raise concern for Ramsay Hunt syndrome (herpes zoster oticus). Shortness of breath and sweating may suggest a panic attack.

Positional maneuvers such as the Dix-Hallpike and supine head roll tests are used to elicit symptoms in patients with BPPV.[35] The Dix-Hallpike maneuver attempts to reproduce vertigo and precipitate torsional and vertical nystagmus in patients with posterior semicircular canal dysfunction. If abnormal, an Epley canalith-repositioning maneuver can be performed for treatment. The supine head roll test is used to diagnose horizontal canal disorder. These maneuvers should not be used in patients with continuous vestibular symptoms because this can lead to false diagnosis of a peripheral cause.

After identifying the category of vestibular syndrome based on the clinical classification discussed earlier, for patients experiencing acute continuous symptoms or those with intermittent spells who are symptomatic at the time of evaluation, a targeted examination can help differentiate between peripheral/otologic and central causes. A focused and expedited neurologic examination with attention to oculomotor findings, presence of a Horner syndrome, and brainstem/cerebellar dysfunction is an essential component of the diagnostic evaluation for patients presenting with vestibular symptoms.

In addition, the HINTS (head impulse, nystagmus, test of skew) test should be performed on every patient suspected to be experiencing central vertigo.[36] This test is a 3-step assessment developed by neuro-otologists and is the best bedside test to distinguish brainstem and cerebellar dysfunction from vestibular neuritis or other peripheral causes of vertigo. Importantly, the test is valid only when the patient is symptomatic with continuous vertigo and is not useful for those who have transient position-related dizziness or TIAs without ongoing dizziness. The 3 components of the HINTS examination are head impulse test (HIT), gaze and nystagmus testing, and alternate cover test for detection of skew deviation, as detailed in **Box 2**. A normal HINTS examination with a positive HIT, absence of skew deviation, and absence of atypical nystagmus features can even outperform brain MRI–diffusion-weighted imaging (DWI) for ruling out acute posterior fossa infarction in the first 48 hours.[36]

Fig. 2 shows a summarized approach to patients presenting with acute dizziness.

Neuroimaging

Noncontrast head CT scan has excellent accuracy for detecting acute intracerebral hemorrhage (ICH) and is therefore useful in promptly diagnosing an acute posterior

---

Box 2
Head impulse, nystagmus, test of skew test[36]

This is a 3-step bedside assessment to differentiate between central and peripheral causes of vertigo. The individual components of HINTS have limitations but the combination of the 3 parts provides accurate information regarding the central or peripheral localization of vestibular symptoms.

The test is only valid when the patient has ongoing symptoms.

HIT
- This is a test of the VOR (described in the text).
- Patient is asked to fix the gaze on the examiner or a distant target. The examiner then firmly holds the patient's head and thrusts it quickly to one side, about 30°.
- Normal response or negative HIT: the eyes remain on the target.[37]
- Abnormal response or positive HIT: the eyes move in the same direction as the head turn, followed by a catch-up saccade back to the target. This response implies a deficient VOR on the side of the head turn, indicating a peripheral vestibular lesion on the ipsilateral side.
- The VOR is preserved in central lesions such as cerebellar infarcts.[a]
- Concomitant hearing loss with an abnormal HIT can be caused by labyrinthitis or an acute labyrinthine and cochlear stroke, structures supplied by the anterior inferior cerebellar artery.

Nystagmus
- Nystagmus is an almost universal finding in vestibular syndromes while symptoms are present.
- Presence of nystagmus alone does not provide adequate differential diagnostic utility. The directional characteristics are more useful in identifying peripheral versus central causes.
- Peripheral causes: nystagmus is generally horizontal and unidirectional, and can be intensified by changing gaze toward the direction of its fast phase.
- Central causes: direction-changing nystagmus, dominant vertical or torsional component.
- Absence of these atypical nystagmus features does not eliminate a central cause but their presence is highly suggestive and warrants further investigation for a posterior fossa lesion.

Skew deviation
- Assessed by alternate cover test of the eyes, assessing for a vertical corrective saccade on the affected side.
- Vertical misalignment or skew occurs as a result of disruption of the efferent vestibular pathway to the oculomotor nuclei and suggests a central cause for vertigo.[38]

Central lesion:
- Negative HIT
- Direction-changing or vertical nystagmus
- Skew deviation present

Peripheral lesion:
- Positive HIT
- Unidirectional nystagmus
- Skew deviation absent

[a]A rare exception is a lateral pontine infarct in which cranial nerve VIII fascicles are affected.

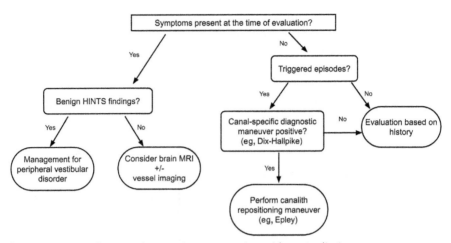

Fig. 2. Summarized approach to patients presenting with acute dizziness.

fossa ICH or to rule out hemorrhage for the purpose of thrombolysis decisions. However, it is exceedingly rare for isolated dizziness to be the chief presenting complaint for an acute brainstem or cerebellar ICH.[39] In addition, head CT has low sensitivity for ischemic changes in the acute phase of a stroke, in particular in the posterior fossa.[40] Therefore, CT studies have been shown to have low accuracy and cost-effectiveness for evaluation of patients presenting to the ED with acute dizziness.[41,42] Despite the shortcomings of this imaging modality, this is still the initial neuroimaging test of choice in about half of the patients presenting to the ED with acute dizziness and is one of the pitfalls in attempting to rule out stroke.

Brain MRI with DWI has superior sensitivity to CT for identification of acute ischemic changes[43] and small brainstem or cerebellar lesions of different causes, such as multiple sclerosis. However, MRI is an expensive and time-consuming test, and there is a nontrivial rate of false-negatives in posterior circulation infarcts, especially within the first 48 hours of symptoms onset. For these reasons, MRI should be the test of choice for patients with a suspected central cause of dizziness, but obtaining MRI on all patients with acute dizziness is not a feasible approach. Therefore, it is of paramount importance to identify patients who need brain imaging based on a focused history regarding symptoms duration and triggers and a neurologic examination targeting oculomotor, brainstem, and cerebellar dysfunction. The underlying clinical suspicion also dictates what imaging study is most appropriate. **Fig. 3** shows the utility of different imaging modalities in the work-up of patients with central vertigo.

TREATMENT

Appropriate management of dizziness and vertigo requires identification of the correct underlying diagnosis. Treatment can then be divided into 3 subgroups: disease-specific treatment, symptomatic treatment, and rehabilitation therapy. Because the list of causes of vestibular syndromes is long, disease-specific therapy only for the conditions most relevant in terms of frequency or severity in an ED setting is briefly discussed here.

Among the peripheral causes, patients with BPPV do not respond well to vestibular suppressants and are best treated with canalith-repositioning maneuvers. Potential treatments for vestibular neuritis and labyrinthitis include corticosteroids and antiviral

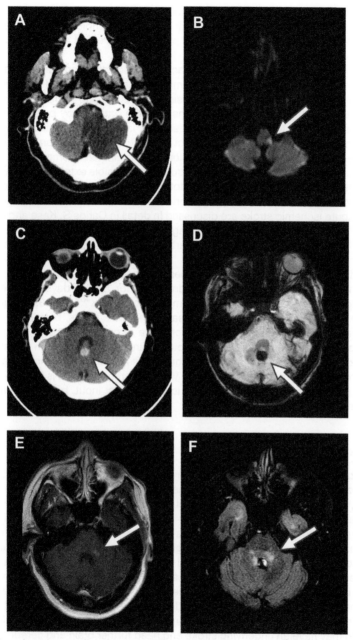

Fig. 3. Neuroimaging studies showing different brainstem and cerebellar lesions (*arrows*) leading to central vertigo. (*A*) Head CT shows subacute infarction of the left cerebellar hemisphere and vermis with surrounding cytotoxic edema leading to effacement of the fourth ventricle, secondary to occlusion of the left posterior inferior cerebellar artery. (*B*) Small area of diffusion restriction in the left lateral medulla on MRI brain indicates Wallenberg syndrome, which in this patient was secondary to atherothrombosis of the left vertebral artery. (*C*) Noncontrast head CT with acute intraparenchymal hemorrhage centered within the cerebellar vermis and (*D*) corresponding susceptibility-weighted imaging on MRI brain. (*E*)

agents, although a meta-analysis of 4 randomized clinical trials comparing corticosteroids with placebo showed no significant effect on complete caloric recovery at 1 year.[44] Ramsay Hunt syndrome should promptly be treated with valacyclovir and corticosteroids.[45]

For acute posterior circulation infarcts, acute revascularization therapies, including thrombolysis with recombinant tissue plasminogen activator and endovascular stroke therapy, should be considered. Thrombolysis is indicated up to 4.5 hours from onset in most patients barring any contraindications, and the patient may be a candidate for mechanical thrombectomy if there is evidence of large-vessel occlusion by neuroimaging. In case of a large cerebellar infarct or posterior fossa hemorrhage, hyperosmolar therapy for intracranial hypertension and brainstem compression may be indicated and neurosurgery should be consulted for possible external ventricular drain placement or decompressive surgery. Endotracheal intubation and mechanical ventilation may be required for airway protection or in comatose patients. Management of ICH and acute ischemic stroke are discussed in detail in Carlos S. Kase and Daniel F. Hanley's article, "Intracerebral Hemorrhage: Advances in Emergency Care"; and Adeel S. Zubair and Kevin N. Sheth's article, "Emergency Care of Patients with Acute Ischemic Stroke," in this issue.

For patients with multiple sclerosis experiencing an acute demyelination, intravenous corticosteroids such as methylprednisolone for 3 to 5 days are used in an attempt to shorten the exacerbation and improve outcome.[46] Vestibular migraine attacks are treated with vestibular suppressants and antiemetics, but do not typically respond as well to triptans unless headache is a strong component. Symptomatic medications to suppress vestibular symptoms are most effective in patients who have dizziness lasting for at least a few hours. These medications include antihistamines, antiemetics, and benzodiazepines. Vestibular rehabilitation is used to improve balance, promote brain adaptation to reduced vestibular input, boost postural confidence, and reduce risk of falls.

SUMMARY

Acute dizziness is one of the most common neurologic presentations in the ED. Most acute dizziness presentations are caused by self-limited conditions, including migraine, hypotension, and peripheral vestibular disorders such as BPPV. However, it is imperative to consider the possibility of high-risk conditions such as ischemic stroke or paroxysmal cardiac arrhythmia as the cause of isolated dizziness. Vestibular symptoms have been associated with a high rate of misdiagnosis or lack of an established underlying diagnosis during the initial clinical encounter, which can be attributed to an overemphasis on the symptom type and relying on head CT imaging for differentiating between benign and dangerous causes of vestibular syndromes. Recent evidence indicates that a clinical approach focusing on symptom timing and triggers supported by a detailed oculomotor examination is highly accurate for identifying patients who may have an underlying stroke and need further brain and cerebrovascular imaging with MRI.

◄──

Small contrast-enhancing lesion in the left middle cerebellar peduncle (MCP) on T1-weighted MRI consistent with acute demyelination in a young woman with multiple sclerosis and (F) previous bilateral MCP involvement present on fluid-attenuated inversion recovery imaging (FLAIR).

CLINICS CARE POINTS

- Dizziness and vertigo are common chief complaints in the ED with a broad differential diagnosis.
- Vertigo is a symptom, not a diagnosis.
- Relying on the character of dizziness is associated with a greater risk of misdiagnosis, and the history should be focused on timing and triggers of symptoms. This change in paradigm still requires that physicians take a detailed and accurate clinical history.
- Central vertigo is much less common than peripheral vertigo, but its recognition is extremely important to improve the outcomes of the patients.
- Dizziness that worsens with movement is not necessarily peripheral in cause.
- Stroke is the most important serious condition presenting with dizziness, and its prompt recognition is critical for treatment.
- In patients presenting with dizziness after trauma, it is important to consider vertebral artery dissection.
- The HINTS examination is the most important bedside clinical test to differentiate peripheral versus central vertigo. This test is valid only when the patient is symptomatic.
- The NIHSS score in posterior circulation infarct can be zero.
- CT should not be used to rule out stroke. Brain MRI is the diagnostic test of choice in appropriately selected patients.

DISCLOSURE

The authors have nothing to disclose.

REFERENCES

1. Newman-Toker DE, Hsieh YH, Camargo CA Jr, et al. Spectrum of dizziness visits to US emergency departments: cross-sectional analysis from a nationally representative sample. Mayo Clin Proc 2008;83(7):765–75.
2. Saber Tehrani AS, Coughlan D, Hsieh YH, et al. Rising annual costs of dizziness presentations to U.S. emergency departments. Acad Emerg Med 2013;20(7):689–96.
3. Royl G, Ploner CJ, Leithner C. Dizziness in the emergency room: diagnoses and misdiagnoses. Eur Neurol 2011;66(5):256–63.
4. Eagles D, Stiell IG, Clement CM, et al. International survey of emergency physicians' priorities for clinical decision rules. Acad Emerg Med 2008;15(2):177–82.
5. Baehr M, Frotscher M. Vestibulocochlear Nerve (CN VIII) – vestibular component and vestibular system. In: Baehrthis M, editor. Topical diagnosis in neurology. 4th edition. Stuttgart (Germany): Thieme; 2005. p. 184–94.
6. Cappello M, di Blasi U, di Piazza L, et al. Dizziness and vertigo in a department of emergency medicine. Eur J Emerg Med 1995;2(4):201–11.
7. Kerber KA, Newman-Toker DE. Misdiagnosing dizzy patients: common pitfalls in clinical practice. Neurol Clin 2015;33(3):565–viii.
8. Newman-Toker DE, Cannon LM, Stofferahn ME, et al. Imprecision in patient reports of dizziness symptom quality: a cross-sectional study conducted in an acute care setting. Mayo Clin Proc 2007;82(11):1329–40.
9. Newman-Toker DE, Edlow JA. TiTrATE: a novel, evidence-based approach to diagnosing acute dizziness and vertigo. Neurol Clin 2015;33(3):577–viii.

10. Edlow JA. Managing patients with acute episodic dizziness. Ann Emerg Med 2018;72(5):602–10.
11. Hotson JR, Baloh RW. Acute vestibular syndrome. N Engl J Med 1998;339(10): 680–5.
12. Dieterich M, Obermann M, Celebisoy N. Vestibular migraine: the most frequent entity of episodic vertigo. J Neurol 2016;263(Suppl 1):S82–9.
13. Lempert T, Olesen J, Furman J, et al. Vestibular migraine: diagnostic criteria. J Vestib Res 2012;22(4):167–72.
14. Headache Classification Committee of the International Headache Society (IHS). The international classification of headache disorders, 3rd edition. Cephalalgia 2018;38:1.
15. Lopez-Escamez JA, Carey J, Chung WH, et al. Diagnostic criteria for Ménière's disease. J Vestib Res 2015;25(1):1–7.
16. Katon WJ. Clinical practice. Panic disorder. N Engl J Med 2006;354(22):2360–7.
17. Paul NL, Simoni M, Rothwell PM, Oxford Vascular Study. Transient isolated brainstem symptoms preceding posterior circulation stroke: a population-based study. Lancet Neurol 2013;12(1):65–71.
18. Voetsch B, DeWitt LD, Pessin MS, et al. Basilar artery occlusive disease in the New England Medical Center Posterior Circulation Registry. Arch Neurol 2004; 61(4):496–504.
19. Newman-Toker DE, Camargo CA Jr. 'Cardiogenic vertigo'–true vertigo as the presenting manifestation of primary cardiac disease. Nat Clin Pract Neurol 2006; 2(3):167–72.
20. Kim JS, Zee DS. Clinical practice. Benign paroxysmal positional vertigo. N Engl J Med 2014;370(12):1138–47.
21. Gilbert VE. Immediate orthostatic hypotension: diagnostic value in acutely ill patients. South Med J 1993;86(9):1028–32.
22. Baloh RW. Superior semicircular canal dehiscence syndrome: Leaks and squeaks can make you dizzy. Neurology 2004;62(5):684–5.
23. Tarnutzer AA, Berkowitz AL, Robinson KA, et al. Does my dizzy patient have a stroke? A systematic review of bedside diagnosis in acute vestibular syndrome. CMAJ 2011;183(9):E571–92.
24. Newman-Toker DE, Stanton VA, Hsieh YH, et al. Frontline providers harbor misconceptions about the bedside evaluation of dizzy patients. Acta Otolaryngol 2008;128(5):601–4.
25. Kim JS, Kim HJ. Inferior vestibular neuritis. J Neurol 2012;259(8):1553–60.
26. Hamed SA. The auditory and vestibular toxicities induced by antiepileptic drugs. Expert Opin Drug Saf 2017;16(11):1281–94.
27. Trevino R. A 19-year-old woman with unexplained weakness and dizziness. J Emerg Nurs 1997;23(5):499–500.
28. Lee H. Audiovestibular loss in anterior inferior cerebellar artery territory infarction: a window to early detection? J Neurol Sci 2012;313(1–2):153–9.
29. Martin-Schild S, Albright KC, Tanksley J, et al. Zero on the NIHSS does not equal the absence of stroke. Ann Emerg Med 2011;57(1):42–5.
30. Tarnutzer AA, Lee SH, Robinson KA, et al. ED misdiagnosis of cerebrovascular events in the era of modern neuroimaging: A meta-analysis. Neurology 2017; 88(15):1468–77.
31. Newman-Toker DE, Moy E, Valente E, et al. Missed Diagnosis of stroke in the emergency department: a cross-sectional analysis of a large population-based sample. Diagnosis 2014;1:155–66.

32. Burns JD, Rindler RS, Carr C, et al. Delay in Diagnosis of Basilar Artery Stroke. Neurocrit Care 2016;24:172–9.
33. Kim HA, Yi HA, Lee H. Apogeotropic central positional nystagmus as a sole sign of nodular infarction. Neurol Sci 2012;33:1189–91.
34. Duan G, Xu J, Shi J, et al. Advances in the pathogenesis, diagnosis and treatment of bow hunter's syndrome: a comprehensive review of the literature. Interv Neurol 2016;5(1–2):29–38.
35. Edlow JA, Newman-Toker D. Using the physical examination to diagnose patients with acute dizziness and vertigo. J Emerg Med 2016;50(4):617–28.
36. Kattah JC, Talkad AV, Wang DZ, et al. HINTS to diagnose stroke in the acute vestibular syndrome: three-step bedside oculomotor examination more sensitive than early MRI diffusion-weighted imaging. Stroke 2009;40(11):3504–10.
37. Newman-Toker DE, Kattah JC, Alvernia JE, et al. Normal head impulse test differentiates acute cerebellar strokes from vestibular neuritis. Neurology 2008;70(24 Pt 2):2378–85.
38. Brodsky MC, Donahue SP, Vaphiades M, et al. Skew deviation revisited. Surv Ophthalmol 2006;51(2):105–28.
39. Kerber KA, Burke JF, Brown DL, et al. Does intracerebral haemorrhage mimic benign dizziness presentations? A population based study. Emerg Med J 2012;29(1):43–6.
40. Hwang DY, Silva GS, Furie KL, et al. Comparative sensitivity of computed tomography vs. magnetic resonance imaging for detecting acute posterior fossa infarct. J Emerg Med 2012;42:559–65.
41. Chalela JA, Kidwell CS, Nentwich LM, et al. Magnetic resonance imaging and computed tomography in emergency assessment of patients with suspected acute stroke: a prospective comparison. Lancet 2007;369(9558):293–8.
42. Wasay M, Dubey N, Bakshi R. Dizziness and yield of emergency head CT scan: Is it cost effective? Emerg Med J 2005;22:312.
43. Simmons Z, Biller J, Adams HP Jr, et al. Cerebellar infarction: Comparison of computed tomography and magnetic resonance imaging. Ann Neurol 1986;19: 291–3.
44. Fishman JM, Burgess C, Waddell A. Corticosteroids for the treatment of idiopathic acute vestibular dysfunction (vestibular neuritis). Cochrane Database Syst Rev 2011;(5):CD008607.
45. Coulson S, Croxson GR, Adams R, et al. Prognostic factors in herpes zoster oticus (Ramsay Hunt syndrome). Otol Neurotol 2011;32(6):1025–30.
46. Murray TJ. Diagnosis and treatment of multiple sclerosis. BMJ 2006;332(7540): 525–7.

Emergency Care of Patients with Acute Ischemic Stroke

Adeel S. Zubair, MD[a,1], Kevin N. Sheth, MD[a,b,*]

KEYWORDS

- Acute stroke • Ischemic stroke • Golden hour • Thrombectomy • Thrombolysis

KEY POINTS

- This article serves to provide an overview of acute stroke care and golden hour management.
- Common work-up and treatment options are discussed.
- Recent pivotal clinical trials in the field of vascular neurology are discussed.

INTRODUCTION

With 26,000,000 people worldwide experiencing a stroke every year, stroke is the second-leading cause of mortality worldwide and a leading cause of long-term disability.[1,2] Ischemic stroke comprises a majority of cerebrovascular disease (two-thirds) and most commonly results from occlusion of cerebral small vessels, cardiac embolism, and atherosclerosis of the cerebral circulation.[3] Great advances have been made in the past decades, transforming acute ischemic stroke (AIS) into a highly treatable neurologic emergency. Yet, despite advances that have expanded the time window of treatment opportunity, diagnosis and subsequent implementation of the correct treatment in the shortest possible time remain essential for optimizing patient outcomes.

The mainstays for treatment of AIS include reperfusion therapy by systemic thrombolysis and/or endovascular therapy (EVT). For patients with AIS, it is crucial to identify patients eligible for acute therapy, in order to potentially reverse a salvageable deficit from brain tissue that is vulnerable but not irreversibly infarcted, known as the penumbra. This review serves to discuss AIS identification and management in the golden hour, starting from prehospital evaluation, followed by acute decision making regarding treatment options, and finally postreperfusion care.

[a] Department of Neurology, Yale School of Medicine, New Haven, CT, USA; [b] Division of Neurocritical Care and Emergency Neurology, Yale School of Medicine, Yale New Haven Hospital, New Haven, CT, USA
[1] Department of Neurology, 15 York St, New Haven CT 06510.
* Corresponding author. 42 Allison Drive, Madison, CT 06443.
E-mail address: Kevin.sheth@yale.edu

Neurol Clin 39 (2021) 391–404
https://doi.org/10.1016/j.ncl.2021.02.001
neurologic.theclinics.com
0733-8619/21/© 2021 Elsevier Inc. All rights reserved.

PREHOSPITAL CONSIDERATIONS

Prehospital factors play a large role in delivery of timely care to patients with AIS. This phase of care, therefore, has been targeted with multiple interventions in order to hasten potential thrombolysis treatment. These interventions have included hospital prenotification, activating the stroke service prior to emergency department arrival for suspected stroke, and multiprofessional workforce training.[4–6]

First responders should evaluate patients with suspected AIS for adequacy of airway, breathing, and circulation and obtain a focused history, focusing especially on the last time patients were known not to have stroke symptoms (last known well [LKW]) from any collateral sources. Important parts of the ideal prehospital history include last known normal time, medication list, vital signs, blood glucose, and recent health issues.[7] These data should be passed on to the hospital team to help expedite care upon arrival. Prehospital notification of a potential incoming stroke allows for activation of critical resources, including preparing imaging machines and immediate assessment by the multidisciplinary stroke team upon patient arrival. This early notification is important in expediting care and can result in increased accessibility to thrombolysis.[8]

An important goal for emergency medical teams is to appropriately triage patients to optimize the chances for reperfusion therapy.[9] In some communities, the emergency medical teams must decide whether to take patients to a closer primary stroke center (PSC) versus a more distant comprehensive stroke center (CSC). A PSC can provide thrombolysis therapy only, whereas a CSC additionally can provide EVT as well as advanced inpatient care in dedicated neuroscience units led by clinical experts. Prehospital scales can help to accurately triage patients to a PSC or CSC by identifying patients who are likely to have a large vessel occlusion (LVO) and, therefore, who would benefit from direct transport to CSC.

The most frequently used scales include the Cincinnati Prehospital Stroke Severity Scale (CPSSS), Los Angeles Motor Scale (LAMS), and Rapid Arterial Occlusion Evaluation (RACE).[9,10] The CPSSS is calculated by assessment of conjugate gaze, arm weakness, and level of consciousness commands and questions and is 89% sensitive and 73% specific in identifying National Institutes of Health Stroke Scale (NIHSS) greater than 15 and LVO.[11] The LAMS is composed of facial droop, arm drift, and grip strength and had a sensitivity of 81% with a specificity of 89% in predicting presence of large vessel occlusion.[12] The RACE score is composed of assessments of facial palsy, arm motor function, leg motor function, gaze, and aphasia/agnosia and has a sensitivity of 85%, with a specificity of 68% in detecting LVO.[13]

Many centers may not have the resources and expertise to perform EVT[14]; in these situations, patients who are eligible for intravenous (IV) tissue plasminogen activator (tPA) should receive treatment and, for those who qualify for thrombectomy, be transferred to a CSC.[15] Time-sensitive treatment of stroke have shaped regionalization of stroke care; between 2006 and 2014, interfacility transfer for ischemic stroke and TIA doubled.[16] Many patients who are not eligible for intra-arterial alteplase still may be eligible for mechanical thrombectomy. Improving communication methods between hospitals as well as improved interhospital systems can result in decreased transfer times.[17] Important consideration should be placed for method of transfer. In many situations, traffic, weather conditions, or distance to a CSC can prolong time to treatment with EVT.

There is a tension between getting all thrombectomy candidates to a CSC as fast as possible and avoiding unnecessarily flooding these centers with non-LVO patients who then have delayed time to IV thrombolysis and also are taken out of their home communities. Two major models exist for dealing with this dilemma. The drip and ship (DS) model is aimed at having a patient arrive as quickly as possible to a PSC for rapid evaluation for and institution of IV thrombolysis therapy (drip) followed by assessment and possible transfer (ship) to a CSC for EVT at a CSC. The mothership (MS) model, on the other hand, is aimed at getting a patient to a CSC as the initial destination regardless of greater travel time to allow for all treatment to occur at the same institution with no need for additional transfer.

The decision whether to transport first to a PSC and then to a CSC versus directly to the CSC is multifactorial.[9] The time since stroke onset (or since LKW) dictates the therapy a patient is eligible to receive, such as thrombolysis and EVT, EVT only, or neither. The primary objective should be to ensure maximal treatment in as quick a time as possible, and implementation of the prehospital scales allows for assessment of stroke severity and helps detect LVOs, which could be better treated at a CSC.

A recent systematic review found that patients (all comers with stroke or those who screen positively for likelihood of LVO) who went directly to a CSC had significantly better outcomes compared with patients who were directed to a PSC followed by transfer, although the studies reviewed were limited and multicenter trials are needed for further clarification.[18] Two clinical trials from Europe, Racecat (Direct Transfer to an Endovascular Center Compared to Transfer to the Closest Stroke Center in Acute Stroke Patients with Suspected Large Vessel Occlusion) and PRESTO (Pre-hospital Evaluation of Sensitive Troponin Study), are investigating prehospital issues and hopefully will shed light on optimal triage options (DS model vs MS model).

Some health systems have developed mobile stroke units to expedite and improve care and obviate the DS versus MS dichotomy. These are ambulances that typically are staffed by paramedics and equipped with a portable computed tomography (CT) scanner and mobile equipment for basic laboratory assessment, facilitating early administration of IV alteplase, frequently prior to arrival to the hospital.[19]

The Pre-Hospital Acute Neurologic Treatment and Optimization of Medical Care in Stroke (PHANTOM-S) study demonstrated that patients who received thrombolysis prior to arrival at the hospital did not have higher risk of mortality and were more likely to be discharged home.[20] Another randomized controlled trial showed that early treatment in a mobile stroke unit substantially reduced time from alarm to therapy decision (35 min vs 76 min).[21] These mobile stroke units can allow for rapid diagnosis and treatment with thrombolysis therapy and can result in patients being taken directly to CSCs for consideration of EVT, resulting in time and cost savings by avoiding further transfer and duplication of testing. CT angiography use in mobile stroke units also can result in decreased door to puncture time for EVT.[22]

INITIAL EVALUATION IN THE EMERGENCY DEPARTMENT

Rapid evaluation for patients presenting with AIS is paramount for clinical care. A door-to-needle time of less than 45 minutes for IV alteplase is a benchmark for treatment, with secondary goals of meeting less than 30 minutes for door-to-needle time.[23] These goals allow for prompt intervention and, for patients requiring transfer to other sites, increased efficiency to allow to optimal care.[23] Patients should be evaluated by a physician within 10 minutes of arrival to the hospital with the stroke team being involved in that timeline as well. Obtaining vital signs and blood work should be done concurrently while conducting the physical examination, because this simple step can result in decreased door to needle times.[24] Critically important information for decision making includes blood pressure (BP), blood sugar, any recent history of anticoagulant use, time of LKW, and any factors that may contraindicate the administration of systemic thrombolytics (**Box 1**). This workup should be done as expeditiously as possible. Finally, door-to-CT time should be under 25 minutes.

Box 1
Absolute contraindication to intravenous alteplase

History of ICH

Severe uncontrolled hypertension—systolic exceeding 185 mm Hg or diastolic 110 mm Hg

Serious head trauma or stroke in previous 3 months

Thrombocytopenia and coagulopathy

Direct thrombin inhibitors

Low-molecular-weight heparin

Factor Xa inhibitors

Severe hypoglycemia or hyperglycemia

Acute intracranial hemorrhage

History

History plays a crucial role in the initial evaluation in the ED. The goal is to piece together a clinical image of a patient and the events leading up to the hospital presentation rapidly. Important points include carefully elucidating the time of last known to be without stroke symptoms, or LKW, from the patient or other collateral sources, including the EMT or family/friends. This information helps guide decision making regarding eligibility for thrombolysis therapy. Additionally, care should be taken to review the past medical history for potential contraindications to therapy, including previous intracerebral hemorrhage (ICH), serious head trauma or stroke in the past 3 months, and anticoagulant use (see **Box 1**). In particular, reviewing a patient's medication list clarifying the last dose of medications, specifically anticoagulants, can help determine if a patient is eligible for thrombolysis therapy.

Examination

Examination of patients should start with an assessment of adequacy of airway, breathing, and circulation, including review of vital signs. To reduce the possibility of post-thrombolysis hemorrhage, the BP should be no greater than 185 mm Hg systolic or 110 mm Hg diastolic prior to administration. Antihypertensives may be given to bring a thrombolytic candidate's BP into this range. Labetalol boluses and continuous infusions of nicardipine or clevidipine are best suited for this purpose. An irregular pulse may help provide potential clues for etiology of stroke.

A key portion of an expedited neurologic assessment includes the NIHSS. The NIHSS serves as an efficient and reliable method for determining stroke severity, following it over time, and conveying it between different providers. The NIHSS is biased toward detection of anterior circulation LVO strokes.[9]

Ruling out Mimics

A variety of different processes can mimic the clinical presentation of AIS and need to be ruled out rapidly to ensure optimal therapy. Chief among these is hypoglycemia, which must be looked for at the beginning of every acute stroke evaluation. Other common diagnoses that can masquerade as AIS include seizures, migraine, and metabolic derangements, including hyponatremia, uremia, hyperammonemia, hyperthyroidism, hypercalcemia, and hypoglycemia.[25] History and clinical evaluation can help sort through these diagnoses. Although seizures and migraine can present acutely, they often have some prodromal event or aura, which can tip off clinicians.

The role of the clinician is to rule out common mimics as best as they are able prior to advancing to treatment considerations. Importantly, this process is not perfect and giving tPA to a patient with a stroke mimic generally is low risk.[26,27]

Imaging

Imaging plays a critical role in golden hour management of patients with AIS. The main goals for imaging are to exclude hemorrhage or large established infarcts and identify potentially treatable LVOs. Stroke imaging can be done using CT or magnetic resonance imaging (MRI). The imaging choice is made based on available resources and stroke team preference.

Most stroke centers utilize CT imaging as a first screen for making decisions regarding thrombolysis. CT images take less time to acquire, are more widely available in the emergency department setting, and do not require the extra time needed to screen patients for MRI-incompatible hardware. An acute ICH typically is seen as a spheroid lesion with high CT density (60–90 Hounsfield units).[28] In addition to ICH, more subtle, low-volume hemorrhagic lesions, such as subarachnoid hemorrhage, subdural hematomas, and intraventricular hemorrhages, should be sought carefully before systemic thrombolysis is given.

The imaging data collected are used overall to guide clinical treatment plans. If there is no evidence of a hemorrhage and patients do not have other contraindications (including large established infarct) to thrombolysis and is within the time window, they should receive therapy immediately. Following this, if there is evidence of LVO on angiography with evidence of a perfusion mismatch, patients are candidates for EVT as well. Even if patients are excluded from receiving thrombolysis, they still may be eligible for thrombectomy.

CT scans also can help with defining the extent and location of ischemic parenchyma irreversibly damaged by hypoperfusion (CBF below 10–12 mL/100 g/min), termed the infarct core. Ischemia results in development of cytotoxic edema, which can be seen as a decrease in tissue density on CT.[29] Early signs of ischemia can be seen in the blurring of the clarity of the internal capsule as well as loss of corticomedullary differentiation.[28] The CT signs have a specificity of 85% and a sensitivity of 40% to 60% in the first 3 hours after symptom onset.[28,30]

The ASPECTS score was developed to provide a reliable method of assessing ischemic changes on head CT in order to assess the extent of ischemia and identify acute stroke patients who are unlikely to make an independent recovery despite treatment.[31] The value is calculated by using 2 standard axial CT cuts, 1 at the level of the thalamus and basal ganglia and 1 just rostral to the basal ganglia.[31,32] A normal CT scan has an ASPECTS value of 10 whereas diffuse ischemic changes throughout the middle cerebral artery (MCA) territory results in a value of 0. This score is used in the context of decision making for thrombectomy; a higher score predicts a more favorable outcome.

MRI uses diffusion-weighted imaging (DWI) to define the ischemic core. DWI uses the restricted motion of the water molecules trapped in the cell to detect cytotoxic edema, which is a bright signal on b1000 DWIs or a low signal on the apparent diffusion coefficient maps.[28,33] DWI is able to detect ischemic as early as 11 minutes after symptom onset and is more sensitive that CT for identification of acute ischemia.[28,34,35]

Given the time constraints and goal to obtain rapid imaging for decision regarding thrombolysis, most centers obtain CT imaging first to rule out hemorrhage. CT scans also are more accessible as they do not require screening of patients for MRI-compatible hardware, a decision point that can slow down imaging times. Following this, advanced imaging techniques, such as perfusion imaging and angiography, may be utilized.

Arterial imaging can be done using CT angiography or magnetic resonance (MR) angiography and should image from the level of the aortic arch to the vertex.[36] It is important for the imaging report to comment on the site of occlusion, details of collateral circulation, tandem occlusions or stenosis, and anatomic peculiarities.[28] In some cases, acute thrombus can be seen on noncontrast CT as a hyperdense artery sign and can have predictive value for outcomes; a study showed a hyperdense MCA longer than 8 mm predicted poor recanalization after IV thrombolysis.[28,37]

Ischemic penumbra is the tissue at risk due to being critically hypoperfused (cerebral blood flow [CBF] 12–20 mL/100 g/min). The damage to the neurons generally can be reversed if timely reperfusion occurs; if not, the penumbra is converted to ischemic core. Perfusion imaging allows for delineation between ischemic core, penumbra, and the surrounding tissue not at risk. Perfusion imaging may be performed by either CT or MR and uses dynamic imaging techniques with IV contrast to yield parameter maps including time maps of tissue-level contrast enhancement (time to maximum [Tmax], time to peak [TTP], and mean transit time [MTT]).[28] Reduced CBF in the penumbra results in energy-dependent autoregulatory mechanisms to keep cerebral blood volume normal and is accompanied by an elevated MTT and TTP. This is distinguished from ischemic core where these compensatory mechanisms fail resulting in a cerebral blood volume drop, which is a measure of infarction and is correlated with restricted diffusion only in hyperacute stroke.[38] CT perfusion uses a mismatch between the cerebral blood volume and MTT or Tmax to define the ischemic penumbra. MR perfusion defines the penumbra as the area of DWI less than perfusion index (PI) mismatch; large trials, such as Diffusion Weighted Imaging Evaluation for Understanding Stroke Evolution Study-2 (DEFUSE-2), used a Tmax with delay of greater than 6 seconds and greater than 10 seconds to define the thresholds for penumbra and ischemic core.[28,39] Postprocessing techniques used for CT perfusion and MR perfusion can vary and are not standardized.[40]

Systemic Thrombolysis

For patients who present with AIS within 3 hours and who have no contraindications, first-line therapy is IV alteplase. Off-label use of tPA may be offered to select patients between 3 hours and 4.5 hours from LKW.[23] tPA results in initiation of local fibrinolysis by binding to fibrin in a thrombus and turning plasminogen to plasmin, breaking up the thrombus.

Multiple clinical trials have assessed long-term neurologic outcomes in patients treated with IV tPA after AIS. A patient-level meta-analysis of these trials showed thrombolysis increased the rate of good neurologic outcomes by 10% (defined as no residual disability) if given within 3 hours of stroke onset.[41] Studies looking at the 3-hour to 4.5-hour window found improved outcomes as well, leading to widespread adoption of the 4.5-hour window. Use in this time window, however, has not been approved by the Food and Drug Administration.[1,41]

Exclusion of contraindications to systemic thrombolysis is a critical part of the management pathway (see **Box 1**). This can be done through a review of the medical record, medication history, patient-provided information, collateral history, and diagnostic testing results. Often, however, patients are unable to add much to the history and there is no other collateral information available. Review of laboratory results and imaging findings can help screen for other underlying conditions or potential contraindications. Discussions with the pharmacy team often can provide a cursory medication list pulled from pharmacy records, which may be useful to gain insight into a patient's medical history.

Patients with an age greater than 80 appear to benefit from thrombolysis despite a higher mortality rate compared with younger patients. Approximately one-third of acute strokes occur among people aged greater than 80 years but data regarding this population initially were limited due to poor representation in early clinical trials of thrombolysis for AIS.[42] Further studies, including the randomized third International Stroke Trial,[43] controlled comparison analyses,[44] and large observational studies, such as the Safe Implementation of Thrombolysis in Upper Time Window Monitoring Study (SITS-UTMOST), however, showed support for use of tPA for AIS in patients aged greater than 80.[45] Guidelines by the American Stroke Association (ASA)/American Heart Association (AHA) and the European Stroke Organisation recommend that alteplase be administered within 4.5 hours of stroke symptoms onset with no upper age limit.[23,46]

The tPA dose is calculated at 0.9 mg/kg of actual body weight, with maximum dose of 90 mg; 10% of the dose is given as an IV bolus over 1 minute whereas the remaining 90% is infused over 1 hour. As discussed previously, prior to administration, BP must be below 185 mm Hg systolic and 110 mm Hg diastolic; for patients with BP above these limits, treatment with IV fast-acting agents, such as labetalol, clevidipine, and nicardipine, should be initiated. If the BP can be controlled in this way, below 185/100 mm Hg, tPA is given. After thrombolytic therapy has been administered, BP should be below 180/105 mm Hg for the following 24 hours.

Issues with consent often arise in patients who present with AIS. Consent is not required to administer tPA as an emergent therapy for otherwise eligible adult patients with a disabling AIS if patient or surrogate consent is not available.[23] All steps should be taken, however, to find a surrogate decision maker rapidly if possible.

Patients who receive tPA for AIS should be monitored for at least 24 hours with dedicated neurologic and cardiac monitoring.[23] Previously, this was done solely in an intensive care unit (ICU) setting; newer research, however, suggests that not all patients require ICU monitoring.[47] For patients with any change in neurologic examination, immediate brain imaging should be done to exclude hemorrhage. Anticoagulant or antithrombotic agents should not be administered for at least 24 hours after infusion is complete.

Complications of Thrombolysis

Neurologic worsening and/or new headache after tPA should alert clinicians to the possibility of hemorrhage. If hemorrhage is found after thrombolysis, steps must be taken to prevent further deterioration. Patients' airway and breathing should be monitored to ensure they do not need assistance with ventilation. Early and sustained reversal of thrombolytic medications are necessary to avoid hematoma expansion. Laboratory tests should be checked, including coagulation factors and fibrinogen. If the fibrinogen level is less than 50 mg/dL, 2 bags of cryoprecipitate should be given with a fibrinogen level checked 60 minutes after completion of transfusion. A stability CT scan should be done after 6 hours of initial deterioration or with any new clinical change. Further intervention, including neurosurgical consultation, should be available.

Orolingual angioedema can occur in 1% to 8% of patients treated with tPA.[48,49] For patients who develop this during treatment, the first step is to halt further infusion. Additionally, it is critically important to monitor the airway and breathing of patients to ensure adequate ventilation. Patients should be treated with antihistamines and steroids and monitored closely for signs of deterioration.[50]

Tenectaplase

A newer fibrinolytic agent, tenecteplase, has been studied for use in AIS. It is a genetically modified variant of alteplase, which has a higher specificity for fibrin.[51] This medication holds promise for improved clinical utility due to the fact that it requires a 1-time bolus for administration, resulting in faster administration and quicker start of subsequent EVT.[52] Tenecteplase has been shown to have similar efficacy and safety outcomes compared with alteplase.[52–54] Tenecteplase can result in decreased costs and has the potential to lead to a shift in treatment paradigm. In particular, it can play a major role in the DS model as it is a 1-time bolus, which facilitates quicker transport.

Thrombectomy

Mechanical thrombectomy is approved for patients with AIS in the anterior circulation within 24 hours of symptom onset. In 2015, 5 randomized trials (ESCAPE, REVASCAT, EXTEND IA, MR CLEAN, and SWIFT PRIME) showed efficacy of EVT over standard medical care with a following meta-analysis (Highly Effective Reperfusion Evaluated in Multiple Endovascular Stroke Trials [HERMES]) showing reduction in disability (**Table 1**).[55–60] In 2018, 2 additional trials, DAWN and DEFUSE-3, demonstrated that thrombectomy can be beneficial in selected patients at up to 24 hours from LKW when there is a mismatch between infarct size on imaging and clinical deficit.[61,62]

The AHA/ASA guidelines specify that thrombectomy is indicated in patients with a prestroke modified Rankin scale score (mRS) of 0 to 1, causative occlusion of the internal carotid artery or MCA (M1), age greater than or equal to age 18, NIHSS score greater than or equal to 6, and treatment initiation within 6 hours.[23]

Oral anticoagulant use frequently is an exclusion to systemic thrombolysis in AIS. Endovascular treatment is a treatment option for this subset of patients. In a subset of the MR CLEAN registry, prior oral anticoagulant use was not associated with increased risk of symptomatic ICH or worse functional outcome in patients treated with EVT for AIS compared with those without prior oral anticoagulant use.[63]

Table 1
Major trials showing efficacy of endovascular thrombectomy over standard medical care

Trial	Intervention
ESCAPE trial: Randomized Assessment of Rapid Endovascular Treatment of Ischemic Stroke	Anterior circulation proximal occlusion randomized to standard care of EVT and standard care
MR CLEAN trial: A Randomized Trial of Intra-arterial Treatment for Acute Ischemic Stroke	Proximal intracranial arterial occlusion randomized to either standard care of intra-arterial treatment (thrombolytic, EVT, or both) and standard care
EXTEND IA Trial: Endovascular Therapy for Ischemic Stroke with Perfusion-Imaging Studies	Proximal intracranial arterial occlusion in patients who received IV tPA plus standard care or IV tPA plus EVT
SWIFT PRIME trial: Stent-retriever thrombectomy after intravenous t-PA vs t-PA alone in stroke	Proximal anterior intracranial arterial occlusion in patients who received IV tPA plus standard care or IV tPA plus EVT
REVASCAT trial: Randomized Trial of Revascularization with Solitaire FR Device vs Best Medical Therapy in the Treatment of Acute Stroke Due to Anterior Circulation Large Vessel Occlusion Presenting Within 8 Hours of Symptom Onset	Large-vessel anterior circulation arterial occlusion in patients who receive medical management alone or those who receive mechanical embolectomy with the Solitaire FR device

The use of EVT in the posterior circulation has not been as vigorously studied. The BEST trial of endovascular treatment of acute vertebrobasilar occlusion was stopped due to slow recruitment and high crossover rate.[64] The Registry on Revascularization in Ischemic Stroke Patients (REVASK) study suggested that mechanical thrombectomy in posterior circulation stroke showed a lower risk of hemorrhage and similar effectiveness compared with anterior circulation.[65] The AHA guidelines suggest level C evidence for causative occlusions of the vertebral artery, basilar artery, or posterior circulation artery.[23] Choosing patients for posterior circulation thrombectomy should be done cautiously and in clinical situations where there is a salvageable penumbra.

Reperfusion routinely is scored with the modified thrombolysis in cerebral infarction grading scale: 0 indicating complete occlusion and 3 indicating complete reperfusion.[66] Grade 2b was shown to be the best cutoff for predicting favorable outcomes at 90 days, so grades 2b, 2c, and 3 are considered successful reperfusion.[67] A large meta-analysis of multiple clinical trials showed that increasing time from admission or first imaging to groin puncture was associated with decreases in rates of successful reperfusion.[68]

Delay in thrombectomy, as shown in the HERMES collaboration, suggested that the likelihood of achieving reperfusion decreases with prolonged admission-to-groin intervals, approximately by 2% per hour.[68,69] Prolonged admission-to-groin intervals results in worse patient outcomes and reducing that time can be a source of improvement of care.[69]

Post-Therapy Care—First 24 Hours

BP elevations are common after stroke and are thought to be a consequence of both neurohumoral activity and a reactive response to ischemia that serves to enhance cerebral perfusion.[70] Within the first hours to days after stroke, there is a natural decline in BP.[70] Current guidelines recommend a BP of less than 180/105 mm Hg for at least 24 hours after EVT but acknowledge that there is a lack of randomized trials on this aspect of management.[71] After successful reperfusion, lower BP targets may be warranted and 1 study showed that noninvasive determination of personalized BP thresholds for stroke patients is feasible.[71] Moreover, deviation from these limits can result in increased risk of further brain injury and poor functional outcome.[71]

Post-tPA and thrombectomy patients need to be monitored closely. For the first hours following treatment, neurovascular checks should be done every 15 minutes. Over the next 6 hours, neurologic checks should be done every 30 minutes and then further liberalized to every hour from 8 hours to 24 hours to monitor for complications to therapy. In many institutions, this level of checks designates an ICU level of care though recent literature, as discussed previously, suggests that many patients may be able to be monitored in a less intense setting, such as an intermediate care unit.[47] With any change in examination or clinical worsening, patients immediately should be evaluated and neuroimaging should be pursued to rule out an ICH.

Following treatment, patients should remain nothing by mouth until dysphagia screening is done and patients prove their ability to safely swallow. In patients receiving IV thrombolysis, deep vein thrombosis prevention should be started immediately upon arrival to the stroke or neurocritical care unit using serial compression devices. Venous thromboembolic pharmacoprophylaxis should wait until 24 hours after tPA with confirmation of lack of significant hemorrhagic transformation.[23] Reperfusion injury and reperfusion edema may reduce the benefit of thrombectomy and necessitates careful selection of patients.[72] Successful reperfusion is associated with reduced mass effect as measured by midline shift.[72]

Future Areas of Study

Further advances in imaging, therapeutic options, and improved preventive care can result in improved outcomes for patients with AIS. Improved perfusion scan techniques as well as new higher-resolution imaging modalities may result in further care improvements. Low-field portable MRI has been shown feasible in a single-center study of patients with critical illness and could be used to help improve stroke care in the future.[73]

Cerebral ischemia–induced cell death activates the immune system and initiates inflammation with early-phase changes exacerbating neurovascular dysfunction by promoting thrombus formation and accumulation of blood components in the cerebral microvasculature.[74,75] As a result of these changes, there is further neural cell death in the penumbra, resulting in extension of infarct, making this inflammatory response an attractive therapeutic target.[76,77] Fingolimod, a medication used in multiple sclerosis, when given with alteplase, showed in a small clinical trial to result in improved clinical outcomes at 24 hours and favorable shift in mRS distribution at day 90.[76] This needs to be further studied, however, in large patient groups.

SUMMARY

AIS is a disease process associated with significant morbidity and mortality. Timely treatment is critical for good clinical outcomes and limited damage to the brain. Significant strides have been made over the past decades to optimize stroke care and provide new therapeutic options. Clinical trials continue and further research progresses forward with the hopes for continuing on current advances.

CLINICS CARE POINTS

- Patients with acute-onset neurologic symptoms should be evaluated as rapidly as possible to enable timely diagnosis and therapy.
- Rapid imaging should be done to rule out ICH prior to treatment with thrombolysis or thrombectomy in patients who meet the criteria.
- Common stroke mimics, such as migraine, seizure, and toxic-metabolic causes, should be considered when evaluating a patient with acute-onset neurologic symptoms.

DISCLOSURE

Dr. Sheth received funding from the NIH (U24NS107215, U24NS107136, U01NS106513, RO1NR018335, R03NS112859, R01NS110721) and AHA (17CSA33550004). Dr. Zubair has nothing to disclose.

REFERENCES

1. Kamel H, Healey JS. Cardioembolic Stroke. Circ Res 2017;120(3):514–26.
2. Krishnamurthi RV, Feigin VL, Forouzanfar MH, et al. Global and regional burden of first-ever ischaemic and haemorrhagic stroke during 1990-2010: findings from the Global Burden of Disease Study 2010. Lancet Glob Health 2013;1(5): e259–81.
3. Adams HP Jr, Bendixen BH, Kappelle LJ, et al. Classification of subtype of acute ischemic stroke. Definitions for use in a multicenter clinical trial. TOAST. Trial of Org 10172 in Acute Stroke Treatment. Stroke 1993;24(1):35–41.

4. Price CI, Shaw L, Islam S, et al. Effect of an enhanced paramedic acute stroke treatment assessment on thrombolysis delivery during emergency stroke care: a cluster randomized clinical trial. JAMA Neurol 2020;77(7):840–8.

5. Wojner-Alexandrov AW, Alexandrov AV, Rodriguez D, et al. Houston paramedic and emergency stroke treatment and outcomes study (HoPSTO). Stroke 2005; 36(7):1512–8.

6. Berglund A, Svensson L, Sjöstrand C, et al. Higher prehospital priority level of stroke improves thrombolysis frequency and time to stroke unit: the Hyper Acute STroke Alarm (HASTA) study. Stroke 2012;43(10):2666–70.

7. Oostema JA, Chassee T, Baer W, et al. Brief Educational Intervention Improves Emergency Medical Services Stroke Recognition. Stroke 2019;50(5):1193–200.

8. Baldereschi M, Piccardi B, Di Carlo A, et al. Relevance of prehospital stroke code activation for acute treatment measures in stroke care: a review. Cerebrovasc Dis 2012;34(3):182–90.

9. Lima FO, Mont'Alverne FJA, Bandeira D, et al. Pre-hospital Assessment of Large Vessel Occlusion Strokes: Implications for Modeling and Planning Stroke Systems of Care. Front Neurol 2019;10:955.

10. Nguyen TTM, van den Wijngaard IR, Bosch J, et al. Comparison of Prehospital Scales for Predicting Large Anterior Vessel Occlusion in the Ambulance Setting. JAMA Neurol 2020;78(2):157–64.

11. Katz BS, McMullan JT, Sucharew H, et al. Design and validation of a prehospital scale to predict stroke severity: Cincinnati Prehospital Stroke Severity Scale. Stroke 2015;46(6):1508–12.

12. Nazliel B, Starkman S, Liebeskind DS, et al. A brief prehospital stroke severity scale identifies ischemic stroke patients harboring persisting large arterial occlusions. Stroke 2008;39(8):2264–7.

13. Pérez de la Ossa N, Carrera D, Gorchs M, et al. Design and validation of a prehospital stroke scale to predict large arterial occlusion: the rapid arterial occlusion evaluation scale. Stroke 2014;45(1):87–91.

14. Josephson SA, Kamel H. The acute stroke care revolution: enhancing access to therapeutic advances. JAMA 2018;320(12):1239–40.

15. Sheth KN, Smith EE, Grau-Sepulveda MV, et al. Drip and ship thrombolytic therapy for acute ischemic stroke: use, temporal trends, and outcomes. Stroke 2015; 46(3):732–9.

16. George BP, Doyle SJ, Albert GP, et al. Interfacility transfers for US ischemic stroke and TIA, 2006-2014. Neurology 2018;90(18):e1561–9.

17. Kansagra AP, Wallace AN, Curfman DR, et al. Streamlined triage and transfer protocols improve door-to-puncture time for endovascular thrombectomy in acute ischemic stroke. Clin Neurol Neurosurg 2018;166:71–5.

18. Ismail M, Armoiry X, Tau N, et al. Mothership versus drip and ship for thrombectomy in patients who had an acute stroke: a systematic review and meta-analysis. J Neurointerv Surg 2019;11(1):14–9.

19. Lachance CC, Ford C. Portable stroke detection devices for patients with stroke symptoms: a review of diagnostic accuracy and cost-effectiveness. Ottawa ON: © 2019 Canadian Agency for Drugs and Technologies in Health; 2019.

20. Ebinger M, Kunz A, Wendt M, et al. Effects of golden hour thrombolysis: a Prehospital Acute Neurological Treatment and Optimization of Medical Care in Stroke (PHANTOM-S) substudy. JAMA Neurol 2015;72(1):25–30.

21. Walter S, Kostopoulos P, Haass A, et al. Diagnosis and treatment of patients with stroke in a mobile stroke unit versus in hospital: a randomised controlled trial. Lancet Neurol 2012;11(5):397–404.

22. Czap AL, Singh N, Bowry R, et al. Mobile stroke unit computed tomography angiography substantially shortens door-to-puncture time. Stroke 2020;51(5):1613–5.

23. Powers WJ, Rabinstein AA, Ackerson T, et al. 2018 Guidelines for the Early Management of Patients With Acute Ischemic Stroke: A Guideline for Healthcare Professionals From the American Heart Association/American Stroke Association. Stroke 2018;49(3):e46–110.

24. Kamal N, Sheng S, Xian Y, et al. Delays in door-to-needle times and their impact on treatment time and outcomes in get with the guidelines-stroke. Stroke 2017; 48(4):946–54.

25. Hosseininezhad M, Sohrabnejad R. Stroke mimics in patients with clinical signs of stroke. Caspian J Intern Med 2017;8(3):213–6.

26. Ali-Ahmed F, Federspiel JJ, Liang L, et al. Intravenous tissue plasminogen activator in stroke mimics. Circ Cardiovasc Qual Outcomes 2019;12(8):e005609.

27. Chernyshev OY, Martin-Schild S, Albright KC, et al. Safety of tPA in stroke mimics and neuroimaging-negative cerebral ischemia. Neurology 2010;74(17):1340–5.

28. El-Koussy M, Schroth G, Brekenfeld C, et al. Imaging of acute ischemic stroke. Eur Neurol 2014;72(5–6):309–16.

29. Unger E, Littlefield J, Gado M. Water content and water structure in CT and MR signal changes: possible influence in detection of early stroke. AJNR Am J Neuroradiol 1988;9(4):687–91.

30. Tissue plasminogen activator for acute ischemic stroke. N Engl J Med 1995; 333(24):1581–7.

31. Barber PA, Demchuk AM, Zhang J, et al. Validity and reliability of a quantitative computed tomography score in predicting outcome of hyperacute stroke before thrombolytic therapy. ASPECTS Study Group. Alberta Stroke Programme Early CT Score. Lancet 2000;355(9216):1670–4.

32. Pexman JH, Barber PA, Hill MD, et al. Use of the Alberta Stroke Program Early CT Score (ASPECTS) for assessing CT scans in patients with acute stroke. AJNR Am J Neuroradiol 2001;22(8):1534–42.

33. Lövblad KO, Baird AE, Schlaug G, et al. Ischemic lesion volumes in acute stroke by diffusion-weighted magnetic resonance imaging correlate with clinical outcome. Ann Neurol 1997;42(2):164–70.

34. Hjort N, Christensen S, Sølling C, et al. Ischemic injury detected by diffusion imaging 11 minutes after stroke. Ann Neurol 2005;58(3):462–5.

35. Barber PA, Darby DG, Desmond PM, et al. Identification of major ischemic change. Diffusion-weighted imaging versus computed tomography. Stroke 1999;30(10):2059–65.

36. von Kummer R, Weber J. Brain and vascular imaging in acute ischemic stroke: the potential of computed tomography. Neurology 1997;49(5 Suppl 4):S52–5.

37. Riedel CH, Zimmermann P, Jensen-Kondering U, et al. The importance of size: successful recanalization by intravenous thrombolysis in acute anterior stroke depends on thrombus length. Stroke 2011;42(6):1775–7.

38. Knash M, Tsang A, Hameed B, et al. Low cerebral blood volume is predictive of diffusion restriction only in hyperacute stroke. Stroke 2010;41(12):2795–800.

39. Lansberg MG, Straka M, Kemp S, et al. MRI profile and response to endovascular reperfusion after stroke (DEFUSE 2): a prospective cohort study. Lancet Neurol 2012;11(10):860–7.

40. Kane I, Carpenter T, Chappell F, et al. Comparison of 10 different magnetic resonance perfusion imaging processing methods in acute ischemic stroke: effect on lesion size, proportion of patients with diffusion/perfusion mismatch, clinical scores, and radiologic outcomes. Stroke 2007;38(12):3158–64.

41. Emberson J, Lees KR, Lyden P, et al. Effect of treatment delay, age, and stroke severity on the effects of intravenous thrombolysis with alteplase for acute ischaemic stroke: a meta-analysis of individual patient data from randomised trials. Lancet 2014;384(9958):1929–35.
42. Marini C, Baldassarre M, Russo T, et al. Burden of first-ever ischemic stroke in the oldest old: evidence from a population-based study. Neurology 2004;62(1):77–81.
43. Sandercock P, Wardlaw JM, Lindley RI, et al. The benefits and harms of intravenous thrombolysis with recombinant tissue plasminogen activator within 6 h of acute ischaemic stroke (the third international stroke trial [IST-3]): a randomised controlled trial. Lancet 2012;379(9834):2352–63.
44. Mishra NK, Ahmed N, Andersen G, et al. Thrombolysis in very elderly people: controlled comparison of SITS International Stroke Thrombolysis Registry and Virtual International Stroke Trials Archive. BMJ 2010;341:c6046.
45. Weber R, Eyding J, Kitzrow M, et al. Distribution and evolution of acute interventional ischemic stroke treatment in Germany from 2010 to 2016. Neurol Res Pract 2019;1(1):4.
46. Ahmed N, Audebert H, Turc G, et al. Consensus statements and recommendations from the ESO-Karolinska Stroke Update Conference, Stockholm 11-13 November 2018. Eur Stroke J 2019;4(4):307–17.
47. Sadaka F, Jadhav A, O'Brien J, et al. Do all acute stroke patients receiving tPA Require ICU Admission? J Clin Med Res 2018;10(3):174–7.
48. Hill MD, Buchan AM. Thrombolysis for acute ischemic stroke: results of the Canadian Alteplase for Stroke Effectiveness Study. CMAJ 2005;172(10):1307–12.
49. Myslimi F, Caparros F, Dequatre-Ponchelle N, et al. Orolingual angioedema during or after thrombolysis for cerebral ischemia. Stroke 2016;47(7):1825–30.
50. Madden B, Chebl RB. Hemi orolingual angioedema after tPA administration for acute ischemic stroke. West J Emerg Med 2015;16(1):175–7.
51. Tanswell P, Modi N, Combs D, et al. Pharmacokinetics and pharmacodynamics of tenecteplase in fibrinolytic therapy of acute myocardial infarction. Clin Pharmacokinet 2002;41(15):1229–45.
52. Burgos AM, Saver JL. Evidence that tenecteplase is noninferior to alteplase for acute ischemic stroke: meta-analysis of 5 randomized trials. Stroke 2019;50(8):2156–62.
53. Parsons M, Spratt N, Bivard A, et al. A randomized trial of tenecteplase versus alteplase for acute ischemic stroke. N Engl J Med 2012;366(12):1099–107.
54. Campbell BCV, Mitchell PJ, Churilov L, et al. Tenecteplase versus alteplase before thrombectomy for ischemic stroke. N Engl J Med 2018;378(17):1573–82.
55. Berkhemer OA, Fransen PS, Beumer D, et al. A randomized trial of intraarterial treatment for acute ischemic stroke. N Engl J Med 2015;372(1):11–20.
56. Goyal M, Menon BK, van Zwam WH, et al. Endovascular thrombectomy after large-vessel ischaemic stroke: a meta-analysis of individual patient data from five randomised trials. Lancet 2016;387(10029):1723–31.
57. Goyal M, Demchuk AM, Menon BK, et al. Randomized assessment of rapid endovascular treatment of ischemic stroke. N Engl J Med 2015;372(11):1019–30.
58. Saver JL, Goyal M, Bonafe A, et al. Stent-retriever thrombectomy after intravenous t-PA vs. t-PA alone in stroke. N Engl J Med 2015;372(24):2285–95.
59. Campbell BC, Mitchell PJ, Kleinig TJ, et al. Endovascular therapy for ischemic stroke with perfusion-imaging selection. N Engl J Med 2015;372(11):1009–18.
60. Jovin TG, Chamorro A, Cobo E, et al. Thrombectomy within 8 hours after symptom onset in ischemic stroke. N Engl J Med 2015;372(24):2296–306.

61. Albers GW, Marks MP, Kemp S, et al. Thrombectomy for Stroke at 6 to 16 Hours with Selection by Perfusion Imaging. N Engl J Med 2018;378(8):708–18.

62. Nogueira RG, Jadhav AP, Haussen DC, et al. Thrombectomy 6 to 24 Hours after Stroke with a Mismatch between Deficit and Infarct. N Engl J Med 2018;378(1): 11–21.

63. Goldhoorn RB, van de Graaf RA, van Rees JM, et al. Endovascular treatment for acute ischemic stroke in patients on oral anticoagulants: results from the MR CLEAN registry. Stroke 2020;51(6):1781–9.

64. Liu X, Dai Q, Ye R, et al. Endovascular treatment versus standard medical treatment for vertebrobasilar artery occlusion (BEST): an open-label, randomised controlled trial. Lancet Neurol 2020;19(2):115–22.

65. Weber R, Minnerup J, Nordmeyer H, et al. Thrombectomy in posterior circulation stroke: differences in procedures and outcome compared to anterior circulation stroke in the prospective multicentre REVASK registry. Eur J Neurol 2019;26(2): 299–305.

66. Higashida RT, Furlan AJ, Roberts H, et al. Trial design and reporting standards for intra-arterial cerebral thrombolysis for acute ischemic stroke. Stroke 2003;34(8): e109–37.

67. Yoo AJ, Simonsen CZ, Prabhakaran S, et al. Refining angiographic biomarkers of revascularization: improving outcome prediction after intra-arterial therapy. Stroke 2013;44(9):2509–12.

68. Bourcier R, Goyal M, Liebeskind DS, et al. Association of time from stroke onset to groin puncture with quality of reperfusion after mechanical thrombectomy: a meta-analysis of individual patient data from 7 randomized clinical trials. JAMA Neurol 2019;76(4):405–11.

69. Kaesmacher J, Maamari B, Meinel TR, et al. Effect of pre- and in-hospital delay on reperfusion in acute ischemic stroke mechanical thrombectomy. Stroke 2020; 51(10):2934–42.

70. Petersen NH, Kodali S, Sheth KN. Towards individualized blood pressure management after stroke. Am J Hypertens 2019;32(3):242–4.

71. Petersen NH, Silverman A, Strander SM, et al. Fixed compared with autoregulation-oriented blood pressure thresholds after mechanical thrombectomy for ischemic stroke. Stroke 2020;51(3):914–21.

72. Kimberly WT, Dutra BG, Boers AMM, et al. Association of reperfusion with brain edema in patients with acute ischemic stroke: a secondary analysis of the MR CLEAN trial. JAMA Neurol 2018;75(4):453–61.

73. Sheth KN, Mazurek MH, Yuen MM, et al. Assessment of brain injury using portable, low-field magnetic resonance imaging at the bedside of critically ill patients. JAMA Neurol 2020. https://doi.org/10.1001/jamaneurol.2020.3263.

74. Liu Q, Jin WN, Liu Y, et al. Brain ischemia suppresses immunity in the periphery and brain via different neurogenic innervations. Immunity 2017;46(3):474–87.

75. Fu Y, Liu Q, Anrather J, et al. Immune interventions in stroke. Nat Rev Neurol 2015;11(9):524–35.

76. Tian DC, Shi K, Zhu Z, et al. Fingolimod enhances the efficacy of delayed alteplase administration in acute ischemic stroke by promoting anterograde reperfusion and retrograde collateral flow. Ann Neurol 2018;84(5):717–28.

77. Kraft P, Göb E, Schuhmann MK, et al. FTY720 ameliorates acute ischemic stroke in mice by reducing thrombo-inflammation but not by direct neuroprotection. Stroke 2013;44(11):3202–10.

Intracerebral Hemorrhage
Advances in Emergency Care

Carlos S. Kase, MD[a],*, Daniel F. Hanley, MD[b],1

KEYWORDS

- Intracerebral hemorrhage • Hematoma expansion • Blood pressure control
- Surgical evacuation

KEY POINTS

- Intracerebral hemorrhage has a mortality of 40% at 1 month, and most survivors have severe disability.
- Hematoma expansion occurs in up to 40% of patients in the first hours after intracerebral hemorrhage onset, and is associated with neurologic deterioration and poor outcome.
- Control of severe hypertension after intracerebral hemorrhage onset is associated with improved outcomes, but specific blood pressure targets have not been defined.
- Platelet transfusions, procoagulant factors, and iron-chelating agents have not been shown to improve outcomes in patients with intracerebral hemorrhage.
- Conventional hematoma drainage by craniotomy does not improve outcomes in patients with intracerebral hemorrhage, but minimally invasive surgery with local thrombolysis is a potentially valuable approach that deserves further evaluation.

Intracerebral hemorrhage (ICH) has a mortality rate of about 40% at 1 month, and 61% to 88% of survivors have high degrees of residual disability.[1] Despite its severity, ICH has fewer scientifically tested therapies than all other stroke subtypes. The initial clinical course and eventual prognosis are dependent on several factors, including age, hematoma volume and location, level of consciousness, associated intraventricular hemorrhage (IVH), and use of anticoagulants before presentation.[2,3]

A major factor that determines the early course of ICH is the dynamic character of the hematoma, which frequently expands in the initial hours after onset: Kazui and colleagues[4] documented hematoma expansion in 36% of 204 patients within 3 hours of onset, and Brott and colleagues[5] showed hematoma expansion in 26% of 103

a Department of Neurology, Emory University School of Medicine, Atlanta, GA, USA; b Division of Brain Injury Outcomes, Johns Hopkins University, Baltimore, MD, USA
1 Present Address: Johns Hopkins University Hospital, BIOS Division, 750 E. Pratt Street, 16th floor, Baltimore, MD 21202.
* Corresponding author. Emory Brain Health Center, 12 Executive Park NE, Atlanta, GA 30329, USA.
E-mail addresses: cskase@bu.edu; cskase@emory.edu

Neurol Clin 39 (2021) 405–418
https://doi.org/10.1016/j.ncl.2021.02.002
0733-8619/21/© 2021 Elsevier Inc. All rights reserved.
neurologic.theclinics.com

patients within 1 hour and in 38% within 20 hours from baseline. The event of hematoma expansion, which is often associated with early neurologic deterioration, has an imaging correlate in the "spot sign," which corresponds to the detection of an ongoing bleeding point within the hematoma on computed tomography angiography,[6–8] as depicted in **Fig. 1**. The identification of risk factors for hematoma expansion has been of interest, as potential determinants of type and intensity of care in the acute phase of ICH. Among the features at presentation with ICH, those independently associated with the probability of expansion were evaluated by Al-Shahi Salman and colleagues,[9] and included: time between symptom onset and baseline imaging (the shorter the interval, the higher the risk of hematoma expansion); volume of ICH in baseline imaging (the higher the ICH volume, the higher the risk of hematoma expansion), with a steep increase in the risk of expansion in hematomas of less than 25 mL volume; and antiplatelet and anticoagulant use at the time of presentation. The inclusion of a positive "spot sign" on computed tomography angiography added slightly to the predictive value of the other factors combined. Several clinical features investigated as potential predictors of hematoma expansion were not consistently associated with it, including sex, age, history of hypertension and diabetes, systolic blood pressure (BP) and blood glucose at presentation, and ICH location.[9]

The management in the acute phase of ICH includes several strategies, directed at decreasing the risk of hematoma expansion, minimizing the detrimental local effects of the blood products in the brain parenchyma, and enhancing hematoma resolution.

MEASURES AIMED AT DECREASING THE RISK OF HEMATOMA EXPANSION

Several measures have been tested for their ability to reduce early ICH growth, including lowering of BP, reversal of anticoagulant or fibrinolytic effect, restoration of platelet function, and use of procoagulant and antifibrinolytic agents.

Lowering of Blood Pressure

Two phase III randomized clinical trials, INTERACT2[10] and ATACH-2,[11] assessed the impact of BP reduction on the outcome of ICH, including its effect on hematoma expansion in the acute phase of the stroke. The trials had similar designs, aiming at

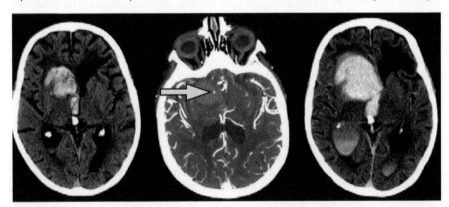

Fig. 1. Demonstration of the "spot sign" (*arrow*) in computed tomography angiography in intracerebral hemorrhage (*center*), along with expansion from volume of 19.6 mL at baseline (*left*) to 110.8 mL (*right*) after 24 hours. (*From* Demchuk et al.,[8] Prediction of haematoma growth and outcome in patients with intracerebral haemorrhage using the CT-angiography spot sign (PREDICT): a prospective observational study. From Lancet Neurol 2012;11:307-314, reprinted with permission.)

comparing two regimens of BP reduction, "intensive" (systolic BP <140 mm Hg) versus "guideline-recommended" (systolic BP <180 mm Hg) in INTERACT2, "intensive" (systolic BP 110–139 mm Hg) versus "standard" (systolic BP 140–179 mm Hg) in ATACH-2, with primary outcomes of modified Rankin Scale (mRS) of 3 to 6 and 4 to 6 (corresponding to death or major disability) at 90 days, respectively. Although both trials achieved the targeted BP reductions, there were no differences in the primary end point between the two levels of intensity of BP reduction in both trials, and a negative impact in renal function was the main adverse event in the intensive group in ATACH-2. In INTERACT2 there was a nonsignificant trend ($P = .06$) in favor of the intensive level of BP control, and a prespecified ordinal analysis of the mRS favored the intensive group, which showed significantly ($P = .04$) lower mRS scores than the guideline-recommended group. The effect on hematoma expansion between baseline and 24 hours in INTERACT2 was evaluated in a subgroup (about one-third) of subjects in each group, with mean baseline hematoma volumes of about 15 mL in both groups, with growth to 18.2 mL in the intensive group and 20.6 mL in the guideline-recommended group, a relative difference of 4.5% and absolute difference of 1.4 mL, which were nonsignificant ($P = .18$). In ATACH-2 the primary end point was reached by 38.7% in the intensive group, and 37.7% in the standard group, a nonsignificant difference ($P = .08$), and the analysis of hematoma expansion between baseline and 24 hours favored the intensive BP control group, with hematoma expansion in 18.9%, versus 24.4% in the standard group, but the difference was not significant ($P = .08$).

These data from two randomized clinical trials did not provide a rationale for specific BP targets in the acute phase of ICH, although INTERACT2 suggested on one hand the safety of the intensive level of systolic BP less than 140 mm Hg, along with possible signal of benefit as measured by the ordinal analysis of the mRS score at 90 days. In ATACH-2, the potential harm of systolic BP reductions was apparent for levels of systolic BP as low as 110 mm Hg. To determine the potential risks of various levels of BP reduction in the acute phase of ICH, Buletko and colleagues[12] conducted an observational study in a single institution to assess the risk of brain ischemic events among patients with ICH treated with a previous institutional protocol of lowering systolic BP less than 160 mm Hg (Group 1), in comparison with an updated institutional protocol of lowering the systolic BP less than 140 mm Hg (Group 2). Acute ischemic events on MRI and neurologic deterioration were more frequent in Group 2 (32% vs 16% [$P = .047$] and 19% vs 5% [$P = .022$], respectively), and all ischemic events occurred in patients who had a minimum systolic BP of less than 130 mm Hg. Although this observational study from a single institution cannot be used as a therapeutic guide, it provides, along with some of the safety data from the randomized trials, potentially useful information for the care of patients with ICH and hypertension, suggesting that systolic BP values of 130 to 140 mm Hg are a safe target, as long as special caution is taken in avoiding minimal systolic BP values less than 130 mm Hg.

Reversal of Anticoagulant or Fibrinolytic Effect

ICH in patients receiving oral anticoagulants is associated with hematomas at high risk of expansion, and high mortality.[13–15] These effects are similar with the use of either warfarin or direct oral anticoagulants (DOACs).[16] The mainstay in the treatment of acute anticoagulant-related ICH is emergency reversal of the coagulopathy, in an attempt at minimizing hematoma expansion. This requires reversal agents that are readily available, rapidly effective, and associated with minimal untoward side effects. In the case of warfarin-associated ICH with elevated international normalized ratio (INR), following the initial use of 10 mg of intravenous (IV) vitamin K, the reversal agent with the best profile is prothrombin complex concentrate (PCC), which contains the vitamin K–dependent coagulation factors II, VII, IX, and X (thus called "four factor" PCC), and the procoagulant proteins C and S. This agent produces a rapid correction of the elevated INR after infusion of small volumes of fluids, thus avoiding the risk of volume overload related to the large-volume infusions required by the alternative treatment, fresh frozen plasma (FFP). A comparison of these two reversal agents in the randomized INCH[17] trial showed superiority of PCC over FFP, because the former normalized the INR at a significantly faster rate, with superior effectiveness in reducing hematoma expansion. The outcome correlates of reduced hematoma expansion suggested a trend toward improved functional status of 90-day survivors, without differences in mortality. A meta-analysis that included 2606 subjects showed evidence of reduced all-cause mortality at 90 days in favor of subjects receiving PCC.[18] Kuramatsu and colleagues[19] showed that the combination of INR reversal to less than 1.3 plus reduction of systolic BP to less than 160 mm Hg within 4 hours of admission resulted in the lowest rates of hematoma enlargement.

In instances of ICH related to use of DOACs, the limited available data on baseline hematoma volume, frequency of expansion, and outcome suggest similar profiles to those of patients with warfarin-related ICH.[16,20,21] Data from two prospective registries in Germany[20,21] showed hematoma expansion in about one-third of subjects, new development of IVH in 18% and 41%, respectively, 90-day mortalities of 28% and 29.5%, respectively, and death or severe disability in two-thirds of the subjects in both studies. Despite high frequency of treatment with PCC, in 57% and 64% of cases, respectively, there was no benefit of this agent in terms of hematoma expansion or unfavorable outcome. In the study by Gerner and coworkers[21] there was a beneficial effect of BP control (<160 mm Hg at 4 hours) with regard to hematoma expansion. These data highlight the severity and poor outcome of ICH in subjects treated with DOACs, in addition showing no benefit of anticoagulation reversal by PCC, suggesting the potential value of alternative treatments, such as antidote-mediated neutralization of anticoagulation. Recently developed antidotes for DOACs include idarucizumab for the thrombin inhibitor dabigatran, and andexanet alpha for the factor X inhibitors apixaban, rivaroxaban, and edoxaban. These agents rapidly neutralize the DOAC effect and reverse the coagulopathy, as measured with the diluted thrombin time for dabigatran, and anti–factor X assays for apixaban, rivaroxaban, and edoxaban.[22] Anticoagulation reversal with these antidotes is recommended in patients with bleeding complications and drug concentration greater than 50 ng/mL, and for those requiring urgent intervention with high risk of bleeding at drug concentration greater than 30 ng/mL.[23] Their dosages and modes of administration are shown in **Table 1**.[15,24]

The complication of ICH after thrombolysis for acute ischemic stroke with tissue plasminogen activator occurs in about 2% to 7% of subjects,[25] usually within 12 hours from tissue plasminogen activator infusion, and is associated with hypofibrinogenemia. The recommended therapy is with 10 U of cryoprecipitate, which is administered until blood fibrinogen reaches greater than 150 mg/dL.[26] If cryoprecipitate is not available, the use of antifibrinolytic agents, such as aminocaproic acid or tranexamic acid, is considered; these agents are associated with thrombotic complications.[15] Other measures that are considered, although their benefit is unclear, include platelet transfusions (only recommended for thrombocytopenia of <100,000 platelets), FFP, PCC, vitamin K, and recombinant activated factor VII (rFVIIa).[26]

Restoration of Platelet Function

The data on the effect of prior treatment with antiplatelet agents on the expansion and progression of ICH have been inconsistent.[27,28] As a result there is controversy about

Table 1
Reversal of anticoagulation for DOAC-related ICH[a]

	Dabigatran	Rivaroxaban, Apixaban, Edoxaban
Reversal agent	Idarucizumab	Andexanet alpha[b]
Dose	5 g IV in 2 doses of 2.5 g	800 mg IV bolus over 15–30 min followed by 960 mg in 2-h infusion if last dose <8 h 400 mg IV bolus over 15–30 min followed by 480 mg in 2-h infusion if last dose ≥8 h
Alternative therapies if reversal agent not available	4-factor PCC, 25–50 U/kg Activated charcoal,[c] 50 g Hemodialysis[e]	4-factor PCC, 25–50 U/kg Activated charcoal,[d] 50 g
Concomitant measures	Systolic BP <140 mm Hg	Systolic BP <140 mm Hg

[a] Modified from Morotti A, Goldstein JN. Anticoagulant-associated intracerebral hemorrhage. Brain Hemorrhages 2020;1:89-94,[15] and Sweidan AJ, Singh NK, Conovaloff JL, et al. Coagulopathy reversal in intracerebral hemorrhage. Stroke & Vascular Neurology 2020;5:e000274.[24]
[b] Food and Drug Administration approved only for apixaban and rivaroxaban.
[c] Recommended if last intake of dabigatran was in the preceding 2 hours.
[d] Recommended if last dose was in the preceding 6-8 hours for rivaroxaban, in the preceding 6 hours for apixaban, in the preceding 2 hours for edoxaban.
[e] Recommended for patients with dabigatran overdose, renal failure.

the value of platelet transfusions in the setting of acute ICH. This issue was addressed in a randomized, phase III, multicenter trial (PATCH),[29] in which subjects previously taking antiplatelet agents who presented with ICH within 6 hours of symptom onset were randomly allocated to standard care versus platelet transfusions within 90 minutes of the imaging diagnosis of ICH. The primary end point was a shift toward death or dependence on the mRS at 3 months, and secondary end points included survival at 3 months and hematoma expansion. The results documented a detrimental effect of platelet transfusions, which were associated with a significantly ($P = .0114$) higher rate of death and dependence at 3 months, and higher frequency of serious adverse events (42% vs 29%), without differences in survival (68% vs 77%) or hematoma expansion (2.01 vs 1.16 mL) at 24 hours from treatment. These data suggest lack of benefit and potential harm from platelet transfusions in the setting of ICH in patients previously treated with antiplatelet agents. Some authors recommend consideration of platelet transfusion in patients with ICH before undergoing neurosurgical intervention.[30]

Use of Procoagulant and Antifibrinolytic Agents

The procoagulant rFVIIa at pharmacologic doses is effective for controlling bleeding at the site of vascular injury by activating factor X on the surface of activated platelets, resulting in a thrombin "burst," which leads to the formation of a stable hemostatic plug.[31] This agent was tested against placebo for its ability to control hematoma expansion in patients with ICH treated within 4 hours from onset in a phase II trial.[32] The rFVIIa arm included doses of 40, 80, and 160 µg/kg, which resulted in a mean increase of hematoma volume (measured at 24 hours) of 16%, 14%, and 11%, respectively, compared with 29% in the placebo group ($P = .01$). Mortality at 90 days was 18% in the rFVIIa group and 29% in the placebo group ($P = .02$). These results led to a phase III trial (FAST),[33] which compared doses of 20 and 80 µg/kg of rFVIIa given within 4 hours of ICH onset against placebo, with the primary efficacy end point of death and severe disability (mRS = 5–6) at 90 days. Although rFVIIa again significantly reduced the degree of hematoma expansion in comparison with placebo (11% for the 80 μg/kg dose; 26% in placebo), the primary efficacy end point showed no differences between the groups, with mRS of 5 to 6 at 90 days in 26% in the rFVIIa 20 μg/kg dose, 30% for the 80 μg/kg dose, and 24% for placebo, along with a significant (P = .04) increase in the rate of arterial thrombotic events in the 80 μg/kg rFVIIa group (9%) as compared with placebo (4%). These results suggested that the potential benefit of rFVIIa with regard to hematoma expansion should be tested in selected groups of patients with ICH at highest risk of hematoma expansion, such as those with the "spot sign," which is associated with high risk of in-hospital mortality and poor outcome in survivors.[34] The SPOTLIGHT (Spot Sign Selection of Intracerebral Hemorrhage to Guide Hemostatic Therapy) and the STOP-IT (The Spot Sign for Predicting and Treating ICH Growth Study) trials tested rFVIIa against placebo in the acute phase of ICH. Because these trials occurred in parallel, in Canada and in the United States, respectively, and used similar protocols, their results were jointly reported.[35] All patients enrolled (n = 69) had "spot sign"–positive ICHs of volumes around 10 mL, with randomization to either rFVIIa (n = 32) at a dose of 80 μg/kg, or placebo (n = 37) via single intravenous bolus within 6.5 hours from onset. The primary outcome was ICH volume expansion measured on computed tomography scan as the difference between the baseline and the 24-hour volume, and the clinical outcome was the proportion of patients with mRS score of 5 to 6 at 90 days. The studies were terminated before achieving the target enrollment of 106 patients. The main results included a low magnitude of hematoma expansion after 24 hours from the baseline computed tomography in both groups, amounting to a median of 2.5 mL in the rFVIIa group and 2.6 mL in the placebo group (P = .89). The clinical outcomes were equally nonsignificant, with mRS scores of 5 to 6 in 30% of the rFVIIa group and 38% in the placebo group (P = .60), with 90-day mortality of 20% and 21% (P = .98), respectively. This neutral clinical trial included a small number of subjects with small ICHs who were treated at a median of approximately 3 (interquartile range, 2–4.5) hours from stroke onset, and who had ICH expansion of small magnitude in both groups. Although the rFVIIa effect was not different from placebo in the overall group, an exploratory analysis of the ICH expansion data on the subgroup of patients treated within 3 hours from onset (n = 9 with rFVIIa; n = 24 with placebo) showed a median volume increase of only 0.9 mL in the rFVIIa group, and 4.3 mL in the placebo group. These data suggest that any further attempts at testing rFVIIa, and possibly other hemostatic agents, should be planned for early treatment windows, ideally with prehospital initiation of diagnostic and treatment protocols, to intervene at a more meaningful, early stage of evolution of the acute ICH. This is the purpose of the NINDS-sponsored phase 3 trial FASTEST (NCT 03496883), designed to test rFVIIa in patients with acute ICH treated within 2 hours of symptom onset.

The antifibrinolytic agent tranexamic acid is safe and effective in the management of traumatic and postpartum hemorrhage,[36,37] because it significantly decreases mortality. Its effect on acute ICH was tested in the Tranexamic acid for hyperacute primary IntraCerebral Haemorrhage (TICH-2) study, an international, randomized, placebo-controlled phase III trial.[38] Patients with ICH were allocated to either tranexamic acid (1 g IV bolus followed by 1 g IV infusion over 8 hours) or placebo within 8 hours of symptom onset. The primary outcome, functional status at 90 days, was measured by shift of the mRS, and secondary outcomes included rate of hematoma expansion, neurologic status at Day 7, and several functional and cognitive scales. The trial results showed no difference in functional status at Day 90, including mortality, despite a decrease in deaths by Day 7 in the tranexamic acid group (9%) compared with

11% in the placebo group (P = .0406). Additional observations in the tranexamic acid group included an interaction with systolic BP less than 170 mm Hg, a lower frequency of adverse events (including venous and arterial thromboembolism), and a reduced rate of hematoma expansion in comparison with placebo. In view of the favorable safety profile of tranexamic acid in the TICH-2 trial, along with evidence of benefit in patients with systemic hemorrhage when used within 3 hours from onset,[39] there are currently ongoing clinical trials in nontraumatic ICH using windows of 2 hours (STOP-MSU, NCT 03385928) and 3 hours (TRANSACT, NCT 03044184).

MEASURES AIMED AT MINIMIZING THE LOCAL EFFECTS OF THE HEMATOMA IN THE BRAIN PARENCHYMA

ICH is associated with surrounding edema and mass effect. The pathogenesis of perihematoma edema is complex, and it includes: initial clot retraction with resulting extrusion of serum at its periphery; a more delayed effect on the blood-brain barrier by thrombin formation; and toxicity from hemoglobin products, especially iron, which contribute to delayed neuronal loss via inflammation and direct cell toxicity.[40] Despite limited supportive data from clinical trials, the mass effect with potential for herniation that results from the ICH with perihematoma edema is managed with short-term use of hyperventilation, mannitol, or hypertonic saline infusions as a way of quickly decreasing intracranial pressure and avoiding/reversing herniation.[41] Other measures that have been tested include iron chelation to reduce its local toxicity, and anti-inflammatory agents aimed at reducing delayed cell death and edema in the perihematoma region.

Iron Chelation

The accumulation of iron that follows red blood cell lysis in the perihematoma region leads to secondary neuronal injury via apoptosis, oxidative stress, inflammation, and autophagy.[42] Iron chelation with deferoxamine mesylate showed imaging and clinical benefits in animal models of ICH,[43] and a pilot study in humans suggested safety of this agent in ICH.[44] These data supported a phase 2, multicenter, randomized, placebo-controlled clinical trial (i-DEF)[45] that tested a deferoxamine infusion of 32 mg/kg/d for 3 days against placebo, within 24 hours of ICH onset. The primary outcome measure was good clinical outcome (mRS = 0–2) at 90 days, which was similar in the two groups (34% for deferoxamine, 33% for placebo). In addition, mortality at 90 days was 7% in both groups, whereas serious adverse events were lower (27%) with deferoxamine than with placebo (33%), a nonsignificant difference. These results suggested futility for advancement to a phase 3 trial. An observed potential benefit for deferoxamine at 6 months raised the possibility of including this longer time for assessment of outcomes in future trials of ICH treatment, in view of data that suggest continuing improvement of patients with ICH up to 1 year from the event.[46]

Anti-inflammatory Agents

Based on the notion that inflammation in the perihematoma area promotes edema and cell death, Fu and colleagues[47] conducted a small (n = 23) proof-of-concept open-label, evaluator-blinded study of the anti-inflammatory immunemodulator fingolimod in patients with small to moderate size (about 15 mL) basal ganglia ICH. They treated 11 subjects with fingolimod (0.5 mg orally for 3 days) within 72 hours from ICH onset, and compared them with 12 control subjects managed with conventional measures for ICH. The clinical status was assessed with Glasgow Coma Score (GCS) and National Institutes of Health Stroke Scale scores, and functional status with mRS and the

Barthel index, all during hospitalization and after 90 days. The results showed a beneficial effect of fingolimod in clinical status at 7 days, and functional status at 90 days. There was also a significant reduction in perihematoma edema in the fingolimod group. These encouraging results justify large-scale studies of fingolimod or similar agents in the acute phase of ICH.

MEASURES AIMED AT ENHANCING HEMATOMA RESOLUTION

The surgical management in patients with ICH includes craniotomy, and a range of minimally invasive surgery (MIS) techniques. End-of-treatment clot volume has been associated with improved outcomes in multiple ICH trials. The mechanisms are currently undefined but may include relieving mass effect and limiting cellular toxicity from residual blood products.

Craniotomy

The University of Texas STICH hyperacute craniotomy trials raised the concern of clot removal-related brain tissue injury occurring after surgery in the first 4 hours after presentation.[48] Stabilization of BP became a more rigorously pursued clinical standard after these small trials. The first large randomized controlled or "pivotal" trial of surgery versus medical care was the Surgical Trial in Intracerebral Haemorrhage (STICH I).[49] It explored the question: "Does a management policy of early surgery in ICH benefit patients by producing improved long term functional outcome?" No difference in either mortality or functional performance as measured by the Glasgow Outcome Scale or the mRS was observed. Subgroup analyses showed that lobar hematomas located within 1 cm from the cortical surface, along with mid-range GCS baseline scores, demonstrated trends of benefit favoring craniotomy. Based on these observations STICH II was designed to test the value of craniotomy for superficial lobar hematomas without IVH.[50] This second trial showed no benefit of craniotomy in the first 24 hours when compared with medical management. Criticism of the trial included a substantial degree of difference in the frequency of craniotomy performed across centers, and a large number (approximately 20%) of crossovers from initially allocated medical care to surgical intervention. These issues may have impacted the ability of the STICH trials to fully address the potential benefits of routine craniotomy.

Minimally Invasive Surgery

The concept of MIS was developed because of the lack of clear benefit from traditional craniotomy and the potential that tissue manipulation promotes rebleeding and requires removal of or damage to tissues not directly involved by the ICH. Multiple similar techniques have evolved in Asia, Europe, and the United States with the greatest initial enthusiasm occurring in Japan, China, and Korea. As techniques have evolved, greater international interest has followed, particularly after the negative STICH trials. MIS has been compared with conventional craniotomy. Meta-analysis of MIS for ICH by Zhou and colleagues[51] included 12 randomized clinical trials and demonstrated that patients who underwent MIS had lower rates of death and functional dependence. These results suggest that a less invasive approach may improve outcomes. A more recent meta-analysis by Scaggiante and colleagues[52] included 15 MIS studies and 2152 patients. The cohort encompassed stereotactic thrombolysis and endoscopic procedures. This analysis demonstrated both interventions decreased the incidence of moderate to severe functional impairment and death at long-term follow-up; this occurred for comparisons with patients who underwent medical management alone or medical management and craniotomy.[52] MIS provides the potential of removing toxic blood products and limiting disruption of healthy brain tissue. The comparison with the operative events in craniotomy seems to account for the current enthusiasm among ICH specialists for MIS.

A US case series evaluated stereotactic aspiration assisted by local thrombolysis with alteplase.[53] This series demonstrated that hematoma volume and perihematomal edema were significantly reduced by MIS. This form of MIS intervention was explored in the randomized controlled trial Minimally Invasive Surgery Plus Alteplase for Intracerebral Hemorrhage Evacuation (MISTIE) II and III. The MISTIE II trial was an open-label phase II clinical trial.[54] The primary end point was a beneficial signal of 10% improved mRS 0 to 3 outcomes at 180 days. This functional improvement was found to be proportional to the amount of blood removed. The safety profile of MISTIE II was encouraging, with no difference in serious bleeding between medical and MIS groups. An increase in asymptomatic bleeding in the MIS group was noted. These findings became the predicate for the next trial, MISTIE III, which evaluated the MIS procedure's ability to reduce the hematoma to a final volume of less than 15 mL, and its correlation with good functional outcome as defined by the proportion of the study population reaching the mRS 0 to 3 status. The study concluded that good functional outcome at 365 days was not significantly different between groups.[55] A small, significant mortality difference favoring MIS was observed. A planned "per protocol

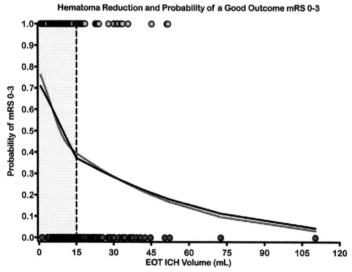

Fig. 2. Cubic spline regression analyses (*blue line*) and linear spline regression analyses (*black line*) showing the relationship of hematoma reduction (end-of-treatment [EOT] ICH volume) to the probability of having a good outcome of mRS 0–3 at 1 year. This is created by classifying dichotomized outcomes as 1 or 0 (*green dots* at 1 = mRS 0–3; *red dots* at 0 = mRS 4–6). Further reduction beyond the 15 mL threshold (odds ratio, 0.09; $P = .002$) increased the chance of having a good outcome by 10% for each additional milliliter of hematoma removed (*green shading* showing statistically significant area of curve). Volume reductions to greater than 15 mL threshold did not significantly impact the likelihood of achieving a good outcome. (*Reprinted from* Awad et al,[56] Surgical performance determines functional outcome benefit in the Minimally Invasive Surgery Plus Recombinant Tissue Plasminogen Activator for Intracerebral Hemorrhage Evacuation (MISTIE) procedure, From Neurosurgery 2019;84:1157–1168, with permission from the Congress of Neurological Surgeons.)

evaluation" of ICH end-of-treatment volume confirmed that clot volume reduction to the threshold of less than or equal to 15 mL correlated with a 10% differential benefit favoring MIS (**Fig. 2**).[56] Other minimally invasive procedures that involve increased manipulation of brain tissues seem to produce similar hematoma volume reductions as the MISTIE procedure,[57] but this has not been confirmed in large randomized clinical trials.

Functional benefit from MIS procedures in patients with ICH at 180 to 365 days will be required to recommend this approach. Current guidelines for surgical evacuation of ICH state that randomized controlled trials do not establish improved outcomes. The expert opinion leaders who author the guidelines write that surgery is considered a lifesaving measure for patients in coma with midline shift or with refractory elevated intracranial pressure.[58] A post hoc evaluation of MISTIE III data does not support this recommendation.[59] Moreover, based on STICH trial data, a policy of early hematoma evacuation does not seem to be beneficial compared with later hematoma evacuation when patients deteriorate. The American Heart Association guidelines do not currently provide recommendations for selecting candidates for surgery, although the European ICH guidelines, based on subgroup analysis, recommend early surgery for patients with a GCS score of 9 to 12.[60] Both guidelines state that MIS (endoscopic or stereotactic thrombolysis) is of uncertain benefit (class IIb, level of evidence B). The best time frame for initiating surgery has not been determined. A meta-analysis of MIS trials found no difference between surgery within 24 hours or within 72 hours.[52] Although another meta-analysis of craniotomy and MIS trials suggests a small benefit of earlier surgery,[61] this analysis does not find an influence of known severity factors, such as GCS, age, and ICH size, bringing the finding into question.[62] MISTIE and perhaps other mechanical extraction MIS techniques are surgical interventions for ICH that should undergo further rigorous clinical trial testing. There remains promise for minimally invasive approaches and the hope is that future trials will eventually clarify the role of these techniques in the acute management of ICH.

CLINICS CARE POINTS

- Control of severe hypertension is essential in the acute phase of intracerebral hemorrhage to control hematoma expansion
- Reversal of the coagulopathy paired with hypertension control improves the outcomes in patients with anticoagulant-related intracerebral hemorrhage
- Procoagulant agents in intracerebral hemorrhage reduce hematoma expansion, but without a concomitant benefit in clinical outcomes
- The iron-chelating agent deferoxamine did not improve functional outcomes in patients with intracerebral hemorrhage
- Conventional craniotomy does not improve outcomes in patients with intracerebral hemorrhage, including those with superficially located hematomas

DISCLOSURE

Dr C.S. Kase reports consulting fees from Bayer Pharmaceuticals and AbbVie Pharmaceuticals, both outside the subjects discussed in the article. Dr D.F. Hanley reports research funding from NIH and the US Department of Defense; personal fees for consulting from Neurotrope and Portola Pharmaceuticals; and medicolegal activities, all outside the submitted work.

REFERENCES

1. van Asch CJJ, Luitse MJA, Rinkel GJE, et al. Incidence, case fatality, and functional outcome of intracerebral hemorrhage over time, according to age, sex, and ethnic origin: a systematic review and meta-analysis. Lancet Neurol 2010; 9:167–76.

2. Thurim S, Dambrosia JM, Price TR, et al. Intracerebral hemorrhage: external validation and extension of a model for prediction of 30-day survival. Ann Neurol 1991;29:658–63.

3. Rosand J, Eckman MH, Knudsen KA, et al. The effect of warfarin and intensity of anticoagulation on outcome of intracerebral hemorrhage. Arch Intern Med 2004; 164:880–4.

4. Kazui S, Naritomi H, Yamamoto H, et al. Enlargement of spontaneous intracerebral hemorrhage: incidence and time course. Stroke 1996;27:1783–7.

5. Brott T, Broderick J, Khotari R, et al. Early hemorrhage growth in patients with intracerebral hemorrhage. Stroke 1997;28:1–5.

6. Wada R, Aviv RI, Fox AJ, et al. CT angiography "spot sign" predicts hematoma expansion in acute intracerebral hemorrhage. Stroke 2007;38:1257–62.

7. Goldstein JN, Fazen LE, Snider R, et al. Contrast extravasation on CT angiography predicts hematoma expansion in intracerebral hemorrhage. Neurology 2007;68:889–94.

8. Demchuk AM, Dowlatshahi D, Rodriquez-Luna D, et al. Prediction of haematoma growth and outcome in patients with intracerebral haemorrhage using the CT-angiography spot sign (PREDICT): a prospective observational study. Lancet Neurol 2012;11:307–14.

9. Al-Shahi Salman R, Frantzias J, Lee RJ, et al. Absolute risk and predictors of the growth of acute spontaneous intracerebral haemorrhage: a systematic review and meta-analysis of individual patient data. Lancet Neurol 2018;17:885–94.

10. Anderson CS, Heeley E, Huang Y, et al. Rapid blood-pressure lowering in patients with acute intracerebral hemorrhage. N Engl J Med 2013;368:2355–65.

11. Qureshi AI, Palesch YY, Barsan WG, et al. Intensive blood-pressure lowering in patients with acute cerebral hemorrhage. N Engl J Med 2016;375:1033–43.

12. Buletko AB, Thaker T, Cho S-M, et al. Cerebral ischemia and deterioration with lower blood pressure target in intracerebral hemorrhage. Neurology 2018;91: e1058–66.

13. Flibotte JJ, Hagan N, O'Donnell J, et al. Warfarin, hematoma expansion, and outcome of intracerebral hemorrhage. Neurology 2004;63:1059–64.

14. Cucchiara B, Messe S, Sansing L, et al. Hematoma growth in oral anticoagulant related intracerebral hemorrhage. Stroke 2008;39:2993–6.

15. Morotti A, Goldstein JN. Anticoagulant-associated intracerebral hemorrhage. Brain Hemorrhages 2020;1:89–94.

16. Wilson D, Seiffge DJ, Traenka C, et al. Intracerebral hemorrhage associated with different oral anticoagulants. Neurology 2017;88:1693–700.

17. Steiner T, Poli S, Griebe M, et al. Fresh frozen plasma versus prothrombin complex concentrate in patients with intracranial haemorrhage related to vitamin K antagonists (INCH): a randomized trial. Lancet Neurol 2016;15:566–73.

18. Hill R, Han TS, Lubomirova I, et al. Prothrombin complex concentrates are superior to fresh frozen plasma for emergency reversal of vitamin K antagonists: a meta-analysis in 2606 subjects. Drugs 2019;79:1557–65.

19. Kuramatsu JB, Gerner ST, Schellinger PD, et al. Anticoagulant reversal, blood pressure levels, and anticoagulant resumption in patients with anticoagulation-related intracerebral hemorrhage. JAMA 2015;313:824–36.

20. Purrucker JC, Haas K, Rizos T, et al. Early clinical and radiological course, management, and outcome of intracerebral hemorrhage related to new oral anticoagulants. JAMA Neurol 2016;73:169–77.

21. Gerner ST, Kuramatsu JB, Sembill JA, et al. Association of prothrombin complex concentrate administration and hematoma enlargement in non-vitamin K antagonist oral anticoagulant-related intracerebral hemorrhage. Ann Neurol 2018;83: 186–96.

22. Steiner T, Weitz JI, Veltkamp R. Anticoagulant-associated intracranial hemorrhage in the era of reversal agents. Stroke 2017;48:1432–7.

23. Levy JH, Ageno W, Chan NC, et al. for the Subcommittee on Control of Anticoagulation. When and how to use antidotes for the reversal of direct oral anticoagulants: guidance from the SSC of the ISTH. J Thromb Haemost 2016;14:623–7.

24. Sweidan AJ, Singh NK, Conovaloff JL, et al. Coagulopathy reversal in intracerebral hemorrhage. Stroke & Vascular Neurology 2020;5:e000274.

25. Seet RC, Rabinstein AA. Symptomatic intracranial hemorrhage following intravenous thrombolysis for acute ischemic stroke: a critical review of case definitions. Cerebrovasc Dis 2012;34:106–14.

26. Yaghi S, Willey JZ, Cucchiara B, et al. Treatment and outcome of hemorrhagic transformation after intravenous alteplase in acute ischemic stroke: a scientific statement for healthcare professionals from the American Heart Association/ American Stroke Association. Stroke 2017;48:e343–61.

27. Saloheimo P, Ahonen M, Juvela S, et al. Regular aspirin use preceding the onset of primary intracerebral hemorrhage is an independent predictor for death. Stroke 2006;37:129–33. 12.

28. Sansing L, Messe S, Cucchiara B, et al. Prior antiplatelet use does not affect hemorrhage growth or outcome after ICH. Neurology 2009;72:1397–402.

29. Baharoglu MI, Cordonnier C, Al-Shahi Salman R, et al. Platelet transfusion versus standard care after acute stroke due to spontaneous cerebral haemorrhage associated with antiplatelet therapy (PATCH): a randomised, open-label, phase 3 trial. Lancet 2016;387:2605–13.

30. Ziai WC, Carhuapoma JR. Intracerebral hemorrhage. Continuum (Minneap Minn) 2018;24:1603–22.

31. Monroe DM, Hoffman M, Oliver JA, et al. Platelet activity of high-dose factor VIIa is independent of tissue factor. Br J Haematol 1997;99:542–7.

32. Mayer SA, Brun NC, Begtrup K, et al. Recombinant activated factor VII for acute intracerebral hemorrhage. N Engl J Med 2005;352:777–85.

33. Mayer SA, Brun NC, Begtrup K, et al. Efficacy and safety of recombinant activated factor VII for acute intracerebral hemorrhage. N Engl J Med 2008;358: 2127–37.

34. Delgado Almandoz JE, Yoo AJ, Stone MJ, et al. The spot sign score in primary intracerebral hemorrhage identifies patients at highest risk of in-hospital mortality and poor outcome among survivors. Stroke 2010;41:54–60.

35. Gladstone DJ, Aviv RI, Demchuk AM, et al. Effect of recombinant activated coagulation factor VII on hemorrhage expansion among patients with spot sign-positive acute intracerebral hemorrhage: the SPOTLIGHT and STOP-IT randomized clinical trials. JAMA Neurol 2019;76:1493–501.

36. The CRASH-2 collaborators. The importance of early treatment with tranexamic acid in bleeding trauma patients: an exploratory analysis of the CRASH-2 randomised controlled trial. Lancet 2011;377:1096–101.
37. WOMAN Trial Collaborators. Effect of early tranexamic acid administration on mortality, hysterectomy, and other morbidities in women with post-partum haemorrhage (WOMAN): an international, randomised, double-blind, placebo-controlled trial. Lancet 2017;389:2105–16.
38. Sprigg N, Flaherty K, Appleton JP, et al. Tranexamic acid for hyperacute primary IntraCerebral Haemorrhage (TICH-2): an international randomized, placebo-controlled, phase 3 superiority trial. Lancet 2018;391:2107–15.
39. Gayet-Ageron A, Prieto-Merino D, Ker K, et al. Effect of treatment delay on the effectiveness and safety of antifibrinolytics in acute severe haemorrhage: a meta-analysis of individual patient-level data from 40 138 bleeding patients. Lancet 2018;391:125–32.
40. Cordonnier C, Demchuk A, Ziai W, et al. Intracerebral haemorrhage: current approaches to acute management. Lancet 2018;392:1257–68.
41. Qureshi AI, Mendelow AD, Hanley DF. Intracerebral haemorrhage. Lancet 2009; 373:1632–44.
42. Wagner KR, Sharp FR, Ardizzone TD, et al. Heme and iron metabolism: role in cerebral hemorrhage. J Cereb Blood Flow Metab 2003;23:629–52.
43. Nakamura T, Keep RF, Hua Y, et al. Deferoxamine-induced attenuation of brain edema and neurological deficits in a rat model of intracerebral hemorrhage. J Neurosurg 2004;100:672–8.
44. Selim M, Yeatts S, Goldstein JN, et al. Safety and tolerability of deferoxamine mesylate in patients with acute intracerebral hemorrhage. Stroke 2011;42:3067–74.
45. Selim M, Foster LD, Moy CS, et al. Deferoxamine mesylate in patients with intracerebral haemorrhage (i-DEF): a multicentre, randomised, placebo-controlled, double-blind phase 2 trial. Lancet Neurol 2019;18:428–38.
46. Sreekrishnan A, Leasure AC, Shi FD, et al. Functional improvement among intracerebral hemorrhage survivors up to 12 months post-injury. Neurocrit Care 2017; 27:326–33.
47. Fu Y, Hao J, Zhang N, et al. Fingolimod for the treatment of intracerebral hemorrhage: a 2-arm proof-of-concept study. JAMA Neurol 2014;71:1092–101.
48. Morgenstern LB, Demchuk AM, Kim DH, et al. Rebleeding leads to poor outcome in ultra-early craniotomy for intracerebral hemorrhage. Neurology 2001;56: 1294–9.
49. Mendelow AD, Gregson BA, Fernandes HM, et al. Early surgery versus initial conservative treatment in patients with spontaneous supratentorial intracerebral haematomas in the International Surgical Trial in Intracerebral Haemorrhage (STICH): a randomised trial. Lancet 2005;365:387–97.
50. Mendelow AD, Gregson BA, Rowan EN, et al. Early surgery versus initial conservative treatment in patients with spontaneous supratentorial lobar intracerebral haematomas (STICH II): a randomised trial. Lancet 2013;382:397–408.
51. Zhou X, Chen J, Li Q, et al. Minimally invasive surgery for spontaneous supratentorial intracerebral hemorrhage: a meta-analysis of randomized controlled trials. Stroke 2012;43:2923–30.
52. Scaggiante J, Zhang X, Mocco J, et al. Minimally invasive surgery for intracerebral hemorrhage. Stroke 2018;49:2612–20.
53. Carhuapoma JR, Barrett RJ, Keyl PM, et al. Stereotactic aspiration-thrombolysis of intracerebral hemorrhage and its impact on perihematoma brain edema. Neurocrit Care 2008;8:322–9.

54. Hanley DF, Thompson RE, Muschelli J, et al. Safety and efficacy of minimally invasive surgery plus alteplase in intracerebral haemorrhage evacuation (MISTIE): a randomised, controlled, open-label, phase 2 trial. Lancet Neurol 2016;15: 1228–37.

55. Hanley DF, Thompson RE, Rosenblum M, et al. Efficacy and safety of minimally invasive surgery with thrombolysis in intracerebral haemorrhage evacuation (MISTIE III): a randomised, controlled, open-label, blinded endpoint phase 3 trial. Lancet 2019;393:1021–32.

56. Awad IA, Polster SP, Carrión-Penagos J, et al. MISTIE III Trial Investigators. Surgical performance determines functional outcome benefit in the Minimally Invasive Surgery Plus Recombinant Tissue Plasminogen Activator for Intracerebral Hemorrhage Evacuation (MISTIE) procedure. Neurosurgery 2019;84:1157–68.

57. Vespa P, Hanley D, Betz J, et al. ICES (intraoperative stereotactic computed tomography-guided endoscopic surgery) for brain hemorrhage. Stroke 2016; 47:2749–55.

58. Hemphill JC, Greenberg SM, Anderson CS, et al. Guidelines for the management of spontaneous intracerebral hemorrhage: a guideline for healthcare professionals from the American Heart Association/American Stroke Association. Stroke 2015;46:2032–60.

59. Menacho ST, Grandhi R, Delic A, et al. Impact of intracranial pressure monitor-guided therapy on neurologic outcome after spontaneous nontraumatic intracranial hemorrhage. J Stroke Cerebrovasc Dis 2020;30:105540.

60. Steiner T, Al-Shahi Salman R, Beer R, et al. European Stroke Organisation (ESO) guidelines for the management of spontaneous intracerebral hemorrhage. Int J Stroke 2014;9:840–55.

61. Sondag L, Schreuder FHBM, Boogaarts HD, et al. Surgical intervention for supratentorial intracerebral hemorrhage. Ann Neurol 2020;88:239–50.

62. Hanley DF, Awad IA, Ziai WC. Role of temporal sequence in treating intracerebral hemorrhage. Ann Neurol 2020;88 with:237–8.

Aneurysmal Subarachnoid Hemorrhage

David Y. Chung, MD, PhD[a,b,c,*], Mohamad Abdalkader, MD[d,e,f],
Thanh N. Nguyen, MD[d,e,f]

KEYWORDS

- Intracranial aneurysm • Subarachnoid hemorrhage • Delayed cerebral ischemia
- Vasospasm • Stroke

KEY POINTS

- Aneurysmal subarachnoid hemorrhage is a neurologic emergency ideally treated in a multidisciplinary comprehensive stroke center.
- Initial management should focus on principles of advanced cardiovascular life support and prompt diagnosis.
- Early complications are aneurysm rebleeding and acute hydrocephalus.
- Most patients have better outcomes after endovascular coiling of the aneurysm, although there are instances when open surgical clipping may be indicated.
- After the aneurysm is treated, survivors require additional monitoring to prevent and manage complications, including a syndrome of delayed neurologic decline known as delayed cerebral ischemia or symptomatic vasospasm.

INTRODUCTION

Aneurysmal subarachnoid hemorrhage (SAH) is a neurologic emergency that requires prompt diagnosis and management to prevent life-threatening rebleeding and optimize patient outcomes. A major challenge lies in the broad range of severity and in continuously tailoring treatments during the complex evolution of the disease. Care of this patient population continues to improve with advances in endovascular therapy and the introduction of dedicated neurocritical care teams. Here, the authors cover the essential approach to the patient with aneurysmal SAH, review current controversies, and discuss ongoing work aimed at improving outcomes in survivors.

[a] Division of Neurocritical Care, Department of Neurology, Boston Medical Center, Boston, MA, USA; [b] Division of Neurocritical Care, Department of Neurology, Harvard Medical School, Massachusetts General Hospital, Boston, MA, USA; [c] Neurovascular Research Unit, Department of Radiology, Harvard Medical School, Massachusetts General Hospital, Boston, MA, USA; [d] Department of Neurology, Boston University School of Medicine, Boston Medical Center, Boston, MA, USA; [e] Department of Neurosurgery, Boston University School of Medicine, Boston Medical Center, Boston, MA, USA; [f] Department of Radiology, Boston University School of Medicine, Boston Medical Center, Boston, MA, USA
* Corresponding author. 72 East Concord Street, Boston, MA 02118.
E-mail addresses: david.chung@bmc.org; dychung@mgh.harvard.edu

Neurol Clin 39 (2021) 419–442
https://doi.org/10.1016/j.ncl.2021.02.006
0733-8619/21/© 2021 Elsevier Inc. All rights reserved.

EVALUATION

The classic chief complaint of the patient presenting with a ruptured aneurysm is the sudden onset of the worst headache of their life or a thunderclap headache. Although a severe headache is a common symptom, presentations can range from no headache to coma.[1] Furthermore, most patients with a headache present to the emergency room, but a subset presents to primary care. A heightened index of suspicion is important when triaging such patients. The emergency management of patients with acute headache, which has a broad differential diagnosis, is covered in a separate article, "Headache Emergencies," in this issue of *Neurologic Clinics*. Other common symptoms of SAH include neck stiffness, photophobia, and vomiting. Transient loss of consciousness has also been described in patients with SAH related to a brief intracranial circulatory arrest.[2] The range of presenting clinical severity is summarized in the Hunt and Hess (HH)[3] and World Federation of Neurological Surgeons scales,[4] which are commonly used to communicate severity of a patient's initial presentation (**Table 1**). The more general terms, high and low grade, or poor and good grade, tend to assume cutoffs of 3 or higher in either severity score.

All patients with a suspected ruptured aneurysm should have a noncontrast head computed tomographic (CT) scan. Subarachnoid blood on head imaging should prompt vessel imaging, usually a CT angiogram (CTA). A ruptured aneurysm is more commonly associated with blood within the basal cisterns (**Fig. 1**A), as opposed to convexal sulcal subarachnoid blood. When the initial noncontrast head CT scan is negative for blood but there is still a clinical suspicion for a ruptured aneurysm, then the traditional approach has been to perform a lumbar puncture (LP).[5] Frank blood and red blood cells (RBC) are commonly seen and are distinguished from a traumatic LP as RBC counts that do not diminish in sequential collecting tubes (**Fig. 1**D, E). An additional classic finding is xanthochromia, due to RBC breakdown products, which is apparent in the cerebrospinal fluid (CSF) on sample collection or after the sample has been spun down in the laboratory.

There have been recent proposals to change practice by foregoing an LP if there is a negative early head CT and certain criteria are met.[6–9] A meta-analysis of a series of studies concluded that a modern head CT 6 hours after ictus can rule out SAH with 98.7% sensitivity in the setting of severe headache if there are no other neurologic symptoms present and the scan is interpreted by an experienced radiologist.[10] In general, when the suspicion for aneurysm rupture remains high, despite an early negative head CT, most clinicians would still carry out an LP, assuming no contraindications. Under specific circumstances when the suspicion for an underlying aneurysm is low, a head CT within 6 hours to rule out a ruptured aneurysm may be reasonable.

When there is documented SAH, either by CT or by LP, initial vessel imaging should be followed by cerebral digital subtraction angiography (DSA) to increase the sensitivity of detecting an aneurysm that was not initially seen or to better characterize an aneurysm for endovascular coiling or surgical clipping.[11–13] Other rarer pathologic conditions, such as dural arteriovenous fistula, arteriovenous malformation, and distal vasculopathy, may also be better characterized on DSA compared with CT imaging.

INITIAL MANAGEMENT

As with most other neurologic emergencies, application of advanced cardiovascular life support in the unstable patient with suspected SAH is the priority, including attention to the airway, breathing, and circulatory status. If the patient is progressing toward coma or there is impending respiratory failure, the patient should be intubated. If the patient is hypotensive, then measures to maintain an adequate blood pressure (BP)

Table 1	
Common aneurysmal subarachnoid hemorrhage scales	
Hunt and Hess	
1	Asymptomatic or minimal headache and slight nuchal rigidity
2	Moderate to severe headache, nuchal rigidity, no neurologic deficit other than cranial nerve palsy
3	Drowsy, confusion, or mild focal deficit
4	Stupor, moderate to severe hemiparesis, possibly early decerebrate rigidity and vegetative disturbances
5	Deep coma, decerebrate rigidity, moribund appearance
World Federation of Neurological Surgeons	
1	GCS 15, absent motor deficits
2	GCS 13/14, absent motor deficits
3	GCS 13/14, motor deficit present
4	GCS 7–12, present or absent motor deficits
5	GCS 3–6, present or absent motor deficits
Fisher	
1	No detectable SAH
2	Diffuse SAH, no localized clot >3 mm thick or vertical layers >1 mm thick
3	Presence of localized clots and/or vertical layers of blood 1 mm or greater in thickness
4	Intraparenchymal or intraventricular hemorrhage with either absent or diffuse SAH
Claassen	
0	No SAH or IVH
1	Minimal/thin SAH, no IVH in both lateral ventricles
2	Minimal/thin SAH, with IVH in both lateral ventricles
3	Thick SAH, no IVH in both lateral ventricles
4	Thick SAH, with IVH in both lateral ventricles
Modified Fisher	
0	No SAH or IVH
1	Minimal/thin SAH, no IVH
2	Minimal/thin SAH, with IVH
3	Thick SAH, no IVH
4	Thick SAH, with IVH

Abbreviation: GCS, Glasgow Coma Scale.

need to be instituted, including the use of vasopressors for a mean arterial pressure (MAP) $\geq$65 mm Hg. There are specialized disease-specific considerations (eg, stress cardiomyopathy [SCM], discussed later), but work up of these potential complications should not delay the initial stabilization of the patient while the differential diagnosis remains broad.

Once the patient is stabilized, initial medical management and evaluation run in parallel. If the pattern of blood on head CT is consistent with SAH (see **Fig. 1**A), then an upper systolic blood pressure (SBP) goal of less than 160 mm Hg is reasonable (**Table 2**). The SBP goal in the setting of SAH should be distinguished from 2 recent randomized clinical trials (RCTs) that suggested a potential benefit of less than

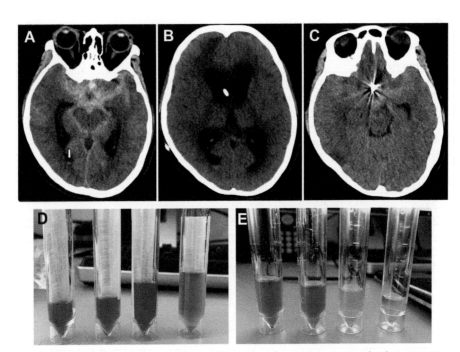

Fig. 1. (*A*) Axial CT scan in a patient with ruptured anterior communicating aneurysm showing diffuse and thick SAH seen in the basal cisterns (quadrigeminal cisterns, perimesencephalic cisterns, and in the Sylvian fissures). Minimal IVH (*arrow*) is also noted layering in the occipital horns of the lateral ventricles, which are significantly dilated. (*B*) Axial CT scan of the same patient showing significant dilatation of the ventricular system consistent with communicating hydrocephalus. A ventricular drain was recently placed with its tip noted in the right lateral ventricle. (*C*) Follow-up CT scan after endovascular coiling of the ruptured anterior communicating aneurysm with resolution of the subarachnoid blood and significant improvement of the ventricular dilatation. Streak artifacts from the coils are noted. (*D*) CSF in a patient with SAH showing the RBCs in the final tube. (*E*) CSF in a patient without SAH with blood clearing in sequential tubes consistent with a traumatic LP.

140 mm Hg in patients with confirmed primary ICH.[14,15] SAH and ICH are not equivalent and, therefore, an SBP goal of less than 140 mm Hg should not be assumed to be beneficial in SAH. There are no high-quality randomized studies of BP goals in SAH patients to guide recommendations. However, the potential for harm in overcorrecting high SBP in this distinct population is not insignificant, especially in comatose patients when intracranial pressure (ICP) may be high and cerebral autoregulation may be dysregulated. In such patients, overtreatment of the BP can lead to diffuse brain hypoperfusion and have significant negative consequences.

The patient should be monitored for signs and symptoms of hydrocephalus or raised ICP that would warrant emergent placement of an external ventricular drain (EVD) (**Fig. 1**B).[16] There should be suspicion for symptomatic hydrocephalus in any high-grade (HH grade 3 or above) patient, including those with progressive lethargy, limited vertical extraocular movements, stupor, hemiparesis, or decerebrate posturing without an alternative cause. If no one is available to emergently place an EVD, then the patient should be treated empirically with bridging osmotherapy and transferred to a higher level of care, ideally a comprehensive stroke center,[17] where a qualified clinician can place an EVD. It is worth noting that some centers place an EVD in all

Table 2
Recommended treatment parameters and orders

Before Aneurysm Securing	
MAP	$\geq$65 mm Hg
SBP	<160 mm Hg
ICP	<20 mm Hg
CPP	$\geq$60 mm Hg
Oxygen saturation	>93%
EVD status	Raised (eg, 20 cm H_2O) or closed, as tolerated
After Aneurysm securing	
MAP	$\geq$65 mm Hg
SBP	Up to 220 mm Hg depending on clinical status
ICP	<20 mm Hg
CPP	$\geq$60 mm Hg
Oxygen saturation	>93%
EVD status	Controversial
TTE	On admission to establish baseline
TCD	Daily when available
Nimodipine	60 mg q4h PO $\times$ 21 d
Fludrocortisone	0.1 mg 1 to 3 times per day for hyponatremia
Head CT	24–48 h following aneurysm securing
Vessel or perfusion imaging	At 4–8 d post-SAH for high-risk patients
Hemoglobin	>7.0 g/dL, consider higher goal for DCI
Temperature management	$\leq$37.5°C
Volume status	Euvolemia with isotonic fluids

Abbreviations: CPP, cerebral perfusion pressure; TTE, transthoracic echocardiography.

patients with SAH for measurement of ICP, for prophylaxis for possible hydrocephalus, and to remove blood from the CSF. In such cases, placement of an EVD would be nonemergent. The authors' recommendation is to place an EVD emergently if the patient is symptomatic or if there are clear signs of hydrocephalus on imaging.

A limited course of seizure prophylaxis is a reasonable approach in the setting of a potentially untreated, ruptured aneurysm because the sequela of seizures is of more potential harm than anticonvulsant side effects in the acute phase. In addition, patients may present with a seizure-like episode at admission, and it would be reasonable to start an anticonvulsant for empiric seizure treatment until further history and work up is obtained. Levetiracetam has become a common first-line agent given its better side-effect profile and pharmacodynamics, compared with phenytoin, which has been associated with worse cognitive and neurologic outcome after SAH.[18] However, there are no high-quality data regarding the use of anticonvulsants, either overall benefit or harm, or for the choice of any specific anticonvulsant over the other in the setting of SAH.

Pain management should take a stepwise approach, starting with nonsedating medications, such as acetaminophen. Nonsteroidal anti-inflammatory drugs are to be avoided given an increased risk of rebleeding before securing of the aneurysm. If pain is persistently severe, then modest doses of opioids, such as oxycodone or hydromorphone, can be added, but given the importance of the clinical examination in the early phase, post–aneurysm rupture expectations should be set with the patient that complete pain freedom may not be the goal.

The patient with aneurysmal SAH should ideally be admitted to an accredited comprehensive stroke center[17] with a neuroendovascular team, neurosurgery, and an intensive care unit (ICU) staffed with clinicians and nurses with specialized training in neurocritical care. This multidisciplinary approach allows for optimal aneurysm treatment and management of potential complications specific to aneurysmal SAH.

ANEURYSM TREATMENT

DSA should be performed in all patients who have a suspected aneurysm seen using other modalities (eg, CTA or magnetic resonance angiography) or in patients in whom noninvasive vessel imaging is negative but there remains a clinical suspicion of an underlying vascular lesion.[19] DSA is important both for aneurysm treatment (**Fig. 2**) and for open surgical planning. The diagnostic approach in patients with nonaneurysmal SAH or patients with an indeterminate diagnosis is variable and has been covered elsewhere.[13]

The International Subarachnoid Aneurysm Trial was a landmark randomized trial that demonstrated better clinical outcomes at 1 year for patients with ruptured aneurysms treated with endovascular coiling compared with surgical clipping (190/801, 24% dependent or dead at 1 year in coiling arm vs 243/793, 31% in clipping arm, $P = .0019$).[20,21] The Barrow Ruptured Aneurysm Trial was another randomized trial of SAH patients treated with alternating clip versus coil strategy. At 1 year, poor outcome was higher in the clip versus the coil group (34% vs. 23%; odds ratio, 1.68, $P = .02$).[22] Furthermore, there is evidence that suggests that coiling is associated with a lower rate of DCI.[23] With advances in endovascular techniques and these recent RCT data, most ruptured aneurysms are being treated by coiling. There are instances whereby open surgical clipping may be favored, such as a patient with a ruptured middle cerebral artery aneurysm with large hematoma and mass effect

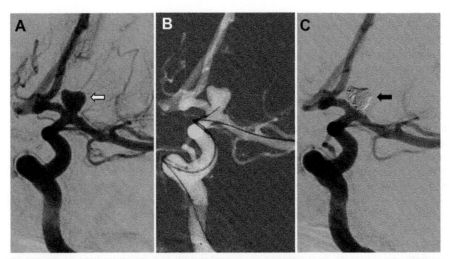

Fig. 2. Anteroposterior angiogram of the left internal carotid artery in a patient with SAH showing a carotid terminus aneurysm (*white arrow*) (A). Balloon-assisted coiling of the carotid terminus aneurysm was performed (B) with complete occlusion of the aneurysm (C, *black arrow*).

requiring evacuation. Still, some surgeons prefer to secure the aneurysm by coiling in such instances followed by immediate craniectomy decompression.[24] There are new endovascular techniques for aneurysm treatment involving a flow diverter device (resembles a stent with more metal surface area) and expandable intrasaccular flow disruption devices, such as the WEB (Woven EndoBridge).[25,26] However, flow diverter and stent-assisted techniques are usually considered a last resort because of obligate dual antiplatelet therapy to prevent stent or flow diverter device thrombosis and risk of hemorrhage.[25,26] Therefore, the patient should be evaluated by a multidisciplinary group experienced in endovascular approaches and/or open neurosurgical clipping to determine the optimal approach for each individual patient.[24]

The timing of aneurysm treatment should be early following aneurysm diagnosis to reduce the risk of aneurysm rerupture. The data on risk of aneurysm rebleeding after SAH trace to studies from the 1970s and 1980s, as most aneurysms are rapidly secured in the modern era.[19,27,28] After SAH, the risk of rerupture is highest in the first day (4%) and then is estimated at 1% to 2% each day in the first month.[29] With conservative management, the risk of aneurysm rebleeding is 20% to 30% in the first month and then ≈3% per year. The mortality associated with aneurysm rerupture is estimated at 67%.[30] Ruptured aneurysms therefore need to be treated early to prevent rerupture.

Ultraearly treatment is considered to be within the first 24 hours after presentation. The question of whether immediate emergent treatment, overnight when needed, is superior to waiting for daytime teams to arrive is controversial but could be considered in cases whereby there is already clinical suspicion or imaging evidence of aneurysm rerupture.[31,32] The current evidence supporting emergent versus within-24-hour treatment is inconclusive, but if there is an effect on rebleed rates, it is likely a very small effect.[32] Therefore, an ultraearly less than 24-hour treatment protocol is a reasonably rapid protocol when taking into account systems of care, resource utilization, and the benefit of proper surgical-endovascular planning.

If there is an unavoidable delay in aneurysm treatment beyond 24 hours, clinicians could consider a limited course of antifibrinolytics, such as aminocaproic acid (Amicar) or tranexamic acid (TXA), to mitigate the risk for aneurysm rebleeding. In the era before early aneurysm treatment several decades ago, these agents were associated with myocardial infarction, pulmonary embolism, and other thrombotic complications. However, in the current period of early ruptured aneurysm treatment, the risk of complications up to 48 to 72 hours remains low to nonexistent.[33–35] One caveat that remains, however, is that antifibrinolytics can cause complications if the agent remains at a therapeutic level during endovascular treatment. Furthermore, a recent RCT found that ultraearly less than 24-hour use of TXA had no detectable effect on long-term functional outcome.[36] Therefore, the authors would reserve the use of antifibrinolytics only for patients in whom a delay of greater than 24 hours is unavoidable and, when used, would hold the medication for at least 2 hours before an aneurysm-securing procedure. It is critical to discuss utilization of antifibrinolytics with the physicians involved in securing the aneurysm (ie, neurointerventionalist or neurosurgeon), as its effect on endovascular or open surgical procedural thrombotic complications is not well established and current clinical practice remains variable.

Finally, there are patients who present with aneurysmal pattern SAH, yet the initial angiogram studies are negative. In these instances, the patient often undergoes repeat angiography in 1 week to look for an underlying lesion that may have been masked by hemorrhage at the initial study. When the repeat study is negative, the cause is often referred to as a venous bleed, as in perimesencephalic SAH.[13] In instances whereby the clinical history points to the onset of pain in the neck or back, or there is a high burden of hemorrhage in the posterior fossa or foramen magnum, a search for a spinal aneurysm may yield the cause of the patient's hemorrhage. Such findings are rare, thought to relate to dissection, and may resolve on their own before securing.[37]

CRITICAL CARE MANAGEMENT

All patients with a suspected or confirmed ruptured aneurysm should be admitted to an ICU, preferably staffed with a clinical and nursing team with specialized training in neurocritical care. The only exception is at some experienced centers where good-grade SAH patients are admitted to an intermediate step-down unit for lack of ICU beds. Studies have demonstrated that patient outcomes are improved when a multidisciplinary neurocritical care service is involved.[38,39] The value of specialized care is underscored by the absence of firm evidence-based recommendations and the complexity of patient management based on time from aneurysm rupture, vasospasm management, and severity of disease. Therefore, there is no substitute for an experienced multidisciplinary neurocritical care team. What follows is an overview of general neurocritical care principles for this patient population to help guide management decisions.

Initial Critical Care Considerations

Before securing the aneurysm, initial management measures described earlier should be continued to prevent aneurysm rerupture, including adequate BP control and anticonvulsants for seizure prophylaxis. If there is an EVD in place, the drain should be kept at a high level (eg, 20 cm H_2O above the tragus of the ear) or closed, as tolerated, to minimize the transmural pressure gradient across the aneurysm wall[40,41] (see **Table 2**).

Once the aneurysm is secured, the focus of care shifts to preventing secondary brain injury and minimizing and treating complications. BP parameters can be liberalized based on medical comorbidities (eg, a lower upper BP limit in the setting of known heart failure). Anticonvulsant medications can be stopped if the clinical suspicion for seizures is low. Important general critical care practice applies to the patient with aneurysmal SAH, such as ventilator liberation strategies, deep venous thromboembolism prophylaxis, infection control, and removing unnecessary lines and catheters on a daily basis. In the era of COVID-19, modified protocols tailored to the management of SAH have been reported to optimize SAH care and protect health care workers.[42] Additional COVID-19–specific recommendations are discussed in the article, "Neurologic Emergencies During the COVID-19 Pandemic," in this issue.

The management of the SAH patient evolves with the time from aneurysm rupture. As such, the authors address potential complications encountered in the ICU and their management strategies as they appear in an approximate chronologic order.

Stress Cardiomyopathy and Neurogenic Pulmonary Edema

An adrenergic surge in the setting of severe SAH can lead to SCM, which is an acute and reversible form of heart failure.[43] The syndrome is also known as takotsubo cardiomyopathy for the characteristic shape of the left ventricle on catheter angiography or echocardiography, which resembles a traditional Japanese octopus trap (tako たこ trans octopus and tsubo つぼ trans pot).[44] The treatment depends on whether there is an associated left ventricular outflow tract obstruction (LVOT).[45] In most cases, there is no LVOT obstruction, and the patient can be treated with vasopressors, inotropes, or in severe cases, mechanical circulatory support. In the less-common case of LVOT obstruction, a beta-agonist can cause a paradoxic worsening of shock, and the approach shifts toward beta-blockers, preload optimization, and, when necessary, careful titration of alpha-agonists, such as phenylephrine. The occurrence of SCM is important to consider, as it influences the differential diagnosis for hypotension and shock in SAH patients. However, available diagnostics are nonspecific, and definitive diagnostics tend to be contraindicated. Therefore, clinical context (ie, pretest probability) is key to the possible diagnosis of SCM. Electrocardiogram and elevation of cardiac enzymes can be indistinguishable from ST-segment elevation myocardial infarction (STEMI). The diagnosis can be supported by the pattern of regional wall motion abnormalities based on TTE in which apical dilation and hypokinesis are more consistent with SCM, and abnormalities in the distribution of a coronary artery could raise additional concern for a STEMI. The gold-standard diagnostic procedure is catheter angiography and the exclusion of coronary artery disease. The incidence of SCM is high enough in SAH patients compared with the general population such that catheter angiography, and the accompanying use of periprocedural heparin, is typically not recommended for most patients, especially in the setting of a ruptured aneurysm. However, there can be concomitant coronary syndromes with SAH, so a primary or concomitant coronary syndrome should not be completely excluded from the differential diagnosis.

Neurogenic pulmonary edema is a related hyperadrenergic syndrome that affects the lungs and should be on the differential diagnosis if there is unexplained early hypoxemia in a patient with severe, high-grade SAH. It can be thought of as a form of acute respiratory distress syndrome (ARDS), which usually resolves within 24 to 48 hours. There can be pulmonary edema exacerbated by concomitant heart failure owing to SCM, but neurogenic pulmonary edema is also seen in the absence of SCM. Treatment is supportive care with lung protective therapy according to current ARDS management strategies.[46–48]

Hyponatremia

Hyponatremia (sodium <135 mmol/L) is common early in the hospital course of patients with SAH. The cause has historically been controversial, but the 2 leading causes are attributed to cerebral salt wasting (CSW)[49] and syndrome of inappropriate antidiuretic hormone secretion (SIADH).[50] The typical treatment of SIADH involves fluid restriction, which can be harmful in the patient with aneurysmal SAH, as it may increase risk for DCI. The treatment of CSW involves fluid administration, which can conflict with SIADH. There are classic urine and blood study values that have been reported to favor 1 diagnosis over the other,[49] but the authors have found that these studies are rarely revealing. Because SIADH tends to occur in the setting of euvolemia or hypervolemia and CSW leads to hypovolemia, volume status may provide insight into cause; however, volume status itself is notoriously challenging to determine in critically ill patients.[51,52] It is also possible that patients have both SIADH and CSW, although it is unclear how such a situation could be proven. Administration of hypertonic saline solutions (typically 1.5%–3% sodium chloride intravenously [IV]) is the most effective treatment in maintaining eunatremia. Some clinicians will administer salt tablets (1–3 g 3 times a day), but this is not always effective and may not be well tolerated in awake patients. Fludrocortisone may have a role prophylactically or in response to hyponatremia[53] to minimize the use of continuous IV infusions (see **Table 2**).

Fever

There are 2 common questions regarding fever following SAH: (1) what is the source of fever, and (2) should fever be controlled? Following SAH, both infectious and noninfectious fever is common. The cause of noninfectious central or neurogenic fever in the setting of SAH is thought to involve hypothalamic irritation from blood products. Within the first 72 hours of admission, the rate of noninfectious fever is higher in SAH,[54] but in practice, empiric antibiotics for possible infection is the usual course of action. Therefore, noninfectious fever remains a diagnosis of exclusion but should be higher on the differential in the SAH population to decrease the rate of unnecessary antibiotic use if an infectious source is ruled out.

Most neurointensivists would treat fever itself (>37.5°C) in SAH patients. Although there are no high-quality data to support the approach, there is a strong rationale that reducing fever might minimize secondary brain injury. Association studies have found a relationship between fever and worse outcomes in SAH,[55,56] but there is an absence of supportive randomized evidence.[57] The reason for debate is that there is a hypothesized role for beneficial effects of fever in the setting of infection.[58] There are also risks associated with implementing fever-control measures, such as intravascular or external cooling devices and their accompanying antishivering medications.[59] What is likely is that the benefit of fever control probably depends on the specific patient population and circumstances that best balance risk and benefit.[60] Therefore, empiric randomized trials are urgently needed. The ongoing INTREPID trial is a randomized study that takes the unique approach of prophylactically preventing fever in brain-injured patients, including SAH patients (INTREPID; ClinicalTrials.gov Identifier #NCT02996266). It is a step toward determining the impact of fever in SAH patients and whether treatment is beneficial. Additional adequately powered randomized trials to treat incident fever are also needed.[61] In the meantime, it is reasonable to treat fever empirically with antibiotics and antipyretic medications (such as acetaminophen) and then escalate to cooling devices for persistent fevers on a case-by-case basis.

Delayed Cerebral Ischemia

The mainstay of critical care management is the prevention and treatment of a syndrome of delayed neurologic deficits that typically occurs 3 to 14 days after aneurysm rupture,[62] with the peak on days 7 to 9 after bleed. The syndrome is variably termed delayed cerebral ischemia (DCI),[63] delayed ischemic neurologic deficits,[64] delayed cerebral infarction,[65] symptomatic vasospasm,[66] or vasospasm.[67] Historically, the cause of delayed neurologic deficits was thought to be related to large-vessel arterial vasospasm (**Fig. 3**). The vasospasm hypothesis led to the practice of fluid administration, permissive or induced hypertension, and administration of vasodilators to increase blood flow. One vasodilator, the calcium channel antagonist, nimodipine, was designed to dilate cerebral blood vessels and has the strongest supportive evidence of any DCI therapy. A pair of randomized trials in the 1980s showed that it reduced the rate of poor outcome or delayed infarcts by as much as 50% when used prophylactically.[68,69] However, nimodipine does not appear to exert its effect solely through dilation of large cerebral arteries given early observations that outcomes could be improved without improvement in angiographic vasospasm and, conversely, that there could be poor outcome even with reversal of vasospasm. Regardless, nimodipine 60 mg every 4 hours used as prophylaxis remains standard of care for most patients with aneurysmal SAH (see **Table 2**). A notable exception exists in Japan, where standard of care is use of the rho kinase inhibitor fasudil, rather than nimodipine, to prevent DCI.[70–73]

Monitoring and delayed cerebral ischemia detection

It is common practice to obtain a head CT 24 to 48 hours following aneurysm securing to distinguish treatment-related infarction from DCI later in the patient's hospital

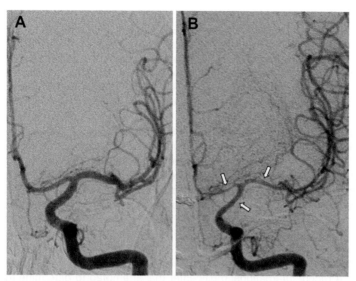

Fig. 3. Anteroposterior angiogram of the left internal carotid artery in a patient with aneurysmal SAH at presentation (*A*) and 8 days later (*B*) showing interval development of severe vasospasm of the left supraclinoid carotid artery, left anterior and middle cerebral arteries (*arrows*).

course (**Fig. 1**C).[74] Furthermore, many centers will use regular monitoring with transcranial Dopplers (TCD) and interval vessel or perfusion imaging 4 to 8 days post-SAH to detect early signs of vasospasm (see **Table 2**). In high grade patients who have a poor exam and are not following commands, these radiographic modalities may be the only triggers to raise a clinical suspicion for DCI. In contrast, for low-grade patients or those with a good examination some clinicians would argue that such monitoring is not necessary. Perfusion imaging may have an advantage over other radiographic modalities in that it can distinguish blood flow (the metric of interest) from velocity and vessel caliber.[75] Therefore, a patient with decreased flow on perfusion imaging but unremarkable large-vessel imaging and TCDs might still be at high risk for impending DCI. Conversely, a patient with a reassuring blood flow perfusion scan but large-vessel vasospasm and elevated TCD velocities may not warrant escalation in their management. However, in practice, there are challenges to implementing perfusion imaging in the SAH patient population and persistent questions about the appropriate timing, modality, and interpretation of the scans.[76] Noninvasive cerebral blood flow (CBF) monitors may address some of these issues, but the technology remains in development.[77] Continuous electroencephalogram (cEEG) is another potential modality that may find use in detecting impending DCI. Although promising, the cEEG approach is resource intensive and requires a reading epileptologist who is specially trained in grading records for DCI risk. Finally, invasive multimodality monitoring using brain tissue oxygenation, microdialysis, and thermal diffusion flow measurement is a promising but complex approach that requires additional development for more widespread use.[78] Regardless of the diagnostics used at any specific institution, the suspicion and triggers for care escalation for DCI should be driven by the patient's clinical examination. Once DCI is suspected, the following measures can be attempted, all with limited supporting evidence.

Hypertension

Strategies to prevent and treat DCI include BP, volume, and hemoglobin optimization. The historical "triple-H" treatment (hypertension, hypervolemia, and hemodilution)[79] approach has been outdated for some time but is worth discussing as a conceptual framework. Of these, only permissive or induced hypertension remains in practice, and even this practice has recently been questioned.[80] The rationale behind elevating BP in the SAH patient is to improve blood flow in the setting of altered cerebrovascular autoregulation that can occur in the setting of brain injury. In normal, uninjured brain, CBF should not vary with changes in MAP within a range of approximately 60 to 150 mm Hg.[81] However, this autoregulation is thought to break down in the setting of acute brain injury, including SAH. Therefore, it may be necessary to modulate CBF through changes in BP. A common practice is to attempt a trial of induced hypertension with vasopressors if there is a clinical neurologic change. A more controversial practice is inducing hypertension for TCD or imaging findings that demonstrate vasospasm as a prophylactic measure in the absence of symptoms. Typically, BP is induced to approximately 20% above baseline BP with MAP or SBP goals, with an upper SBP limit of 220 mm Hg (see **Table 2**). The choice of MAP or SBP is not standardized, and there is limited high-quality evidence supporting specific targets or protocols. A recent international multicenter trial attempted to determine the benefit of a protocolized induced hypertension approach in patients with clinical symptoms of DCI but was not able to reach their enrollment goal of 240 patients, did not find a benefit to prophylactic hypertension in their analyzed patients, and found a higher rate of serious adverse effects in the induced hypertension group, which was further supported in a systematic literature review.[80] Therefore, there is a disconnect between the practice of induced hypertension and the current level of evidence.

Cardiac output

Cardiac output enhancement is related to induced hypertension but is a distinct and independent strategy to increase CBF to prevent or treat DCI. Titrating supranormal cardiac output with inotropes, such as dobutamine, and a pulmonary artery catheter used to be practiced but has now largely fallen out of favor. Trials have thus far failed to show benefit of such therapy, and many clinicians are wary of adverse effects, such as cardiac arrhythmia and central venous line complications related to dobutamine titration with a pulmonary artery catheter. Various device-based strategies have been designed to enhance CBF through increasing cardiac output (eg, aortic balloon pumps) or diverting flow to the brain by occluding flow within the descending aorta.[82] However, these devices have a large potential for morbidity with no clear demonstration of benefit. Therefore, the authors would not recommend routine guided pharmacologic or device-based cardiac output therapy given an unfavorable risk-benefit ratio in most patients. Such therapy may be considered for a poor-grade patient who has failed more conservative approaches.

Vasodilators

One promising, less-invasive approach that may act through a combination of enhanced cardiac output and cerebral vasodilation is the administration of IV milrinone.[83] As a phosphodiesterase inhibitor, IV milrinone has inotropic properties and causes peripheral and cerebral vasodilation. It is also used by angiographers intra-arterially as a cerebral vasodilator. A protocol developed by clinicians at the Montreal Neurological Institute has proven safe and suggests favorable outcomes in a single-center retrospective cohort without the need for invasive hemodynamic monitoring.[83,84] This approach has been adapted by other centers, again with a good safety profile, but further study is likely required to meet the evidence threshold to incorporate or reject widespread milrinone therapy in clinical practice.[85]

Volume
A longstanding cornerstone in prevention and management of DCI is volume optimization.[86] The current practice is for goal euvolemia. Hypervolemia is no longer favored and likely leads to increased complications and increased length of stay. A single-center randomized study comparing euvolemia versus hypervolemia demonstrated an effect on cardiac filling pressures but did not find a difference in CBF or blood volumes.[87] Hypovolemia could lead to low cardiac output, hypotension, and potential precipitation or exacerbation of DCI. Therefore, current practice focuses on avoiding hypovolemia and maintaining euvolemia through clinical assessment of volume status and administration of PO and isotonic IV fluids as needed.

Hemoglobin
The optimal hemoglobin concentration in SAH patients remains unclear, although there is agreement that the hemoglobin concentration should be at least 7.0 g/dL. Patients with SAH tend to develop a relative anemia, which is thought to be due to hospitalization-associated anemia and fluid administration. One prospective study transfused 1 unit of RBCs in patients with a hemoglobin concentration less than 11 g/dL and found improvements in oxygen delivery, as measured with PET imaging, that were superior to induced hypertension or an equivalent fluid bolus.[88] On the other hand, blood transfusions have known complications in general (eg, greater infection rate, acute lung injury, transfusion reactions) and in SAH patients have been found to have a greater risk of thrombotic complications.[89] The best hemoglobin goal is unknown and requires further study. In the meantime, when there is a concern for active cerebral ischemia, it is reasonable to aim for a transfusion hemoglobin goal of greater than 8.0 g/dL or even higher depending on the clinical scenario.[90]

Hemodilution and viscosity
Hemodilution (from classic triple-H therapy) should not be a goal. A related strategy is attempting to improve blood viscosity through a continuous low-dose infusion of mannitol. The rationale is to improve CBF by making it easier for RBCs to transit the capillary bed.[91,92] There is evidence that a continuous low-dose mannitol infusion can improve CBF in SAH patients independent of its effect on ICP and without causing a decrease in BP.[93] Mannitol in SAH patients was more common in the past but has largely fallen out of clinical practice, perhaps out of a concern for its diuretic effects. The historical papers demonstrate safety,[91–93] however, and the effect of continuous mannitol after SAH may warrant further study.

Future work
DCI remains an important problem with a sizable proportion of patients that could benefit from new therapies to prevent and fully treat the disease. The focus of these therapies should be on long-term functional outcome, minimizing procedures and complications, and decreasing length of stay so that all patients with ruptured aneurysms might benefit from new approaches.

There have been several additional investigational therapies that target the prevention and treatment of DCI.[82,94,95] One of these promising therapies involves use of the phosphodiesterase inhibitor, cilostazol, which exerts its effects through cerebral vasodilation and inhibition of platelet aggregation.[96] In a single-center randomized trial, cilostazol administration was associated with less symptomatic vasospasm compared with placebo.[97] A subsequent single-center randomized trial from an independent group found that cilostazol use was associated with fewer sequelae of spreading depolarizations,[73] a phenomenon thought to be part of the pathophysiological pathway leading to secondary brain injury in SAH.[98–101] These studies were conducted in Japan, where fasudil, rather than nimodipine, is used for DCI prophylaxis. Therefore, they are not generalizable, and additional studies are required.

Another promising approach involves targeting arterial vasospasm. SAH leads to elevated levels of the potent endogenous vasoconstrictor endothelin 1 (ET-1). A phase 3 randomized trial of the ET-1 receptor antagonist clazosentan demonstrated a reduced rate of rescue therapy, but did not meet the threshold for statistically significant improvement in the primary composite outcome of all-cause mortality, rescue therapy, DCI-related cerebral infarcts, and neurologic deficits in patients undergoing surgical clipping.[102] As a result, a related phase 3 randomized trial in patients undergoing endovascular coiling of their aneurysm was stopped early.[103] Regardless, the study in coiled patients demonstrated that at higher doses, clazosentan led to a decreased rate in the primary composite outcome. Neither study met their predefined secondary outcome of functional improvement, possibly because of underpowering owing to better than expected outcomes in placebo groups. A major caveat is that clazosentan led to an increased rate of pulmonary edema. An ongoing follow-up study called REACT (ClinicalTrials.gov Identifier #NCT03585270) will determine if clazosentan can decrease the incidence of clinical deterioration due to DCI in high-risk patients and to address remaining concerns.

Finally, work toward predicting which patients develop DCI is ongoing. Publication of the original Fisher scale was an important step toward using an early head CT to predict the risk of vasospasm and poor outcome.[104] However, it was designed as preliminary scale and does not take into account the additive effect that intraventricular hemorrhage (IVH) may have on risk for DCI (see **Table 1**). The modified Fisher (mF) scale was developed as an ordinal radiological scale that built on Fisher's work and incorporates the amount of SAH and presence of IVH in any ventricle. An increase in the scale from 0 to 4 is associated with an approximately stepwise increased risk of developing DCI.[105] The Claassen scale is very similar to the mF scale but requires IVH in both lateral ventricles rather that blood in any ventricle[106]; given this specificity for blood in both lateral ventricles, it is not as widely used as the mF scale. There has been increasing acknowledgment of issues with interrater reliability with the different Fisher scales.[107] For research purposes, it is important that raters are using the same scoring criteria and that the different versions of the scales are not conflated with each other. In clinical practice, the mF and Claassen scales are the most helpful and commonly used scales to communicate the amount and distribution of intracranial blood, when used consistently within an institution. Aside from the Fisher scales, there are other potential predictors of DCI that are being explored. The Hijdra scale is another CT-based scale that quantifies the amount of blood in several basal cisterns in greater detail than the Fisher scales.[108] Investigators have reported increased sensitivity in early prediction and detection of DCI or secondary brain injury by supplementing clinical and CT data with TCD,[109] cEEG,[110,111] inflammatory biomarkers,[112,113] and common laboratory values.[114] Future work will determine how such approaches can influence interventions and impact outcomes.

Seizures

Seizures should remain on the differential diagnosis for hospitalized SAH patients in a coma or for patients with more subtle changes in mental status. The only way to confirm a suspicion of nonconvulsive seizures is through cEEG. Convulsive seizures can be treated empirically but should also be followed up with cEEG to capture subsequent convulsive or nonconvulsive events. The duration of monitoring remains controversial, but a good rule of thumb is 24 hours in awake patients and at least 48 hours in comatose patients.[115] The exception may be in patients in whom there is not a high clinical suspicion of seizures and who have an absence of epileptiform abnormalities on cEEG in the first 4 hours of recording.[116]

If seizures are detected, clinically or electrographically, then they should be treated according to local practice, which varies considerably. There is no evidence that seizure control in SAH leads to improved outcomes; however, given the likelihood that seizures on top of SAH could lead to even worse neurologic injury, the authors advocate for seizure detection and control measures in the ICU. Following control of confirmed seizures, they recommend maintenance or careful slow down-titration of anticonvulsants, to reduce the risk of seizure recurrence in the resolution phase of the disease.

It is worth commenting on whether anticonvulsants should be continued in the common instance of isolated seizurelike episodes on presentation. Nonepileptic convulsions in the setting of syncope are very common. One study found no association between seizurelike episodes and the risk of developing subsequent seizures.[117] Therefore, if there are no concerning features of presenting abnormal movements (eg, development of status epilepticus), it is reasonable to defer anticonvulsants in patients in whom there is only an isolated seizurelike episodes on presentation.

Hydrocephalus and External Ventricular Drain Management

Hydrocephalus is a clear indication for EVD placement and CSF diversion. A controversial area of post–aneurysm treatment involves how to manage the EVD once it is in place.[41] The issue is important, as it can impact ICU length of stay and is thought to influence patient outcomes. There are prospective randomized and retrospective studies that have suggested that keeping the EVD closed and only opening intermittently when needed can prevent EVD-related complications, specifically reducing the rate of drain malfunction and ventriculostomy-associated infection.[118,119] However, surveys of actual practice patterns have revealed that most institutions take the opposite approach of keeping the EVD open and draining continuously by default once the aneurysm is treated.[120,121] The rationale is that draining CSF might help to clear RBCs and breakdown products that are thought to contribute to neuroinflammation. However, if the goal is to drain blood products from the CSF, then lumbar drainage is likely more effective and leads to fewer complications than EVD drainage.[122] Regardless, there are currently no high-quality data to suggest that CSF drainage either improves or worsens functional outcomes.[41,123]

Another controversial aspect of EVD management is how to discontinue the drain once the clinical decision has been made that it is no longer needed. The choice in discontinuation strategies is typically between what is referred to as a gradual wean versus rapid wean. The most common approach is a gradual wean, whereby the drain is raised in steps every 24 hours and then clamped (closed), usually over the course of 3 to 4 days.[82] A typical gradual wean scenario is a patient with an EVD open and continuously draining at 10 cm H_2O above the tragus of the ear. When the decision is made to attempt drain discontinuation, the drain is raised to 15 cm H_2O for 24 hours, then 20 cm H_2O, and then closed. A wean failure is typically defined as the patient developing symptoms (eg, headache or drowsiness), an elevated ICP, CSF leakage from around the EVD site, or signs of radiographic hydrocephalus at any point during the process. Once the EVD has been closed for 24 to 48 hours and repeat imaging does not show radiographic hydrocephalus, then the EVD is discontinued. In contrast, a typical rapid wean consists of the EVD being closed for 24 to 48 hours regardless of the starting height of the drain. A single-center randomized trial of rapid versus gradual

EVD weaning found that a rapid wean led to shorter ICU length of stay without a detectable effect on the rate of vasospasm.[124] A more recent single-center before-and-after retrospective study also found that a rapid wean was associated with shorter ICU length of stay and additionally found that patients undergoing a rapid EVD wean had a lower rate of permanent CSF diversion in the form of a ventriculoperitoneal shunt.[119] A prospective multicenter study would be helpful to determine the generalizability of the rapid versus gradual wean findings.

SUMMARY

Aneurysmal SAH is a neurologic emergency that requires prompt patient stabilization, diagnosis, and treatment. Although the classic presentation of a severe headache is common, there are a wide range of presentations, including mild pain and coma. Treatment advances have moved toward early endovascular coiling of the ruptured aneurysm in most cases, based on 2 RCTs. Following securing of the aneurysm, there is evidence that patients are best served at centers employing multidisciplinary teams with specialized training in neurocritical care. The critical care management of the SAH patient is essential for treatment and mitigation of complications, in particular, a syndrome of delayed neurologic decline. Further study is essential for optimizing the acute care and improving outcomes in patients with aneurysmal SAH.

CLINICS CARE POINTS

Preaneurysm securing

- After the initial airway, breathing, and circulation assessments, the patient should be evaluated for symptomatic hydrocephalus or a clinical presentation concerning for elevated intracranial pressure (ie, high-grade SAH) and considered for an external ventricular drain.
- The patient should be evaluated by cerebral angiography for consideration for endovascular coiling versus open surgical clipping to secure the culprit aneurysm.
- When there is equipoise between securing the aneurysm with coiling versus clipping, more patients have better outcomes at 1 year after coiling compared with clipping.

Postaneurysm securing

- The patient should be monitored and treated for potential medical complications of subarachnoid hemorrhage.
- Delayed neurologic decline is a common occurrence after aneurysmal subarachnoid hemorrhage, typically arising day 5 to 12 after SAH. If clinically evident, this is termed delayed cerebral ischemia or symptomatic vasospasm.
- The tenets of medical therapy for the prevention and treatment of symptomatic cerebral vasospasm, or delayed cerebral ischemia, are nimodipine administration and euvolemia.
- Patients with persistent symptomatic vasospasm refractory to medical management should be considered for endovascular therapy with intra-arterial vasodilators or balloon angioplasty. This can be bridged with intravenous vasodilator infusion in the neurointensive care unit.

ACKNOWLEDGMENTS

Dr D.Y. Chung has received support from the National Institutes of Health (KL2TR002542 and K08NS112601), the American Heart Association and American

Stroke Association (18POST34030369), the Andrew David Heitman Foundation, the Brain Aneurysm Foundation's Timothy P. Susco and Andrew David Heitman Foundation Chairs of Research, and the Aneurysm and AVM Foundation. The authors thank Kazutaka Sugimoto, MD for helpful discussions regarding the treatment of SAH patients in Japan.

DISCLOSURES

Dr D.Y. Chung and Dr M. Abdalkader have no disclosures. Dr T.N. Nguyen is Principal Investigator of the CLEAR study (CT for Late Endovascular Reperfusion) funded by Medtronic and serves on the Data Safety Monitoring Board for TESLA (Thrombectomy for Emergent Salvage of Large Anterior Circulation Ischemic Stroke), ENDOLOW (Endovascular Therapy for Low NIHSS Ischemic Strokes), and SELECT 2 (a randomized controlled trial to optimize patient's selection for endovascular treatment in acute ischemic stroke), and CREST-2 trials.

REFERENCES

1. Bassi P, Bandera R, Loiero M, et al. Warning signs in subarachnoid hemorrhage: a cooperative study. Acta Neurol Scand 1991;84(4):277–81.
2. Rautalin I, Korja M. Transient intracranial circulatory arrest evidenced at the time of intracranial aneurysm rupture: case report. Neurocrit Care 2020. https://doi.org/10.1007/s12028-020-00948-w.
3. Hunt WE, Hess RM. Surgical risk as related to time of intervention in the repair of intracranial aneurysms. J Neurosurg 1968;28(1):14–20.
4. Teasdale GM, Drake CG, Hunt W, et al. A universal subarachnoid hemorrhage scale: report of a committee of the World Federation of Neurosurgical Societies. J Neurol Neurosurg Psychiatry 1988;51(11):1457.
5. Edlow JA, Malek AM, Ogilvy CS. Aneurysmal subarachnoid hemorrhage: update for emergency physicians. J Emerg Med 2008;34(3):237–51.
6. Perry JJ, Stiell IG, Sivilotti ML, et al. Sensitivity of computed tomography performed within six hours of onset of headache for diagnosis of subarachnoid haemorrhage: prospective cohort study. BMJ 2011;343:d4277.
7. Backes D, Rinkel GJ, Kemperman H, et al. Time-dependent test characteristics of head computed tomography in patients suspected of nontraumatic subarachnoid hemorrhage. Stroke 2012;43(8):2115–9.
8. Blok KM, Rinkel GJ, Majoie CB, et al. CT within 6 hours of headache onset to rule out subarachnoid hemorrhage in nonacademic hospitals. Neurology 2015; 84(19):1927–32.
9. Edlow JA, Fisher J. Diagnosis of subarachnoid hemorrhage: time to change the guidelines? Stroke 2012;43(8):2031–2.
10. Dubosh NM, Bellolio MF, Rabinstein AA, et al. Sensitivity of early brain computed tomography to exclude aneurysmal subarachnoid hemorrhage: a systematic review and meta-analysis. Stroke 2016;47(3):750–5.
11. Kallmes DF, Layton K, Marx WF, et al. Death by nondiagnosis: why emergent CT angiography should not be done for patients with subarachnoid hemorrhage. AJNR Am J Neuroradiol 2007;28(10):1837–8.
12. Westerlaan HE, Eshghi S, Oudkerk M, et al. Re: Death by nondiagnosis: why emergent CT angiography should not be done for patients with subarachnoid hemorrhage. AJNR Am J Neuroradiol 2008;29(6):e43, author reply e46–47.

13. Heit JJ, Pastena GT, Nogueira RG, et al. Cerebral angiography for evaluation of patients with CT angiogram-negative subarachnoid hemorrhage: an 11-year experience. AJNR Am J Neuroradiol 2016;37(2):297–304.

14. Anderson CS, Heeley E, Huang Y, et al. Rapid blood-pressure lowering in patients with acute intracerebral hemorrhage. N Engl J Med 2013;368(25): 2355–65.

15. Qureshi AI, Palesch YY, Barsan WG, et al. Intensive blood-pressure lowering in patients with acute cerebral hemorrhage. N Engl J Med 2016;375(11):1033–43.

16. Kusske JA, Turner PT, Ojemann GA, et al. Ventriculostomy for the treatment of acute hydrocephalus following subarachnoid hemorrhage. J Neurosurg 1973; 38(5):591–5.

17. McKinney JS, Cheng JQ, Rybinnik I, et al. Myocardial infarction data acquisition system study G. Comprehensive stroke centers may be associated with improved survival in hemorrhagic stroke. J Am Heart Assoc 2015;4(5):e001448.

18. Naidech AM, Kreiter KT, Janjua N, et al. Phenytoin exposure is associated with functional and cognitive disability after subarachnoid hemorrhage. Stroke 2005; 36(3):583–7.

19. Eskey CJ, Meyers PM, Nguyen TN, et al. Indications for the performance of intracranial endovascular neurointerventional procedures: a scientific statement from the American Heart Association. Circulation 2018;137(21):e661–89.

20. Molyneux AJ, Kerr RS, Yu LM, et al. International Subarachnoid Aneurysm Trial (ISAT) of neurosurgical clipping versus endovascular coiling in 2143 patients with ruptured intracranial aneurysms: a randomised comparison of effects on survival, dependency, seizures, rebleeding, subgroups, and aneurysm occlusion. Lancet 2005;366(9488):809–17.

21. Darsaut TE, Findlay JM, Magro E, et al. Surgical clipping or endovascular coiling for unruptured intracranial aneurysms: a pragmatic randomised trial. J Neurol Neurosurg Psychiatry 2017;88(8):663–8.

22. McDougall CG, Spetzler RF, Zabramski JM, et al. The barrow ruptured aneurysm trial. J Neurosurg 2012;116(1):135–44.

23. Gross BA, Rosalind Lai PM, Frerichs KU, et al. Treatment modality and vasospasm after aneurysmal subarachnoid hemorrhage. World Neurosurg 2014; 82(6):e725–30.

24. Connolly ES Jr, Rabinstein AA, Carhuapoma JR, et al. Guidelines for the management of aneurysmal subarachnoid hemorrhage: a guideline for healthcare professionals from the American Heart Association/American Stroke Association. Stroke 2012;43(6):1711–37.

25. Kallmes DF, Hanel R, Lopes D, et al. International retrospective study of the pipeline embolization device: a multicenter aneurysm treatment study. AJNR Am J Neuroradiol 2015;36(1):108–15.

26. Arthur AS, Molyneux A, Coon AL, et al. The safety and effectiveness of the Woven EndoBridge (WEB) system for the treatment of wide-necked bifurcation aneurysms: final 12-month results of the pivotal WEB Intrasaccular Therapy (WEB-IT) Study. J Neurointerv Surg 2019;11(9):924–30.

27. Rosenorn J, Eskesen V, Schmidt K, et al. The risk of rebleeding from ruptured intracranial aneurysms. J Neurosurg 1987;67(3):329–32.

28. Eskesen V, Rosenorn J, Schmidt K. The impact of rebleeding on the life time probabilities of different outcomes in patients with ruptured intracranial aneurysms. A theoretical evaluation. Acta Neurochir (Wien) 1988;95(3–4):99–101.

29. Kassell NF, Torner JC. Aneurysmal rebleeding: a preliminary report from the cooperative aneurysm study. Neurosurgery 1983;13(5):479–81.

30. Winn HR, Richardson AE, Jane JA. The long-term prognosis in untreated cerebral aneurysms: I. The incidence of late hemorrhage in cerebral aneurysm: a 10-year evaluation of 364 patients. Ann Neurol 1977;1(4):358–70.

31. Park J, Woo H, Kang DH, et al. Formal protocol for emergency treatment of ruptured intracranial aneurysms to reduce in-hospital rebleeding and improve clinical outcomes. J Neurosurg 2015;122(2):383–91.

32. Linzey JR, Williamson C, Rajajee V, et al. Twenty-four-hour emergency intervention versus early intervention in aneurysmal subarachnoid hemorrhage. J Neurosurg 2018;128(5):1297–303.

33. collaborators C-t, Shakur H, Roberts I, et al. Effects of tranexamic acid on death, vascular occlusive events, and blood transfusion in trauma patients with significant haemorrhage (CRASH-2): a randomised, placebo-controlled trial. Lancet 2010;376(9734):23–32.

34. collaborators C-, Roberts I, Shakur H, et al. The importance of early treatment with tranexamic acid in bleeding trauma patients: an exploratory analysis of the CRASH-2 randomised controlled trial. Lancet 2011;377(9771):1096–101, 1101 e1091-1092.

35. collaborators C-t. Effects of tranexamic acid on death, disability, vascular occlusive events and other morbidities in patients with acute traumatic brain injury (CRASH-3): a randomised, placebo-controlled trial. Lancet 2019;394(10210): 1713–23.

36. Post R, Germans MR, Tjerkstra MA, et al. Ultra-early tranexamic acid after subarachnoid haemorrhage (ULTRA): a randomised controlled trial. Lancet 2021; 397(10269):112–8.

37. Abdalkader M, Samuelsen BT, Moore JM, et al. Ruptured spinal aneurysms: diagnosis and management paradigms. World Neurosurg 2020. https://doi.org/10.1016/j.wneu.2020.10.098.

38. Samuels O, Webb A, Culler S, et al. Impact of a dedicated neurocritical care team in treating patients with aneurysmal subarachnoid hemorrhage. Neurocrit Care 2011;14(3):334–40.

39. Diringer MN, Bleck TP, Claude Hemphill J 3rd, et al. Critical care management of patients following aneurysmal subarachnoid hemorrhage: recommendations from the neurocritical care society's multidisciplinary consensus conference. Neurocrit Care 2011;15(2):211–40.

40. Nornes H. The role of intracranial pressure in the arrest of hemorrhage in patients with ruptured intracranial aneurysm. J Neurosurg 1973;39(2):226–34.

41. Chung DY, Olson DM, John S, et al. Evidence-based management of external ventricular drains. Curr Neurol Neurosci Rep 2019;19(12):94.

42. Nguyen TN, Jadhav AP, Dasenbrock HH, et al. Subarachnoid hemorrhage guidance in the era of the COVID-19 pandemic - an opinion to mitigate exposure and conserve personal protective equipment. J Stroke Cerebrovasc Dis 2020;29(9): 105010.

43. Ibrahim MS, Samuel B, Mohamed W, et al. Cardiac dysfunction in neurocritical care: an autonomic perspective. Neurocrit Care 2019;30(3):508–21.

44. Samuels MA. The brain-heart connection. Circulation 2007;116(1):77–84.

45. Medina de Chazal H, Del Buono MG, Keyser-Marcus L, et al. Stress cardiomyopathy diagnosis and treatment: JACC state-of-the-art review. J Am Coll Cardiol 2018;72(16):1955–71.

46. Davison DL, Terek M, Chawla LS. Neurogenic pulmonary edema. Crit Care 2012;16(2):212.

47. Vespa PM, Bleck TP. Neurogenic pulmonary edema and other mechanisms of impaired oxygenation after aneurysmal subarachnoid hemorrhage. Neurocrit Care 2004;1(2):157–70.

48. Fan E, Brodie D, Slutsky AS. Acute respiratory distress syndrome: advances in diagnosis and treatment. JAMA 2018;319(7):698–710.

49. Yee AH, Burns JD, Wijdicks EF. Cerebral salt wasting: pathophysiology, diagnosis, and treatment. Neurosurg Clin N Am 2010;21(2):339–52.

50. Hannon MJ, Behan LA, O'Brien MM, et al. Hyponatremia following mild/moderate subarachnoid hemorrhage is due to SIAD and glucocorticoid deficiency and not cerebral salt wasting. J Clin Endocrinol Metab 2014;99(1):291–8.

51. Marik PE, Cavallazzi R. Does the central venous pressure predict fluid responsiveness? An updated meta-analysis and a plea for some common sense. Crit Care Med 2013;41(7):1774–81.

52. Rass V, Gaasch M, Kofler M, et al. Fluid intake but not fluid balance is associated with poor outcome in nontraumatic subarachnoid hemorrhage patients. Crit Care Med 2019;47(7):e555–62.

53. Shah K, Turgeon RD, Gooderham PA, et al. Prevention and treatment of hyponatremia in patients with subarachnoid hemorrhage: a systematic review. World Neurosurg 2018;109:222–9.

54. Rabinstein AA, Sandhu K. Non-infectious fever in the neurological intensive care unit: incidence, causes and predictors. J Neurol Neurosurg Psychiatry 2007;78(11):1278–80.

55. Fernandez A, Schmidt JM, Claassen J, et al. Fever after subarachnoid hemorrhage: risk factors and impact on outcome. Neurology 2007;68(13):1013–9.

56. Badjatia N, Fernandez L, Schmidt JM, et al. Impact of induced normothermia on outcome after subarachnoid hemorrhage: a case-control study. Neurosurgery 2010;66(4):696–700 [discussion 700–691].

57. Greer DM, Funk SE, Reaven NL, et al. Impact of fever on outcome in patients with stroke and neurologic injury: a comprehensive meta-analysis. Stroke 2008;39(11):3029–35.

58. Drewry AM, Ablordeppey EA, Murray ET, et al. Antipyretic therapy in critically ill septic patients: a systematic review and meta-analysis. Crit Care Med 2017;45(5):806–13.

59. Choi HA, Ko SB, Presciutti M, et al. Prevention of shivering during therapeutic temperature modulation: the Columbia anti-shivering protocol. Neurocrit Care 2011;14(3):389–94.

60. Young PJ, Prescott HC. When less is more in the active management of elevated body temperature of ICU patients. Intensive Care Med 2019;45(9):1275–8.

61. Marehbian J, Greer DM. Normothermia and stroke. Curr Treat Options Neurol 2017;19(1):4.

62. Macdonald RL. Delayed neurological deterioration after subarachnoid haemorrhage. Nat Rev Neurol 2014;10(1):44–58.

63. Vergouwen MD, Vermeulen M, van Gijn J, et al. Definition of delayed cerebral ischemia after aneurysmal subarachnoid hemorrhage as an outcome event in clinical trials and observational studies: proposal of a multidisciplinary research group. Stroke 2010;41(10):2391–5.

64. Kramer A, Fletcher J. Do endothelin-receptor antagonists prevent delayed neurological deficits and poor outcomes after aneurysmal subarachnoid hemorrhage?: a meta-analysis. Stroke 2009;40(10):3403–6.

65. Zafar SF, Westover MB, Gaspard N, et al. Interrater agreement for consensus definitions of delayed ischemic events after aneurysmal subarachnoid hemorrhage. J Clin Neurophysiol 2016;33(3):235–40.
66. Frontera JA, Fernandez A, Schmidt JM, et al. Defining vasospasm after subarachnoid hemorrhage: what is the most clinically relevant definition? Stroke 2009;40(6):1963–8.
67. Fisher CM, Roberson GH, Ojemann RG. Cerebral vasospasm with ruptured saccular aneurysm–the clinical manifestations. Neurosurgery 1977;1(3):245–8.
68. Allen GS, Ahn HS, Preziosi TJ, et al. Cerebral arterial spasm–a controlled trial of nimodipine in patients with subarachnoid hemorrhage. N Engl J Med 1983; 308(11):619–24.
69. Pickard JD, Murray GD, Illingworth R, et al. Effect of oral nimodipine on cerebral infarction and outcome after subarachnoid haemorrhage: British aneurysm nimodipine trial. BMJ 1989;298(6674):636–42.
70. Shibuya M, Suzuki Y, Sugita K, et al. Effect of AT877 on cerebral vasospasm after aneurysmal subarachnoid hemorrhage. Results of a prospective placebo-controlled double-blind trial. J Neurosurg 1992;76(4):571–7.
71. Suzuki Y, Shibuya M, Satoh S, et al. A postmarketing surveillance study of fasudil treatment after aneurysmal subarachnoid hemorrhage. Surg Neurol 2007; 68(2):126–31 [discussion 131–22].
72. Zhao J, Zhou D, Guo J, et al. Efficacy and safety of fasudil in patients with subarachnoid hemorrhage: final results of a randomized trial of fasudil versus nimodipine. Neurol Med Chir (Tokyo) 2011;51(10):679–83.
73. Sugimoto K, Nomura S, Shirao S, et al. Cilostazol decreases duration of spreading depolarization and spreading ischemia after aneurysmal subarachnoid hemorrhage. Ann Neurol 2018;84(6):873–85.
74. Muehlschlegel S. Subarachnoid hemorrhage. Continuum (Minneap Minn) 2018; 24(6):1623–57.
75. Malinova V, Dolatowski K, Schramm P, et al. Early whole-brain CT perfusion for detection of patients at risk for delayed cerebral ischemia after subarachnoid hemorrhage. J Neurosurg 2016;125(1):128–36.
76. Nelson S, Edlow BL, Wu O, et al. Default mode network perfusion in aneurysmal subarachnoid hemorrhage. Neurocrit Care 2016;25(2):237–42.
77. Selb J, Wu KC, Sutin J, et al. Prolonged monitoring of cerebral blood flow and autoregulation with diffuse correlation spectroscopy in neurocritical care patients. Neurophotonics 2018;5(4):045005.
78. Hanggi D. Participants in the International Multi-disciplinary Consensus Conference on the critical care management of subarachnoid H. Monitoring and detection of vasospasm II: EEG and invasive monitoring. Neurocrit Care 2011;15(2): 318–23.
79. Sen J, Belli A, Albon H, et al. Triple-H therapy in the management of aneurysmal subarachnoid haemorrhage. Lancet Neurol 2003;2(10):614–21.
80. Gathier CS, van den Bergh WM, van der Jagt M, et al. Induced hypertension for delayed cerebral ischemia after aneurysmal subarachnoid hemorrhage: a randomized clinical trial. Stroke 2018;49(1):76–83.
81. Paulson OB, Strandgaard S, Edvinsson L. Cerebral autoregulation. Cerebrovasc Brain Metab Rev 1990;2(2):161–92.
82. Francoeur CL, Mayer SA. Management of delayed cerebral ischemia after subarachnoid hemorrhage. Crit Care 2016;20(1):277.

83. Lannes M, Teitelbaum J, del Pilar Cortes M, et al. Milrinone and homeostasis to treat cerebral vasospasm associated with subarachnoid hemorrhage: the Montreal Neurological Hospital Protocol. Neurocrit Care 2012;16(3):354–62.

84. Abulhasan YB, Ortiz Jimenez J, Teitelbaum J, et al. Milrinone for refractory cerebral vasospasm with delayed cerebral ischemia. J Neurosurg 2020;1–12. https://doi.org/10.3171/2020.1.JNS193107.

85. Bernier TD, Schontz MJ, Izzy S, et al. Treatment of subarachnoid hemorrhage-associated delayed cerebral ischemia with milrinone: a review and proposal. J Neurosurg Anesthesiol 2021. https://doi.org/10.1097/ANA. 0000000000000755.

86. Kassell NF, Peerless SJ, Durward QJ, et al. Treatment of ischemic deficits from vasospasm with intravascular volume expansion and induced arterial hypertension. Neurosurgery 1982;11(3):337–43.

87. Lennihan L, Mayer SA, Fink ME, et al. Effect of hypervolemic therapy on cerebral blood flow after subarachnoid hemorrhage: a randomized controlled trial. Stroke 2000;31(2):383–91.

88. Dhar R, Scalfani MT, Zazulia AR, et al. Comparison of induced hypertension, fluid bolus, and blood transfusion to augment cerebral oxygen delivery after subarachnoid hemorrhage. J Neurosurg 2012;116(3):648–56.

89. Kumar MA, Boland TA, Baiou M, et al. Red blood cell transfusion increases the risk of thrombotic events in patients with subarachnoid hemorrhage. Neurocrit Care 2014;20(1):84–90.

90. Raya AK, Diringer MN. Treatment of subarachnoid hemorrhage. Crit Care Clin 2014;30(4):719–33.

91. Ogilvy CS, Carter BS, Kaplan S, et al. Temporary vessel occlusion for aneurysm surgery: risk factors for stroke in patients protected by induced hypothermia and hypertension and intravenous mannitol administration. J Neurosurg 1996; 84(5):785–91.

92. Suzuki J, Fujimoto S, Mizoi K, et al. The protective effect of combined administration of anti-oxidants and perfluorochemicals on cerebral ischemia. Stroke 1984;15(4):672–9.

93. Jafar JJ, Johns LM, Mullan SF. The effect of mannitol on cerebral blood flow. J Neurosurg 1986;64(5):754–9.

94. Maher M, Schweizer TA, Macdonald RL. Treatment of spontaneous subarachnoid hemorrhage: guidelines and gaps. Stroke 2020;51(4):1326–32.

95. Sugimoto K, Chung DY. Spreading depolarizations and subarachnoid hemorrhage. Neurotherapeutics 2020;17(2):497–510.

96. Goto S. Cilostazol: potential mechanism of action for antithrombotic effects accompanied by a low rate of bleeding. Atheroscler Suppl 2005;6(4):3–11.

97. Matsuda N, Naraoka M, Ohkuma H, et al. Effect of cilostazol on cerebral vasospasm and outcome in patients with aneurysmal subarachnoid hemorrhage: a randomized, double-blind, placebo-controlled trial. Cerebrovasc Dis 2016; 42(1–2):97–105.

98. Dreier JP. The role of spreading depression, spreading depolarization and spreading ischemia in neurological disease. Nat Med 2011;17(4):439–47.

99. Chung DY, Oka F, Ayata C. Spreading depolarizations: a therapeutic target against delayed cerebral ischemia after subarachnoid hemorrhage. J Clin Neurophysiol 2016;33(3):196–202.

100. Chung DY, Ayata C. Spreading Depolarizations. In: Caplan LR, Biller J, Leary MC, et al, editors. Primer on Cerebrovascular Diseases, Second Edition. San Diego: Academic Press; 2017. p. 149–53.

101. Oka F, Chung DY, Suzuki M, et al. Delayed cerebral ischemia after subarachnoid hemorrhage: experimental-clinical disconnect and the unmet need. Neurocrit Care 2019. https://doi.org/10.1007/s12028-018-0650-5.
102. Macdonald RL, Higashida RT, Keller E, et al. Clazosentan, an endothelin receptor antagonist, in patients with aneurysmal subarachnoid haemorrhage undergoing surgical clipping: a randomised, double-blind, placebo-controlled phase 3 trial (CONSCIOUS-2). Lancet Neurol 2011;10(7):618–25.
103. Macdonald RL, Higashida RT, Keller E, et al. Randomized trial of clazosentan in patients with aneurysmal subarachnoid hemorrhage undergoing endovascular coiling. Stroke 2012;43(6):1463–9.
104. Fisher CM, Kistler JP, Davis JM. Relation of cerebral vasospasm to subarachnoid hemorrhage visualized by computerized tomographic scanning. Neurosurgery 1980;6(1):1–9.
105. Frontera JA, Claassen J, Schmidt JM, et al. Prediction of symptomatic vasospasm after subarachnoid hemorrhage: the modified Fisher scale. Neurosurgery 2006;59(1):21–7 [discussion 21–7].
106. Claassen J, Bernardini GL, Kreiter K, et al. Effect of cisternal and ventricular blood on risk of delayed cerebral ischemia after subarachnoid hemorrhage: the Fisher scale revisited. Stroke 2001;32(9):2012–20.
107. Melinosky C, Kincaid H, Claassen J, et al. The modified Fisher scale lacks interrater reliability. Neurocrit Care 2020. https://doi.org/10.1007/s12028-020-01142-8.
108. Hijdra A, Brouwers PJ, Vermeulen M, et al. Grading the amount of blood on computed tomograms after subarachnoid hemorrhage. Stroke 1990;21(8):1156–61.
109. Otite F, Mink S, Tan CO, et al. Impaired cerebral autoregulation is associated with vasospasm and delayed cerebral ischemia in subarachnoid hemorrhage. Stroke 2014;45(3):677–82.
110. Kim JA, Rosenthal ES, Biswal S, et al. Epileptiform abnormalities predict delayed cerebral ischemia in subarachnoid hemorrhage. Clin Neurophysiol 2017;128(6):1091–9.
111. Rosenthal ES, Biswal S, Zafar SF, et al. Continuous electroencephalography predicts delayed cerebral ischemia after subarachnoid hemorrhage: a prospective study of diagnostic accuracy. Ann Neurol 2018;83(5):958–69.
112. Takase H, Chou SH, Hamanaka G, et al. Soluble vascular endothelial-cadherin in CSF after subarachnoid hemorrhage. Neurology 2020;94(12):e1281–93.
113. Lissak IA, Zafar SF, Westover MB, et al. Soluble ST2 is associated with new epileptiform abnormalities following nontraumatic subarachnoid hemorrhage. Stroke 2020;51(4):1128–34.
114. Savarraj JP, Hergenroeder GW, Zhu L, et al. Machine learning to predict delayed cerebral ischemia and outcomes in subarachnoid hemorrhage. Neurology 2020. https://doi.org/10.1212/WNL.0000000000011211.
115. Claassen J, Mayer SA, Kowalski RG, et al. Detection of electrographic seizures with continuous EEG monitoring in critically ill patients. Neurology 2004;62(10):1743–8.
116. Shafi MM, Westover MB, Cole AJ, et al. Absence of early epileptiform abnormalities predicts lack of seizures on continuous EEG. Neurology 2012;79(17):1796–801.
117. Rhoney DH, Tipps LB, Murry KR, et al. Anticonvulsant prophylaxis and timing of seizures after aneurysmal subarachnoid hemorrhage. Neurology 2000;55(2):258–65.

118. Olson DM, Zomorodi M, Britz GW, et al. Continuous cerebral spinal fluid drainage associated with complications in patients admitted with subarachnoid hemorrhage. J Neurosurg 2013;119(4):974–80.

119. Rao SS, Chung DY, Wolcott Z, et al. Intermittent CSF drainage and rapid EVD weaning approach after subarachnoid hemorrhage: association with fewer VP shunts and shorter length of stay. J Neurosurg 2019;132(5):1–6.

120. Olson DM, Batjer HH, Abdulkadir K, et al. Measuring and monitoring ICP in neurocritical care: results from a national practice survey. Neurocrit Care 2014; 20(1):15–20.

121. Chung DY, Leslie-Mazwi TM, Patel AB, et al. Management of external ventricular drains after subarachnoid hemorrhage: a multi-institutional survey. Neurocrit Care 2016. https://doi.org/10.1007/s12028-016-0352-9.

122. Klimo P Jr, Kestle JR, MacDonald JD, et al. Marked reduction of cerebral vasospasm with lumbar drainage of cerebrospinal fluid after subarachnoid hemorrhage. J Neurosurg 2004;100(2):215–24.

123. Chung DY, Mayer SA, Rordorf GA. External ventricular drains after subarachnoid hemorrhage: is less more? Neurocrit Care 2018;28(2):157–61.

124. Klopfenstein JD, Kim LJ, Feiz-Erfan I, et al. Comparison of rapid and gradual weaning from external ventricular drainage in patients with aneurysmal subarachnoid hemorrhage: a prospective randomized trial. J Neurosurg 2004; 100(2):225–9.

Blunt and Penetrating Severe Traumatic Brain Injury

Courtney E. Takahashi, MD, MCR[a],*, Deepti Virmani, MD[b],
David Y. Chung, MD, PhD[b,c,d], Charlene Ong, MD, MPHS[b],
Anna M. Cervantes-Arslanian, MD[e]

KEYWORDS

- Severe traumatic brain injury • Penetrating brain injury • Intensive care management
- Review article • Summary

KEY POINTS

- Early resuscitation, initiated the moment that first responders arrive and continued into the trauma bay, is important to patient outcomes and survival.
- Intensive care treatment includes seizure prophylaxis, antibiotic stewardship, and evaluating patients for invasive monitor placement.
- External ventricular drains and intraparenchymal tissue monitors may be used to measure intracranial pressure and monitor for crises in severe traumatic brain injury (sTBI).
- Brain tissue oxygenation monitors and cerebromicrodialysis provide ways to directly monitor intraparenchymal oxygen pressures and the surrounding molecular environment.
- Serial transcranial Doppler velocities, optic nerve sheath diameter, pupillometry, cerebral oximetry, and diffuse correlation spectroscopy are novel tools that may advance the ability to care for sTBI patients.

INTRODUCTION

Traumatic brain injury (TBI) is a common problem worldwide, with 69 million people affected annually.[1] Severe TBI (sTBI) is defined as TBI with Glasgow Coma Scale (GCS) score less than or equal to 8.[2] Although sTBI only represents 4% to 5% of all TBI patients, these cases require expert care and often have prolonged

[a] Department of Neurology, Boston Medical Center, 72 East Concord Street, Collamore, C-3, Boston, MA 02118, USA; [b] Department of Neurology, Boston University School of Medicine and Boston Medical Center, 72 East Concord Street, Collamore, C-3, Boston, MA 02118, USA; [c] Division of Neurocritical Care, Department of Neurology, Harvard Medical School, Massachusetts General Hospital, Boston, MA, USA; [d] Neurovascular Research Unit, Department of Radiology, Harvard Medical School, Massachusetts General Hospital, Boston, MA, USA; [e] Boston University School of Medicine and Boston Medical Center, 72 East Concord Street, Collamore, C-3, Boston, MA 02118, USA
* Corresponding author.
E-mail address: Courtney.takahashi@bmc.org

Neurol Clin 39 (2021) 443–469
https://doi.org/10.1016/j.ncl.2021.02.009
0733-8619/21/© 2021 Elsevier Inc. All rights reserved.

hospitalizations.[1,3] Favorable functional recovery (ie, community reintegration and high scores on functional independence scales) is possible for a majority (70%–80%) of patients[4]; however, it requires experienced hospital providers and intensive rehabilitation.[5]

Penetrating brain injury (PBI) is a subset of patients with sTBI, with distinct needs due to retained foreign bodies, tissue maceration, and thermal burn due to kinetic energy transfer. PBI patients have much higher mortality, with 85% to 90% of patients dying before reaching a hospital. The majority of PBI is the result of gunshot wounds.[6] Due to the mechanism of injury, PBI patients may suffer from specific complications, such as meningitis and vascular injuries.

Advances in prehospital management, surgical approaches, and neuromonitoring offer new opportunities to improve patient outcomes. This article reviews contemporary prehospital and intensive care management strategies and their applications.

PART 1: PREHOSPITAL MANAGEMENT
Airway, Oxygenation, and Ventilation

Many sTBI patients require an airway device or intubation because they are unable to protect their airway due to neurologic injury.[7] There is no standard approach, however, to intubation in the field by emergency medical services (EMS), and practice usually is dictated by regional hospital protocols.[7] For example, in some geographic regions, orotracheal intubation is performed only in the field in comatose patients without a gag reflex and neither induction agents nor neuromuscular blockade is administered,[8] whereas other regions have rapid sequence intubation protocols and/or use neuromuscular blockade.[9,10] In patients with suspected cervical spine injury, direct laryngoscopy with manual in-line stabilization is a commonly adapted approach to intubation, although supporting evidence quality is low.[11] Selecting patients for in-field intubation can be challenging because data on patient outcomes are conflicting. In several studies, patients with GCS score less than or equal to 8 are more likely to survive if they are intubated by EMS prior to hospital arrival.[8] Yet, failed intubation attempts result in higher mortality.[12] It may be that failed attempts delay access to hospital care sooner, affecting patient outcomes. Overall, the data suggest that if intubation can be performed quickly, they may improve patient outcomes.

Brain Trauma Foundation (BTF) guidelines emphasize the importance of maintaining adequate perfusion and oxygen delivery to the injured brain. Maintenance of oxygen saturation as measured by pulse oximetry (Spo_2) greater than 90% is associated with lower morbidity and mortality.[13] Additionally, normocarbia (Pco_2 35–45 mm Hg) is desirable for most patients because it maintains normal cerebral artery diameter and, therefore, normal cerebral perfusion.[14,15] There is a tendency to over-ventilate sTBI patients, which is associated with increased mortality.[16] Hence, there is no role for preventive hyperventilation and it should be reserved for herniation crises.[17]

In summary, if intubation can be performed quickly, it should be completed in the field. Every effort should be made to maintain Spo_2 greater than 90% and normocarbia.

Circulation

Hypotension is an independent risk factor for mortality.[18] Intravenous fluid administration in the prehospital setting is encouraged. Systolic blood pressure (SBP) greater than 110 is recommended for patients aged 15 to 49 and over 70, whereas SBP greater than 100 is recommended for patients aged 50 to 69.[19,20] Although the SBP goal is supported by guidelines, there are emerging data that blood pressure goals may be dynamic. Currently, this is an active area of development.

In the future, instead of focusing on SBP, newer data may target optimal cerebral perfusion pressure (CPP). Instead of a population-based target (eg, CPP 50–70 mm Hg), optimized CPP focuses on an individuals' perfusion through a pressure-reactivity index (PRx). PRx is the correlation coefficient between intracranial pressure (ICP) and arterial pressure readings. When PRx is compared with spontaneous fluctuations in CPP over time, it forms a U-shaped curve. When PRx on this curve is minimized, CPP is optimized.[21] A CPP consistently at or higher than the optimal value is an independent predictor of good functional outcomes and higher GCS in 1 study.[22] Despite initial promising results, the association was absent in larger, prospective studies evaluating Extended Glasgow Outcome Scale scores at 6 months and 12 months.[23] Current guidelines for targeted CPP management are vague. The BTF recommends monitoring of CPP to decrease 2-week mortality.[20] The Trauma Quality Improvement Program (TQIP) recommends maintaining CPP at greater than or equal to 60 mm Hg.[24] Given the controversial results in the current literature, dynamic CPP goal targets may be a future intervention with more supporting data. For now, there is insufficient evidence to recommend a specific mean arterial pressure (MAP) or CPP target during early resuscitation because the association is inconsistent.

Isotonic fluids are first-line treatment of hypotension, followed by vasopressors.[25] Although resuscitation with any isotonic fluid is better than none,[26] there are insufficient data to recommend a specific fluid. Studies evaluating resuscitation with hypertonic saline show an increase osmolarity but no effect on mortality.[25] Despite the purported volume expanding effects of albumin, when compared with saline, post hoc analyses reported increased mortality in albumin-treated sTBI patients.[27] Larger studies of hemorrhagic shock in general trauma patients (sTBI inclusive but not the target population) have shown some beneficial effects of 1:1:1 transfusions of platelets, plasma, and blood but the primary outcomes were not focused on neurologic performance.[28] A retrospective trial specifically evaluating blood product resuscitation in sTBI found lower mortality rates in patients with high fresh frozen plasma–to–packed red blood cell ratio tranfusions.[29] Although the retrospective data are encouraging, additional prospective studies need to be completed before a specific fluid can be recommended.

If fluid resuscitation alone does not achieve SBP greater than or equal to 90 mm Hg, a vasopressor should be started. In a randomized controlled trial in general trauma patients, vasopressin decreased the number of blood product transfusions needed in the setting of shock but did not alter requirement for crystalloids or impact mortality.[30] A retrospective single-center study of pediatric TBI looked at effects of specific single vasopressors (phenylephrine, norepinephrine, epinephrine, and dopamine) on MAP and CPP at 3 hours postinjury and found no statistically significant difference between vasopressors but a trend toward increased CPP and lower ICP with norepinephrine.[31] Another single-center retrospective study in adults, however, showed higher MAPs with phenylephrine use than dopamine and higher CPP than with norepinephrine 3 hours after vasopressor start.[32]

All considered, initial expeditious fluid resuscitation is strongly encouraged. Isotonic fluids (eg, normal saline or balanced crystalloids) or blood products in a 1:1 ratio are recommended. Data on vasopressor selection for hemorrhagic shock in TBI are inconclusive but it is the authors' preference to use norepinephrine for its beneficial effects on cardiac output and limited data supporting improved CPP.

Transport

After initial stabilization, EMS should triage patient to a high volume (>40 sTBI cases/year), level 1 trauma center. Level 1 trauma designation means that these centers have

24-hour specialist coverage (including orthopedics, neurosurgery, radiology, anesthesiology, and critical care), patient education resources, provider educational requirements, and a referral basis from other hospitals and meet minimum case number requirements annually.[33] Studies have demonstrated that sTBI patients admitted to level 1 trauma centers have better functional outcomes.[34,35]

If patients cannot be safely transported to a level 1 center because of distance, they may be stabilized in a level 2 or level 3 center and transferred later to a level 1 center after initial stabilization. Non–level 1 centers with head computerized tomography (HCT) capability and airway support are preferred.[36] Hospitals should jointly create transfer protocols with EMS to predetermine transfer routes and plans because protocol-driven care is associated with higher rates of survival to hospital admission.[37]

PART 2: EMERGENCY DEPARTMENT/TRAUMA BAY MANAGEMENT

Upon hospital arrival, respiratory management, circulatory support, and intravenous fluid resuscitation should continue. During the period of immediate stabilization, intracranial imaging also should be obtained. Early collaboration between trauma/surgical critical care, emergency medicine, neurosurgery, and neurocritical care is essential.

Empiric Use of Hyperosmolar Therapy

During the initial neurologic evaluation, providers may find evidence of herniation or elevated ICP. These include headache, nausea, vomiting, and encephalopathy in early stages. Later signs include sixth nerve palsy, third nerve palsy (initial anisocoria that progresses to a fully dilated pupil), bradycardia, hypertension and irregular respirations (Cushing triad).[38] Papilledema, a classic marker of elevated ICP, may not develop early on and is present in only 3.5% of all sTBI patients.[39] In particular, signs, such as GCS score less than 4 and anisocoria, justify immediate treatment with hyperosmolar therapy without imaging studies.[40] In patients without signs of clear herniation or ICP crisis, there are fewer data to support empiric treatment. Studies comparing mannitol and hypertonic saline are compared and have not shown differences in mortality, ICP, or functional outcomes.[41] Because many sTBI patients arrive in hypovolemic shock (eg, hemorrhagic shock), urgent hypertonic saline administration serves dually as fluid resuscitation and cerebral edema treatment. In contrast, mannitol could be chosen in the less frequent context of a volume overloaded patient. Overall, providers should feel empowered to treat initial signs of elevated ICP aggressively, based on examination, with hyperosmolar agents chosen based on practical considerations, such as intravenous access, overall volume status, and known comorbidities. There is not enough evidence however, to recommend a prophylactic approach to ICP management besides attempts to maintain normal physiology (eg, euvolemia, euthermia, perfusing blood pressure, and euglycemia).

Computerized Tomography of the Head

In sTBI, HCT often is the first imaging evaluation because it is widely available, fast, and sensitive for identifying blood.[42] HCT readily identifies common patterns associated with sTBI.

- Epidural hematomas are collections of blood in the potential space between the dura mater and the inner table of the skull[43] (**Box 1**). Typically, if an epidural hematoma meets the following characteristics—volume less than 30 mL, clot diameter less than 15 mm, and midline shift less than 5 mm—then it may be managed conservatively with close observation. If a patient develops a GCS

Box 1
Modified Denver criteria for screening blunt cerebrovascular injury

Signs and symptoms

- Arterial hemorrhage
- Cervical bruit
- Expanding cervical hematoma
- Focal neurologic deficit
- Neurologic examination incongruous with HCT findings
- Ischemic stroke on HCT

Risk factors

- Le Fort II or III fracture
- Cervical spine fracture patterns: subluxation, fractures extending into transverse foramen of CI-3
- Basilar skull fracture with carotid canal involvement
- DAI with GCS $\leq$6
- Hanging or anoxic brain injury

---

score less than 8, focal neurologic signs, or progression on imaging, urgent evaluation for possible surgical intervention is indicated.[44,45]

- Subdural hematomas (SDHs) are collections of blood beneath the dura mater (**Box 2**). Among sTBI patients, 10% to 20% have an acute SDH.[46] If an SDH is causing less than 5 mm of midline shift and its greatest diameter is less than 10 mm, then usually it may be managed initially with observation as long as the patient lacks focal neurologic deficits attributable to the SDH.[47]

- Subarachnoid hemorrhage (SAH) results from damage to small cortical veins as they pass through the subarachnoid space[43] (**Box 3**). Although rare, the presence of SAH may lead to complications, such as vasospasm and hydrocephalus. Patients with large-volume SAH with extension into the basilar cisterns are at particularly high risk.[48]

- Cerebral contusions are the result of direct contact between the inner table of the skull and the brain parenchyma. The force from the contact causes capillary injury and edema, in turn damaging underlying tissue.[49] Cerebral contusions may progress because small capillary bleeds coalesce into intraparenchymal hematomas.

Box 2
Eastern Trauma Association: level 3 screening criteria for blunt cerebrovascular injury

- GCS less than or equal to 8
- Petrous bone fracture
- DAI
- Cervical spine fracture
- C spine fracture with subluxation or rotational component
- Le fort II or III fractures

Box 3
Descriptive summary of intracranial invasive monitoring devices

Monitor Type	Description
EVD	A temporary system that allows CSF to drain from the ventricles into a closed container outside the body. In sTBI, an EVD may be placed as a means to monitor ICP, shunt off CSF, treat hydrocephalus, and drain ventricular blood.[97] Depending on the region of the world, EVDs are used most commonly to treat hydrocephalus or for ICP monitoring.[91]
IPM	Pressure sensors placed into frontal brain parenchyma that measure ICP. Both EVDs and IPMs have the ability to measure ICP, but only an EVD has the ability to remove CSF.[98,99]
Invasive parenchymal catheter brain tissue oxygenation monitors	Monitors are similar to IPMs. They are equipped with sensors to measure $Pbto_2$.[100] Normal $Pbto_2$ range is documented as 20–35 mm Hg.[101]
CM	Artificial CSF dialysate runs through a catheter semipermeable membrane. The change along the concentration gradient is analyzed to determine the concentration of extracellular substrates. Commonly analyzed substrates include lactate, pyruvate, glucose, glutamate, and glycerol.

- PBI patients need urgent imaging to characterize the object trajectory, to visualize retained foreign object fragments, and to evaluate intracranial hemorrhages. The initial HCT helps to refine surgical needs and approach.[50,51]

Computerized Tomography Angiography

Computerized tomography angiography (CTA) is a highly accurate screening tool to detect cerebrovascular injuries, such as dissection or pseudoaneurysm.[52] Urgent acquisition is recommended in patients with any of the following signs or injury patterns:

- PBI patients have high rates of cerebrovascular injury (50%–75%), especially with transverse object trajectories.[53]
- Focal neurologic deficit or ischemic stroke can be signs of acute traumatic dissection. CTA of both head and neck may be indicated.[54]
- Arterial hemorrhage/cervical bruit/cervical hematoma all can be signs of direct arterial injury of the carotid artery. Delays in intervention can lead to airway compromise and uncontrolled hemorrhage.[54,55]

The Denver and Eastern Trauma Association have produced protocols to screen asymptomatic patients for blunt cerebrovascular injury based on other clinical findings (see **Boxes 1** and **2**). Research supports both a protocol-driven approach to asymptomatic patients[52] and broad screening for all TBI patients.[16,56] Both approaches are safe and report an approximately 9% rate of identifying asymptomatic injuries.

Magnetic Resonance Imaging

Although brain magnetic resonance imaging (MRI) often shows lesions missed on admission HCTs, its role in emergency settings is not well defined.[57] MRI is superior at detecting diffuse axonal injury (DAI), particularly in the brainstem, but detection of such injuries should not dictate early critical care interventions.[58] There is some association between DAI and outcomes; however, this relationship is not strong enough to change standard clinical care.[59] Factors, such as ICP crisis, that prevent supine positioning, retained metal fragments, and hemodynamic instability limit hyperacute MRI acquisition. Recent introduction of portable MRI scanners may allow for wider testing of the utility of acute-phase MRI.

Tranexamic Acid and Severe Traumatic Brain Injury

Expansion of intracranial hemorrhage may greatly worsen neurologic outcomes and increase mortality. This is seen in 30% of cases.[60] Thus, facilitating hemostasis with antifibrinolytic medications may be a way to prevent poor outcomes. Tranexemic acid (TXA) is a synthetic derivative of lysine that binds to plasminogen and stops plasmin formation on the fibrin surface, allowing for faster and more effective clot formation.[61] Although there were initial concerns that TXA would induce increased rates of thrombotic events, comparison studies demonstrated rates were no different between treatment and control groups.[62,63] Small trials showed blunted hematoma expansion with TXA.[64,65] Based on initially promising results, CRASH-3 was a randomized controlled trial developed to compare the rates of death and disability between TBI patients who received TXA versus placebo. In mild and moderate TBI patients, rates of head injury related mortality were lower in the TXA group compared with placebo. Unfortunately, there was no difference in mortality in the sTBI group. Secondary safety analyses reported no differences in rates of thromboses between groups.[66] Ultimately, the proposed benefit of TXA from CRASH-3 is not significant enough to mandate a change in guidelines or national practice standards.[67–69]

PART 3: INTENSIVE CARE/INPATIENT MANAGEMENT
Seizure Prophylaxis

Posttraumatic seizures are common and affect 5% to 7% of all sTBI patients.[70] Prophylaxis with phenytoin is associated with lower rates of seizures in the 7 days after injury; hence, it is recommended by the BTF for the 7 days following injury.[13] Although the rates of early (<7 days) posttraumatic seizures are higher in PBI, the rates of new epilepsy development are the same in both blunt and penetrating injury.[71] Administration for more than 7 days does not change the likelihood of developing epilepsy from chronic injury and may be associated with worsened neurocognitive outcomes.[72–74] The predictors of long-term epilepsy are poorly defined, although there may be some association between retained metal and bone fragments and the development of epilepsy.[75] Unfortunately, there is no evidence that seizure prophylaxis changes rates of mortality, functional outcomes, or the development of long-term epilepsy.[76]

More recently, there is a trend toward utilizing levetiracetam for seizure prophylaxis. It has the benefit of fewer drug interactions and adverse systemic effects in comparison to phenytoin. Overall, levetiracetam does not have clear superiority or inferiority compared with phenytoin.[77,78] Valproic acid, popular for its mood-stabilizing effects, also has been used for seizure prophylaxis for sTBI. An early report concluded that valproic acid may have a trend toward increased mortality but these findings were not reproducible.[79] Valproic acid prevents early seizures in small studies of TBI patients and is noninferior to other antiseizure medications.[80,81]

Because the data are not strong enough to recommend a specific antiepileptic medication for prophylaxis, drug selection depend largely on side-effect profiles and patient-specific factors. For patients with liver dysfunction or multiple medications metabolized by the P_{450} system, levetiracetam may be the superior choice. For patients with injury secondary to suicide attempt, known psychiatric disease, or agitation. valproic acid may be the preferred agent.

Antibiotic Prophylaxis

In PBI, tissues, such as skin, hair, bone, and foreign bodies, frequently enter the intracranial space. Penetrating wounds can destroy the ear canal, sinuses, and nasal passages. Intuitively, these types of injuries seem to carry high risk for meningitis, cerebritis, brain abscess, osteomyelitis, and epidural abscess. Incidence of infection following PBI varies but appears to be in the range as low as 4% to 11% in modern studies to 58.8% during World War II. Overall infection risk is higher from military PBI than civilian.[82] There are retrospective data suggesting that central nervous system (CNS) infections are much less common after antibiotic prophylaxis, 1% to 14%.[82,83] The British Society for Antimicrobial Chemotherapy in 2000 performed a systematic review of both civilian and military literature over the past 25 years and 50 years, respectively.[84] Despite acknowledgment of unsatisfactory level of evidence, based on the perceived high risk of infection and potentially high mortality (up to 50%) associated with superimposed infection extrapolated from military data, they recommend a 5-day course of broad spectrum antibiotics after wound débridement.[85]

More recent data, however, have not supported the use in all cases. A group in Colombia in 2013 performed a prospective observational study of 160 patients with craniocerebral gunshot wounds. Infection occurred in 20 of the 59 (33.9%) who received antibiotic prophylaxis, which targeted skin flora, and in 20 of the 101 (19.8%) who did not receive prophylaxis. They found 3 factors associated with increased risk for intracranial infection: presence of osseous or metallic fragments on CT postoperatively, projectile trajectory through natural orifices, and prolonged hospital stay (>12.5 days). Based on their findings, the investigators of this study could not recommend empiric use of antibiotics in all cases of PBI but acknowledged that the study was limited and more robust data from randomized controlled trials were necessary.[86]

Data on the use of antibiotic prophylaxis for basilar skull fractures in non-PBI are slightly more robust. Because basilar skull fractures increase risk for cerebrospinal fluid (CSF) leak (12%–30% of cases with basilar fracture vs 2% of TBI cases without basilar fracture),[87,88] practitioners may be inclined to initiate antibiotic prophylaxis to prevent meningitis. CSF leaks frequently spontaneously resolve after TBI, but persistence greater than 1 week is associated with increased risk of meningitis.[89] A Cochrane systematic review, including 5 randomized control trials and 17 nonrandomized trials, examined the role of antibiotic prophylaxis in patients with basilar skull fractures. Outcomes varied between studies and included reduction in the frequency of meningitis, all-cause mortality, and meningitis-related mortality. Antibiotic prophylaxis did not change the frequency of any outcome compared with controls.[90]

In summary, there is insufficient evidence of the benefit to uniform use of antibiotic prophylaxis for prevention of CNS infection in all TBI cases and thus they are not recommended by the Infectious Diseases Society of America. CNS infection may be diagnostically challenging. Studies have shown that neither peripheral leukocyte count or a rise greater than 10% nor fever (>38°C) is a reliable indicator of meningitis in TBI.[87,91] Thus, it is important to maintain a high index of suspicion, particularly in patients with declining neurologic examination without other explanation. In the authors' practice, there may be some cases where a lowered threshold is used for the use of antibiotics to treat potential CNS infection, namely in cases of significant pneumoce-phalus occurring due to persistent open intracranial wounds; presence of substantial foreign bodies or bone fragments that cannot be débrided, especially in those with wounds clearly contaminated by soil, where risk of anerobic infection is high; or ongoing CSF leaks or other situations where CSF sampling for testing may not be ob-tained, such as contraindication to lumbar puncture.

Ventilator-Associated Pneumonia

Ventilator-associated pneumonia (VAP) is a frequent concern for intubated sTBI pa-tients, and pneumonia is the most common infection occurring in TBI patients, up to 44% of patients in 1 study.[92] Patients younger than 40 seem to be at higher risk with an estimated incidence of 20%.[93] Prophylactic antibiotics have been proposed as a possible means to decrease rates of VAP. There is limited evidence that prophy-lactic antibiotics (both single-dose and course-limited ampicillin-sulbactam) may decrease the rate of early pneumonia.[94,95] Neither regimen, however, decreased the rates of late pneumonia development or mortality. In contrast, other single-center retrospective trials of single-dose prophylactic antibiotics did not show any difference in the rates of VAP, intubation days, or hospital length of stay.[96,97] A Cochrane review suggests when the quality of the data is considered, there may be a small advantage favoring prophylactic antibiotic administration.[90] Regardless, given the limited data, a larger randomized trial likely would help guide future therapy.

The authors' view is that the evidence on prophylactic antibiotics to prevent VAP is weak. Given the importance of antibiotics stewardship with increasing rates and new strain introduction of *Clostridium difficile* worldwide, antibiotics for VAP prevention should not be implemented routinely.[98] The best strategies for VAP prevention include consistent hand hygiene by health care workers, head of bed between 30° and 45°, regular spontaneous breathing trials, and oral care with chlorhexidine.[99–101]

Vascular Complications of Severe Traumatic Brain Injury

Vascular injuries (arterial and venous) complicate approximately 60% of all PBIs and 9% of all blunt sTBIs.[16] Risk factors for vascular injuries include bihemispheric wound trajectory, damage near the circle of Willis, subarachnoid hemorrhage, and intraven-tricular hemorrhage.[102]

- Arterial pseudoaneurysms of the anterior and middle cerebral arteries are the most common PBI injury and comprise slightly more than half of all vascular in-juries.[103] Arterial pseudoaneurysms may be treated with standard strategies to prevent rupture, such as endovascular coil placement and surgical clipping.[104]
- Venous thromboses, in particular sigmoid sinus thromboses, are the second most common injury pattern. They are more common with PBI than with blunt injury (11% vs 2%, respectively). Venous thromboses are associated with higher rates of hemorrhage, increased mortality, and higher odds of nursing home discharge.[105] Systemic anticoagulation and aggressive fluid hydration are first-line therapy but may be contraindicated in patients with active bleeding or substantial intracranial hemorrhage. Limited evidence supports mechanical thrombectomy for those who progress on anticoagulation or cannot receive it.[106] Retrospective data do not report increased risk of mortality or poor func-tional outcome with either treatment.[107]
- Dissections (both cervical and intracranial) result from intimal tears in the arte-rial endothelium. Younger age (18–24 years) is the largest risk factor for blunt injury dissection. The risk of dissection is higher in the immediate postinjury

period, then decreases after a month.[108] Although either CTA or digital subtraction angiography (DSA) may be obtained, DSA remains the gold standard. Vascular injury detection is 76% specific and 93% sensitive on CTA compared with DSA.[53]

- Carotid cavernous fistula result from an abnormal connection between the arteries and veins in the cavernous sinus.[109] Direct fistulas connect the internal carotid artery to the dural sinuses. Indirect fistulas connect meningeal branches from the internal carotid artery, the external carotid artery, or both to the dural sinuses. Direct fistulas are more common overall and associated with TBI, whereas indirect fistulas are not.[110,111] The precise pathophysiology underlying formation is unclear. Researchers hypothesize that carotid cavernous fistula may form when venous thromboses forces alternative routes of blood flow or that direct injury to previously weakened veins forces blood flow through abnormal direct arterial channels.[110,112] Symptoms include bruit, tearing, conjunctival injection, proptosis, blurred vision, and headache.[113,114] CTA, magnetic resonance angiography (MRA), and DSA all are diagnostically accurate. Once diagnosed, endovascular treatment with coil embolization, balloon embolization, and ethylene vinyl alcohol copolymer (eg, Onyx) all are acceptable treatment options.[115] Specific treatment approaches and techniques depend on arterial vascular supply and venous drainage.[116]

- Vasospasm—the presence of SAH may lead to vasospasm. Larger overall blood volumes (reflected in Fisher scores) increase vasospasm risk.[117,118] Other factors that increase risk of vasospasm include age less than 30 and GCS score less than 9 on admission.[119] Neurologic examination and transcranial Dopplers (TCDs) are appropriate screening tools for traumatic vasospasm. Follow-up imaging by CT angiogram or DSA may be performed when confirmatory imaging or treatment is necessary.[120] Newer technologies that may detected vasospasm include repeated CT perfusion scanning, black blood MRA, and quantitative electroencephalogram (EEG). CT perfusion showing increased mean times to drain have high sensitivity and specificity in predicting clinical vasospasm.[121] Black blood MRA may help to detect changes in arterial caliber and can be compared with the clinical standards of CTA and DSA.[122] Decreases in alpha power in quantitative EEG over a 4-hour period also are associated with vasospasm.[123]

Introduction: Invasive Devices and Neuromonitoring

Patients with lower GCS are at a higher risk for secondary neurologic decline, yet intubation, sedating medications, and a limited baseline neurologic examination may delay identification. In comatose TBI patients, invasive monitoring techniques may help provide adjunct measures to assess neurologic function. ICP monitors are the most common invasive devices used in sTBI care,[124,125] although more advanced catheters are being adopted, which provide data on brain tissue oxygenation (partial pressure of oxygen in brain tissue [Pbto$_2$]), brain temperature, and markers of tissue metabolism. Data support placement of ICP monitors in patients with GCS less than or equal to 8, abnormal HCT, or concern for possible ICP crisis.[126,127] Although estimates vary based on study criteria, ICP measurements 20 mm Hg to 25 mm Hg generally are considered elevated and require intervention.[128,129] Uncontrolled intracranial hypertension is associated with increased morbidity and mortality and should be treated aggressively.[130] Therefore, ICP monitors have the advantage of providing real-time data to providers for therapeutic decision makin[131,132] (see **Box 3**).

Intracranial Pressure Monitoring

Intracranial hypertension is common (54% of sTBI), but, as discussed previously, but may not always be detectable on bedside examination. Although HCT monitoring can show midline shift and compressed basilar cisterns, they also can be normal during the first 24 hours in 15% of patients with ICP crisis.[133] Prompt diagnosis and treatment of ICP crisis are critical because there are effective interventions for lowering ICP. Hyperosmolar therapy and sedation are administered widely and are effective in lowering ICP.[134,135] Interventions for refractory ICP, such as induced barbiturate coma and surgical decompression, also are effective in lowering ICP, but it is unclear if they produce better long-term outcomes.[136–138] Regardless, cases should be evaluated on an individual basis and aggressive early intervention for elevated ICP pursued. The authors refer readers to Aleksey Tadevosyan and Joshua Kornbluth article, "Brain Herniation and Intracranial Hypertension" in this issue.

The routine use of ICP monitors came into question after publication of the BEST TRIP trial. In this South American study, 324 patients were randomized to an intracranial hypertension treatment protocol based on either a combination of clinical and imaging findings or ICP monitoring, with a threshold of 20 mm Hg. The primary outcome was a composite score essentially representing functional outcome at 6 months and there was no difference seen between the groups.[139] There are many criticisms about the generalizability of the study to other health care systems, because there may have been exclusion of some of the sickest patients due to poor availability of prehospital care. Similarly, inclusion of less ill patients may have mitigated any effect of the protocol based on ICP monitoring. More hyperosmolar therapy was given to the group without ICP monitors, suggesting that ICP monitoring may have a benefit in reducing unnecessary therapy. Other investigators have interpreted the study and determined that perhaps a threshold of 20 mm Hg for treatment was too low. ICP monitors still are recommended by the most recent update of the BTF and TQIP[13,140] but guidance now suggests using a threshold of 20 mm Hg to 25 mm Hg.

Both external ventricular drains (EVDs) and IPMs perform approximately equally in their ability to capture ICP data.[141] Rates of EVD associated hemorrhage and infection are operator dependent and typically much higher than those associated with IPM.[142] Infection rates in EVDs vary, however, depending on institution; high rates range from 30% to 45% whereas lower rates are approximately 10%.[63,143,144] Infection control protocols help reduce infection rates to 0 to 10% but they still remain higher than IPM.[145,146] EVDs may seem preferable because they have the dual advantage of CSF removal during ICP crisis and do not need replacement for calibration. The disadvantages of IPMs include false upward drift of measured ICP over time with inability to recalibrate values.[147]

In the authors' practice, EVD placement is recommended in patients at risk for hydrocephalus, such as those with intraventricular hemorrhage, despite higher infection risks. If intracranial hypertension is suspected but other considerations for a patient's poor neurologic examination (eg, DAI) are suspected, IPM placement may be preferable[148]

Brain Tissue Oxygenation Monitoring

Increased brain tissue hypoxia is associated with worsened outcomes.[149,150] Hence, there are many diagnostic tools focused on the ascertainment of cerebral oxygenation. The use of jugular bulb monitoring is 1 measure of global cerebral oxygenation.[151] By comparison, local cerebral oximetry now can be monitored through parenchymal catheters.

In America, the Licox Brain Oxygen Monitor (Integra Neuroscience, Plainsboro, New Jersey) is a Food and Drug Administration approved, commonly available device utilizing the polarographic method.[152] Licox catheters are placed directly into the brain parenchyma. Location selection can be challenging. Placing the monitor adjacent to a damaged area can provide important information about penumbral brain tissue oxygen tension (Pbto$_2$) but these areas can be difficult to identify with HCT alone for a guide.[153] If there are bihemispheric or scattered injuries, monitors generally are placed in the right frontal lobe because it is relatively ineloquent cortex.[154] The normal range for Pbto$_2$ is 20 mm Hg to 35 mm Hg in non-lesioned tissue.[155]

Low Pbto$_2$ and very low Pbto$_2$ (<10 mm Hg) are associated with increased morbidity and mortality.[156] To treat cerebral hypoxia, providers must increase cerebral blood flow (CBF) or increase the oxygen content within arterial blood. Increasing CBF often entails CPP. Initiation of vasopressors or lowering of ICP both increase CPP and may help to correct cerebral hypoxia.[157] Packed red blood cell transfusion has been evaluated in small observational studies for its effects on cerebral metabolism. In the setting of anemia (hemoglobin <8), transfusion results in a transient rise in PbtO$_2$ for 57% of patients, but the clinical significance of this rise is unclear.[158,159]

Although increasing the arterial oxygen content initially may appear straightforward, solutions may not be intuitive. Pathologies that impair oxygenation (eg, lung injury) are associated with lower Pbto$_2$.[160] Yet, correcting these pathologies through strategies, such as increasing fraction of inspired oxygen (Fio$_2$), positive end-expiratory pressure, and proning, do not always result in the higher Pbto$_2$ levels.[161] Hyperoxia may induce vasoconstriction and this may explain in part why higher Fio$_2$ does not translate to target Pbto$_2$ levels.[162] Alternatively, low flow states or other perturbations in physiology may change brain cellular function, such that it oxygen cannot diffuse efficiently or it cannot be utilized.[163]

Clinical applications for Pbto$_2$ are in a developmental phase. A large retrospective trial at a level 1 trauma center demonstrated low brain tissue oxygen tension (Pbto$_2$ <20 mm Hg) in the majority of TBI patients at the time of placement, despite normal peripheral oxygen saturation. It suggests a possible mismatch between peripheral oxygen saturation and brain tissue uptake. In the same study, there was linear correlation between Pbto$_2$ and outcome until 33 mm Hg, when higher Pbto$_2$ did not yield additional clinical benefit.[151] A separate systematic review yielded similar findings with extreme brain hypoxia (Pbto$_2$ <10 mm Hg) associated with increased mortality.[156] The Brain Oxygen Optimization in Severe TBI Phase II (BOOST-II) study was a randomized prospective clinical trial performed at 10 level I trauma centers, where Licox catheters were placed in 119 sTBI patients. The study investigated a treatment protocol using either ICP or ICP plus Pbto$_2$ monitoring. The results showed similar ICP in both groups but the group treated under the ICP plus Pbto$_2$ monitoring had a shorter proportion of time with brain tissue hypoxia. The study was not powered for clinical efficacy but there was a trend toward more favorable outcomes in the ICP plus Pbto$_2$ monitoring group.[164] Despite these small pilot and observational studies, ideal management approaches are largely unknown. Practical clinical targets, such as probe placement, minimum Pbto$_2$ levels, target Pbto$_2$ levels, and maximum Pbto$_2$ levels, have not been established robustly.[165]

Cerebral Microdialysis

The blood-brain barrier and its selective permeability create a unique cellular environment within brain tissue. Cerebral microdialysis (CM) utilizes the principles of diffusion as a means to gain information about brain metabolism by analyzing the interstitial fluid of this environment.[166,167] The technology consists of 2 adjacent catheters. An artificial fluid similar to CSF flows at a constant rate through the first catheter. A semi-permeable dialysis membrane covers the catheter tip. There are 2 common permeability sizes: 20 kDa and 100 kDa. The fluid then passes through the second collecting catheter to yield dialysate. The dialysate may be analyzed subsequently for particles that have diffused inward and particles lost to the extracellular fluid space.[168,169] The 20-kDa membrane may be preferred because it allows clinically meaningful substrates, such as glycerol, glucose, lactate, and pyruvate, to pass through for analysis.[170] Among the biomarkers, glycerol is the most straightforward. Glycerol detection implies cell wall breakdown. When elevated levels are detected in CM, cellular destruction is assumed.[171]

The brain preferentially utilizes glucose for its cellular energy source.[172–174] Cerebral hypoglycemia may not be detected by serum glucose measurements and it is associated with worsened outcomes in sTBI. In the first 24 hours following sTBI, glucose uptake increases but oxygen consumption typically remains unchanged.[175] The metabolic shift implies that glucose is being utilized for hyperglycolysis and the pentose phosphate pathway.[176,177] Glucose may be shifted to energy production (pentose phosphate creates NADPH) during this acute period to help restore cellular homeostasis. By detecting these dynamic cellular metabolic changes, providers may change their systemic treatment strategies. Dextrose administration, insulin adjustments, and feeding all may be changed in response to intracranial glucose needs.

Traditionally, elevations in lactate, pyruvate, and the lactate-to-pyruvate ratio (LPR) have been associated with ischemia.[178] Elevated LPR is common in sTBI; it is detected in 20% to 25% of patients, depending on the study population, yet only a fraction of patients (2.4%) have the expected ischemic findings.[179,180] Elevated LPR without associated ischemia may be termed, *metabolic crisis without ischemia*. These metabolic crises are associated with increased mortality, cortical atrophy, and worsened long-term outcomes.[181,182] Mitochondrial dysfunction may be the underlying pathophysiology driving the elevated LPR.[183]

In summary, brain tissue oxygenation monitoring and CM are exciting, emerging technologies in sTBI. This is an area of active research because ideal placement and individual patient target values are unknown. The biggest drawback with the current monitors is data application. For instance, cerebral hypoglycemia can be tracked, but if exogenous glucose administration and feeding are ineffective, then it is unclear how to intervene. The volume of brain tissue accessible for monitoring is relatively very small and may not represent global cerebral dysfunction. Considering the volumes, the overall utility of monitoring may be questioned. Larger, prospective multicenter trials, such as the follow-up BOOST-III study; BOOST-III is ongoing and designed to evaluate 6-month outcomes.[184] Both brain tissue oxygen monitoring and CM may influence future care but still in a phase of active research.

PART 4: FUTURE DIRECTIONS

Noninvasive ways to monitor ICP are actively being investigated. Noninvasive technology could expand the use of ICP monitoring to moderate and noncomatose TBI patients. Furthermore, it would avoid complications, such as infectious risk and hemorrhage.

- TCD is a noninvasive way to measure changes in cerebral blood velocities. Most practitioners are familiar with TCD technology as a way to detect vasospasm in subarachnoid hemorrhage and emboli detection.[185] TCD also can calculate pulsatility index (PI) which correlates with ICP measurements.[186,187] PI is calculated as $(FV_{[systolic]} - FV_{[diastolic]})/(FV_{[mean]})$, in which FV represents flow velocity.[188] There are 2 forces acting on intracranial arteries: external pressure from the acquired pathology (eg, hemorrhage) and internal tensile pressure from the blood within the lumen. The external pressure is ICP. Because arteries are elastic and distensible, changes in PI may represent changes in ICP. Changes in flow velocity and TCD wave form correlate with high ICP; hence, PI may be a proxy for ICP measurements.[189] Individually, each parameter (FV and PI) can give an estimate of ICP but, when used together, the gauge of ICP is close to that of traditional invasive methods.[189] TCD is promising as a noninvasive means to measure ICP, but it has limitations. TCDs cannot be performed continuously, data are operator dependent, and 15% of patients have bone windows that preclude the use of TCD.[190]

- Optic nerve sheath diameter (ONSD) relies on the neuroanatomical structure of the optic nerve sheath as a proxy for ICPs. The optic nerve subarachnoid space is contiguous with the intracranial space and is covered by a dural sheath. Hence, changes in ICP can be transmitted and measured within the optic nerve.[191] Recent studies have used ultrasound of the eye to create an estimate of ICP. In 2 studies, ICP determined by ultrasound ONSD had 90% sensitivity and specificity compared with values determined by the EVD.[192,193] Meta-analyses and systematic reviews also have promising results, with pooled sensitivity of 95% and specificity 92% and 81% to 90% accuracy in another.[193,194] Despite this early promise, a reliable cutoff ONSD value that is predictive of intracranial hypertension has yet to be determined, limiting the present utility of this technique.[194] ONSD cannot be used in patients with severe orbital injuries or in those with presumed compromised ONSD (eg, Graves disease).[195]

- Quantitative pupillometry is the assessment of pupil size and reactivity using portable devices that automatically measure multiple components of the pupillary response to standardized light stimuli. Recent exploratory work has been done to characterize the relationship of quantitative pupil characteristics, elevated ICP, and outcome in patients with sTBI. Jahns and colleagues[196] studied 54 patients with intracranial hypertension secondary to TBI and found that episodes of sustained ICP were associated with concomitant decreased neurologic pupil index. They also found that cumulative abnormal pupil reactivity burden was associated with an unfavorable 6-month outcome. A prospective pilot study enrolled 36 patients with TBI and used abnormal pupil reactivity to predict whether a patient would need an intervention for intracranial hypertension, including ICP monitor placement and craniectomy. Normal neurologic pupil index may indicate that invasive monitoring is not necessary, based on this small cohort of sTBI.[197] More definitive work is needed to verify and standardize how quantitative pupillometry can best be used as a diagnostic and triage tool in TBI, but as an adjunct to the clinical examination it holds promise of improving noninvasive clinical monitoring.

- Cerebral oximetry using near-infrared spectroscopy (NIRS) is a promising noninvasive approach to determine continuous oxygen saturation in the brain. Several studies have demonstrated the feasibility of employing NIRS in patients following TBI.[198] Sensors typically are placed on the forehead, although there have been reports of more posterior lead placement after shaving parts of the head using commercial devices[199] or without head shaving in custom devices.[200] The potential advantages of NIRS over $Pbto_2$ monitoring is noninvasiveness and more flexibility in the number and placement of leads, leading to the ability to monitor a much larger portion of the brain. Furthermore, NIRS not only collects oxygen saturation but also can determine relative changes in total hemoglobin concentration, which potentially could be used to assess expansion of frontal contusions. Limitations of the modality are that it cannot distinguish between venous and arterial blood oxygenation and that despite corrections the brain signal can be contaminated by scalp and skull interference. Nonetheless, NIRS remains a promising modality that requires additional validation in the TBI patient population.

- Diffuse correlation spectroscopy is a promising modality to determine continuous relative CBF noninvasively. With the possible exception of the invasive Hemedex Bowman Perfusion Monitor, a reliable and continuous CBF monitor has proved elusive. Diffuse correlation spectroscopy relies on the effect of moving red blood cells on measured variability in detected infrared laser light.[201] It has been applied in animal models of TBI[202] and in hemorrhagic stroke patients in the intensive care unit.[203] Future work will focus on developing the approach in the critically ill TBI patient population.

SUMMARY

TBI is common problem worldwide. Current practices focus on the importance of early resuscitation, transfer to high-volume centers, and provider expertise across multiple specialties. HCT provides important information for sTBI management and urgent CTA is the preferred study to evaluate for vascular injury. Close observation in the neurological intensive care unit helps identify problems, such as seizure, ICP crisis, and injury progression. In addition to traditional neurologic examination, there is a focus on using real-time, intracranial monitors to gather physiologic data at a cellular level. $Pbto_2$ monitoring and CM are modern technologies that show immense promise in translational and pilot studies. Both technologies have the potential for many future applications that will help spare neurons during secondary injury cascades. Noninvasive ICP measurement devices are poised to become superior technologies. Reliable ways to monitor ICP without risk are the next frontier in TBI and there will be more opportunities for prospective and randomized research.

DISCLOSURE

The authors have nothing to disclose.

REFERENCES

1. Dewan MC, Abbas R, Saksham G, et al. Estimating the global incidence of traumatic brain injury. J Neurosurg 2019;130:1080–97.
2. Teasdale G, Jennett B. Assessment of coma and impaired consciousness. A practical scale. Lancet 1974;2:81–4.
3. CDC Traumatic Brain Injury & Concussion. Centers for Disease Control, Traumatic Brain Injury & Concussion. 2020. Available at: https://www.cdc.gov/traumaticbraininjury/index.html.
4. Lu J, Roe C, Sigurdardottir S, et al. Trajectory of functional independent measurements during first five years after moderate and severe traumatic brain injury. J Neurotrauma 2018;35:1596–603.
5. Khan F, Bhasker A, Rodney J, et al. Factors associated with long-term functional and psychological outcomes in persons with moderate to severe traumatic brain injury. J Rehabil Med 2016;48:442–8.

6. Joseph B, Hassan A, Viraj P, et al. Improving survival rates after civilian gunshot wounds to the brain. J Am Coll Surg 2014;218:58–65.

7. Bossers SM, Lothar AS, Stephan AL, et al. Experience in prehospital endotracheal intubation significantly influences mortality of patients with severe traumatic brain injury: a systematic review and meta-analysis. PLoS One 2015;10: e0141034.

8. Winchell RJ, Hoyt DB. Endotracheal intubation in the field improves survival in patients with severe head injury. Trauma Research and Education Foundation of San Diego. Arch Surg 1960;132:592–7 (1997).

9. Bulger EM, Copass MK, Sabath DR, et al. The use of neuromuscular blocking agents to facilitate prehospital intubation does not impair outcome after traumatic brain injury. J Trauma 2005;58:718–23 [discussion 723-724].

10. Sloane C, Vilke GM, Chan TC, et al. Rapid sequence intubation in the field versus hospital in trauma patients. J Emerg Med 2000;19:259–64.

11. Manoach S, Paladino L. Manual in-line stabilization for acute airway management of suspected cervical spine injury: historical review and current questions. Ann Emerg Med 2007;50:236–45.

12. Davis DP, Kent MK, Craig DN, et al. The Relationship between out-of-hospital airway management and outcome among trauma patients with glasgow coma scale scores of 8 or less. Prehosp Emerg Care 2011;15:184–92.

13. The brain trauma foundation. The American association of neurological surgeons. The joint section on neurotrauma and critical care. Glasgow coma scale score. J Neurotrauma 2000;17:563–71.

14. Diringer MN, Tom OV, Kent Y, et al. Regional cerebrovascular and metabolic effects of hyperventilation after severe traumatic brain injury. J Neurosurg 2002; 96:103–8.

15. Rangel-Castilla L, Lara LR, Gopinath S, et al. Cerebral hemodynamic effects of acute hyperoxia and hyperventilation after severe traumatic brain injury. J Neurotrauma 2010;27:1853–63.

16. Esnault P, Johanna R, Mickael C, et al. Spontaneous hyperventilation in severe traumatic brain injury: incidence and association with poor neurological outcome. Neurocrit Care 2019;30:405–13.

17. Thomas SH, Orf J, Wedel SK, et al. Hyperventilation in traumatic brain injury patients: inconsistency between consensus guidelines and clinical practice. J Trauma 2002;52:47–52 [discussion 52-53].

18. Chesnut RM, et al. Early and Late systemic hypotension as a frequent and fundamental source of cerebral ischemia following severe brain injury in the traumatic coma data bank. In: Unterberg AW, Schneider G-H, Lanksch WR, editors. Monitoring of cerebral blood flow and metabolism in intensive care. 121–125. . Springer Vienna; 1993. https://doi.org/10.1007/978-3-7091-9302-0_21.

19. Bullock R, Chesnut RM, Clifton G, et al. Guidelines for the management of severe head injury. Brain Trauma Foundation. Eur J Emerg Med 1996;3:109–27.

20. Hawryluk GWJ, Rubiano AM, Totten AM, et al. Guidelines for the management of severe traumatic brain injury: 2020 update of the decompressive craniectomy recommendations. Neurosurgery 2020;87:427–34.

21. Donnelly J, Czosnyka M, Adams H, et al. Pressure reactivity-based optimal cerebral perfusion pressure in a traumatic brain injury cohort. Acta Neurochir Suppl 2018;126:209–12.

22. Svedung Wettervik T, Howells T, Enblad P, et al. Temporal neurophysiological dynamics in traumatic brain injury: role of pressure reactivity and optimal

cerebral perfusion pressure for predicting outcome. J Neurotrauma 2019;36: 1818–27.

23. Zeiler FA, Ari E, Manuel C, et al. Comparison of performance of different optimal cerebral perfusion pressure parameters for outcome prediction in adult traumatic brain injury: a collaborative european neurotrauma effectiveness research in traumatic brain injury (CENTER-TBI) Study. J Neurotrauma 2019;36:1505–17.

24. Cryer, H. & FACS, & Manley, Geoffrey & Adelson, P., et al (2015). American College of Surgeons Trauma Quality Improvement Program Guidelines, Traumatic Brain Injury. Committee on trauma expert panel 1/2015, American College of Surgeons.

25. Cooper DJ, Myles PS, McDermott FT, et al. Prehospital hypertonic saline resuscitation of patients with hypotension and severe traumatic brain injury: a randomized controlled trial. JAMA 2004;291:1350–7.

26. Pinto FCG, Capone-Neto A, Prist R, et al. Volume replacement with lactated Ringer's or 3% hypertonic saline solution during combined experimental hemorrhagic shock and traumatic brain injury. J Trauma 2006;60:758–63 [discussion 763-764].

27. SAFE Study Investigators, Australian and New Zealand Intensive Care Society Clinical Trials Group, Australian Red Cross Blood Service, et al. Saline or albumin for fluid resuscitation in patients with traumatic brain injury. N Engl J Med 2007;357:874–84.

28. Holcomb JB, Charles EW, Michalek JE, et al. Increased plasma and platelet to red blood cell ratios improves outcome in 466 massively transfused civilian trauma patients. Ann Surg 2008;248:447–58.

29. Peiniger S, Nienaber U, Lefering R, et al. Balanced massive transfusion ratios in multiple injury patients with traumatic brain injury. Crit Care Lond Engl 2011; 15:R68.

30. Sims CA, et al. Effect of low-dose supplementation of arginine vasopressin on need for blood product transfusions in patients with trauma and hemorrhagic shock: a randomized clinical trial. JAMA Surg 2019;154:994.

31. Di Gennaro JL, Mack CD, Malakouti A, et al. Use and effect of vasopressors after pediatric traumatic brain injury. Dev Neurosci 2010;32:420–30.

32. Sookplung P, Siriussawakul A, Malakouti A, et al. Vasopressor use and effect on blood pressure after severe adult traumatic brain injury. Neurocrit Care 2011;15: 46–54.

33. American Trauma Society. Trauma Center Levels Explained - American Trauma Societ. Available at: https://www.amtrauma.org/page/traumalevels.

34. Tepas JJ, Pracht EE, Orban BL, et al. High-volume trauma centers have better outcomes treating traumatic brain injury. J Trauma Acute Care Surg 2013;74: 143–7 [discussion 147-148].

35. Brown JB, Stassen NA, Cheng JD, et al. Trauma center designation correlates with functional independence after severe but not moderate traumatic brain injury. J Trauma 2010;69:263–9.

36. Sugerman DE, Xu L, Pearson WS, et al. Patients with severe traumatic brain injury transferred to a Level I or II trauma center: United States, 2007 to 2009. J Trauma Acute Care Surg 2012;73:1491–9.

37. Spaite DW, Bentley JB, Samuel MK, et al. Association of statewide implementation of the prehospital traumatic brain injury treatment guidelines with patient survival following traumatic brain injury: the excellence in prehospital injury care (EPIC) Study. JAMA Surg 2019;154:e191152.

38. Stevens RD, Shoykhet M, Cadena R. Emergency neurological life support: intracranial hypertension and herniation. Neurocrit Care 2015;23(Suppl 2):S76–82.

39. Selhorst JB, Gudeman SK, Butterworth JF 4th, et al. Papilledema after acute head injury. Neurosurgery 1985;16:357–63.

40. Chesnut RM, Nancy T, Sureyya D, et al. A method of managing severe traumatic brain injury in the absence of intracranial pressure monitoring: the imaging and clinical examination protocol. J Neurotrauma 2018;35:54–63.

41. Burgess S, Abu-Laban RB, Slavik RS, et al. A Systematic review of randomized controlled trials comparing hypertonic sodium solutions and mannitol for traumatic brain injury: implications for emergency department management. Ann Pharmacother 2016;50:291–300.

42. Provenzale JM. Imaging of traumatic brain injury: a review of the recent medical literature. Am J Roentgenol 2010;194:16–9.

43. Kubal WS. Updated imaging of traumatic brain injury. Radiol Clin North Am 2012;50:15–41.

44. Sullivan TP, Jarvik JG, Cohen WA. Follow-up of conservatively managed epidural hematomas: implications for timing of repeat CT. AJNR Am J Neuroradiol 1999;20:107–13.

45. Khairat A, Waseem M. Epidural hematoma. StatPearls: StatPearls Publishing; 2018.

46. Karibe H, Toshiaki H, Takayuki H, et al. Surgical management of traumatic acute subdural hematoma in adults: a review. Neurol Med Chir (Tokyo) 2014;54: 887–94.

47. Fomchenko EI, Gilmore EJ, Matouk CC, et al. Management of subdural hematomas: Part II. Surgical management of subdural hematomas. Curr Treat Options Neurol 2018;20:34.

48. Zubkov AY, Lewis AI, Raila FA, et al. Risk factors for the development of post-traumatic cerebral vasospasm. Surg Neurol 2000;53:126–30.

49. Gentry LR, Godersky JC, Thompson B. MR imaging of head trauma: review of the distribution and radiopathologic features of traumatic lesions. AJR Am J Roentgenol 1988;150:663–72.

50. Levi L, Borovich B, Guilburd JN, et al. Wartime neurosurgical experience in Lebanon, 1982-85. I: Penetrating craniocerebral injuries. Isr J Med Sci 1990; 26:548–54.

51. Chaudhri KA, Choudhury AR, al Moutaery KR, et al. Penetrating craniocerebral shrapnel injuries during 'Operation Desert Storm': early results of a conservative surgical treatment. Acta Neurochir (Wien) 1994;126:120–3.

52. Tso MK, Myunghyun ML, Chad GB, et al. Clinical utility of a screening protocol for blunt cerebrovascular injury using computed tomography angiography. J Neurosurg 2017;126:1033–41.

53. Bodanapally UK, Kathirkamanathan S, Alexis RB, et al. Vascular complications of penetrating brain injury: comparison of helical CT angiography and conventional angiography: Clinical article. J Neurosurg 2014;121:1275–83.

54. Bromberg WJ, Bryan CC, Larry ND, et al. Blunt cerebrovascular injury practice management guidelines: the Eastern Association for the Surgery of Trauma. J Trauma 2010;68:471–7.

55. Eastman AL, Chason DP, Perez CL, et al. Computed tomographic angiography for the diagnosis of blunt cervical vascular injury: is it ready for primetime? J Trauma 2006;60:925–9 [discussion 929].

56. Wang AC, Michael AC, Jayesh PT, et al. Evaluating the use and utility of noninvasive angiography in diagnosing traumatic blunt cerebrovascular injury. J Trauma Acute Care Surg 2012;72:1601–10.

57. Malak W. Contribution of Brain MRI after Head CT in the evaluation of acute, hospitalized traumatic brain injury patients: an under-utilized resource? Biomed J Sci Tech Res 2020;26.

58. Mannion RJ, Justin C, Peter B, et al. Mechanism-based MRI classification of traumatic brainstem injury and its relationship to outcome. J Neurotrauma 2007;24:128–35.

59. Henninger N, Rebecca AC, Muhammad WK, et al. 'Don't lose hope early': Hemorrhagic diffuse axonal injury on head computed tomography is not associated with poor outcome in moderate to severe traumatic brain injury patients. J Trauma Acute Care Surg 2018;84:473–82.

60. Rodriguez-Luna D, Pilar C, Marta R, et al. Ultraearly hematoma growth in active intracerebral hemorrhage. Neurology 2016;87:357–64.

61. Reed MR, Woolley LT. Uses of tranexamic acid. Contin Educ Anaesth Crit Care Pain 2015;15:32–7.

62. Myles PS, Smith JA, Forbes A, et al. Tranexamic acid in patients undergoing coronary-artery surgery. N Engl J Med 2017;376:136–48.

63. Chornenki NLJ, Kevin JU, Pablo AM, et al. Risk of venous and arterial thrombosis in non-surgical patients receiving systemic tranexamic acid: A systematic review and meta-analysis. Thromb Res 2019;179:81–6.

64. Zehtabchi S, Abdel Baki SG, Falzon L, et al. Tranexamic acid for traumatic brain injury: a systematic review and meta-analysis. Am J Emerg Med 2014;32:1503–9.

65. Chen H, Chen M. The efficacy of tranexamic acid for brain injury: a meta-analysis of randomized controlled trials. Am J Emerg Med 2020;38:364–70.

66. CRASH-3 trial collaborators. Effects of tranexamic acid on death, disability, vascular occlusive events and other morbidities in patients with acute traumatic brain injury (CRASH-3): a randomised, placebo-controlled trial. Lancet 2019;394:1713–23.

67. Weng S, Wanqi W, Quantang W, et al. Effect of tranexamic acid in patients with traumatic brain injury: a systematic review and meta-analysis. World Neurosurg 2019;123:128–35.

68. Jokar A, Ahmadi K, Salehi T, et al. The effect of tranexamic acid in traumatic brain injury: A randomized controlled trial. Chin J Traumatol 2017;20:49–51.

69. Yutthakasemsunt S, Warawut K, Parnumas P, et al. Tranexamic acid for patients with traumatic brain injury: a randomized, double-blinded, placebo-controlled trial. BMC Emerg Med 2013;13:20.

70. Torbic H, Forni AA, Anger KE, et al. Use of antiepileptics for seizure prophylaxis after traumatic brain injury. Am J Health Syst Pharm 2013;70:759–66.

71. Loggini A, Valentina IV, Ali M, et al. Management of civilians with penetrating brain injury: a systematic review. J Crit Care 2020;56:159–66.

72. Dikmen SS, Machamer JE, Powell JM, et al. Outcome 3 to 5 years after moderate to severe traumatic brain injury11No commercial party having a direct financial interest in the results of the research supporting this article has or will confer a benefit upon the author(s) or upon any organization with which the author(s) is/are associated. Arch Phys Med Rehabil 2003;84:1449–57.

73. Bhullar IS, Donald J, Julia PP, et al. More harm than good: Antiseizure prophylaxis after traumatic brain injury does not decrease seizure rates but may inhibit functional recovery. J Trauma Acute Care Surg 2014;76:54–61.

74. Wilson CD, Josh DB, Richard BR, et al. Early and late posttraumatic epilepsy in the setting of traumatic brain injury: a meta-analysis and review of antiepileptic management. World Neurosurg 2018;110:e901–6.

75. Englander J, Tamara B, Thao TD, et al. Analyzing risk factors for late posttraumatic seizures: a prospective, multicenter investigation. Arch Phys Med Rehabil 2003;84:365–73.

76. Temkin NR, Dikmen SS, Wilensky AJ, et al. A randomized, double-blind study of phenytoin for the prevention of post-traumatic seizures. N Engl J Med 1990;323:497–502.

77. Inaba K, Jay M, Bernardino CB, et al. A prospective multicenter comparison of levetiracetam versus phenytoin for early posttraumatic seizure prophylaxis. J Trauma Acute Care Surg 2013;74:766–71 [discussion 771-773].

78. Yang Y, Zheng F, Xu X, et al. Levetiracetam Versus Phenytoin for Seizure Prophylaxis Following Traumatic Brain Injury: A Systematic Review and Meta-Analysis. CNS Drugs 2016;30:677–88.

79. Dikmen SS, Machamer JE, Winn HR, et al. Neuropsychological effects of valproate in traumatic brain injury: a randomized trial. Neurology 2000;54:895–902.

80. Thompson K, Pohlmann-Eden B, Campbell LA, et al. Pharmacological treatments for preventing epilepsy following traumatic head injury. Cochrane Database Syst Rev 2015;CD009900. https://doi.org/10.1002/14651858.CD009900.pub2.

81. Ma C, Xue Y, Li M, et al. Sodium valproate for prevention of early posttraumatic seizures. Chin J Traumatol 2010;13:293–6.

82. Benzel EC, Day WT, Kesterson L, et al. Civilian craniocerebral gunshot wounds. Neurosurgery 1991;29:67–71 [discussion 71-72].

83. Stuehmer C, Katrin SB, Horst K, et al. Influence of different types of guns, projectiles, and propellants on patterns of injury to the viscerocranium. J Oral Maxillofac Surg 2009;67:775–81.

84. Rish BL, Caveness WF, Dillon JD, et al. Analysis of brain abscess after penetrating craniocerebral injuries in Vietnam. Neurosurgery 1981;9:535–41.

85. Bayston R, J de Louvois, E M Brown, et al. Use of antibiotics in penetrating craniocerebral injuries. 'Infection in Neurosurgery' Working Party of British Society for Antimicrobial Chemotherapy. Lancet 2000;355:1813–7.

86. Jimenez CM, Polo J, España JA. Risk factors for intracranial infection secondary to penetrating craniocerebral gunshot wounds in civilian practice. World Neurosurg 2013;79:749–55.

87. La Russa R, Maiese A, Di Fazio N, et al. Post-traumatic meningitis is a diagnostic challenging time: a systematic review focusing on clinical and pathological features. Int J Mol Sci 2020;21:4148.

88. Prosser JD, Vender JR, Solares CA. Traumatic cerebrospinal fluid leaks. Otolaryngol Clin North Am 2011;44:857–873, vii.

89. Sonig A, Thakur JD, Chittiboina P, et al. Is posttraumatic cerebrospinal fluid fistula a predictor of posttraumatic meningitis? A US Nationwide Inpatient Sample database study. Neurosurg Focus 2012;32:E4.

90. Poole D, Arturo C, Martin L, et al. Systematic review of the literature and evidence-based recommendations for antibiotic prophylaxis in trauma: results from an italian consensus of experts. PLoS One 2014;9:e113676.

91. Khalili H, YadollahiKhales G, Isaee M. Diagnostic accuracy of peripheral white blood cell count, fever and acute leukocutosis for bacterial meningitis in patients with severe traumatic brain injury. Bull Emerg Trauma 2015;3:53–8.

92. Kourbeti IS, John AP, Christodoulos N, et al. Infections in patients with traumatic brain injury who undergo neurosurgery. Br J Neurosurg 2011;25:9–15.

93. Robba C, Paola R, Erika B, et al. Incidence, risk factors, and effects on outcome of ventilator-associated pneumonia in patients with traumatic brain injury: analysis of a large, multicenter, prospective, observational longitudinal study. Chest 2020. https://doi.org/10.1016/j.chest.2020.06.064.

94. Vallés J, Raquel P, Jose Burgueño M, et al. Efficacy of single-dose antibiotic against early-onset pneumonia in comatose patients who are ventilated. Chest 2013;143:1219–25.

95. Acquarolo A, Urli T, Perone G, et al. Antibiotic prophylaxis of early onset pneumonia in critically ill comatose patients. A randomized study. Intensive Care Med 2005;31:510–6.

96. McMillian WD, Bednarik JL, Aloi JJ, et al. Utility of ampicillin-sulbactam for empiric treatment of ventilator-associated pneumonia in a trauma population. J Trauma 2010;69:861–5.

97. Lewis TD, Dehne KA, Morbitzer K, et al. Influence of single-dose antibiotic prophylaxis for early-onset pneumonia in high-risk intubated patients. Neurocrit Care 2018;28:362–9.

98. Sartelli M, Malangoni MA, Abu-Zidan FM, et al. WSES guidelines for management of Clostridium difficile infection in surgical patients. World J Emerg Surg 2015;10:38.

99. Munro CL, Grap MJ, Jones DJ, et al. Chlorhexidine, toothbrushing, and preventing ventilator-associated pneumonia in critically ill adults. Am J Crit Care 2009; 18:428–37 [quiz 438].

100. Hua F, Xie H, Worthington HV, et al. Oral hygiene care for critically ill patients to prevent ventilator-associated pneumonia. Cochrane Database Syst Rev 2016; 10:CD008367.

101. Yokoe DS, Leonard AM, Deverick JA, et al. A compendium of strategies to prevent healthcare-associated infections in acute care hospitals. Infect Control Hosp Epidemiol 2008;29(Suppl 1):S12–21.

102. Bodanapally UK, Saksobhavivat N, Shanmuganathan K, et al. Arterial injuries after penetrating brain injury in civilians: risk factors on admission head computed tomography. J Neurosurg 2015;122:219–26.

103. Mansour A, Loggini A, El Ammar F, et al. Cerebrovascular complications in early survivors of civilian penetrating brain injury. Neurocrit Care 2020. https://doi.org/10.1007/s12028-020-01106-y.

104. Haddad FS, Haddad GF, Taha J. Traumatic intracranial aneurysms caused by missiles: their presentation and management. Neurosurgery 1991;28:1–7.

105. Qureshi AI, Sahito S, Liaqat J, et al. Traumatic injury of major cerebral venous sinuses associated with traumatic brain injury or head and neck trauma: analysis of national trauma data bank. J Vasc Interv Neurol 2020;11:27–33.

106. Ilyas A, Ching-Jen C, Daniel MR, et al. Endovascular mechanical thrombectomy for cerebral venous sinus thrombosis: a systematic review. J Neurointerv Surg 2017;9:1086–92.

107. Liao C-H, Nien-Chen L, Wen-Hsien C, et al. Endovascular mechanical thrombectomy and on-site chemical thrombolysis for severe cerebral venous sinus thrombosis. Sci Rep 2020;10:4937.

108. McFarlane TD, Love J, Hanley S, et al. Increased risk of stroke among young adults with serious traumatic brain injury. J Head Trauma Rehabil 2020;35: E310–9.

109. Barrow DL, Spector RH, Braun IF, et al. Classification and treatment of spontaneous carotid-cavernous sinus fistulas. J Neurosurg 1985;62:248–56.
110. Taki W, Nakahara I, Nishi S, et al. Pathogenetic and therapeutic considerations of carotid-cavernous sinus fistulas. Acta Neurochir (Wien) 1994;127:6–14.
111. Houser OW, Campbell JK, Campbell RJ, et al. Arteriovenous malformation affecting the transverse dural venous sinus–an acquired lesion. Mayo Clin Proc 1979;54:651–61.
112. Robert T, Philippe S, Raphaël B, et al. Thrombosis of venous outflows of the cavernous sinus: possible aetiology of the cortical venous reflux in case of indirect carotid-cavernous fistulas. Acta Neurochir (Wien) 2017;159:835–43.
113. Nomura M, Kentaro M, Akira T, et al. Cavernous sinus dural arteriovenous fistula patients presenting with headache as an initial symptom. J Clin Med Res 2016; 8:342–5.
114. Pashapour A, Reza M, Firooz S, et al. Long-term endovascular treatment outcome of 46 patients with cavernous sinus dural arteriovenous fistulas presenting with ophthalmic symptoms. A non-controlled trial with clinical and angiographic follow-up. Neuroradiol J 2014;27:461–70.
115. Debrun GM, Viñuela F, Fox AJ, et al. Indications for treatment and classification of 132 carotid-cavernous fistulas. Neurosurgery 1988;22:285–9.
116. Andrade G, Ponte De Souza ML, Marques R, et al. Endovascular treatment of traumatic carotid cavernous fistula with balloon-assisted sinus coiling. A technical description and initial results. Interv Neuroradiol 2013;19:445–54.
117. Servadei F, Picetti E. Traumatic subarachnoid hemorrhage. World Neurosurg 2014;82:e597–8.
118. Lin T-K, Tsai H-C, Hsieh T-C. The impact of traumatic subarachnoid hemorrhage on outcome: a study with grouping of traumatic subarachnoid hemorrhage and transcranial Doppler sonography. J Trauma Acute Care Surg 2012;73:131–6.
119. Al-Mufti F, Krishna A, Abhinav C, et al. Traumatic brain injury and intracranial hemorrhage-induced cerebral vasospasm: a systematic review. Neurosurg Focus 2017;43:E14.
120. Al-Mufti F, Krishna A, Megan L, et al. Low glasgow coma score in traumatic intracranial hemorrhage predicts development of cerebral vasospasm. World Neurosurg 2018;120:e68–71.
121. Vulcu S, Wagner F, Fernandes Santos A, et al. Repetitive computed tomography perfusion for detection of cerebral vasospasm-related hypoperfusion in aneurysmal subarachnoid hemorrhage. World Neurosurg 2019;121:e739–46.
122. Takano K, Hida K, Iwaasa M, et al. Three-dimensional spin-echo-based black-blood MRA in the detection of vasospasm following subarachnoid hemorrhage. J Magn Reson Imaging 2019;49:800–7.
123. Gollwitzer S, Groemer T, Rampp S, et al. Early prediction of delayed cerebral ischemia in subarachnoid hemorrhage based on quantitative EEG: A prospective study in adults. Clin Neurophysiol 2015;126:1514–23.
124. Badri S, Jasper C, Jason B, et al. Mortality and long-term functional outcome associated with intracranial pressure after traumatic brain injury. Intensive Care Med 2012;38:1800–9.
125. Narayan RK, Kishore PR, Becker DP, et al. Intracranial pressure: to monitor or not to monitor? A review of our experience with severe head injury. J Neurosurg 1982;56:650–9.
126. Stocchetti N, Zoerle T, Carbonara M. Intracranial pressure management in patients with traumatic brain injury: an update. Curr Opin Crit Care 2017;23:110–4.

127. on behalf of the CENTER-TBI investigators, Maryse CC, Jilske AH, van der Jagt M, et al. Variation in monitoring and treatment policies for intracranial hypertension in traumatic brain injury: a survey in 66 neurotrauma centers participating in the CENTER-TBI study. Crit Care 2017;21:233.

128. Adams H, Donnelly J, Czosnyka M, et al. Temporal profile of intracranial pressure and cerebrovascular reactivity in severe traumatic brain injury and association with fatal outcome: An observational study. PLoS Med 2017;14:e1002353.

129. Miller JD, Becker DP, Ward JD, et al. Significance of intracranial hypertension in severe head injury. J Neurosurg 1977;47:503–16.

130. Treggiari MM, Schutz N, Yanez ND, et al. Role of intracranial pressure values and patterns in predicting outcome in traumatic brain injury: a systematic review. Neurocrit Care 2007;6:104–12.

131. Lundberg N. Continuous recording and control of ventricular fluid pressure in neurosurgical practice. J Neuropathol Exp Neurol 1962;21:489.

132. Lundberg N, Troupp H, Lorin H. Continuous recording of the ventricular-fluid pressure in patients with severe acute traumatic brain injury: a preliminary report. J Neurosurg 1965;22:581–90.

133. Kishore PR, Lipper MH, Becker DP, et al. Significance of CT in head injury: correlation with intracranial pressure. AJR Am J Roentgenol 1981;137:829–33.

134. Gu J, Huang H, Huang Y, et al. Hypertonic saline or mannitol for treating elevated intracranial pressure in traumatic brain injury: a meta-analysis of randomized controlled trials. Neurosurg Rev 2019;42:499–509.

135. Alnemari AM, Krafcik BM, Mansour TR, et al. A comparison of pharmacologic therapeutic agents used for the reduction of intracranial pressure after traumatic brain injury. World Neurosurg 2017;106:509–28.

136. Andrews PJD. Hypothermia for intracranial hypertension after traumatic brain injury. N Engl J Med 2015;373:2403–12.

137. Cooper DJ, Rosenfeld JV, Murray L, et al. Decompressive craniectomy in diffuse traumatic brain injury. N Engl J Med 2011;364:1493–502.

138. Dereeper E, Berré J, Vandesteene A, et al. Barbiturate coma for intracranial hypertension: clinical observations. J Crit Care 2002;17:58–62.

139. Chesnut RM, Nancy T, Nancy C, et al. A trial of intracranial-pressure monitoring in traumatic brain injury. N Engl J Med 2012;367:2471–81.

140. American College of Surgeons. Management of Traumatic Brain Injury. 2015. Available at: https://www.facs.org/-/media/files/quality-programs/trauma/tqip/tbi_guidelines.ashx.

141. Le Roux P, Menon DK, Citerio G, et al. The international multidisciplinary consensus conference on multimodality monitoring in neurocritical care: a list of recommendations and additional conclusions: a statement for healthcare professionals from the neurocritical care society and the european society of intensive care medicine. Neurocrit Care 2014;21(Suppl 2):S282–96.

142. Bauer DF, Razdan SN, Bartolucci AA, et al. Meta-analysis of hemorrhagic complications from ventriculostomy placement by neurosurgeons. Neurosurgery 2011;69:255–60.

143. Kitchen WJ, Navneet S, Sharon H, et al. External ventricular drain infection: improved technique can reduce infection rates. Br J Neurosurg 2011;25:632–5.

144. Sieg EP, Schlauderaff AC, Payne RA, et al. Impact of an external ventricular drain placement and handling protocol on infection rates: a meta-analysis and single institution experience. World Neurosurg 2018;115:e53-e58.

145. Hepburn-Smith M, Irina D, Marina S, et al. Establishment of an external ventricular drain best practice guideline: the quest for a comprehensive, universal standard for external ventricular drain care. J Neurosci Nurs 2016;48:54–65.

146. Talibi SS, Adikarige Hd S, Fardad TA, et al. The implementation of an external ventricular drain care bundle to reduce infection rates. Br J Neurosurg 2020; 34:181–6.

147. Bekar A, Doğan S, Abaş F, et al. Risk factors and complications of intracranial pressure monitoring with a fiberoptic device. J Clin Neurosci 2009;16:236–40.

148. Chung DY, DaiWai MO, Sayona J, et al. Evidence-based management of external ventricular drains. Curr Neurol Neurosci Rep 2019;19:94.

149. Meixensberger J, Albert V, Matthias J, et al. Monitoring of brain tissue oxygenation following severe subarachnoid hemorrhage. Neurol Res 2003;25:445–50.

150. Kett-White R, Hutchinson PJ, Al-Rawi PG, et al. Adverse cerebral events detected after subarachnoid hemorrhage using brain oxygen and microdialysis probes. Neurosurgery 2002;50:1213–22.

151. Gupta AK, Hutchinson PJ, Al-Rawi P, et al. Measuring brain tissue oxygenation compared with jugular venous oxygen saturation for monitoring cerebral oxygenation after traumatic brain injury. Anesth Analg 1999;88:549–53.

152. Stewart C, Iain H, Zsolt Z, et al. The new Licox combined brain tissue oxygen and brain temperature monitor: assessment of in vitro accuracy and clinical experience in severe traumatic brain injury. Neurosurgery 2008;63:1159–64 [discussion 1164-1165].

153. Coles JP. Defining ischemic burden after traumatic brain injury using [15] O PET imaging of cerebral physiology. J Cereb Blood Flow Metab 2004;24:191–201.

154. Sarrafzadeh AS, Kiening KL, Bardt TF, et al. Cerebral oxygenation in contusioned vs. nonlesioned brain tissue: monitoring of PtiO2 with Licox and Paratrend. Acta Neurochir Suppl 1998;71:186–9.

155. Longhi L, Francesca P, Valerio V, et al. Monitoring brain tissue oxygen tension in brain-injured patients reveals hypoxic episodes in normal-appearing and in peri-focal tissue. Intensive Care Med 2007;33:2136–42.

156. Maloney-Wilensky E, Vicente G, Arthur I, et al. Brain tissue oxygen and outcome after severe traumatic brain injury: a systematic review. Crit Care Med 2009;37: 2057–63.

157. Stocchetti N, et al. High Cerebral Perfusion Pressure Improves Low Values of Local Brain Tissue O2 Tension (PtiO2) in Focal Lesions. In: Marmarou A, et al, editors. Intracranial pressure and neuromonitoring in brain injury. Springer Vienna; 1998. p. 162–5. https://doi.org/10.1007/978-3-7091-6475-4_47.

158. Zygun DA, Jurgens N, Peter JH, et al. The effect of red blood cell transfusion on cerebral oxygenation and metabolism after severe traumatic brain injury. Crit Care Med 2009;37:1074–8.

159. McCredie VA, Simone P, Marlene S, et al. The impact of red blood cell transfusion on cerebral tissue oxygen saturation in severe traumatic brain injury. Neurocrit Care 2017;26:247–55.

160. Oddo M, Edjah N, Suzanne F, et al. Acute lung injury is an independent risk factor for brain hypoxia after severe traumatic brain injury. Neurosurgery 2010;67: 338–44.

161. Reinprecht A, Manfred G, Stefan W, et al. Prone position in subarachnoid hemorrhage patients with acute respiratory distress syndrome: effects on cerebral tissue oxygenation and intracranial pressure. Crit Care Med 2003;31:1831–8.

162. Nakajima S, Meyer JS, Amano T, et al. Cerebral vasomotor responsiveness during 100% oxygen inhalation in cerebral ischemia. Arch Neurol 1983;40:271–6.

163. Diringer MN, Aiyagari V, Zazulia AR, et al. Effect of hyperoxia on cerebral metabolic rate for oxygen measured using positron emission tomography in patients with acute severe head injury. J Neurosurg 2007;106:526–9.

164. Okonkwo DO, Lori AS, Carol M, et al. Brain oxygen optimization in severe traumatic brain injury phase-II: a phase II randomized trial. Crit Care Med 2017;45:1907–14.

165. Lazaridis C, Andrews CM. Brain tissue oxygenation, lactate-pyruvate ratio, and cerebrovascular pressure reactivity monitoring in severe traumatic brain injury: systematic review and viewpoint. Neurocrit Care 2014;21:345–55.

166. Bito L, Davson H, Levin E, et al. The concentrations of free amino acids and other electrolytes in cerebrospinal fluid, in vivo dialysate of brain, and blood plasma of the dog. J Neurochem 1966;13:1057–67.

167. Delgado JM, DeFeudis FV, Roth RH, et al. Dialytrode for long term intracerebral perfusion in awake monkeys. Arch Int Pharmacodyn Ther 1972;198:9–21.

168. Benveniste H, Hüttemeier PC. Microdialysis–theory and application. Prog Neurobiol 1990;35:195–215.

169. Chen KC, Höistad M, Kehr J, et al. Theory relating in vitro and in vivo microdialysis with one or two probes. J Neurochem 2002;81:108–21.

170. Hutchinson PJ, O'Connell MT, Nortje J, et al. Cerebral microdialysis methodology–evaluation of 20 kDa and 100 kDa catheters. Physiol Meas 2005;26:423–8.

171. Merenda A, Marinella G, Rebecca H, et al. Validation of brain extracellular glycerol as an indicator of cellular membrane damage due to free radical activity after traumatic brain injury. J Neurotrauma 2008;25:527–37.

172. Harris JJ, Jolivet R, Attwell D. Synaptic energy use and supply. Neuron 2012;75:762–77.

173. Howarth C, Gleeson P, Attwell D. Updated energy budgets for neural computation in the neocortex and cerebellum. J Cereb Blood Flow Metab 2012;32:1222–32.

174. Vespa PM, McArthur D, O'Phelan K, et al. Persistently low extracellular glucose correlates with poor outcome 6 months after human traumatic brain injury despite a lack of increased lactate: a microdialysis study. J Cereb Blood Flow Metab 2003;23:865–77.

175. Bergsneider M, Hovda DA, Shalmon E, et al. Cerebral hyperglycolysis following severe traumatic brain injury in humans: a positron emission tomography study. J Neurosurg 1997;86:241–51.

176. Jalloh I, Carpenter KLH, Grice P, et al. Glycolysis and the pentose phosphate pathway after human traumatic brain injury: microdialysis studies using 1,2-(13)C2 glucose. J Cereb Blood Flow Metab 2015;35:111–20.

177. Bartnik BL, Richard LS, Masamichi F, et al. Upregulation of pentose phosphate pathway and preservation of tricarboxylic acid cycle flux after experimental brain injury. J Neurotrauma 2005;22:1052–65.

178. Carre E, Michael O, Henry B, et al. Metabolic crisis in severely head-injured patients: is ischemia just the tip of the iceberg? Front Neurol 2013;4:146.

179. Merino MA, Sahuquillo J, Borrull A, et al. Is lactate a good indicator of brain tissue hypoxia in the acute phase of traumatic brain injury? Results of a pilot study in 21 patients. Neurocirugia (Astur) 2010;21:289–301.

180. Timofeev I, Carpenter KLH, Nortje J, et al. Cerebral extracellular chemistry and outcome following traumatic brain injury: a microdialysis study of 223 patients. Brain 2011;134:484–94.

181. Wright MJ, McArthur DL, Alger JR, et al. Early metabolic crisis-related brain atrophy and cognition in traumatic brain injury. Brain Imaging Behav 2013;7: 307–15.

182. Xu Y, McArthur DL, Alger JR, et al. Early nonischemic oxidative metabolic dysfunction leads to chronic brain atrophy in traumatic brain injury. J Cereb Blood Flow Metab 2010;30:883–94.

183. Vespa P, Marvin B, Nayoa H, et al. Metabolic crisis without brain ischemia is common after traumatic brain injury: a combined microdialysis and positron emission tomography study. J Cereb Blood Flow Metab 2005;25:763–74.

184. Barsan W. Brain Oxygen Optimization in Severe TBI, Phase 3 (BOOST). Available at: https://clinicaltrials.gov/ct2/show/NCT03754114.

185. Bonow RH, Young CC, Bass DI, et al. Transcranial Doppler ultrasonography in neurological surgery and neurocritical care. Neurosurg Focus 2019;47:E2.

186. Homburg AM, Jakobsen M, Enevoldsen E. Transcranial Doppler recordings in raised intracranial pressure. Acta Neurol Scand 1993;87:488–93.

187. Bellner J, Romner B, Reinstrup P, et al. Transcranial Doppler sonography pulsatility index (PI) reflects intracranial pressure (ICP). Surg Neurol 2004;62:45–51 [discussion 51].

188. de Riva N, Budohoski KP, Smielewski P, et al. Transcranial Doppler pulsatility index: what it is and what it isn't. Neurocrit Care 2012;17:58–66.

189. Cardim D, Chiara R, Joseph D, et al. Prospective study on noninvasive assessment of intracranial pressure in traumatic brain-injured patients: comparison of four methods. J Neurotrauma 2016;33:792–802.

190. Rasulo FA, Rita B, Chiara R, et al. The accuracy of transcranial Doppler in excluding intracranial hypertension following acute brain injury: a multicenter prospective pilot study. Crit Care 2017;21:44.

191. Hansen HC, Helmke K. The subarachnoid space surrounding the optic nerves. An ultrasound study of the optic nerve sheath. Surg Radiol Anat 1996;18:323–8.

192. Rajajee V, Vanaman M, Fletcher JJ, et al. Optic nerve ultrasound for the detection of raised intracranial pressure. Neurocrit Care 2011;15:506–15.

193. Ohle R, McIsaac SM, Woo MY, et al. Sonography of the optic nerve sheath diameter for detection of raised intracranial pressure compared to computed tomography: a systematic review and meta-analysis. J Ultrasound Med 2015;34: 1285–94.

194. Robba C, Gregorio S, Marek C, et al. Optic nerve sheath diameter measured sonographically as non-invasive estimator of intracranial pressure: a systematic review and meta-analysis. Intensive Care Med 2018;44:1284–94.

195. Ballantyne SA, O'Neill G, Hamilton R, et al. Observer variation in the sonographic measurement of optic nerve sheath diameter in normal adults. Eur J Ultrasound 2002;15:145–9.

196. Jahns F-P, Paul Miroz J, Messerer M, et al. Quantitative pupillometry for the monitoring of intracranial hypertension in patients with severe traumatic brain injury. Crit Care 2019;23:155.

197. El Ahmadieh TY, Bedros N, Stutzman SE, et al. Automated pupillometry as a triage and assessment tool in patients with traumatic brain injury. World Neurosurg 2020. https://doi.org/10.1016/j.wneu.2020.09.152. S1878875020321719.

198. Davies DJ, Zhangjie S, Michael TC, et al. Near-infrared spectroscopy in the monitoring of adult traumatic brain injury: a review. J Neurotrauma 2015;32: 933–41.

199. Chung DY, Claassen J, Agarwal S, et al. Assessment of noninvasive regional brain oximetry in posterior reversible encephalopathy syndrome and reversible cerebral vasoconstriction syndrome. J Intensive Care Med 2016;31:415–9.
200. Muehlschlegel S, Selb J, Patel M, et al. Feasibility of NIRS in the neurointensive care unit: a pilot study in stroke using physiological oscillations. Neurocrit Care 2009;11:288–95.
201. Boas DA, Sava S, Juliette S, et al. Establishing the diffuse correlation spectroscopy signal relationship with blood flow. Neurophotonics 2016;3:031412.
202. Zhou C, Stephanie AE, Turgut D, et al. Diffuse optical monitoring of hemodynamic changes in piglet brain with closed head injury. J Biomed Opt 2009;14:034015.
203. Selb J, Wu KC, Sutin J, et al. Prolonged monitoring of cerebral blood flow and autoregulation with diffuse correlation spectroscopy in neurocritical care patients. Neurophotonics 2018;5:045005.

Acute Traumatic Spinal Cord Injury

Ilyas Eli, MD[a,b], David P. Lerner, MD[c], Zoher Ghogawala, MD[b,*]

KEYWORDS

- Spinal cord injury • Apoptosis • Corticosteroids • Mean arterial pressure
- Quantitative magnetic resonance imaging

KEY POINTS

- Traumatic spinal cord injury is a common occurrence throughout the world with significant morbidity, including permanent disability from motor, sensory, and autonomic dysfunction.
- Hyperacute management of suspected or confirmed spinal cord injury includes maintaining airway, breathing, and circulation with special consideration for early airway stabilization via intubation while maintaining spinal precautions. Further management involves avoidance of hypotension and external spinal stabilization with cervical collar and backboard as appropriate.
- Computed tomography scan and MRI are necessary to assess the extent of bony, ligamentous, and spinal cord injury to assist with surgical planning.
- Intensive care unit management with close monitoring of airway and blood pressure with vigilant monitoring for complications, including bowel and bladder dysfunction, pressure ulceration, and infection, is required.

INTRODUCTION

Acute traumatic spinal cord injury (SCI) is typically associated with devastating outcomes. The injury to the spinal cord results in damage to motor, sensory, and autonomic functions of the spinal cord but also takes a toll on a patient's well-being, including their physical and psychological state.

The literature provides many descriptions of the pathophysiology and management of acute SCI, yet there continue to be controversies regarding the overall management. Numerous guidelines have been published, by the American Association of Neurological Surgeons/Congress of Neurological Surgeons (AANS/CNS) in 2002 and 2013, The Paralyzed Veterans of America in 2008, and AO Spine in 2017, which provide sufficient framework to reference in the management of SCI.[1–5] This review

^a Department of Neurosurgery, Clinical Neurosciences Center, University of Utah, Salt Lake City, UT, USA; ^b Department of Neurosurgery, Lahey Hospital and Medical Center, Burlington, MA, USA; ^c Department of Neurology, Lahey Hospital and Medical Center, Burlington, MA, USA
* Corresponding author. Department of Neurosurgery, Lahey Hospital and Medical Center, 41 Mall Road, Burlington, MA 01805.
E-mail address: zoher.ghogawala@lahey.org

Neurol Clin 39 (2021) 471–488
https://doi.org/10.1016/j.ncl.2021.02.004
0733-8619/21/© 2021 Elsevier Inc. All rights reserved.

neurologic.theclinics.com

focuses on a comprehensive overview of SCI as it relates to current understanding, acute management, and promising investigational treatment modalities.

EPIDEMIOLOGY

The incidence of SCI in the United States is 54 cases per 1 million people, resulting in approximately 17,810 new cases per year.[6-8] Worldwide incidence ranges from 10.4 to 83 cases per million persons per year.[9,10] SCI results in major morbidity and mortality and is associated with lifetime health care costs ranging from $1.1 to $5.4 million and innumerable costs to the community and society.[11] SCI typically affects men more often than women, with 78% of new cases being in male individuals.[12] The average age of patients at the time of injury is approximately 43 years, but there is a bimodal distribution with a peak in adolescents/young adults and a second peak in the elderly population (older than 65 years of age).[13] Motor vehicle accidents account for 38.6% of SCIs, whereas falls account for 32.2% of cases, violent activity (eg, gunshots) accounts for 14.0%, sports-related activity accounts for 7.8%, surgery accounts for 4.2%, and 3.2% accounts for all other causes (**Fig. 1**).[11]

ANATOMY AND PATHOPHYSIOLOGY

Management and treatment of SCI require a firm understanding of the pathophysiological process involved. The initial insult in SCI is a direct result of a mechanical traumatic injury to the spinal cord. Burst fracture, facet dislocation, and other more extensive fractures, such as flexion-distraction injuries, can result in a forceful damage to the vertebral column, intervertebral disc, ligaments, and the spinal cord.[14] The acute SCI that ensues has 2 phases: primary and secondary. The primary phase is a result of the blunt trauma, which results in shearing and laceration of spinal cord fibers owing to an acceleration-deceleration mechanism.[15] The impact can result in a contused spinal cord and rarely in full transection. The overall primary phase consists of axonal injury, disruption of blood vessels, and disruption of cellular membranes.

The secondary phase is the physiologic response to the initial trauma, which results in inflammation, ischemia, vascular dysfunction, free-radical formation, impaired neuronal hemostasis, and apoptosis/necrosis. The secondary phase can be classified into the immediate, acute, intermediate, and chronic stages.[16] The immediate phase occurs during the first 2 hours after injury and results in the death of neurons and glia; it is associated clinically with "spinal shock,"[17,18] reversible reduction in sensory, motor,

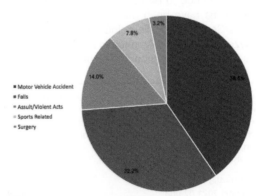

Fig. 1. Causes of acute traumatic SCI in the United States.

and reflexes in the hyperacute setting of SCI. The immediate phase is also associated with cellular necrosis owing to the mechanical injury to cell membranes and microhemorrhages owing to the vascular injury.[19,20]

The acute phase occurs from 2 hours to 2 weeks after injury. The early acute phase (2–48 hours) comprises increasing inflammation, edema, and hemorrhage. Acute phase injuries are caused by free-radical generation, ionic dysregulation, excitotoxicity (owing to glutamate-mediated pathways), immune-related neurotoxicity, and further vascular disruption that all result in progression of axonal injury and cellular necrosis.[21–26] The subacute phase, which occurs from approximately day 2 to 2 weeks after injury, refers to the phagocytic response to clear cellular debris and initiate early axonal growth. During this phase, damaged astrocytes undergo cellular edema and necrosis, whereas astrocytes on the periphery of the injured tissue proliferate and function to reestablish ionic hemostasis and the blood-brain barrier and to restrict immune cell inflow. A deleterious consequence of astrocytic proliferation is scar formation, which prevents axonal regeneration because the scar functions as a physical and chemical barrier.[16,27,28]

The intermediate phase occurs after week 2, lasts up to 6 months, and includes continual maturation of the astrocytic scar and the beginning of axonal sprouting.[29] The chronic phase starts at 6 months after injury and continues through the lifetime of the patient. During the chronic phase, there are further scar maturation and the formation of syrinxes. The process of Wallerian degeneration persists and requires several years for the injured axons to be fully eliminated.[30] Furthermore, maturation of the lesion is evidenced by the presence of myelomalacia and cystic cavitations.[21,31] Potential therapeutic interventions target these primary and secondary phases to optimize recovery and spinal cord regeneration.

MANAGEMENT
Hyperacute Management

Initial management of patients with SCI is started at the scene of the injury. Nearly 25% of SCI cooccurs with brain, chest/abdomen, or major extremity injury.[32] As with all medical emergencies, the first evaluation focuses on ABCs (airway, breathing, and circulation) and then comprehensive emergency management of the injured patient as indicated by Advanced Traumatic Life Support guidelines. Patients with the following should be considered for spinal immobilization[33]:

- Blunt trauma
- Spinal tenderness or pain
- Patients with an altered level of consciousness
- Neurologic deficits
- Obvious anatomic deformity of the spine
- High-energy trauma
- Presence of a distracting injury or intoxication from drugs or alcohol

Patients with suspected fractures of the thoracic and lumbar regions should undergo thoracolumbar precautions and immobilization using a backboard and logroll techniques for turning and transfers.[34]

Patients with SCI benefit from being transferred directly to a level 1 trauma center equipped with specialized physicians (emergency medicine, trauma surgeons, neuroradiologists, neurosurgeons, spine surgeons, and intensivists), nurses with experience and skill in managing acute SCI patients, and imaging (computed tomography [CT] and MRI) capabilities that allow for immediate evaluation. Early transfer of SCI patients to specialized SCI centers has been proven to yield improved patient outcomes.[35] The mode of transport to higher-level care centers, either by ground or by air, has not been shown to produce a difference in outcomes.[36]

On arrival to an emergency department, the primary survey requires focused attention and stabilization of ABCs. Next, a rapid neurologic examination should be performed, consisting of a Glasgow Coma Scale assessment with attention to movement of all 4 extremities, as well as pupil size and reactivity. In the secondary survey for suspected SCI, the entire spinal column and paravertebral musculature should be examined for deformity and focal tenderness, and a neurologic examination as detailed in later discussion should occur. During this assessment, cervical and thoracolumbar spine precautions should be maintained.

Airway/Breathing

Patients with suspected or confirmed cervical SCI require close respiratory monitoring. Patients with injury rostral to C5 are more likely to require intubation and ventilator support.[1] Patients in respiratory distress should undergo immediate controlled intubation while cervical spine precautions are taken. Exaggerated bradycardia can occur during intubation because of an abnormal, unopposed parasympathetic response to tracheal stimulation during suctioning and endotracheal tube insertion.[37] Subjective complaint of dyspnea should be taken seriously because early neuromuscular respiratory failure results in hypoventilation with normal oxygen saturation. For patients able to participate in examination, bedside assessment with a single breath count test can provide an indirect evaluation of forced vital capacity, and a value less than 12 is concerning for imminent respiratory failure.[38] As noted above, the temporal progression of SCI can result in worsening spinal cord edema and perfusion, which may worsen respiratory status in a delayed fashion.[39] Focus should then be directed toward hemodynamic monitoring. Resuscitation is initiated with the goal of preventing hypotension, which can occur with blood loss and neurogenic shock.

Circulation

As noted above, polytrauma is common with SCI. Shock may be present and is of particular concern in patients with SCI because periods of hypotension can worsen neurologic outcome.[40,41] Hemorrhagic, cardiogenic, and restrictive shock should all be considered in trauma patients, but neurogenic shock can also develop in those with SCI above the T4 level.[42] Neurogenic shock results from effective sympathectomy and unopposed parasympathetic activity, which manifests as hypotension and bradycardia.[43] Bradycardia is a characteristic finding in neurogenic shock and should raise suspicion, although its presence is not invariable. Initial management includes fluid resuscitation followed rapidly by vasopressor or inotrope addition.[44] Vasopressor and inotropes are discussed in more detail later.

Disability

A full clinical examination should be performed to determine the level of SCI using the American Spinal Injury Association (ASIA) International Standards for Neurological Classification of SCI.[45] The ASIA injury score involves a detailed examination of motor and sensory functions, including rectal sensation, which provides the best description of a person's neurologic status after injury (**Fig. 2**).[46] The strength score is based on the MRC (Medical Research Council) scale of 0 to 5 for motor strength in all 20 muscle groups in the entire body. Sensation assessment is based on whether it is absent (0 points), altered (1 point), normal (2 points), or untestable. The ASIA scale also records the degree of injury (complete or incomplete) on a 5-element scale (**Table 1**). Practitioners should be aware that the ASIA scale can be inaccurate in the hyperacute

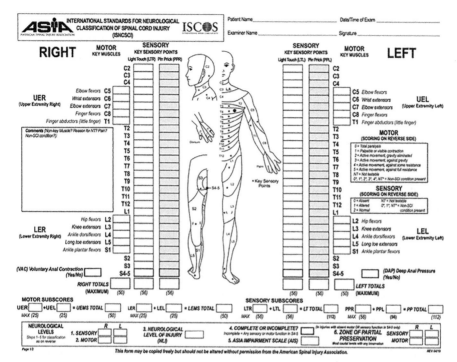

Fig. 2. ASIA classification of SCI. (© 2020 American Spinal Injury Association. Reprinted with permission.)

setting because of "spinal shock." The overall identification of baseline functional abilities and impairments is essential in determining recovery, prognostication, and eligibility for clinical trials.[34]

IMAGING AND DIAGNOSTIC TESTING

Imaging plays an essential role in the diagnosis and guidance of management in SCI. Early imaging allows for the identification of the structural injury to the spinal column, which will determine surgical and nonsurgical treatment. The injury can then be classified using the AO Spine thoracolumbar or subaxial cervical spine injury classification systems or the thoracolumbar injury classification system (TLICS).[47–49] The TLICS classification system is based on 3 categories: morphology of injury, integrity of the

Table 1	
American spinal injury association scale	
Grade A Complete	No motor or sensory function below the level of injury
Grade B Incomplete	Sensory function is preserved below the level of injury, but not motor function. Sensation is preserved in some of the sacral segments S4-S5
Grade C Incomplete	More than half of the key muscles below the neurologic level have a muscle grade <3
Grade D Incomplete	At least half of the key muscles below the neurologic level have a muscle grade of 3 or more
Grade E None	Normal motor and sensory function

posterior ligamentous complex, and neurologic status (**Table 2**).[50] The total sum of points based on severity in each category determines whether the patient is likely or not to benefit from surgical intervention. CT scans provide a clear radiographic image of the bony destruction to the spinal column (**Fig. 3**). CT serves as an initial imaging modality, as it is fast and reliable. Subsequently, MRI provides further understanding of the injury, which may or may not involve the disc space and ligaments and can show whether an epidural or subdural hematoma exists (**Fig. 4**).

SURGICAL MANAGEMENT

Numerous studies have evaluated whether early decompressive surgery improves outcomes after SCI. The Surgical Timing in Acute Spinal Cord Injury Study, which was a prospective multicenter study published in 2012, assessed 6-month outcomes after early (<24 hours) versus late (>24 hours) surgery in a total of 313 patients with cervical SCI.[51] The results showed that patients who had early decompressive surgery had a higher rate of a 2-grade improvement in the ASIA impairment scale (AIS) score at 6-month follow-up when compared with patients who underwent late surgical decompression. However, critics of the study mention that a power calculation was not stated in the study, which could have led to an inadequate sample size.[9] In addition, because the timing of surgical decompression was not randomized, there might be significant surgeon bias in selecting patients for early surgery. In addition, when the analysis was limited to patients with initial ASIA grade A, B, and C (for whom a 2-grade improvement is possible), the results are no longer statistically significant.[9] In another prospective study, Jug and colleagues[52] evaluated the role of early surgical decompression of cervical SCI ASIA grade A, B, or C within 8 hours versus 8 to 24 hours after injury. Their results showed that at 6-month follow-up, there was an improvement of at

Table 2	
Thoracolumbar injury classification and severity score system	
Injury Category	**Point Value**
Injury morphology	
Compression	1
Burst	2
Translation or rotation	3
Distraction	4
Posterior ligamentous complex status	
Intact	0
Injury suspected or indeterminate	2
Injured	3
Neurologic status	
Intact	0
Nerve root involvement	2
Spinal cord or conus medullaris injury	
Incomplete	3
Complete	2
Cauda equina syndrome	3

Scores: <4, nonoperative; 4, nonoperative or operative; >4, operative.

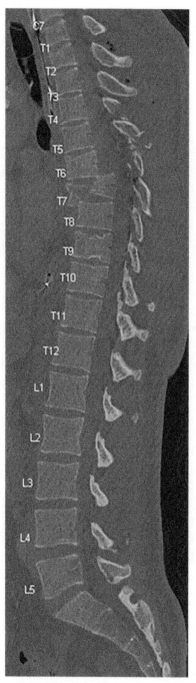

Fig. 3. CT scan demonstrating the bony destruction in a T6-T7 fracture dislocation injury.

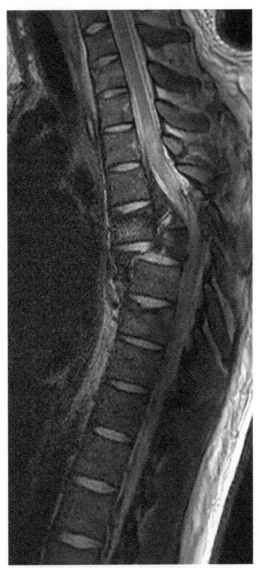

Fig. 4. T2-weighted MRI demonstrating complete disruption of the posterior ligamentous complex and anterior longitudinal ligament. A large ventral epidural hematoma at the level of the fracture is also shown.

least 2 AIS grades in 5.5% of patients in the early group and 10% in the late group (P = .017). A meta-analysis of 18 studies from 1996 to 2012 demonstrated that early surgery was associated with a higher total motor score improvement in 7 studies, neurologic improvement in 6 studies, and shorter hospital length of stay in 6 studies. The studies pooled in the meta-analysis were heterogeneous in nature, and the studies were concerning for publication biases.[53] A Canadian multicenter cohort study[54] looked at 84 patients with cervical, thoracic, or lumbar SCI who underwent either early, defined as less than 24 hours from injury (35 patients), or late (49 patients) surgery. The results showed that a greater portion of patients who underwent early surgery had at least a 2-grade AIS improvement ($P = .01$).

Many of the studies evaluating the timing of surgical decompression demonstrate benefit from early decompressive surgery, despite the criticisms of the biases and study designs. Further studies, such as the multicenter prospective, observational European study (SCI-POEM), are currently in process. On the basis of existing data, the AO Spine guidelines currently suggest early decompressive surgery when possible.[55]

MEDICAL MANAGEMENT
Role of Corticosteroids

The use of steroids remains controversial in the treatment of acute SCI. Initial interest in the use of steroids was based on a rationale of augmenting anti-inflammatory mechanisms and thus promoting cell survival by limiting inflammation-mediated secondary injury. Although early data suggested a benefit for steroid administration, multiple subsequent studies investigating the role of steroids have found no benefit for their use.[56–58] The National Acute Spinal Cord Injury Study investigated the role of very-high-dose methylprednisolone (bolus of methylprednisolone 30 mg/kg followed by an infusion of 5.4 mg/kg/h for 48 hours) in acute SCI. It showed no improvement of outcomes as assessed by its primary endpoints among patients treated with steroids. Secondary subgroup analysis showed significant motor recovery in patients who received methylprednisolone within 8 hours of injury, but the study also demonstrated the major adverse effects of high-dose steroids.[42] In the study, 48-hour administration of high-dose steroids resulted in increased risk of pneumonia and sepsis, whereas lower complication rates were observed with a shorter (24-hour) course of high-dose steroids.[56–58] A Cochrane Review analyzing 6 studies of methylprednisolone in acute SCI found an overall 4-point increase in ASIA motor score when steroids were administered within 8 hours of injury.[59] The AANS/CNS guidelines from 2013 do not recommend the use of methylprednisolone for the treatment of SCI.[60] The rationale for this exclusion was the lack of level I and II evidence in support of the treatment and the presence of level III evidence that demonstrated possible deleterious effects. However, the AO Spine guidelines from 2017 state that high-dose methylprednisolone given intravenously for 24 hours should be offered within 8 hours of SCI in patients without medical contraindications.[2] Thus, the role of steroids in acute SCI remains controversial, with no level I or II evidence to suggest its benefit.

Blood Pressure Management

Blood pressure management plays an important role in acute SCI. It is widely accepted that hypotension in the setting of SCI results in poor outcomes[40]; however, there are only limited low-quality data to suggest that augmenting mean arterial pressure (MAP) results in improved outcomes.[61–63] As noted above, the secondary phase of SCI results in cord edema and ischemia. The edema can result in relative hypoperfusion of the injured spinal cord by limiting local blood flow. In attempts to perfuse the injured spinal cord, increasing MAP may overcome relative increases in spinal cord pressure and disrupted spinal cord autoregulation. Two prospective studies demonstrated that higher MAP goals, 85 to 90 mm Hg, after SCI resulted in better outcomes.[61,62]

On the basis of those studies and numerous retrospective studies, the AANS/CNS guidelines from 2002 and 2013 recommended avoiding hypotension (systolic blood pressure <90 mm Hg) and maintaining MAP goal of greater than 85 to 90 mm Hg.[3,55] Thus, an MAP goal of greater than 85 mm Hg is currently the standard of care for management of SCI despite being supported by only a lower body of evidence. The duration of MAP augmentation is variable in practice and ranges from 5 days to 7 days after injury.[64] The current AANS/CNS guidelines recommend maintaining MAP goals for 7 days.[5] The recommendation is based on study protocols from studies in the 1990s based on animal study results measuring spinal cord swelling at 5 days after injury.[62,65] Other studies have MAP goal duration up to 7 days, but no randomized studies exist to compare different MAP goal duration with outcomes. Studies whereby MAP goals were augmented for 5 days only after SCI did not show any decline in neurologic findings.[66–69]

Close blood pressure monitoring and augmentation require the placement of an arterial line, and previously used pulmonary artery catheterization for cardiac output optimization in the intensive care unit setting.[61,62] Pulmonary artery catheterization is less common than previously practiced, and only those with training and practice should use the invasive monitoring. Because the MAP goal of greater than 85 mm Hg may be greater than an individual's baseline blood pressure, augmentation with vasopressors may be required. The AANS/CNS guidelines do not have recommendations on preferred vasopressor or inotrope, but the Consortium for Spinal Cord Medicine recommends the use of norepinephrine and dopamine for SCI in the cervical and upper thoracic regions.[1,55] These medications have both alpha-adrenergic and beta-adrenergic effects, which counter the potential neurogenic shock associated with these levels of SCI. For lower thoracic SCI whereby the mechanism of hypotension is due to vasodilation, phenylephrine, a purely alpha-agonist, is recommended.

Although use of vasopressors can help achieve MAP goals and improve spinal cord perfusion, there are risks (**Table 3**). Dopamine has been associated with a 10% major complication rate compared with a 3% major complication rate with the use of phenylephrine. The major complications include ST segment elevation, elevated troponins, atrial fibrillation, and ventricular tachycardia.[68] Dobutamine is not used because of vasodilatation and reflex bradycardia. Epinephrine is also not used, as it can result in arrhythmias.[68] Norepinephrine has been commonly used for blood pressure

Table 3
Commonly used vasopressors/inotropes physiologic response and complications

Medication	Mean Arterial Pressure	Heart Rate	Cardiac Output	Systemic Vascular Resistance	Activity	Complications
Norepinephrine	Increase	Increase	Increase	Increase	A > β	Arrhythmia; peripheral ischemia
Phenylephrine	Increase	Decrease	Decrease	Increase	α	Reflex bradycardia; peripheral ischemia
Epinephrine	Increase	Increase	Increase	Increase	α > β	Tachyarrhythmia; stress cardiomyopathy/ cardiac ischemia
Dopamine	Increase	Increase	Increase	Increase	α = β	Low dose can cause hypotension; tachyarrhythmias; tissue ischemia
Dobutamine	Similar	Increase	Increase	Decrease	β > α	Tachyarrhythmias; cardiac ischemia
Milrinone	Similar	Increase	Increase	Decrease	cAMP > inotropic	Vasodilation; can decrease blood pressure

Abbreviation: cAMP, cyclic adenosine monophosphate.

augmentation because of its mixed alpha and beta effects, which decreases vasoconstriction and bradycardias. One study showed that administration of norepinephrine in SCI increased spinal cord blood flow and Pao_2 compared with phenylephrine.[70] Overall, optimal medication for blood pressure augmentation depends on the level of injury and patient risk factors (namely underlying cardiac function), but close monitoring of hemodynamics and potential complications is necessary regardless of choice.

SUBACUTE TO CHRONIC MANAGEMENT
General Critical Care

Traumatic SCI may not occur in isolation, and critical care management for additional injuries is important. Management of additional specific traumatic injury is beyond the scope of this discussion, but there are common principles that should guide the critical care management of these patients. SCI and resultant immobilization place the patient at risk for multiple complications. Some degree of bladder dysfunction is reported in up to 84% of patients with SCI.[71] Initially, this is treated with early insertion of a Foley catheter. For those that require long-term management, the use of intermittent clean catheterization is recommended.[72] Acute respiratory failure owing to SCI can result from diminished vital capacity, impairment of clearance of pulmonary secretions, and atelectasis/pneumonia; it may require prolonged mechanical ventilation and is directly related to the spinal level and degree of motor weakness.[73]

Deep Vein Thrombosis/Pulmonary Embolism Prophylaxis

Pulmonary embolism (PE) was the leading cause of death after SCI until effective use of thromboprophylaxis was achieved.[74] The balance of deep vein thrombosis (DVT) and PE prevention is tempered by the risk of ongoing posttraumatic or postoperative bleeding resulting in recurrent spinal cord compression. Prophylactic inferior vena cava filter placement in severely injured patients did not decrease the incidence of symptomatic PE or death and is not recommended.[75] The risk-benefit analysis of bleeding versus prevention of DVT and PE should be made on an individual and daily basis, and prophylactic-dose anticoagulation should be initiated as soon as it is deemed safe. The Neurocritical Care Society recommends initiation of DVT prophylaxis as early as possible, and within 72 hours of injury.[76] The Consortium of Spinal Cord Injury does not specify specific timing but does recommend use of low-molecular-weight heparin use for the prevention of DVT in the acute-care phase, and if there is delay because of bleeding concerns, daily assessment of bleeding risk should be carried out.[1] Enoxaparin appears to have benefit over unfractionated heparin in prevention of PE in SCI.[77]

LATEST THERAPIES
Quantitative MRI

MRI is a critical diagnostic tool used to understand the extent of injury in the setting of SCI. Emerging advances in MRI modalities serve to improve the understanding of SCI. Quantitative MRI techniques, such as magnetization transfer, magnetic resonance relaxation mapping, and diffusion imaging, all have the utility of evaluating the microstructural neural features, which allows for a better understanding of the myelination status and axonal degeneration/regeneration.[78–80]

Diffusion tensor imaging (DTI) measures the direction and amplitude of diffusion of water molecules inside tissue. In axons, the diffusion of water is restricted by cell membrane and myelin sheath, which results in a high diffusion gradient in the direction that is parallel to the white matter tracts and lower diffusion perpendicular to the white matter tracts. In SCI, whereby there is disruption of the normal architecture, this results in increased radial diffusivity because a new perpendicular pathway for water diffusion exists. Two metrics used in DTI allow for user-friendly display for interpretation: fractional anisotropy evaluates the extent to which diffusion is limited in a direction and mean diffusivity assesses overall diffusion.[81] Changes seen after SCI using DTI metrics can be used to correlate with clinical function and can be monitored throughout the diagnosis and recovery phases of patients with SCI.

The measurement of relaxation and magnetization transfer parameters is a way to connect imaging modality with histologic myelin content, iron deposition, and neuronal mapping. Pending further development, this modality feature can provide insight and serve as an imaging biomarker for tracking glial cells and neural structures in SCI.[82]

Using DTI data, a diffusion tensor tractography (DTT) can be derived using a computational method that reconstructs major nerve bundles in 3-dimensional spaces based on the anisotropy properties. DTT can distinguish the distorted and injured nerve fibers from intact areas. DTT can thus be used in the preoperative planning of surgical intervention by providing insight into the degree of damage and a view of the shape of the contused spinal cord.[83]

Invasive Spinal Cord Monitoring

Emerging invasive options offer new modalities for evaluating and treating SCI. For example, the placement of an epidural or intrathecal pressure monitoring device may allow a better understanding of spinal cord perfusion pressure parameters after various interventions. Other interventions that can be tailored toward reducing intrathecal pressure by decreasing production or increasing drainage of cerebrospinal fluid could, in turn, improve perfusion of the spinal cord.[84] Much of this research is in its early stages, but ongoing efforts will enhance the understanding of the importance of spinal cord perfusion on outcomes after SCI.[85]

CLINICAL TRIALS

There are numerous clinical trials currently ongoing for the treatment of acute SCI that targets the primary and secondary phases of injury focusing on neuroprotection and neuro-regeneration.

Multiple pharmacologic agents are being investigated in clinical trials (**Table 4**).

Table 4
Ongoing clinical trials

Neuroprotective	Regenerative	Anti-inflammatory
Zoledronic acid	Mesenchymal stem cells	Minocycline
Riluzole	Autologous bone marrow derived stem cells	Mometasone furoate
Antirepulsive guidance antibody	Adipose derived stem cells	Selenium
C3 transferase	Hepatocyte growth factor	Vitamin E
Buspirone	Growth hormone	D-Cycloserine
Nimodipine	Anti-Nogo antibody	Elezanumab
Magnesium		Solvatelide (PMZ-1620)
		Glyburide

Pharmacologic agents involved in clinical trials include nimodipine, naloxone, minocycline, riluzole, magnesium, C3 transferase (Cethrin), Gacyclidine, anti-Nogo-A antibody, GM-1 ganglioside, fibroblast growth factor, hepatocyte growth factor, and granulocyte colony-stimulating factors.[86–88] Cell-based therapies are also being investigated for potential benefits in SCI. Cell-based treatments include transplantation of autologous Schwann cell, olfactory ensheathing cells, mesenchymal stem cells, neural precursor cells, oligodendrocyte progenitor cells, and macrophages.[86,87] In addition, biomaterials, such as scaffolds, have been tested in SCI to provide a structural environment that facilitates regenerative axonal growth.[89] Scaffolds are implantable biomaterial that contains biological molecules and cells. They provide a vehicle for structural support and delivery of stem cells to alter the microenvironment and influence nerve regeneration.[90] Most of the pharmacologic agents, cell-based therapies, and biomaterials have demonstrated positive results; however, further trials are currently underway before bringing any therapies to the market.

SUMMARY

Acute SCI results in devastating outcomes with significant disability to the patient and is associated with significant ongoing health and societal costs. Acute management is geared toward preventing hypotension, early identification of injury level, and early decompression with stabilization of the spinal column. The role of steroids continues to remain controversial with no evidence to suggest a benefit. Blood pressure augmentation is currently the standard practice for up to 7 days after injury. Emerging technologies include quantitative imaging modalities and invasive spinal cord monitoring, which promise to improve the understanding of SCI. Finally, numerous ongoing clinical trials are focused on neuroprotection and neuro-regeneration. Although acute hospital management allows for the greatest possible recovery, rehabilitation serves an important role in improving functional outcome.

CLINICAL CARE POINTS

- Early management of traumatic spinal cord injury follows common airway, breathing, and circulation assessment. Disability evaluation during the secondary survey should include assessment of spinal level involved using a standardized approach. The authors advocate for using the American Spinal Injury Association grading system.

- The American Academy of Neurological Surgery does not recommend the use of high-dose methylprednisolone in the setting of acute spinal cord injury. Other medical management includes blood pressure augmentation to maintain a mean arterial pressure of greater than 85 mm Hg for 7 days after the acute injury.

- AO Spine recommends early spinal stabilization when possible. Although there is potential bias in prior trials, early (<24 hours from injury) decompression may result in improved motor and functional status of patients.

DISCLOSURE

Dr I. Eli has no disclosures. Dr D. Lerner has no disclosures. Dr Z. Ghogawala is a shareholder and IP ownership for Nidus.

REFERENCES

1. Consortium for Spinal Cord M. Early acute management in adults with spinal cord injury: a clinical practice guideline for health-care professionals. J Spinal Cord Med 2008;31:403–79.
2. Fehlings MG, Wilson JR, Tetreault LA, et al. A clinical practice guideline for the management of patients with acute spinal cord injury: recommendations on the use of methylprednisolone sodium succinate. Global Spine J 2017;7:203S–11S.
3. Hadley MN, Walters BC, Grabb PA, et al. Guidelines for the management of acute cervical spine and spinal cord injuries. Clin Neurosurg 2002;49:407–98.
4. O'Toole JE, Kaiser MG, Anderson PA, et al. Congress of Neurological Surgeons systematic review and evidence-based guidelines on the evaluation and treatment of patients with thoracolumbar spine trauma: executive summary. Neurosurgery 2019;84:2–6.
5. Walters BC, Hadley MN, Hurlbert RJ, et al. Guidelines for the management of acute cervical spine and spinal cord injuries: 2013 update. Neurosurgery 2013; 60:82–91.
6. Devivo MJ. Epidemiology of traumatic spinal cord injury: trends and future implications. Spinal Cord 2012;50:365–72.
7. Jain A, Brooks JT, Rao SS, et al. Cervical fractures with associated spinal cord injury in children and adolescents: epidemiology, costs, and in-hospital mortality rates in 4418 patients. J Child Orthop 2015;9:171–5.
8. Sherrod B, Karsy M, Guan J, et al. Spine trauma and spinal cord injury in Utah: a geographic cohort study utilizing the National Inpatient Sample. J Neurosurg Spine 2019;31:93–102.
9. Karsy M, Hawryluk G. Modern medical management of spinal cord injury. Curr Neurol Neurosci Rep 2019;19:65.
10. Wyndaele M, Wyndaele JJ. Incidence, prevalence and epidemiology of spinal cord injury: what learns a worldwide literature survey? Spinal Cord 2006;44: 523–9.
11. Center NSCIS. Spinal cord injury facts and figures at a glance, in, ed 2020. Birmingham (AL): University of Alabama at Birmingham; 2020.
12. McDonald JW, Sadowsky C. Spinal-cord injury. Lancet 2002;359:417–25.
13. Jabbour P, Fehlings M, Vaccaro AR, et al. Traumatic spine injuries in the geriatric population. Neurosurg Focus 2008;25:E16.
14. Sekhon LH, Fehlings MG. Epidemiology, demographics, and pathophysiology of acute spinal cord injury. Spine (Phila Pa 1976) 2001;26:S2–12.
15. Baptiste DC, Fehlings MG. Pharmacological approaches to repair the injured spinal cord. J Neurotrauma 2006;23:318–34.
16. Rowland JW, Hawryluk GW, Kwon B, et al. Current status of acute spinal cord injury pathophysiology and emerging therapies: promise on the horizon. Neurosurg Focus 2008;25(E2).
17. Ditunno JF, Little JW, Tessler A, et al. Spinal shock revisited: a four-phase model. Spinal Cord 2004;42:383–95.
18. Norenberg MD, Smith J, Marcillo A. The pathology of human spinal cord injury: defining the problems. J Neurotrauma 2004;21:429–40.
19. Kakulas BA. Neuropathology: the foundation for new treatments in spinal cord injury. Spinal Cord 2004;42:549–63.
20. Tator CH, Koyanagi I. Vascular mechanisms in the pathophysiology of human spinal cord injury. J Neurosurg 1997;86:483–92.

21. Beattie MS, Hermann GE, Rogers RC, et al. Cell death in models of spinal cord injury. Prog Brain Res 2002;137:37–47.
22. Fleming JC, Norenberg MD, Ramsay DA, et al. The cellular inflammatory response in human spinal cords after injury. Brain 2006;129:3249–69.
23. Lipton SA, Rosenberg PA. Excitatory amino acids as a final common pathway for neurologic disorders. N Engl J Med 1994;330:613–22.
24. Park E, Velumian AA, Fehlings MG. The role of excitotoxicity in secondary mechanisms of spinal cord injury: a review with an emphasis on the implications for white matter degeneration. J Neurotrauma 2004;21:754–74.
25. Tator CH, Fehlings MG. Review of the secondary injury theory of acute spinal cord trauma with emphasis on vascular mechanisms. J Neurosurg 1991;75: 15–26.
26. Xiong Y, Rabchevsky AG, Hall ED. Role of peroxynitrite in secondary oxidative damage after spinal cord injury. J Neurochem 2007;100:639–49.
27. Hagg T, Oudega M. Degenerative and spontaneous regenerative processes after spinal cord injury. J Neurotrauma 2006;23:264–80.
28. Herrmann JE, Imura T, Song B, et al. STAT3 is a critical regulator of astrogliosis and scar formation after spinal cord injury. J Neurosci 2008;28:7231–43.
29. Hill CE, Beattie MS, Bresnahan JC. Degeneration and sprouting of identified descending supraspinal axons after contusive spinal cord injury in the rat. Exp Neurol 2001;171:153–69.
30. Ehlers MD. Deconstructing the axon: Wallerian degeneration and the ubiquitin-proteasome system. Trends Neurosci 2004;27:3–6.
31. Coleman MP, Perry VH. Axon pathology in neurological disease: a neglected therapeutic target. Trends Neurosci 2002;25:532–7.
32. Saboe LA, Reid DC, Davis LA, et al. Spine trauma and associated injuries. J Trauma 1991;31:43–8.
33. Feller R, Furin M, Alloush A, et al. EMS immobilization techniques. Treasure Island (FL): StatPearls; 2020.
34. Hachem LD, Ahuja CS, Fehlings MG. Assessment and management of acute spinal cord injury: from point of injury to rehabilitation. J Spinal Cord Med 2017;40: 665–75.
35. Ahn H, Singh J, Nathens A, et al. Pre-hospital care management of a potential spinal cord injured patient: a systematic review of the literature and evidence-based guidelines. J Neurotrauma 2011;28:1341–61.
36. Burney RE, Waggoner R, Maynard FM. Stabilization of spinal injury for early transfer. J Trauma 1989;29:1497–9.
37. Stein DM, Roddy V, Marx J, et al. Emergency neurological life support: traumatic spine injury. Neurocrit Care 2012;17(Suppl 1):S102–11.
38. Durga P, Sahu BP, Mantha S, et al. Development and validation of predictors of respiratory insufficiency and mortality scores: simple bedside additive scores for prediction of ventilation and in-hospital mortality in acute cervical spine injury. Anesth Analg 2010;110:134–40.
39. Velmahos GC, Toutouzas K, Chan L, et al. Intubation after cervical spinal cord injury: to be done selectively or routinely? Am Surg 2003;69:891–4.
40. Piepmeier JM, Lehmann KB, Lane JG. Cardiovascular instability following acute cervical spinal cord trauma. Cent Nerv Syst Trauma 1985;2:153–60.
41. Resnick DK. Updated guidelines for the management of acute cervical spine and spinal cord injury. Neurosurgery 2013;72(Suppl 2):1.
42. Consortium for Spinal Cord Medicine. "Early Acute Management in Adults with Spinal Cord Injury: A Clinical Practice Guideline for Health-Care Providers."

[Online]. 2008. Available at: pvasamediaprd.blob.core.windows.net. Paralyzed Veterans of America. Accessed on: Mar 2021.

43. Bilello JF, Davis JW, Cunningham MA, et al. Cervical spinal cord injury and the need for cardiovascular intervention. Arch Surg 2003;138:1127–9.

44. Stevens RD, Bhardwaj A, Kirsch JR, et al. Critical care and perioperative management in traumatic spinal cord injury. J Neurosurg Anesthesiol 2003;15:215–29.

45. Hadley MN, Walters BC, Aarabi B, et al. Clinical assessment following acute cervical spinal cord injury. Neurosurgery 2013;72(Suppl 2):40–53.

46. Kirshblum SC, Biering-Sorensen F, Betz R, et al. International standards for neurological classification of spinal cord injury: cases with classification challenges. Top Spinal Cord Inj Rehabil 2014;20:81–9.

47. Park HJ, Lee SY, Park NH, et al. Modified thoracolumbar injury classification and severity score (TLICS) and its clinical usefulness. Acta Radiol 2016;57:74–81.

48. Pizones J, Alvarez-Gonzalez P, Sanchez-Mariscal F, et al. AOSpine thoracolumbar spine injury classification system. Fracture description, neurological status, and key modifiers. Spine 2013;38:2028–37. Spine (Phila Pa 1976) 39:783, 2014.

49. Vaccaro AR, Koerner JD, Radcliff KE, et al. AOSpine subaxial cervical spine injury classification system. Eur Spine J 2016;25:2173–84.

50. Lee JY, Vaccaro AR, Lim MR, et al. Thoracolumbar injury classification and severity score: a new paradigm for the treatment of thoracolumbar spine trauma. J Orthop Sci 2005;10:671–5.

51. Fehlings MG, Vaccaro A, Wilson JR, et al. Early versus delayed decompression for traumatic cervical spinal cord injury: results of the Surgical Timing in Acute Spinal Cord Injury Study (STASCIS). PLoS One 2012;7:e32037.

52. Jug M, Kejzar N, Vesel M, et al. Neurological recovery after traumatic cervical spinal cord injury is superior if surgical decompression and instrumented fusion are performed within 8 hours versus 8 to 24 hours after injury: a single center experience. J Neurotrauma 2015;32:1385–92.

53. van Middendorp JJ, Hosman AJ, Doi SA. The effects of the timing of spinal surgery after traumatic spinal cord injury: a systematic review and meta-analysis. J Neurotrauma 2013;30:1781–94.

54. Wilson JR, Singh A, Craven C, et al. Early versus late surgery for traumatic spinal cord injury: the results of a prospective Canadian cohort study. Spinal Cord 2012;50:840–3.

55. Fehlings MG, Tetreault LA, Wilson JR, et al. A clinical practice guideline for the management of patients with acute spinal cord injury and central cord syndrome: recommendations on the timing (</=24 hours versus >24 hours) of decompressive surgery. Global Spine J 2017;7:195S–202S.

56. Bracken MB, Collins WF, Freeman DF, et al. Efficacy of methylprednisolone in acute spinal cord injury. JAMA 1984;251:45–52.

57. Bracken MB, Shepard MJ, Collins WF, et al. A randomized, controlled trial of methylprednisolone or naloxone in the treatment of acute spinal-cord injury. Results of the second national acute spinal cord injury study. N Engl J Med 1990;322:1405–11.

58. Bracken MB, Shepard MJ, Holford TR, et al. Administration of methylprednisolone for 24 or 48 hours or tirilazad mesylate for 48 hours in the treatment of acute spinal cord injury. Results of the third National Acute Spinal Cord Injury randomized controlled trial. National Acute Spinal Cord Injury Study. JAMA 1997;277:1597–604.

59. Bracken MB. Steroids for acute spinal cord injury. Cochrane Database Syst Rev 2012;1:CD001046.
60. Hurlbert RJ, Hadley MN, Walters BC, et al. Pharmacological therapy for acute spinal cord injury. Neurosurgery 2015;76(Suppl 1):S71–83.
61. Levi L, Wolf A, Belzberg H. Hemodynamic parameters in patients with acute cervical cord trauma: description, intervention, and prediction of outcome. Neurosurgery 1993;33:1007–16 [discussion 1016–07].
62. Vale FL, Burns J, Jackson AB, et al. Combined medical and surgical treatment after acute spinal cord injury: results of a prospective pilot study to assess the merits of aggressive medical resuscitation and blood pressure management. J Neurosurg 1997;87:239–46.
63. Wilson JR, Forgione N, Fehlings MG. Emerging therapies for acute traumatic spinal cord injury. CMAJ 2013;185:485–92.
64. Saadeh YS, Smith BW, Joseph JR, et al. The impact of blood pressure management after spinal cord injury: a systematic review of the literature. Neurosurg Focus 2017;43:E20.
65. Yashon D, Bingham WG Jr, Faddoul EM, et al. Edema of the spinal cord following experimental impact trauma. J Neurosurg 1973;38:693–7.
66. Dakson A, Brandman D, Thibault-Halman G, et al. Optimization of the mean arterial pressure and timing of surgical decompression in traumatic spinal cord injury: a retrospective study. Spinal Cord 2017;55:1033–8.
67. Hawryluk G, Whetstone W, Saigal R, et al. Mean arterial blood pressure correlates with neurological recovery after human spinal cord injury: analysis of high frequency physiologic data. J Neurotrauma 2015;32:1958–67.
68. Inoue T, Manley GT, Patel N, et al. Medical and surgical management after spinal cord injury: vasopressor usage, early surgerys, and complications. J Neurotrauma 2014;31:284–91.
69. Kepler CK, Schroeder GD, Martin ND, et al. The effect of preexisting hypertension on early neurologic results of patients with an acute spinal cord injury. Spinal Cord 2015;53:763–6.
70. Streijger F, So K, Manouchehri N, et al. A direct comparison between norepinephrine and phenylephrine for augmenting spinal cord perfusion in a porcine model of spinal cord injury. J Neurotrauma 2018;35:1345–57.
71. Manack A, Motsko SP, Haag-Molkenteller C, et al. Epidemiology and healthcare utilization of neurogenic bladder patients in a US claims database. Neurourol Urodyn 2011;30:395–401.
72. Linsenmeyer TA. Update on bladder evaluation recommendations and bladder management guideline in patients with spinal cord injury. Curr Bladder Dysfunct Rep 2008;2:134.
73. Hou YF, Lv Y, Zhou F, et al. Development and validation of a risk prediction model for tracheostomy in acute traumatic cervical spinal cord injury patients. Eur Spine J 2015;24:975–84.
74. DeVivo MJ, Krause JS, Lammertse DP. Recent trends in mortality and causes of death among persons with spinal cord injury. Arch Phys Med Rehabil 1999;80:1411–9.
75. Ho KM, Rao S, Honeybul S, et al. A multicenter trial of vena cava filters in severely injured patients. N Engl J Med 2019;381:328–37.
76. Nyquist P, Bautista C, Jichici D, et al. Prophylaxis of venous thrombosis in neurocritical care patients: an evidence-based guideline: a statement for healthcare professionals from the neurocritical care society. Neurocrit Care 2016;24:47–60.

77. Prevention of venous thromboembolism in individuals with spinal cord injury: clinical practice guidelines for health care providers, 3rd ed.: Consortium for Spinal Cord Medicine. Top Spinal Cord Inj Rehabil 2016;22:209–40.
78. Cohen-Adad J. Microstructural imaging in the spinal cord and validation strategies. Neuroimage 2018;182:169–83.
79. Freund P, Seif M, Weiskopf N, et al. MRI in traumatic spinal cord injury: from clinical assessment to neuroimaging biomarkers. Lancet Neurol 2019;18:1123–35.
80. Stroman PW, Wheeler-Kingshott C, Bacon M, et al. The current state-of-the-art of spinal cord imaging: methods. Neuroimage 2014;84:1070–81.
81. Zaninovich OA, Avila MJ, Kay M, et al. The role of diffusion tensor imaging in the diagnosis, prognosis, and assessment of recovery and treatment of spinal cord injury: a systematic review. Neurosurg Focus 2019;46:E7.
82. Wang F, Li K, Mishra A, et al. Longitudinal assessment of spinal cord injuries in nonhuman primates with quantitative magnetization transfer. Magn Reson Med 2016;75:1685–96.
83. Li XH, Li JB, He XJ, et al. Timing of diffusion tensor imaging in the acute spinal cord injury of rats. Sci Rep 2015;5:12639.
84. Jones CF, Newell RS, Lee JH, et al. The pressure distribution of cerebrospinal fluid responds to residual compression and decompression in an animal model of acute spinal cord injury. Spine (Phila Pa 1976) 2012;37:E1422–31.
85. Kwon BK, Curt A, Belanger LM, et al. Intrathecal pressure monitoring and cerebrospinal fluid drainage in acute spinal cord injury: a prospective randomized trial. J Neurosurg Spine 2009;10:181–93.
86. Donovan J, Kirshblum S. Clinical trials in traumatic spinal cord injury. Neurotherapeutics 2018;15:654–68.
87. Hawryluk GW, Rowland J, Kwon BK, et al. Protection and repair of the injured spinal cord: a review of completed, ongoing, and planned clinical trials for acute spinal cord injury. Neurosurg Focus 2008;25:E14.
88. Witiw CD, Fehlings MG. Acute spinal cord injury. J Spinal Disord Tech 2015;28:202–10.
89. Sakiyama-Elbert S, Johnson PJ, Hodgetts SI, et al. Scaffolds to promote spinal cord regeneration. Handb Clin Neurol 2012;109:575–94.
90. Zhang Q, Shi B, Ding J, et al. Polymer scaffolds facilitate spinal cord injury repair. Acta Biomater 2019;88:57–77.

Acute Myelopathy
Vascular and Infectious Diseases

Caleb R. McEntire, MD[a], Richard S. Dowd, MD[b],
Emanuele Orru', MD[c], Carlos David, MD[b,d], Juan E. Small, MD[e],
Anna Cervantes-Arslanian, MD[f], David P. Lerner, MD[g,h,*]

KEYWORDS

- Spinal cord infarction • Myelopathy • Hematomyelia • Arteriovenous malformation
- Dural fistula • Artery of Adamkiewicz • Epidural abscess • Acute flaccid myelopathy

KEY POINTS

- Acute spinal cord infarction can present with a variety of clinicoanatomic patterns depending on the vascular territory and craniocaudal level affected. It is common that patients will have a subacute progressive presentation over the course of hours and commonly do not reach the nadir of the symptoms for 12 to 24 hours. Back pain is a common symptom that should raise clinical suspicion for spinal cord infarction.
- There are limited data to guide management of acute spinal cord infarction. It is therefore paramount to exclude other diagnoses with effective, specific treatments, such as spinal cord compression, for which prompt management can preserve neurologic function. Common management of cord infarction includes appropriate intravascular volume resuscitation, blood pressure augmentation with vasopressors, and vigilant monitoring for and prevention of potential medical complications, such as respiratory insufficiency/failure, pneumonia, deep vein thrombosis, pressure ulcerations, urinary retention, and constipation.
- Vascular malformations of the spine can be a cause of congestive or hemorrhagic myelopathy, with a variety of clinical manifestations. These manifestations include arteriovenous shunts (arteriovenous malformations or fistulae), cavernous malformations, or aneurysms and are diagnosed via a combination of cross-sectional and conventional angiographic imaging. Treatment is tailored to the single patient and can be conservative, surgical, endovascular, or a combination thereof.

Continued

---

[a] Department of Neurology, Massachusetts General Hospital and Brigham & Women's Hospital, Harvard Medical School, Boston, MA, USA; [b] Department of Neurosurgery, Tufts University School of Medicine, Boston, MA 02111, USA; [c] Department of Radiology, Neurointerventional Radiology Division, Lahey Hospital and Medical Center, Burlington, MA 01805, USA; [d] Department of Neurosurgery, Lahey Hospital and Medical Center, Burlington, MA 01805, USA; [e] Department of Radiology, Neuroradiology Section, Lahey Hospital and Medical Center, Burlington, MA 01805, USA; [f] Department of Neurology, Boston University School of Medicine, Boston, MA 02118, USA; [g] Division of Neurology, Lahey Hospital and Medical Center, Burlington, MA 01805, USA; [h] Department of Neurology, Tufts University School of Medicine, Boston, MA 02111, USA
* Corresponding author. 41 Mall Road, Burlington, MA 01805.
E-mail address: david.lerner@lahey.org

Neurol Clin 39 (2021) 489–512
https://doi.org/10.1016/j.ncl.2021.01.011
0733-8619/21/© 2021 Elsevier Inc. All rights reserved.

neurologic.theclinics.com

Continued

- Infectious causes of acute myelopathy have a variety of pathologic conditions, including cord compression, intrinsic cord injury, and cord ischemia. Rapid imaging will assist with diagnosing the pathologic process and guide early antimicrobial and additional medical and potentially surgical management.

ACUTE VASCULAR MYELOPATHY
Background

Vascular spinal cord injury is an uncommon cause of acute myelopathy (5%–8%) and comprises 1.2% of all strokes.[1,2] This form of neurologic injury is potentially devastating and requires a multidisciplinary approach to management in both the acute and chronic phases. Ischemic spinal cord injury more commonly affects women, and when compared with cerebral infarction, patients are younger and have a lower rate of associated cardiovascular disease.[3] Acute spinal cord infarction can present in varied fashion depending on the tracts and rostrocaudal section of the cord involved. The most common level for spinal cord infarction is the lower thoracic region.[4] The most common vascular territory affected is that of the anterior spinal artery.[5] Commonly, there is sudden onset of neurologic symptoms, but these can progress over 12 to 24 hours following the initial insult.[1–3,6] An additional common symptom is radicular neck or back pain referred to the dermatome associated with the level of infarction.[7]

Spontaneous spinal cord infarction is an uncommon entity, and in such cases, no definitive cause is determined in 33% to 74%.[2,8] On the other hand, there is a clear risk of spinal cord infarction associated with aortic surgical and endovascular procedures. Following open thoracoabdominal aortic surgery, the reported rate of spinal cord ischemia is 4% to 33%, and following endovascular surgery, the rate is 3% to 12%, depending on the procedure performed.[9–12] Risk factors for perioperative spinal cord ischemia during open vascular surgery include systemic hypotension and longer duration of aortic clamp time, especially when exceeding 60 minutes.[9–12]

Although spinal cord infarcts typically present with rapid symptom onset, many other vascular abnormalities of the spinal cord, including dural arteriovenous shunts, spinal arteriovenous malformations (AVMs), and cavernous malformations, can have more variable time courses of presentation. These conditions can result in spinal cord injury because of venous hypertensive myelopathy without or with infarction, compression, or acute hemorrhage. Again, clinical signs and symptoms are determined by the tracts and rostrocaudal sections of the cord involved. However, the temporal evolution of the clinical syndromes associated with these conditions is quite variable, with some presenting relatively rapidly over the course of minutes, as with the rupture of a cavernous malformation, whereas others evolve in a more insidious fashion over years.[13–15]

Anatomy

The cross-sectional anatomy of the spinal cord varies with the rostrocaudal level, but the tracts remain in similar ventral/dorsal and medial/lateral orientation. The dorsal, or posterior, spinal cord contains the dorsal columns (fasciculus gracilis more medial and fasciculus cuneatus more lateral), which carry tactile and proprioceptive information from the legs and arms, respectively. This region receives blood supply from the paired posterior spinal arteries, and infarction here results in loss of tactile, proprioceptive, and vibratory sensation. The dorsolateral tract (also known as fasciculus of Lissauer) is a common region of posterior and anterior spinal circulation overlap. The anterior and lateral tracts of the spinal cord, namely the lateral spinothalamic tract, ventral and dorsal spinocerebellar tracts, and lateral and medial corticospinal tracts, are supplied by the anterior spinal artery. Complete infarction of the anterior spinal artery territory results in loss of pain and temperature sensation and weakness.

Understanding the vascular anatomy of the spinal cord is essential to understanding the potential mechanism of vascular injury. The vascular supply of the spinal cord is composed of an extensive ventral-dorsal and central-peripheral anastomotic network. The ventral-dorsal network comprises the single anterior and paired posterior spinal arteries. The anterior spinal artery supplies the ventrolateral cord, comprising approximately two-thirds to three-fourths of the cord at any particular level. The anterior spinal artery commonly arises from the fourth (intracranial) segment of the vertebral arteries. Although commonly thought of as a single vessel, it is actually a longitudinal network of vessels and receives additional supply from the deep cervical arteries, thyrocervical trunk, and posterior inferior cerebellar arteries.[16] More caudal portions of the anterior spinal artery receive input from radiculomedullary arteries, the largest and most important being the great vertebral or dominant vertebral radicular artery of Adamkiewicz, which commonly enters the spinal canal between thoracic levels 8 to 12.[17] The midthoracic region, commonly T4-T6, is accordingly a longitudinal watershed region owing to small arterial input from radicular arteries in the cervical and higher thoracic cord. The paired posterior spinal arteries run longitudinally along the length of the spinal cord and receive supplemental vascular supply from the posterior radicular arteries. Multiple sulcocommissural arteries traverse the anterior median fissure of the spinal cord to supply the central cord. These arteries then spread from the most central portions of the cord out laterally, while peripheral branches from the longitudinal, single anterior and paired posterior, spinal arteries supply the lateral aspects of the cord and then penetrate into the deeper portions of cord. The central cord and anterior horn cells are common vascular watershed zones owing to the small penetrating vessels.

Discussion

Spinal cord ischemia

Spinal cord infarction can be the result of systemic low-flow state, as can be seen after cardiac arrest; a combination of hypotension and surgical aortic manipulation; or selective occlusion of a particular radiculomedullary, anterior, or posterior, spinal artery. Common causes of cerebral infarction, such as atherosclerotic disease, embolization, vasculitis, aortic dissection, and coagulopathy, can result in focal ischemic cord injury, but there are additional uncommon considerations, including decompression sickness (DCS), fibrocartilaginous embolization (FCE), and surfer's myelopathy (**Table 1**).[7,18,19] Between 14% and 33% of spinal cord ischemia is idiopathic.[7,18,19]

Spinal cord infarction occurs more frequently in women and at younger ages than brain infarction. The average age at the time of spinal cord infarction is 56 years.[20] Patients with spinal cord infarction also have fewer cardiovascular risk factors than those with brain infarction.[21] Nonetheless, because the same diseases that cause brain infarction can cause infarction of the spinal cord, the diagnostic evaluation for both includes evaluation of vascular risk factors, including hyperlipidemia and diabetes

Table 1			
Cause of spinal cord ischemia			
Embolic	Cardioembolic Aortic atheroembolism Fibrocartilaginous Decompression sickness	*Hypercoagulability*	Malignancy DIC[b] Antiphospholipid syndrome Sickle cell disease
Dissection	Aortic Subclavian Vertebral	*Vasculitis*	Systemic vasculitis VZV Primary angiitis of the central nervous system Syphilis
Iatrogenic	Aortic surgery (open and endovascular) Renal artery embolization Cardiac catheterization ECMO[a] Catheter angiogram (rare)	*Hypotension*	Cardiac arrest Profound Shock/hypotension

[a] Extracorporeal membrane oxygenation.
[b] Disseminated intravascular coagulopathy.

mellitus, as well as transthoracic, and commonly, transesophageal echocardiography. Transesophageal echocardiography should be strongly considered in this group of patients because it provides excellent visualization of the proximal aorta, which can be a source of embolization. In the appropriate clinical context, laboratory evaluation can be expanded to include testing for hypercoagulability, vasculitis, and other causes of myelopathy, such as inflammatory myelitis (**Table 2**). As noted above, spinal cord ischemia is uncommon and can have varying clinical presentations and time course, making it a difficult diagnosis. Therefore, consideration and testing for other causes of myelopathy are important. Imaging can demonstrate spinal cord infarction and differentiate it from other causes of acute myelopathy and thus should be completed when this diagnosis is suspected as discussed later.

Fibrocartilaginous embolization

An uncommon but often discussed cause of spinal cord infarction is fibrocartilaginous embolization (FCE). It is reported to be the cause of 5.5% of all spinal cord infarction, and some think this may be an underrepresentation given the difficulty of definitive diagnosis.[22] There are histopathologically confirmed cases that demonstrate fibrocartilaginous disc material in the arteries of the spinal cord thought to be due to herniation of nucleus pulposus material into radicular arteries that supply the longitudinal spinal arteries.[7,23] Additional theoretic pathophysiology includes retrograde migration of nucleus pulposa material through venous plexus resulting in venous infarction.[7,23] FCE commonly affects younger patients, with nearly half of reported cases in patients younger than 40 years of age. It typically affects the anterior spinal artery territory and is commonly associated with physical exertion, trauma (such as fall from standing onto the gluteal region), and Valsalva maneuvers.[7,23]

Surfer's myelopathy

First defined in 2004, surfer's myelopathy is a rare nontraumatic cause of acute spinal cord infarction.[24] The underlying pathophysiology has not been definitively demonstrated, but is thought to be due to hyperextension of the spine, as occurs while the surfer is paddling prone while peering over waves, leading to increased tension on

Table 2
Diagnostic evaluation for spinal cord ischemia

Standard Evaluation	Lumbar Puncture
Lipid panel	Cell count
Hemoglobin A1c	Protein
TTE and TEE	Glucose
Electrocardiogram	IgG Index
Complete blood count	Oligoclonal bands
Coagulation profile (PTT/PT/INR)[a]	VZV PCR[b]
	VRDL (syphilis)[c]
Hypercoagulability	
Lupus anticoagulant, antiphospholipid antibody, anticardiolipin antibody	*Vasculitis/Autoimmune*
Malignancy screening	Antinuclear antibody
Hemoglobin electrophoresis	Extractable nuclear antigens (ENA, eg, anti-Ro)
Antithrombin	Antineutrophil cytoplasm antibodies
Protein C and protein S	Rheumatoid factor/anticitrullinated protein antibodies
Factor V Leiden	Erythrocyte sedimentation rate/C-reactive protein
Immunoglobulin electrophoresis	Behcets disease[d]

[a] Partial thromboplastin time/prothrombin time/international normalized ratio.
[b] Varicella zoster virus polymerase chain reaction.
[c] Venereal Disease Research Laboratory.
[d] There is no specific or sensitive laboratory test for Behcet but clinical history of ocular, oral, genital, and skin lesions.

the cord and surrounding vasculature, ultimately causing avulsion of perforating vessels.[18,24] Other proposed mechanisms include increased inferior vena cava compression owing to prolonged prone positioning or embolization of spinal disc material similar to FCE.[18]

Decompression sickness

Myelopathy caused by DCS is a rare entity described in the literature mainly through case reports. DCS type I includes joint pain, rash, and localized edema, whereas DCS type II involves injury to the central nervous system with the spinal cord affected in 30% to 50% of cases.[25] DCS occurs as the result of intravascular and extravascular gas bubble formation during rapid decompression from hyperbaric exposure, most commonly after rapid decompression from diving to depths of approximately 40 m.[25] The clinical syndrome can present with minimal symptoms of paresis and sphincter dysfunction to complete paraplegia and permanent disability.[25] The proposed pathophysiologic mechanism is bubble formation in small arterioles and venules as the surrounding pressure decreases during decompression resulting in obstruction of venous drainage.[26] There are conflicting data on appropriate recompression therapy, but the most common procedure is to recompress to 2.8 atm using 100% oxygen in a hyperbaric chamber.[25,27–29]

Imaging

The diagnosis of spinal cord infarction depends on clinical symptoms and MRI findings (**Table 3**). The primary purpose of early imaging is to exclude other diagnoses.[30] Acute myelopathy without trauma can be due to a wide array of causes of which some,

Table 3
MRI sequences for spinal cord infarction

Imaging Sequence	Common Radiographic Finding
T2	Hyperintensity, focal cord enlargement (typically 48 h from onset)
T1 with and without contrast	Contrast enhancement, focal cord enlargement (typically 48 h from onset)
Diffusion-weighted imaging (DWI)	Restricted diffusion at the area of ischemia
Echo planar imaging-DWI	Small segment MRI, increased spatial quality compared with DWI
Short tau inversion recovery	Fat-suppression imaging allows for improved resolution of cord edema and focal cord enlargement
Time resolved MRA (TWIST or TRICK)	Series of images displaying contrast movement. They can sometimes identify a fistulous point or a cutoff in an artery in case of ischemic infarct
Gradient echo or susceptibility-weighted image	Imaging of blood products within the spinal cord. Blood products and hemosiderin appear as a characteristic "blooming" on these sequences

such as infectious (see section Spinal Cord Abscess later in this section) and tumor compression, require rapid diagnosis and treatment. Rapid imaging with computed tomography (CT) scan and computed tomography arteriogram (CTA) of the spinal cord and chest/abdomen will diagnose many of these causes of myelopathy. CTA is of utility, as the artery of Adamkiewicz can be visualized as well as the ascending and descending aorta.

Although CT and CTA are unlikely to demonstrate the acute spinal cord infarct itself, high-resolution MRI can demonstrate acute ischemic changes in up to 67% of cases.[6] MRI may be insensitive in the hyperacute setting because of delayed evolution of imaging changes owing to infarction and limitation in spatial resolution even with 3-T MRI. As with the anticipated temporal evolution of cerebral infarction on MRI, there is commonly evolution of MRI signal abnormalities as spinal cord infarction progresses. MRI within the first 24 hours of symptom onset may yield normal results in up to 80% of cases.[31] Within 2 days of symptom onset, MRI can reveal T2 hyperintensity, focal cord enlargement, and contrast enhancement at the level of infarction.[6,31,32] The most commonly described MRI findings include "pencil-like" hyperintensities on sagittal T2-weighted images and "owl-eyes" hyperintensities on axial T2-weight images (**Fig. 1**).[33,34] The characteristic "owl-eyes" appearance, although not pathognomonic for anterior spinal cord ischemia, is due to the anterior horn cells lying within the watershed territory.[34] Because the vertebral bodies also receive vascular supply from radicular arteries, there can also be concomitant bony infarction at the level of spinal cord ischemia.[32,35,36]

Commonly obtained MRI sequences include short tau inversion recovery (STIR), which suppresses fat signal, fast spin-echo, diffusion-weighted image (DWI), and time-resolved contrast-enhanced magnetic resonance arteriogram (MRA) (TWIST), which will provide vascular imaging. To combat spatial resolution limitations, echo planar imaging (EPI) sequences can provide short-segment, zoomed-in views.[37] Although TWIST and additional MRA sequences can provide information on spinal vasculature, if there are abnormal findings, digital subtraction angiogram with selective spinal injections is the gold standard for diagnosis and can simultaneously provide the opportunity for therapeutic interventions.[33,34]

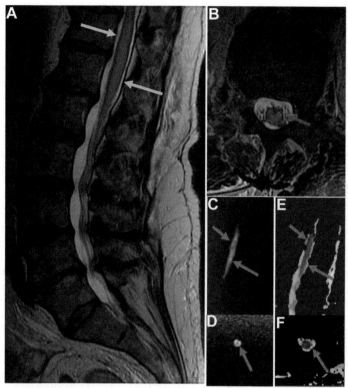

Fig. 1. Acute spinal cord infarct. Sagittal (*A*) and axial (*B*) T2 images through the conus demonstrate conus edema (blue arrows) with "owl-eyes" appearance (*red arrow*) suggesting infarction. Sagittal and axial DWI (*C, D*) and ADC (*E, F*) images through the conus confirm restricted diffusion (*orange arrows*) diagnostic of acute infarction. There are no abnormal dorsal flow voids to suggest an occult arteriovenous fistula.

Treatment

There are no published guidelines for the acute management of spontaneous spinal cord infarction. As noted above, exclusion of diagnoses that require rapid surgical management (eg, compression) is of utmost importance. Inflammatory and infectious intrinsic cord lesions (eg, transverse myelitis) can appear similar on early MRI, although they are more likely to demonstrate early contrast enhancement and tend to have less abrupt symptom onset. For patients in whom inflammatory and infectious causes are considered, lumbar puncture can be pursued. In spinal cord infarction, cerebrospinal fluid (CSF) is typically normal but can have mild elevation in protein concentration.[38] There are a few case reports of management of acute spinal cord ischemia with intravenous (IV) thrombolysis, but its efficacy has not been clearly demonstrated.[39,40] In addition, many patients will be excluded from systemic thrombolysis because of recent trauma, dissection, surgery, and delayed timing of presentation.

Infarct-related cytotoxic edema can cause secondary cord injury by way of focal cord compression and venous congestion, resulting in regional spinal cord hypoperfusion adjacent to the infarct. Appropriate volume resuscitation and blood pressure augmentation with vasopressors are therefore the mainstays of acute management.[7,41] Small case series report the use of systemic steroids and lumbar drains, but the data supporting these interventions are mixed.[5,30] Although there are limited data on use of lumbar drain and CSF diversion in spontaneous spinal cord infarction, the potential benefit demonstrated in thoracoabdominal aortic surgery permit consideration and use in spontaneous spinal cord infarction.

Spinal cord infarction following endovascular or open thoracoabdominal aortic surgery has more robust data supporting the beneficial effect of lumbar drainage. Theoretically, by decreasing the CSF volume within the spinal column, the intraspinal pressure is decreased, thereby allowing for increased spinal cord perfusion (spinal perfusion pressure = mean arterial pressure − intraspinal pressure). Augmentation of blood pressure with appropriate volume resuscitation and use of vasopressors is also recommended, with a goal mean arterial pressure greater than 80 mm Hg.[5,41] If a lumbar drain is used, the goal intraspinal pressure is 8 to 12 mm Hg, and CSF diversion is used for 24 to 48 hours.[5,7,41]

Although specific acute management is somewhat limited for acute spinal cord infarction, these patients may experience significant medical complications during their hospitalization and recovery, making meticulous supportive care essential. Depending on the craniocaudal level of injury, patients can experience respiratory insufficiency/failure because of weakness from the chest wall musculature and diaphragm; gastrointestinal motility issues, including gastroparesis, constipation, and ileus; urinary retention; deep vein thrombosis and pulmonary emboli; and pressure-related deep tissue injury. Early recognition and fastidious preventive measures for these potential complications will ensure the best possible outcome. Early physical and occupational rehabilitation is important to prevent long-term disability.[42]

Prognosis

Long-term prognosis after spinal cord infarction is variable, but improvement is common. Patients who present with American Spinal Injury Association (ASIA) A (complete loss of sensory and motor function below the level of injury) and B (incomplete, with preservation of sensory but no motor function below the level of injury) patterns have a worse prognosis than ASIA C, D, and E.[5,38] Additional clinical and radiographic findings at the time of presentation concerning for worse outcomes include the presence of extensor plantar response, bladder dysfunction, and the longitudinal extent of spinal cord infarction on MRI.[5,38] Of the patients who are wheelchair bound at the time of hospital discharge, 41% are able to walk without or with minimal assistance at mean follow-up of 3 years.[38] In addition, 33% of patients who required chronic catheterization at hospital discharge was able to urinate at mean follow-up of 3 years.[38] Although motor, sensory, and autonomic function can improve, upwards of 33% is left with chronic pain.[43] Importantly, ongoing functional improvement can occur even several years out from spinal cord infarction.[38]

Spinal hemorrhage

Spinal cord hemorrhage (hematomyelia) is a rare cause of myelopathy. The typical presentation is similar to spinal cord ischemia with sudden, severe back pain and associated neurologic deficit.[44,45] However, hematomyelia can present in subacute, chronic, or stepwise fashion.[46] The most common cause of hematomyelia is spinal cord trauma (discussed in Traumatic Spinal Cord Injury in Clinics: Neurologic Emergencies) followed by vascular abnormalities like spinal AVMs and cavernous malformations, which will be discussed in detail later.[46] MRI with gradient-echo (GRE) and susceptibility-weighted sequences provide optimal sensitivity for detecting hemorrhage. Although no guidelines exist for acute management, surgical hematoma evacuation can be considered. Before surgical intervention, the cause of hemorrhage should be discerned, as certain vascular abnormalities may require alterations to the surgical approach. Digital subtraction angiography is more sensitive in determining the anatomy of vascular abnormalities and should be considered in all cases of hematomyelia.

Spinal Cord Vascular Malformations

There are several different spinal vascular lesions, and it is important to precisely determine the type, anatomy, and severity/grade of a lesion, as this information is crucial for planning the treatment approach. As a general concept, spinal arteriovenous shunts and aneurysms can potentially be visualized on cross-sectional imaging (CT or MRI), but invariably need spinal digital subtraction angiography (SpDSA) to be completely characterized, whereas cavernous malformations are best studied with MRI [47,48]. Surgical and endovascular management of spinal vascular malformations is beyond the scope of this article, but commonly, a multidisciplinary approach with endovascular, open surgery, and radiosurgery can be considered depending on the specific patient and lesion characteristics.

Spinal arteriovenous shunts

There have been multiple classification systems presented throughout the literature for spinal arteriovenous shunts from 1971 to 2016. The authors adopted the category system proposed by Doppman and colleagues[49] (**Table 4**).

Type I: dural arteriovenous fistula. Dural arteriovenous fistulas (dAVF) are the most common type of spinal vascular malformation, making up approximately 60% to 80% of all spinal vascular lesions (**Figs. 2–4**).[50] They consist of a direct connection between a radicular dural artery and radicular veins without an intervening capillary bed. The fistulous point is most commonly located within the dural sleeve of a nerve root at the level of the neural foramen, but it can also be in the spinal epidural space, in which case the fistula is defined as epidural. Over time, the long-standing dural venous hypertension secondary to the shunt extends from meningeal to perimedullary veins that drain the spinal cord, resulting in progressive perimedullary venous engorgement and enlargement with hypertensive congestive myelopathy.[13,50] dAVF are more common in men and typically present in the fifth decade of life.[13,14,50] Given the relatively low flow that characterizes these shunts, congestive myelopathy takes a variably long amount of time to develop, accounting for the insidious and slowly progressive nature of the symptoms. The most common clinical manifestation is progressive myelopathy with early asymmetric symptoms involving the lower thoracic cord.[14] As the venous congestion worsens, progressive weakness, sensory changes, and sphincter dysfunction can occur.[14] Because of the insidious onset, the diagnosis is commonly delayed by 1 to 3 years from the initial symptoms.[13,14] On MRI, dilated and engorged

Type	Name	Shunt Location	Pressure	Flow
Table 4				
Types of spinal arteriovenous shunts				
I	Dural/epidural fistula	Extramedullary	High	Low
II	Intramedullary glomus arteriovenous malformation	Intramedullary	High	High
III	Juvenile arteriovenous malformation	Intramedullary/metameric	High	High
IV	Perimedullary fistula	Extramedullary (pial)	High	Low/high

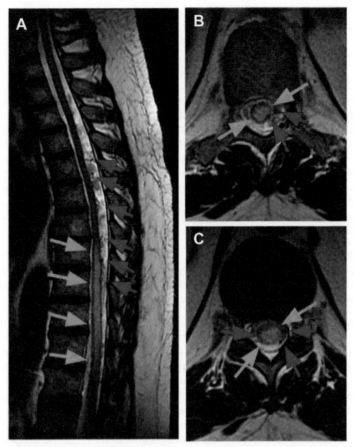

Fig. 2. Spinal dAVF. Sagittal (*A*) and axial (*B, C*) T2 images of the thoracic spinal cord clearly demonstrate mid to distal thoracic spinal cord edema (*blue arrows*) with numerous subtle dorsal vascular flow voids (*red arrows*) highly suspicious for an underlying dAVF.

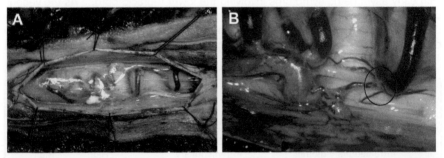

Fig. 3. Intraoperative pictures of a type I dAVF of the spinal cord. (*A*) This is a posterior approach to the spinal cord with the dura mater open and the arachnoid intact. There is a serpiginous arterialized vein visible on the dorsal surface of the spinal cord. (*B*) Higher magnification view of the dAVF with the arachnoid removed; the circle highlights the fistulous connection between the artery and vein.

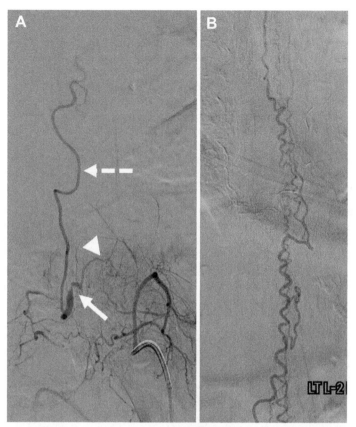

Fig. 4. Spinal dAVF in a 78-year-old woman with progressive paraplegia and decreased sphincter tone. Anteroposterior view of a selective angiography of the left L2 intersegmental artery. Early arterial phase (*A*) demonstrates an arteriovenous fistula at the level of the right L2-L3 intervertebral foramen. The left L2 intersegmental artery feeds the fistula through a retrocorporeal arterial anastomosis (*arrowhead*). An enlarged, elongated dural draining vein is directed cranially toward the perimedullary venous system (*dotted arrow*). Late angiographic venous phase (*B*) demonstrates retrograde drainage along the entire length of the spinal cord, with enlargement of the perimedullary veins.

perimedullary veins can be visualized as flow voids in T2 sequences and as serpiginous-enhancing structures on the surface of the spinal cord on T1 postcontrast images. These findings are highly specific, but they become detectable only in dAVF with advanced venous hypertension. The overall sensitivity of MRI can be as low as 40% if the fistula is not in its late stages. Nonspecific T2 hyperintense cord signal changes are present in about 75% of cases, often leading to a misdiagnosis of transverse myelitis[48]. Given the overall low sensitivity of cross-sectional imaging, a complete SpDSA should be performed if the clinical suspicion is high. Conventional MRA is of limited value and only correctly identifies the culprit spinal level ± 1 level in 73% of cases.[14,51] Treatment is surgical or endovascular, with the goal being to disconnect the draining vein from the arterial supply.[52,53] Despite the typical delay in diagnosis, 65% of those who undergo successful treatment will experience improvement in gait and 33% will have improvement in bladder control.[52,54]

Type II and III: arteriovenous malformation. Arteriovenous malformations are high-flow lesions with a nidus that is completely or partially intramedullary.[55,56] Because of the involvement of spinal cord parenchyma and of the large flow voids, MRI without and with contrast has excellent sensitivity and specificity and is the best imaging modality for detection of the location of the nidus and for determining the extension of medullary involvement. SpDSA is then required to delineate the vascular anatomy and the flow characteristics of the lesion.[56] Spinal AVMs are the most common cause of hematomyelia and comprise approximately 10% of all spinal vascular shunt lesions.[55] These lesions are normally evident on MRI because of the prominent flow voids of the nidus and draining veins on T2-weighted sequences. MRI is fundamental to determine the intramedullary location of the shunt and to quantify the damage to the adjacent cord parenchyma. Vascular anatomy and the hemodynamics of spinal AVMs are fully characterized by SpDSA.

- Type II: Glomus type AVM (**Fig. 5**) are usually localized to the ventral spinal cord and supplied by a radiculomedullary feeder or by the anterior spinal artery itself. The nidus is intramedullary and does contain intervening neural tissue. Although these patients can present with acute severe "dagger stab" back pain with weakness, 80% remains independent 5 years from initial diagnosis.[55] The annual hemorrhage rate is 4% but can be as high as 10% in patients with a history of prior

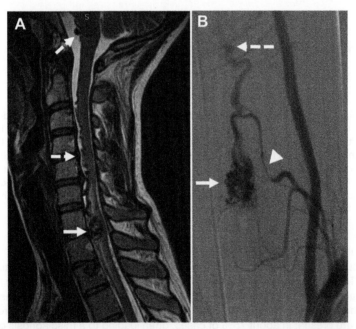

Fig. 5. Spinal AVM in a 29-year-old woman with cervical pain. Sagittal T2-weighted image (*A*) shows intramedullary flow voids suggestive of the nidus of an AVM within the anterior portion of the lower cervical spinal cord. Serpiginous flow voids along the anterior surface of the cord, also seen intracranially at the level of the bulb (*dotted arrows*), represent dilated perimedullary veins. Anteroposterior left subclavian artery angiogram (*B*) demonstrates the lesion is an AVM with a compact nidus (*arrow*) fed by a spinal radiculomedullary feeder originating from the ascending cervical artery (*arrowhead*). The lesion drains into an enlarged cervical perimedullary vein directed cranially (*dotted arrow*).

hemorrhage.[57] Treatment of these lesions is complex and often requires a combined endovascular and open surgical approach.

- Type III: Juvenile-type AVMs are extremely rare (<5% of spinal AVMs), high-flow and high-pressure lesions whose nidus is located in the spinal cord with intervening neural tissue and variable extension into extramedullary soft tissues and bones. These lesions are commonly fed by multiple medullary arteries, making surgical resection nearly impossible.[49] Because of the anatomic complexity of the AVM, curative therapy is exceedingly rare, and treatment involves endovascular and radiosurgical approaches.

Type IV: perimedullary arteriovenous fistula. These fistulas are located on the spinal cord pial surface and are fed by spinal arteries, most commonly the anterior one (**Fig. 6**). The shunt drains directly into perimedullary veins, and they are most often found in children and young adults. Symptoms can be secondary to congestive myelopathy or hemorrhage from venous rupture. These lesions are normally

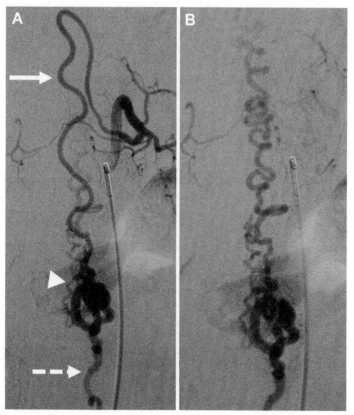

Fig. 6. Perimedullary arteriovenous fistula (subtype C) in a 30-year-old man with progressive myelopathy. Anteroposterior angiogram of the left T11 intersegmental artery in the early arterial phase (*A*) demonstrates a significantly enlarged radiculomedullary feeder, and anterior spinal artery (*arrow*) that feeds a high-flow fistula with multiple ectatic venous structure at the level of the fistulous point (*arrowhead*). The lesion drains in enlarged perimedullary veins directed both caudally (*dotted arrow*) and cranially along the entire length of the spinal cord (*B*).

detectable on MRI because of the presence of large flow voids on the surface of the cord, but SpDSA is needed for complete characterization. Treatment is based on exclusion of the shunt and can be carried out either surgically or endovascularly. Depending on size of the fistula, shunt entity, and number of feeding vessels, they can be subdivided into 3 subtypes [55,58,59]:

- ○ Subtype A: Single fistula of the conus medullaris or filum terminalis fed by the anterior spinal artery with slow perimedullary drainage
- ○ Subtype B: Multiple small fistulae of the conus or filum fed by both anterior and posterior spinal arterial feeders with slow retrograde perimedullary drainage
- ○ Subtype C: Single fistula fed by single or multiple, both anterior and posterior spinal feeders. These are high-flow shunts with fast retrograde drainage in significantly ectatic or aneurysmatic perimedullary veins

Cavernous malformations

Cavernous malformations are low-flow lesions that do not involve arteriovenous shunting and are often small (**Fig. 7**).[55] They are constituted by thin-walled, dilated sinusoidal vessels.[15] Pathologically, there is commonly a ring of hemosiderin and gliosis surrounding the malformation, resulting from multiple, subsequent hemorrhages over a prolonged time. MRI commonly demonstrates hypodense margin on T2-weighted sequences and as blooming on susceptibility weighted imaging.[55] Although more commonly encountered in the brain, cavernous malformations comprise up to 12% of spinal vascular abnormalities.[60] Symptoms often present in the third to sixth (most commonly fourth) decade of life in a slowly progressive fashion because of intralesional microhemorrhages, although there is variability in the acuity and severity of the clinical manifestations.[15,61] Following initial hemorrhage, the recurrent hemorrhage rate is 2.1% to 3.9% annually.[15] These lesions are better diagnosed with MRI and are angiographically occult.[55]

Conservative management with surveillance imaging may be appropriate for those with asymptomatic or nonprogressive symptoms, but surgical intervention is indicated for those with progressive neurologic deficits.[55] Ventral lesions are associated with poor outcomes.[62]

Aneurysm

Spinal arterial aneurysms are uncommon and account for less than 1% of all cases of subarachnoid hemorrhage [63,64]. Aneurysm formation is most commonly related to high-flow arteriovenous shunts (both malformations and fistulae), but additional causes include infectious, noninfectious inflammatory, and collagen vascular disorders (especially Ehlers-Danlos type IV and fibromuscular dysplasia).[65] Although aneurysms can enlarge and cause compressive myelopathy, rupture with subarachnoid hemorrhage is the most common clinical manifestation, typically presenting as acute onset headache, back/neck pain, and nausea/vomiting. Uncommonly (<15% of patients), a ruptured spinal artery aneurysm may cause acute myelopathy.62 SpDSA is the diagnostic modality of choice and can be followed by endovascular treatment in the same session.

ACUTE INFECTIOUS MYELOPATHY
Background

Acute infectious myelopathy may be caused by bacterial, fungal, parasitic, and viral pathogens. Although infectious myelopathy is rare, identification and early treatment with antimicrobial therapy and source control are paramount to management. The list of possible specific causes of infectious myelopathy is extensive, and this section

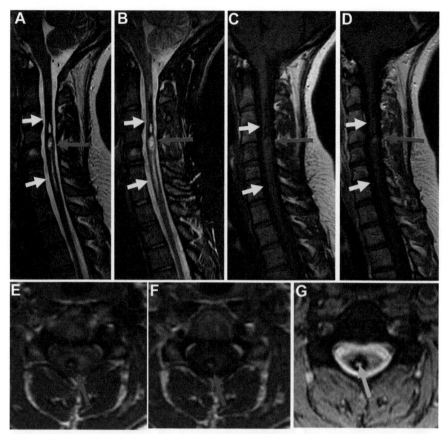

Fig. 7. Spinal cord cavernous malformation with hematomyelia. Sagittal T2 (*A*), STIR (*B*), T1 (*C*), and T1 post contrast (*D*) images of the cervical spine demonstrate a subtly enhancing intramedullary lesion (red arrows) with associated hematomyelia (*yellow arrows*). Axial T1 (*E*), T1 post contrast (*F*) confirm the presence of a subtly enhancing intramedullary lesion. Axial GRE (*G*) image demonstrates prominent associated susceptibility blooming and a complete rim of hypointensity consistent with a hemorrhagic lesion such as a cavernous malformation (*blue arrow*).

highlights 3 different pathophysiologic mechanisms and syndromes by which infections can cause acute myelopathy:

- Infections around the spinal cord can result in extrinsic compression, as seen in extramedullary abscess.
- Pathogens can directly invade neurons, causing intrinsic cord dysfunction owing to axonal and/or neuronal death, as seen in poliovirus.
- Spinal cord ischemia owing to infectious vasculitis can occur, as seen in varicella-zoster virus (VZV) vasculitis.

As discussed in the vascular myelopathy section of this article, the clinical manifestations of acute myelopathy owing to an infection vary depending on the particular parts of the cord that are involved in both terms of the tracts and cell types as well as the rostrocaudal spinal level. It is important to note that intrinsic spinal cord and intradural infections may not present with typical systemic infectious symptoms, such as fever, chills, and fatigue, because the central nervous system is immunologically isolated by the blood-cord barrier. A thorough history can provide clues, such as recent travel, exposures, illicit drug use, chronic infections, or immunosuppression. An exhaustive discussion of infectious causes of myelopathy is beyond the scope of this review.

Spinal cord abscess

Extramedullary abscess. The incidence of spinal epidural abscess (SEA) (**Fig. 8**) is increasing as risk factors, including aging population, prevalence of IV drug use, and increase in volume of invasive spinal procedures for pain control or anesthesia, increases.[66] The classic triad of fever, back pain, and neurologic deficits is present in only a small minority of patients at the time of presentation. Fever may be present in one-half to two-thirds of patients.[67] Neurologic deficits may be present in fewer than half of patients. The most common presenting symptom is back pain, which may be accompanied by localized spinal tenderness in a minority of patients, leading to a delay in presentation to medical care.[66,68] Thus, by the time an individual does present to care, their disease may have reached an advanced stage, making prompt diagnosis and management particularly important.[69]

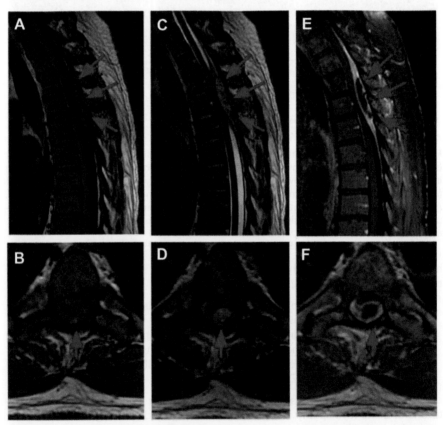

Fig. 8. SEA. Thoracic spine sagittal and axial images, including T1 (*A, B*), T2 (*C, D*), and T1 postcontrast (*E, F*) sequences, demonstrate a dorsal, peripherally enhancing upper thoracic epidural abscess compressing the spinal cord (*arrows*).

SEA is an extramedullary lesion in the epidural space, where it can appear as a result of hematogenous seeding from nearby structures, such as the psoas muscle or vertebral body, or by introduction directly to the epidural compartment after injury or medical procedures. Individuals with bacteremia from IV drug use or long-term vascular access, or those with immune suppression, such as human immunodeficiency virus (HIV)/AIDS, can also present with the syndrome, and any of the above risk factors should raise suspicion for SEA. However, up to one-third of individuals with SEA can present without known risk factors, and their absence cannot exclude the condition.[70]

The causative organism of SEA is *Staphylococcus aureus* in approximately two-thirds of cases, gram-negative bacilli in 16%, and streptococci in 9%.[71] Nonbacterial causes are vanishingly rare at less than 1%. As such, empiric treatment should include gram-positive, including methicillin-resistant *S aureus*, and gram-negative organisms. Adjunctive surgical evacuation for decompression and source control is crucial. CT-guided abscess biopsy to guide definitive antimicrobial regimen is indicated when surgical treatment is not planned.[72]

Acute flaccid paralysis

Acute flaccid paralysis (AFP) is a syndrome of spinal anterior horn cell dysfunction that leads to rapid onset of weakness in one or more limbs. Although it was historically caused most commonly by myelitis from poliovirus infection, other infectious and parainfectious causes are now more commonly seen. Presentation can occur rapidly over 48 hours, and the syndrome often has extremely poor outcomes, including death.[73] These days it is rare, occurring in fewer than 1 person per million in the United States, although it can occur in clusters following seasonal outbreaks of viral illnesses, such as enterovirus D68.[74,75]

Enterovirus. Enteroviruses D68 and D71 have been associated with acute flaccid myelitis (AFM) in the United States and abroad. Enterovirus D68 specifically appears to present with characteristic biennial outbreaks, occurring most recently in the United States in 2014, 2016, and 2018, which is driven by a combination of serotype specific herd immunity and seasonal factors.[76,77] Enterovirus and poliovrius are picornavirusess, which ave neurotropic antigens.[77] It is most common in the fall months regardless of geographic location, occurring approximately in August to November in the northern hemisphere and in April to June in the southern hemisphere.[78–80]

Studies have found high levels of antienterovirus antibodies in the CSF of individuals with AFM compared with controls, although it remains unclear whether the illness is the direct result of enterovirus infection or a parainfectious immune response.[81] Weakness can involve from 1 to 4 limbs, and cranial nerve abnormalities can be present in approximately one-third of patients. Symptoms typically progress subacutely over days but can progress rapidly to neurologic nadir in a matter of hours in some patients. Approximately 20% to 35% of patients will require intubation for respiratory support.[82,83]

Diagnosis should be pursued with spinal cord MRI and CSF analysis. MRI of the spine typically shows T2-hyperintense lesions that are gray matter–predominant in more than half of patients. Nerve root enhancement in the cauda equina can be seen in one-third of patients.[84] However, imaging performed within 72 hours of symptom onset may show no signal abnormality or ill-defined signal abnormality of the entire central spinal cord gray matter.[85] CSF analysis generally demonstrates a lymphocytic pleocytosis in up to 81% of patients, mild or no protein elevation, and mild decrease to normal CSF-to-serum glucose ratio.[86]

There is a paucity of data on treatment of AFM available for systematic analysis, as most studies on this are retrospective. No evidence significantly supports the efficacy of high-dose steroids, intravenous immunoglobulin (IVIg), or plasmaphresis or plasma exhange (PLEX).[83,87] Inpatient hospitalization largely focuses on supportive care, including intubation for respiratory failure, which has been reported in 9% to 34% of patients.[82]

West Nile virus. Neurologic manifestations of West Nile virus (WNV)-associated neurologic disease can include encephalitis as well as several neuromuscular syndromes, including brachial plexopathy and postinfectious demyelinating neuropathy. Estimated to occur in about 10% of individuals with neuroinvasive WNV, or less than 1% of those infected with WNV overall, WNV-AFP is the most emergent presentation of the disease. More than 80% of patients in whom paralysis occurs appears to be otherwise healthy without other significant medical history.[88,89] Thus, it is imperative that appropriate diagnostic testing, including lumbar puncture, electromyography, and nerve conduction studies, be obtained before initiating therapy for Guillain-Barré syndrome or other inflammatory neuropathies that can mimic WNV-AFP.

Although no acute treatment of WNV-AFP is supported by substantial evidence, there is a single report of IVIg used to successfully treat it as well as another case report of high-dose corticosteroids.[90,91] There are not enough data to draw a clear conclusion of benefit, but these treatments are safe and can be considered.

Acute infectious vasculitis

Infectious vasculitis and parainfectious vasculitis are exceedingly rare causes of acute myelopathy.[92] Potential causes include Epstein-Barr virus, cytomegalovirus, hepatitis A and B, coxsackievirus, Rickettsia, HIV, VZV, and herpes simplex virus, bacterial, fungal, and parasitic, but many of these are only described in case reports or small case series.[92,93]

Varicella zoster virus. VZV vasculitis can affect many vascular locations, including the spinal cord. The typical presentation is similar to spinal cord infarction because of other causes, with back pain, sensory loss, and paraparesis or paraplegia. Perhaps the most robust evidence to support infectious vasculitis causing spinal cord infarction comes from postmortem-verified pathologic condition of VZV-associated vasculitis causing spinal cord infarction.[94,95] Pathologic specimens demonstrate hemorrhagic necrosis in the leptomeninges and hemorrhagic spinal cord necrosis.[94] CSF virologic analysis and MRI are used to diagnose VZV vasculitis. Detection of anti-VZV immunoglobulin G (IgG) antibody in the CSF is more sensitive for VZV vasculitis than detection of VZV DNA.[96] The synthesis of intrathecal anti-VZV antibodies can be assessed, and a decreased serum:CSF ratio of anti-VZV IgG is indicative of intrathecal synthesis of anti-VZV antibodies and infection.[97] MRI of the spinal cord can demonstrate acute spinal cord infarction (as discussed above).[98] The recommended treatment of VZV vasculitis is 10 to 15 mg/kg IV acyclovir 3 times a day for at least 14 days.[97]

SUMMARY

Vascular and infectious causes of acute myelopathy are rare but important causes of spinal cord injury. A high level of suspicion for these processes is necessary, as early symptoms can be nonspecific and may progress over hours to days, resulting in delayed presentation and diagnosis. History and clinical examination findings can assist with localization of potential vascular territory and spinal level affected, which will assist with focusing spinal imaging. Rapid CT/CTA and MRI/MRA are necessary to exclude compressive lesions that may require abrupt surgical management. There are limited data for management of spinal cord infarction, but blood pressure augmentation and lumbar CSF drainage can be beneficial, and prevention of and close monitoring for systemic complications are important. Infectious myelopathy treatment consists of targeted antimicrobial therapy, infection source control, and again, prevention of and close monitoring for systemic complications.

CLINICS CARE POINTS

- Acute myelopathy, regardless of the underlying cause, will present with clinical symptoms determined by the longitudinal tracts and rostrocaudal levels affected. Because the differential diagnosis is broad, and presentation of vascular or infectious myelopathy can be insidious over hours to days, a high degree of suspicion for these entities and rapid imaging of the spinal cord are necessary.

- Although there are multiple anterior-to-posterior and cranial-to-caudal vascular anastomoses, the anterior spinal artery supplies most of the spinal cord, and there are watershed areas at high risk for ischemic injury, including the anterior horn cells and central spinal cord, and classically the T4-T6 spinal level.

- Imaging in the hyperacute phase of vascular myelopathy may be normal, even when specialized imaging is performed. Nonetheless, spinal diffusion-weighted imaging and echo planar imaging can provide additional insight into spinal cord ischemia.

- Infectious causes of myelopathy do not always present with typical systemic signs and symptoms of infection, such as fever and leukocytosis. A high degree of suspicion; thorough history aimed at discovering risk factors for infection, including exposures, immunosuppression, intravenous drug abuse, and travel; and imaging directed by the clinical findings are therefore essential.

DISCLOSURE

The authors have nothing to disclose.

REFERENCES

1. Rigney L, Cappetin-Smith C, Sebire D, et al. Nontraumatic spinal cord ischaemic syndrome. J Clin Neurosci 2015;22(10):1544–9.
2. Masson C, Pruvo JP, Meder JF, et al. Spinal cord infarction: clinical and magnetic resonance imaging findings and short term outcome. J Neurol Neurosurg Psychiatry 2004;75(10):1431–5.
3. Naess H, Romi F. Comparing patients with spinal cord infarction and cerebral infarction: clinical characteristics and short-term outcome. Vasc Health Risk Manag 2011;7:497–502.
4. Nasr DM, Rabinstein A. Spinal cord infarcts: risk factors, management and prognosis. Curr Treat Options Neurol 2017;19:28.
5. Novy J, Carruzzo A, Maeder P, et al. Spinal cord ischemia: clinical and imaging patterns, pathogenesis and outcomes in 27 patients. Arch Neurol 2006;63(8):1113–20.
6. Vargas MI, Garieni J, Sztajzel R, et al. Spinal cord ischemia: practical imaging tips, pearls and pitfalls. AJNR Am J Neuroradiol 2015;36(5):825–30.
7. Mateen FJ, Monrad PA, Hunderfund AN, et al. Clinically suspected fibrocartilaginous embolism: clinical characteristics, treatments and outcomes. Eur J Neurol 2001;18(2):218–25.

8. Nedeltchev K, Loher JT, Stepper F, et al. Long-term outcome of acute spinal cord ischemia syndrome. Stroke 2004;35(2):560–5.

9. McCarvey ML, Cheung AT, Szeto W, et al. Management of neurologic complications of thoracic aortic surgery. J Clin Neurophysiol 2007;24(4):336–43.

10. But J, Harris PL, Hobo R, et al. Neurologic complications associated with endovascular repair of thoracic aortic pathology: incidence and risk factors. A study from the European Collaborators on Stent/Graft Techniques for Aortic Aneurysm Repair (EUROSTAR) registry. J Vasc Surg 2007;46(6):1103–10.

11. Makaroun MS, Dillavous ED, Kee ST, et al. Endovascular treatment of thoracic aortic aneurysms: results of the phase II multicenter trial of the GORE TAG thoracic endoprothesis. J Vasc Surg 2005;41(1):1–9.

12. Stone DH, Brewster DC, Kwoleck CJ, et al. Stent-graft versus open-surgical repair of the thoracic aorta mid-term results. J Vasc Surg 2006;44(6):1188–97.

13. Narvid J, Hetts SW, Larsen D, et al. Spinal dural arteriovenous fistulae: clinical features and long-term results. Neurosurgery 2008;62(1):159–66.

14. Lee J, Lim YM, Suh DC, et al. Clinical presentation, imaging findings and prognosis of spinal dural arteriovenous fistula. J Clin Neurosci 2016;26:105–9.

15. Badhiwala JH, Farrokhyar F, Alhazzani W, et al. Surgical outcomes and natural history of intramedullary spinal cord cavernous malformations: a single-center series and meta-analysis of individual patient data: clinical article. J Neurosurg Spine 2014;21(4):662–76.

16. Bosnia AN, Tubbs RS, Hogan E, et al. Blood supply to the shaman spinal cord: part III. Imaging and Pathology. Clin Anat 2015;28(1):65–74.

17. Biglioli P, Roberto M, Cannata A, et al. Upper and lower spinal cord blood supply: the continuity of the anterior spinal artery and the relevance of the lumbar arteries. J Thorac Cardiovasc Surg 2004;127(4):1188–92.

18. Freedman BA, Malone CG, Rasmussen PA, et al. Surfer's myelopathy: a rare form of spinal cord infarction in novice surfers: a systemic review. Neurosurgery 2016; 78(5):602–11.

19. Hsu CY, Cheng CY, Lee JD, et al. Clinical features ant outcomes of spinal cord infarction following vertebral artery dissection: a systemic review of the literature. Neurol Res 2013;35(7):676–83.

20. Sullivan TM, Sundt TM. Complications of thoracic aortic endografts: spinal cord ischemia and stroke. J Vasc Surg 2006;43(Suppl A):85A–8A.

21. Sandson TA, Friedman JH. Spinal cord infarction. Report of 8 cases and review of the literature. Medicine 1989;68(5):282.

22. Mateen FJ, Monrad PA, Hunderfund AN, et al. Clinically suspected fibrocartilaginous embolism: clinical characteristics, treatments and outcomes. Eur J Neurol 2011;18(2):218–25.

23. AbdelRazek MA, Mowla A, Farooq S, et al. Fibrocartilaginous embolism: a comprehensive review of an understudied cause of spinal cord infarction and proposed diagnostic criteria. J Spinal Cord Med 2016;39(2):146–54.

24. Thompson TP, Pearce J, Chang G, et al. Surfer's myelopathy. Spine (Phila Pa 1976) 2004;29:E353–6.

25. Gempp E, Blatteau JE. Risk factors and treatment outcomes in scuba divers with spinal cord spinal cord decompression sickness. J Crit Care 2010;25(2):236–42.

26. Francis TJR, Mitchell SJ. Pathophysiology of decompression sickness. In: Brubback AO, Neuman TS, editors. The Bennett and Elliot's physiology and medicine of diving. 5th edition. London (United Kingdom): WB Saunders; 2003. p. 530–6.

27. Thalmann ED. Principles of US Navy recompression treatments for decompression sickness. In: Moon RE, Sheffields PJ, editors. Diving accident management. Bethesda (MD): Undersea and Hyperbaric Medical Society; 1996. p. 75–95.

28. Weaver LK. Monoplace hyperbaric chamber use of US Navy Table 6: a 25-year experience. Undersea Hyperb Med 2006;33:85–8.

29. Bond JG, Moon RE, Morris DL. Initial table treatment of decompression sickness and arterial gas embolism. Aviat Space Environ Med 1990;61:738–43.

30. Kister I, Johnson E, Raz E, et al. Specific MRI findings help distinguish acute transverse myelitis of neuromyelitis optical from spinal cord infarction. Mult Scler Relat Disord 2016;9:62–7.

31. Alblas CL, Bouvy WH, Lycklama A, et al. Acute spinal-cord ischemia: evolution of MRI findings. J Clin Neurol 2012;8(3):218–23.

32. Thurnher MM, Bammer R. Diffusion-weighted MR imaging (DWI) in spinal cord ischemia. Neuroradiology 2006;48(11):795–801.

33. Weidauer S, Nichtweiss M, Lanfermann H, et al. Spinal cord infarction: MR imaging and clinical features in 16 cases. Neuroradiology 2002;44(10):851–7.

34. Friedman DP, Tartaglino LM, Fisher AR, et al. MR imaging in the diagnosis of intramedullary spinal cord diseases that involve specific neural pathways or vascular territories. AJR Am J Roentgenol 1995;165(3):515–23.

35. Bosmia AN, Hogan E, Loukas M, et al. Blood supply to the human spinal cord part 1. Anatomy and hemodynamics. Clin Anat 2015;28(1):52–64.

36. Mawad ME, Rivera V, Crawford S, et al. Spinal cord ischemia after resection of thoracoabdominal aortic aneurysms. Am J Neuroradiol 1990;11:987–91.

37. Andre JB, Bammer R. Advanced diffusion-weighted magnetic resonance imaging techniques of the human spinal cord. Top Magn Reson Imaging 2010; 21(6):367–78.

38. Robertson CE, Brown RD Jr, Wijdicks EF, et al. Recovery after spinal cord infarcts: long-term outcomes in 115 patients. Neurology 2012;78(2):114–21.

39. Etgen T, Hocherl C. Repeated early thrombosis in cervical spinal cord ischemia. J Thromb Thrombolysis 2016;42(1):142–5.

40. Muller JI, Steffensen LJ, Johnsen SH. Thrombolysis in anterior spinal artery syndrome. BMJ Case Rep 2012;2012. bcr2012006862.

41. Fedorow CA, Moon MC, Mutch AC, et al. Lumbar cerebrospinal fluid drainage for thoracoabdominal aortic surgery: rationale and practical considerations for management. Anesth Analg 2010;111:46–58.

42. Nas K, Yazmalar L, Sah V, et al. Rehabilitation of spinal cord injuries. World J Orthop 2015;6(1):8–16.

43. Romi F, Naess H. Spinal cord infarction in clinical neurology: a review of characteristics and long-term prognosis in comparison to cerebral infarction. Eur Neurol 2016;76(3–4):95–8.

44. Zevgaridis D, Medele RJ, Hamburger C, et al. Cavernous haemangiomas of the spinal cord. A review of 117 cases. Acta Neurochir (Wien) 1999;141:237–45.

45. Matsumura A, Ayuzawa S, Doi M, et al. Chronic progressive hematomyelia: case reports and review of the literature. Surg Neurol 1999;51:559–63.

46. Hunderfund ANL, Wijdicks EFM. Intramedullary spinal cord hemorrhage (hematomyelia). Rev Neurol Dis 2009;6(2):E53–61.

47. Krings T. Vascular malformations of the spine and spinal cord: anatomy, classification and treatment. Clin Neuroradiol 2010;20:5–24.

48. El Mekabaty A, Pardo CA, Gailloud P. The yield of initial conventional MRI in 115 cases of angiographically confirmed spinal vascular malformations. J Neurol 2017;264(4):733–9.

49. Doppman JL, Dichiro G, Oldfield EH. Origin of spinal arteriovenous malformation and normal cord vasculature from a common segmental artery: angiographic and therapeutic considerations. Radiology 1985;154(3):687–9.

50. Jellema K, Tijssen CC, can Gijn J. Spinal dural arteriovenous fistulas: a congestive myelopathy that initially mimics a peripheral nerve disorder. Brain 2016;129: 3150–64.

51. Saraf-Lavi E, Bowen BC, Quencer RM, et al. Detection of spinal dural arteriovenous fistulae with MR imaging and contrast-enhanced MR angiography: sensitivity, specificity and prediction of vertebral level. AJNR Am J Neuroradiol 2002; 23:858–67.

52. Sasamori T, Hida K, Yano S, et al. Long-term outcomes after surgical and endovascular treatment of spinal dural ateriovenous fistulae. Eur Spine J 2016;25(3): 748–54.

53. Koch MJ, Stapleton CJ, Agarwalla PK, et al. Open and endovascular treatment of spinal dural arteriovenous fistulas: a 1-year experience. J Neurosurg Spine 2017; 26(4):519–23.

54. Jellema K, Tijssen CC, van Rooij WJ, et al. Spinal dural arteriovenous fistulas: long-term follow-up of 44 treated patients. Neurology 2004;25:1839–41, 62(10).

55. Singh R, Lucke-Wold B, Gyure K, et al. A review of vascular abnormalities of the spine. Ann Vasc Med Res 2016;3(4):1045.

56. Unsrisong K, Taphey S, Oranratanachai K. Spinal arteriovenous shunts accuracy of shunt detection, localization, and subtype discrimination using spinal magnetic resonance angiography and manual contrast injection using a syringe. J Neurosurg Spine 2016;24:664–70.

57. Gross BA, Du R. Spinal glomus (type II) arteriovenous malformations: a pooled analysis of hemorrhage risk and results of intervention. Neurosurgery 2013; 72(1):25–32.

58. Rosenblum B, Oldfield EH, Doppman JL, et al. Spinal arteriovenous malformations: a comparison of dural arteriovenous fistulas and intradural AVM's in 81 patients. J Neurosurg 1987;67:795–802.

59. Mourier KL, Gobin YP, George B, et al. Intradural perimedullary arteriovenous fistulae: results of surgical and endovascular treatment in a series of 35 cases. Neurosurgery 1993;32(6):885–91.

60. Killeen T, Czaplinski A, Cesnulis E. Extradural spinal cavernous malformation: a rare but important mimic. Br J Neurosurg 2014;28:340–6.

61. Scherman DB, Rao PJ, Varikatt W, et al. Clinical presentation and surgical outcomes of an intramedullary C2 spinal cord cavernoma: a case report and review of the relevant literature. J Spine Surg 2016;2:139–42.

62. Liang JT, Bao YH, Zhang HQ, et al. Management and prognosis of symptomatic patients with intramedullary spinal cord cavernoma: clinical article. J Neurosurg Spine 2011;15:447–56.

63. Berlis A, Scheufler KM, Schmahl C, et al. Solitary spinal artery aneurysms as a rare source of spinal subarachnoid hemorrhage: potential etiology and treatment strategy. AJNR Am J Neuroradiol 2005;26:405–10.

64. Abdalkader M, Samuelsen BT, Moore J, et al. Ruptured spinal aneurysms: diagnosis and management paradigms. World Neurosurgery 2020;146:e368–77.

65. Madhugirl VS, Ambelcars S, Roopesh Kumar VR, et al. Spinal aneurysms: clincoradiological paradigms and management paradigms. J Neurosurg Spine 2013; 19(1):34–48.

66. Reihsaus E, Waldbaur H, Seeling W. Spinal epidural abscess: a meta-analysis of 915 patients. Neurosurg Rev 2000;23(4):175–204.

67. Curry WT Jr, Hoh BL, Amin-Hanjani S, et al. Spinal epidural abscess: clinical presentation, management, and outcome. Surg Neurol 2005;63(4):364–71.

68. Bond A, Manian FA. Spinal epidural abscess: a review with special emphasis on earlier diagnosis. Biomed Res Int 2016.

69. Wang VY, Chou D, Chin C. Spine and spinal cord emergencies: vascular and infectious causes. Neuroimaging Clin N Am 2010;20(4):639–50.

70. Patel AR, Timothy BA, Richard JB, et al. Spinal epidural abscesses: risk factors, medical versus surgical management, a retrospective review of 128 cases. Spine J 2014;14(2):326–30.

71. Scheld WM, Whitley RJ, Durack DT. Infections of the central nervous system. Philadelphia, PA: Lippincott Williams & Wilkins; 1997.

72. Darouiche RO. Spinal epidural abscess. N Engl J Med 2006;355(19):2012–20.

73. Petersen LR, Brault AC, Nasci RS. West Nile virus: review of the literature. JAMA 2013;310(3):308–15.

74. Stelzer-Braid S, Rawlinson W. Outbreaks of acute flaccid myelitis in the US. British Medical Journal Publishing Group; 2018.

75. Lopez A, Adria L, Angela G, et al. Vital signs: surveillance for acute flaccid myelitis - United States, 2018. MMWR Morb Mortal Wkly Rep 2019;68(27): 608–14.

76. Pons-Salort M, Grassly NC. Serotype-specific immunity explains the incidence of diseases caused by human enteroviruses. Science 2018;361(6404):800–3.

77. Pons-Salort M, Oberste MS, Pallansch MA, et al. The seasonality of nonpolio enteroviruses in the United States: patterns and drivers. Proc Natl Acad Sci U S A 2018;115(12):3078–83.

78. Messacar K, Abzug MJ, Dominguez SR. Acute flaccid myelitis surveillance: a signal through the noise. Pediatrics 2019;144(5):e20192492.

79. Carballo CM, García Erro M, Sordelli N, et al. Acute flaccid myelitis associated with enterovirus D68 in children, Argentina, 2016. Emerg Infect Dis 2019; 25(3):573.

80. Chong PF, Kira R, Mori H, et al. Clinical features of acute flaccid myelitis temporally associated with an enterovirus D68 outbreak: results of a nationwide survey of acute flaccid paralysis in Japan, August–December 2015. Clin Infect Dis 2018; 66(5):653–64.

81. Schubert RD, Isobel AH, Prashanth SR, et al. Pan-viral serology implicates enteroviruses in acute flaccid myelitis. Nat Med 2019;25(11):1748–52.

82. Messacar K, Schreiner TL, Van Haren K, et al. Acute flaccid myelitis: a clinical review of US cases 2012–2015. Ann Neurol 2016;80(3):326–38.

83. Van Haren K, Patrick A, Emmanuelle W, et al. Acute flaccid myelitis of unknown etiology in California, 2012-2015. JAMA 2015;314(24):2663–71.

84. Elrick MJ, Gordon-Lipkin E, Crawford TO, et al. Clinical subpopulations in a sample of North American children diagnosed with acute flaccid myelitis, 2012-2016. JAMA Pediatr 2019;173(2):134.

85. Maloney JA, Mirsky DM, Messacar K, et al. MRI findings in children with acute flaccid paralysis and cranial nerve dysfunction occurring during the 2014 enterovirus D68 outbreak. AJNR Am J Neuroradiol 2015;36(2):245–50.

86. Ayers T, Adriana L, Adria L, et al. Acute flaccid myelitis in the United States: 2015–2017. Pediatrics 2019;144(5):e20191619.

87. Greninger AL, Samia NN, Kevin M, et al. A novel outbreak enterovirus D68 strain associated with acute flaccid myelitis cases in the USA (2012-14): a retrospective cohort study. Lancet Infect Dis 2015;15(6):671–82.

88. Sejvar JJ, Amy VB, Anthony AM, et al. West Nile virus-associated flaccid paralysis. Emerg Infect Dis 2005;11(7):1021–7.
89. Patriarca PA, Sutter RW, Oostvogel PM. Outbreaks of paralytic poliomyelitis, 1976-1995. J Infect Dis 1997;175(Suppl 1):S165–72.
90. Walid MS, Mahmoud FA. Successful treatment with intravenous immunoglobulin of acute flaccid paralysis caused by West Nile virus. Perm J 2009;13(3):43–6.
91. Pyrgos V, Younus F. High-dose steroids in the management of acute flaccid paralysis due to West Nile virus infection. Scand J Infect Dis 2004;36(6–7):509–12.
92. Gilden D, Cohrs RJ, Mahalingam R, et al. Varicella zoster virus vasculopathies: diverse clinical manifestations, laboratory features, pathogenesis and treatment. Lancet Neurol 2008;8(8):731. Varicella Zoster Virus (VZV) Associated Spinal Cord Infarction.
93. Belizna CC, Hamidou MA, Levesque H, et al. Infection and vasculitis. Rheumatology 2009;48(5):475–82.
94. Devinsky O, Cho ES, Petito CK, et al. Herpes zoster myelitis. Brain 1991;114: 1181–96.
95. Kenyon LC, Dulaney E, Montone KT, et al. Varicella-zoster ventriculoencephalitis and spinal cord infarction in a patient with AIDS. Acta Neuropathol 1996;92: 202–5.
96. Nagel MA, Forghani B, Mahalingam R, et al. The value of detecting anti-VZV antibody in CSF to diagnose VZV vasculopathy. Neurology 2007;68:1069–73.
97. Nagel MA, Gilden D. Update on varicella zoster virus vasculopathy. Curr Infect Dis Rep 2014;16(6):407.
98. Orme HT, Smight AG, Nagel MA, et al. VZV spinal cord infarction identified by diffuse-weighted MRI (DWI). Neurology 2007;69(4):398–400.

Evaluation and Management of Seizures and Status Epilepticus

Pouya Alexander Ameli, MD, MS[a,b],
Abdalla A. Ammar, PharmD, BCCCP, BCPS[c],
Kent A. Owusu, PharmD, BCCCP, BCPS, FCCM[c,d],
Carolina B. Maciel, MD, MSCR[a,b,e,f,*]

KEYWORDS

- Status epilepticus • Nonconvulsive status epilepticus • Electroencephalogram
- EEG • Antiseizure drug • Antiepileptic drug • Neurocritical care

KEY POINTS

- Imbalances between excitatory and inhibitory synapses underlie the pathobiology of seizures, which tend to cease spontaneously and within 5 minutes. Failure of physiologic mechanisms of seizure termination lead to status epilepticus.
- Status epilepticus can be classified according to time domains, age, electroencephalographic features, etiology, and semiology. Operational definitions based on seizure duration thresholds are most used: 5 minutes for tonic-clonic seizures, 10 minutes for focal seizures with impaired awareness.
- Management priorities include implementing cardiorespiratory monitoring, maintaining airway and oxygenation, identification and prompt treatment of hypoglycemia, and use of antiseizure therapy in a manner that considers risks of treatment.
- Mechanisms of seizure refractoriness are time-dependent. Therefore, prompt implementation of a stepwise therapeutic algorithm is the cornerstone of status epilepticus management.
- First-line pharmacologic therapy for status epilepticus comprises prompt and adequately dosed parenteral benzodiazepine administration. Second-line therapy includes appropriately selected and dosed parenteral antiseizure drugs (eg, fosphenytoin, valproic acid, levetiracetam). Intravenous anesthetic administration targeting therapeutic coma is considered third-line therapy.

---

[a] Department of Neurology, University of Florida McKnight Brain Institute, 1149 Newell Drive, Gainesville, FL 32610, USA; [b] Department of Neurosurgery, University of Florida McKnight Brain Institute, 1149 Newell Drive, Gainesville, FL 32610, USA; [c] Department of Pharmacy, Yale New Haven Health, 55 Park Street, New Haven, CT 06511, USA; [d] Care Signature, Yale New Haven Health, 20 York Street, New Haven, CT, 06510, USA; [e] Department of Neurology, Yale University, 20 York Street, New Haven, CT, 06510, USA; [f] Department of Neurology, University of Utah, 383 Colorow Drive, Salt Lake City, UT, 84132, USA
* Corresponding author.
E-mail address: carolina.maciel@neurology.ufl.edu

Neurol Clin 39 (2021) 513–544
https://doi.org/10.1016/j.ncl.2021.01.009
0733-8619/21/© 2021 Elsevier Inc. All rights reserved.

INTRODUCTION

Status epilepticus (SE) is a common neurologic emergency affecting 18.3 to 41.0 per 100,000 people yearly in the United States, and is associated with direct hospitalization costs surpassing $4 billion.[1–3] The incidence of SE follows a U-shaped curve with regard to patient age, with highest frequencies of occurrence among 0-year-old to 4-year-old children and adults older than 60.[1] Estimated 30-day mortality is 21%, but surpasses 30% across all age groups in the 10-year period following an SE episode[1] and spans 24.5% to 37.9% in refractory cases.[4] The prognosis of SE is heavily influenced by the underlying SE etiology, type and duration of seizures, history of seizures, age, and electroencephalogram (EEG) features.[4–12] Seizure termination mechanisms weaken over time and contribute to refractoriness of treatment.[13] As such, much of the focus in management of SE is rapid seizure control.

Improving our ability to prevent and treat SE, the past few decades brought a flurry of new anti-seizure drugs (ASDs),[14] advanced monitoring abilities with continuous EEG (cEEG) and quantitative EEG (qEEG) have decreased time to treatment decisions,[15–17] and standardized intensive care unit (ICU) EEG terminology to forge better understanding of rhythmic and periodic patterns.[18] This incredible pace of advancement has made it difficult to remain abreast of new developments and to determine how they should be implemented in routine care, if at all. We summarize recent advances in the field of SE with the goal of providing a concise resource focusing on SE management.

BACKGROUND
The Basics: Conceptualizing Seizure and Status Epilepticus

To fully understand SE management, it is helpful to have a working concept of seizure as a phenomenon. In the simplest terms, seizure is the dysregulated propagation of electrical activity from hyperexcitable cortical neurons, which can also be conceptualized as excessive synchrony within a cluster of neurons. By studying the voltage required for electroconvulsive therapy, we know that all humans have a seizure threshold that varies among individuals,[19] modified by inherited and acquired factors, commonly lowered by genetic influences, electrolyte abnormalities, infections, toxins, or structural lesions, and raised by ASDs, ketosis, and hypothermia.[20,21]

Importantly, even correctable causes of seizure can lead to SE or epilepsy if severe enough.[22] Prolonged and/or repetitive seizure burden may cause reorganization of neural networks that facilitates further seizures, which may have ramifications in the short-term (ie, controlling SE) and the long-term (ie, likelihood of developing epilepsy).[23,24] Furthermore, persistent SE causes excitotoxic neuronal injury, occurring when neurons are continuously activated to the point of energy failure, which prompts neuronal apoptosis or necrosis.[25] Excitotoxic injury is frequently exacerbated by a cascade of secondary injury resulting from dysregulation of cerebral blood flow, hypoxia, hypoglycemia, and fever.[26] Hence, prompt identification of SE with rapid seizure control and supportive care are the pillars of management.

Defining Status Epilepticus

In 1962, Gastaut and colleagues[27] defined SE as "seizures persisting for sufficient time or repeated frequently enough to produce a fixed or enduring epileptic condition." By 1993, the American Epilepsy Society Working Group on Status Epilepticus defined a "sufficient time" as 30 minutes based on animal models demonstrating severe metabolic derangements and enduring neuronal injury beyond this threshold.[28,29] Subsequently, the link between seizure duration and outcomes, in particular the occurrence of systemic complications with prolonged seizures,[12,30,31] challenged the 30-minute threshold. Further, typical seizures rarely last longer than 5 minutes.[31,32] As such, in 1999, grounds were established to treat patients earlier by defining SE with a time threshold of greater than 5 minutes.[31]

The 2015 International League Against Epilepsy definition of SE followed suit by defining 2 operational time domains for each major category of SE (**Table 1**). T1 represents the timepoint at which a seizure is abnormally prolonged with usual seizure termination mechanisms having failed, rendering it unlikely to spontaneously cease. T2 is the timepoint at which continued seizure activity is expected to cause long-term consequences via neuronal injury or network reorganization.[33] The T1 timepoint is when clinical criteria for SE have been met and intervention is recommended; it is defined with consideration to the risk of continued seizure and the risk associated with aggressive interventions.[33]

Refractory SE (RSE) may be defined as SE that persists despite administration of 2 appropriately-dosed ASDs, including benzodiazepine as first line. Super-refractory SE (SRSE) consists of ongoing seizures persisting for $\geq$24 hours despite third-line therapy with anesthetic treatment, or when seizures reemerge on attempted anesthetic wean.[34] SRSE frequently occurs in the setting of acute brain injury or new-onset SE in a patient with no history of seizure.[35] The latter scenario is known as new-onset RSE (NORSE), and is commonly precipitated by infectious, autoimmune, and paraneoplastic causes.[36] Febrile infection-related epilepsy syndrome (FIRES) is a subcategory of NORSE consisting of RSE occurring in close temporal relationship with a febrile illness (between 24 hours and 2 weeks) before the SE onset. Although FIRES can occur at any age, the syndrome is better characterized in the pediatric population.[36]

Prolonged RSE (PRSE) is SE that persists for 7 days despite appropriate treatment, but without the use of anesthetic agents.[36] This may occur in the setting of repetitive focal seizures without generalization, thus meeting criteria for PRSE, but in which the risk of anesthetic coma may be thought to outweigh the benefit. Prolonged SRSE (PSRSE) is SRSE that persists for 7 days including ongoing need for anesthetics.[36]

Defining Nonconvulsive Status Epilepticus, Identifying Status Epilepticus in the Critically Ill, and Using Electroencephalogram Monitoring

Nonconvulsive SE (NCSE) can be defined as SE with or without impaired consciousness and without overt motor phenomena.[33] As patients with NCSE are often clinically indistinguishable from patients with other causes of altered mentation, the diagnosis

Table 1
Status epilepticus definition according to time domain and seizure type

Seizure Type	Timepoint t1: Clinical Criteria for SE Are Met, Treat as SE	Timepoint t2: Continued SE May Cause Long-Term Consequences
Tonic-clonic	5 min	30 min
Focal with impaired awareness	10 min	>60 min
Absence	10–15 min	Unknown

Abbreviation: SE, status epilepticus.
Adapted from (Trinka and colleagues 2015) Trinka, E., H. Cock, D. Hesdorffer, A. O. Rossetti, I. E. Scheffer, S. Shinnar, S. Shorvon, and D. H. Lowenstein. 2015. 'A definition and classification of status epilepticus–Report of the ILAE Task Force on Classification of Status Epilepticus', Epilepsia, 56: 1515-23.

of NCSE relies on EEG. Following the American Clinical Neurophysiology Society Terminology for ICU EEG, the Salzburg criteria were proposed for the diagnosis of electrographic SE, summarized in **Table 2**.[37] The criteria for RSE, SRSE, and prolonged SE remain unchanged with NCSE; however, to apply the Salzburg Criteria, one first needs to identify which patients require EEG.

In a cohort comprising 570 patients connected to cEEG for decreased consciousness, nonconvulsive seizures without SE were more likely in patients with convulsive seizures before cEEG hook-up (43%), age younger than 18 years (36%), history of epilepsy (41%), central nervous system infection (29%), brain tumor (23%), or recent neurosurgical procedure (23%).[38] NCSE was most common in those with history of epilepsy (20%), central nervous system infection (17%), subarachnoid hemorrhage (13%), hypoxic-ischemic encephalopathy (12%), and brain tumor (12%).[38] Each of these factors has had fairly consistent predictive value for seizure across multiple studies.[39]

Nonconvulsive seizures occur in nearly half of comatose patients.[38,40] Nonetheless, because EEG is a limited resource, uncertainty surrounding patient selection for monitoring among critically ill patients exists.[15] The CERTA trial showed that cEEG, compared with repeated routine EEG, detected more ictal and interictal discharges and resulted in more frequent ASD adjustments, but did not result in a change in mortality or functional outcome.[41] However, larger-scale retrospective data have shown mortality benefit with cEEG when compared with routine EEG or no EEG, despite increased illness severity in the cEEG group.[42]

The first hour of EEG monitoring may fail to detect nonconvulsive seizures in 40% to 50% of monitored patients.[39,43] The first 24 hours of cEEG monitoring detects more than 90% of all nonconvulsive seizures when all use cases are considered. In comatose patients, the overall sensitivity of EEG for seizure detection only approaches 90% by 48 hours.[38,44] However, the absence of any epileptiform discharges in the first 2 hours of monitoring is associated with 5% seizure risk in the subsequent 72 hours of recording, regardless of level of consciousness.[39] Seizure risk stratification using early EEG findings may help guide resource allocation. The time-dependent electroclinical risk stratification for electrographic seizures (TERSE) algorithm, factoring in clinical and electrographic features to guide duration of EEG monitoring, detected

Table 2	
Diagnostic criteria for electrographic status epilepticus	
No Known Epileptic Encephalopathy	**Known Epileptic Encephalopathy**
Repetitive epileptiform discharges sustaining >2.5 Hz	Electroclinical response to parenteral ASD trial
Repetitive epileptiform discharges ≤2.5 Hz or rhythmic delta activity >0.5 Hz WITH at least one: • Electroclinical response to parenteral ASD trial • Clear evolution on frequency of discharges (speeding up or slowing down) or location (spreading) • Consistent clinical correlate (albeit subtle)	Notable change in clinical state associated with worsened rhythmic or periodic pattern on EEG when compared with baseline

Abbreviation: ASD, antiseizure drug.

Adapted from (Beniczky and colleagues 2013) Beniczky, S., L. J. Hirsch, P. W. Kaplan, R. Pressler, G. Bauer, H. Aurlien, J. C. Brogger, and E. Trinka. 2013. 'Unified EEG terminology and criteria for nonconvulsive status epilepticus', *Epilepsia*, 54 Suppl 6: 28-9.

97% of SE in a critically ill cohort while reducing cEEG monitoring duration by two-thirds.[45] The recently validated 2HELPS2B score (**Table 3**), can be calculated after 1 hour of EEG to accurately stratify patients with regard to risk of seizure in the following 72 hours, providing a practical tool to determine appropriate duration of EEG when extending limited resources to an ever-growing population meeting criteria for monitoring.[46–48] In addition, where there is a lack of manpower or expertise to interpret traditional EEG, quantitative EEG has been shown to facilitate seizure detection and treatment, as well as potentially make possible a bedside seizure monitor that could be followed by nursing staff with appropriate training.[49,50]

Pitfalls: Selected Seizure Mimics

Especially when SE is being managed in an emergency setting, it is important to consider common or potentially devastating mimics before anchoring to a diagnosis of seizure. The seizure mimic placing patients at highest risk of iatrogenic complications are psychogenic non-epileptic attacks (PNEA). The prevalence of PNEA is estimated to be as high as 33 per 100,000 and prolonged nonepileptic attacks (mimicking SE) occur in up to 78% of patients with PNEA.[51–53] The duration of psychogenic attacks tends to be longer than usual epileptic seizures, and a spell lasting >5 minutes increases the likelihood of PNEA 24-fold.[54] Hence, it should be no surprise that prolonged PNEA is the most frequently seen SE mimic,[51–53] accounting for up to 10% of patients in therapeutic SE trials.[55]

Table 3 Seizure stratification with 2HELPS2B score	
Clinical or Electrographic Feature? Yes/No	**Points if Yes**
Frequency of discharges in any rhythmic or periodic pattern >2 Hz	1
Sporadic epileptiform discharges	1
Lateralized periodic discharges or rhythmic delta activity, or bilateral independent periodic discharges	1
Patterns with "plus" modifiers • Associated fast activity for periodic discharges or rhythmic delta activity • Associated rhythmicity in periodic discharges • Embedded sharp waves or sharp contour in rhythmic delta activity	1
History of epilepsy or seizure preceding monitoring?	1
Brief potentially ictal rhythmic discharges	2
Seizure Risk According to Total Score, %	
<5	0
12	1
27	2
50	3
73	4
88	5
>95	>6

Data from Struck, A. F., B. Ustun, A. R. Ruiz, J. W. Lee, S. M. LaRoche, L. J. Hirsch, E. J. Gilmore, J. Vlachy, H. A. Haider, C. Rudin and M. B. Westover (2017). "Association of an Electroencephalography-Based Risk Score With Seizure Probability in Hospitalized Patients." JAMA Neurol 74(12): 1419-1424.

Given the potential for harm and unnecessary resource utilization, all providers who treat SE should have familiarity with PNEA. Psychogenic attacks typically present with autonomic, sensorimotor, and affective manifestations provoked by emotional distress.[56] Patients with PNEA tend to be young women with a history of psychiatric disease, and frequently a childhood history of abuse.[57,58] Psychogenic attacks tend to evolve more gradually and be less stereotyped than epileptic seizures, with episodes more likely to display a number of features, including eye closure, side-to-side head movements, opisthotonos, random asynchronous movement, and full-body shaking with preserved awareness, whereas the presence of micturition, self-injury, or post-event somnolence do not rule out PNEA.[56,59] Notably, many patients with PNEA have comorbid epilepsy,[60] so previous diagnosis of one does not rule out the other. Determining the correct diagnosis and treatment are nonetheless paramount, as PNEA without epilepsy portends a mortality 2.5 times that of the general population.[61] Importantly, there is extensive literature illustrating imperfect specificity of all reported historical or clinical indicators of PNEA, emphasizing the importance of evaluation by an experienced provider and employment of video cEEG for clarification.[58,59] Ultimately, if there remains concern for SE, it is prudent to treat aggressively until a more definitive diagnosis can be made.

Another SE mimic with high morbidity potential is the cerebellar (or basilar) fit. Reported in patients with cerebellar mass lesions, rapid rise in intracranial pressure, lesions causing brainstem compression, brainstem encephalitis, and sudden cerebral hypoxia or basilar artery occlusion, episodes involve sudden spells of neck extension, back arching, and extensor posturing, thought to result from disconnection of brainstem motor tracts from cortical inhibition. EEG tends to reveal diffuse asynchronous and polymorphic slow waves.[62–65] Often intermittent or asymmetric, episodes frequently evolve to sustained extensor posturing and eventual flexor posturing, commonly with respiratory insufficiency.[63] Index of suspicion is key to identifying cerebellar fits, and emergent brain imaging with angiography should be considered in all patients presenting with unexplained episodes meeting this description.[63–65]

Several movement disorders frequently confused for seizure include tremor, ballismus, and myoclonus. However, these conditions are relatively less likely to be confused for SE and thus are out of the scope of this review.

STATUS EPILEPTICUS TREATMENT APPROACH AND MITIGATING COMPLICATIONS

The management of SE centers on mitigation of secondary injury and prevention of systemic complications.[26,66] Managing providers should titrate the aggressiveness of their treatment approach to the risk of continued seizure as well as the risks of treatment. Treatment of generalized SE should begin at 5 minutes (T1 timepoint), whereas it is typically recommended to begin treatment for focal SE at 10 minutes, and absence SE at 10 to 15 minutes.[33] The relative delay in treatment for focal and absence SE is based on studies suggesting these conditions do not cause neuronal injury as quickly as typical generalized SE, and may not cause lasting injury at all in the case of absence SE.[67–69] In addition to considerations regarding the type of SE, the seizure burden may be a useful tool to help gauge the risks and benefits of additional treatment. Especially in scenarios in which seizure freedom is not achievable, either from lack of treatment efficacy or risk of additional aggressive treatment, it may be clinically and prognostically helpful to note that seizure burden less than 20% per hour has not been associated with significantly increased risk of enduring neurologic injury.[70]

When treatment begins, like other medical emergencies, the first steps in management of SE are the assessment of airway, breathing, and circulation, while also establishing intravenous (IV) access and evaluating for and promptly treating hypoglycemia. SE can cause many systemic ramifications that frequently require urgent attention and/or confound management, including catecholamine-induced hypertension and arrhythmia, lactic acidosis, and respiratory failure.[71] Notably, although hyperoxia can prolong seizure, hypoxia and hypotension can worsen brain and systemic injury, therefore, normoxia and normotension should be targeted.[26] These systemic aberrations should be quickly identified and addressed to maximize success in SE management. **Fig. 1** summarizes the main systemic treatment considerations when managing SE in a stepwise approach.[26] A comprehensive list with pharmacologic considerations for ASDs is provided in **Table 4**.

While stabilization occurs, the first doses of medication should already be ordered and en route to the patient, as mortality in SE correlates with time to treatment and duration of seizure activity.[9,72] The initial treatment of choice is an appropriately dosed benzodiazepine, most commonly intravenous lorazepam at 0.1 mg/kg; we suggest dividing this dose into 2-mg to 4-mg boluses given over 60 to 90 seconds, and repeat every 3 to 5 minutes until seizure cessation. Alternatively, midazolam 5 to 10 mg via intramuscular, buccal, intranasal, or intravenous routes is acceptable. Benzodiazepine underdosing is common and is associated with more than eightfold increase in risk of airway compromise, whereas overdosing can increase respiratory depression without improving outcome.[73–75] Appropriately aggressive treatment is particularly important as SE tends to become self-sustaining and pharmacoresistant as it continues: benzodiazepine resistance ensues in vitro models in the first 30 minutes, suggesting a 20-fold decrease in efficacy[76] due to trafficking of GABA receptors.[77] Phenytoin and barbiturates also lose potency at a slower rate, whereas animal models have shown that N-methyl-D-aspartate (NMDA)-receptor antagonists tend to remain effective into later stages.[78,79]

Because it is often difficult to predict individual response to a specific ASD, and responsiveness may change as SE evolves, the ASD choice in the acute setting is typically based on the side-effect profile of the drugs and consideration of receptors being targeted, based on limited data that a polytherapy approach with varying targets may increase the likelihood of interrupting the mechanisms driving SE.[80,81] The best current evidence in second-line therapy for benzodiazepine-resistant convulsive SE, the Established Status Epilepticus Treatment Trial, demonstrated that 20 mg/kg of fosphenytoin, 40 mg/kg of valproate sodium, and 60 mg/kg of levetiracetam had similar success rates in terminating SE (nearly 50%).[55] Prior studies have shown similar results with lacosamide 400 mg and fosphenytoin 20 mg/kg.[80]

If convulsive SE persists despite administration of first-line and second-line therapy (ie, RSE), a consideration for therapeutic coma with intravenous anesthetics titrated according to cEEG is warranted. Insufficient data exist supporting the benefits of targeting burst suppression over seizure suppression with anesthetics[82]; thus, careful risk-benefit assessment of deeper anesthesia (and consequent systemic complications) must occur when targeting burst suppression. The choice of anesthetic in the acute setting is also commonly based on the side-effect profile of the agent, which renders ketamine, modulating the NMDA/glutamate pathway, and typically with less hemodynamic side effects than GABAergic anesthetics, a growingly favored choice by many neurointensivists, despite commonly being listed as a rescue anesthetic choice after GABAergic anesthetics in guidelines. A recent study of ketamine in 68 patients with SRSE showed seizure cessation in 63%, and a 50% reduction in seizure burden in 81%.[83] The duration of therapeutic coma is commonly 24 to 48 hours based on current guidelines; however, recent studies have suggested greater success with

Medications		Medical Management
With Established IV Access	**If No IV Access**	• Circulation, airway, breathing, obtain IV access, check finger stick glucose
< 10 minutes **Lorazepam:** 4 mg IV push over 2 min. If still seizing after 5 min, repeat x 1 Do not administer IM or SC **Consult Neurology** → If seizures continue →	**Diazepam:** 20 mg PR (using IV solution or rectal gel) **OR** **Midazolam:** 10 mg IN/buccal/IM	• Continuous monitoring: O₂, HR, BP, EKG, ETCO₂ • Obtain labs: CBC, BMP, Ca, Mg, P, Troponin, LFTs, ABG, ASD levels, toxicology screen, HCG, lactic acid, CK • Administer thiamine 100mg IVx1 prior to dextrose • Administer D50W 50 mL IV if low/unknown glucose • Consider administering pyridoxine 250 mg IV x 1 followed by 100 mg PO daily (unless suspicion of isoniazid toxicity then administer 5 g IV); obtain pyridoxine level • Consider head CT scan
10 – 30 minutes **Levetiracetam:** 60 mg/kg IV (over 15 min); max 4500 mg. If still seizing give an additional 20 mg/kg IV (max 1500 mg) over 5 min **OR** **Valproate:** 40 mg/kg IV (over 5 – 10 min); max 4000 mg. If still seizing, give additional 20 mg/kg IV (max 2000 mg) over 5 min **OR** **Fosphenytoin:** 20 mg PE/kg IV at 150 mg/min; max 2000 mg. If still seizing, give additional 5 mg/kg IV (max 500 mg) at 150 mg/min **If still seizing after administering one of the above, either: Administer a second agent from the above list OR intubate and initiate continuous anesthetic infusion:** **Midazolam** **Load dose:** 0.2 mg/kg IV (push over 1 – 2 min); max 20 mg. Repeat 0.2 – 0.4 mg/kg boluses (max 40 mg per bolus) q5min until seizures cessation; max total load of 2mg/kg **Maintenance Infusion Dose:** initial 0.1 mg/kg/hr; 0.1– 2.9 mg/kg/hr; titrate to seizure suppression **OR** **Propofol** (consider simultaneous benzodiazepine infusion) **Load Dose:** 1 – 2 mg/kg IV bolus (intubated patients only) Max dose 200 mg. Repeat q3-5min until seizures cessation; max total load of 10 mg/kg. **Maintenance Infusion Dose:** initial 30 mcg/kg/min; maintenance 30 – 200 mcg/kg/min ; titrate to seizure suppression → If seizures continue →		• Continuous anesthetic infusions: before initiating maintenance infusion, repeat boluses until seizures cessation; for refractory seizures, re-bolus and increase infusion rates • Short-acting neuromuscular blockade is preferred for intubation • Avoid continuous anesthetic infusions if unable to intubate **Alternative therapies to levetiracetam/valproate/fosphenytoin:** **Lacosamide:** 10 mg/kg, max 500 mg IV (over 5 –10 min). If still seizing, give an additional 5 mg/kg; max 250 mg IV over 5 min **OR** **Brivaracetam:** 6 mg/kg IV (over 5 min); max 400 mg. If still seizing, give an additional 200 mg IV over 5 min **OR** **Phenytoin:** 20 mg/kg IV up to 50 mg/min (give at a slower rate of 25 mg/min in elderly patients or with pre-existing cardiovascular conditions); max dose 2000 mg. Infuse through dedicated line with 0.22-micron filter. If still seizing, give additional 5 mg/kg IV (not compatible with dextrose-containing fluids) *If other ASD are contraindicated, consider:* **Phenobarbital:** 15 mg/kg IV, may give up to 60 mg/min; max dose 1500 mg. If still seizing, give an additional 5-10 mg/kg
> 30 minutes **Ketamine** (recommend simultaneous benzodiazepine infusion) **Load dose:** 1.5 mg/kg IV (push over 3 – 5 min); max 150 mg. Repeat until seizures cessation; max total load of 4.5 mg/kg **Maintenance Infusion Dose:** initial 1.2 mg/kg/hr; maintenance 0.3 – 7.5 mg/kg/hr; titrate to seizure suppression **OR** **Pentobarbital** **Load dose:** 5 mg/kg IV at 50 mg/min; max dose 500 mg. Repeat until seizures cessation; max total load of 25 mg/kg **Maintenance Infusion Dose:** initial 1 mg/kg/hr; maintenance 0.5 – 10 mg/kg/hr; titrate to seizure suppression		• If patient is still seizing after 30 min, administer at least 1 continuous anesthetic infusion with boluses • Begin continuous EEG if patient does not awaken rapidly or if continuous anesthetic infusion is being used • Treat fever aggressively • Consider lumbar puncture and/or antibiotics if there is clinical suspicion of infection • Check autoimmune and paraneoplastic antibodies in serum and CSF, if clinical suspicion for autoimmune disorders

Fig. 1. Tiered therapeutic and diagnostic approach to status epilepticus. ABG, arterial blood gas; ASD, antiseizure drug; BMP, basic metabolic profile; Ca, calcium; CBC, complete blood count; CK, creatine kinase; CSF, cerebrospinal fluid; CT, computed tomography; EKG, electrocardiogram; ETCO2, end-tidal carbon dioxide; HCG, human chorionic gonadotropin; HR, heart rate; IM, intramuscular; IN, intranasal; IV, intravenous; LFTs, liver function tests; Mg, magnesium; P, phosphorus; PO, per oral route; PR, per rectum. (*Adapted from* the Yale New Haven Hospital status epilepticus protocol.)

shorter and deeper therapeutic coma as brief as 90 minutes.[84,85] Furthermore, quantitative EEG markers of functional connectivity may predict successful anesthetic wean with 75% accuracy, suggesting the possibility for personalized duration of therapeutic coma in the future.[86]

Table 4
Pharmacologic therapy in status epilepticus

Drug	Dosing	Approximate Half-Life (h) in Non-Critically Ill Patients	Protein Binding	Clinically Relevant Drug-Drug Interactions with Other Drugs	Consideration for Dose Adjustments in Renal Impairment	Consideration for Dose Adjustment in Hepatic Impairment	Comments
Injectable anesthetic agents							
Ketamine	LD: 1.5 mg/kg IV push over 3–5 min (max 150 mg); repeat until seizure suppression; max total load of 4.5 mg/kg MD: initial 1.2 mg/kg/h, range 0.3–7.5 mg/kg/h; titrate to seizure suppression	2.5	27%		None	Consider dose reduction.	NMDA antagonist; provides an infusion with a different mechanism of action (non-GABA). May have sympathomimetic properties, but can also cause hypotension when HR/SBP > 0.9.
Midazolam	LD: 0.2 mg/kg IV (push over 1–2 min); max 20 mg. Repeat 0.2–0.4 mg/kg boluses (max 40 mg per bolus) q5min until seizures suppression; max total load of 2 mg/kg. MD: 0.05–2.9 mg/kg/h; titrate to seizure suppression	7	97%		Consider dose reduction: risk of active metabolite accumulation (1-hydroxy-midazolam)	Consider dose reduction.	Rapid redistribution Active metabolites [1-hydroxy-midazolam (or alpha-hydroxymidazolam)]. May be administered via alternate routes: 0.2 mg/kg (up to 10 mg) IM, intranasal, or buccal routes; all well absorbed rapidly.

(continued on next page)

Table 4
(*continued*)

Drug	Dosing	Approximate Half-Life (h) in Non–Critically Ill Patients	Protein Binding	Clinically Relevant Drug-Drug Interactions with Other Drugs	Consideration for Dose Adjustments in Renal Impairment	Consideration for Dose Adjustment in Hepatic Impairment	Comments
Pentobarbital	LD: 5 mg/kg IVP (up to 50 mg/min); max 500 mg. Repeat until seizures suppression; max total load of 25 mg/kg. MD: 0.5–10 mg/kg/h; titrate to seizure suppression	22	45%–75%		None	Consider dose reduction.	Prolonged half-life (up to 50 h; dose dependent). May cause hypotension, ileus, myocardial suppression, immunosuppression, and thrombocytopenia. IV formulation contains 40% propylene glycol; may cause metabolic acidosis.

| Propofol | LD: 1–2 mg/kg IV over 5 min; max 200 mg. Repeat until seizures cessation up to total LD of 10 mg/kg. MD: 30–200 μg/kg/min (1.8–12 mg/kg/h); titrate to seizure suppression | 0.6 (extended with prolonged use) Terminal half-life: 4–7 | 90% | None | None | None | May cause respiratory depression, hypotension, hypertriglyceridemia, pancreatitis, and PRIS (metabolic acidosis, bradycardia, cardiac arrest, rhabdomyolysis, renal failure). Contraindicated in patients with hypersensitivity to egg or soy products. Monitor pH, bicarbonate, triglycerides, creatine kinase, lipase with prolonged therapy (>48 h) or high doses (>80 μg/kg/min or 5 mg/kg/h). |

Injectable nonanesthetic agents

| Brivaracetam | LD: 100–400 mg. MD: 50–600 mg/d divided q12h or q8h | 9 | <20% | Increase concentrations of carbamazepine and phenytoin | None | Consider dose reduction. | No added therapeutic benefit when coadministered with levetiracetam. |

(continued on next page)

Table 4
(continued)

Drug	Dosing	Approximate Half-Life (h) in Non–Critically Ill Patients	Protein Binding	Clinically Relevant Drug-Drug Interactions with Other Drugs	Consideration for Dose Adjustments in Renal Impairment	Consideration for Dose Adjustment in Hepatic Impairment	Comments
Carbamazepine	LD: 400–800 mg MD: 400–600 mg/d divided q12h	24 8 (with prolonged use due to auto-induction; 2–4 wk)	75%–90%	Major CYP3A4 substrate; major CYP2C19/3A4 inducer. Phenytoin and other CYP3A4 inducers decrease carbamazepine levels. Valproic acid and other CYP3A4 inhibitors increase carbamazepine levels	Consider dose reduction in severe renal impairment (CrCl < 10 mL/min): reduce dose by 25%	Consider dose reduction: undergoes extensive hepatic metabolism.	Strong association between the risk of developing Stevens-Johnson syndrome/TEN and the presence of HLA-B*1502 allele (documented mostly in Asian descent). Dose-dependent hyponatremia; decreased incidence compared with oxcarbazepine.

Diazepam	LD: 0.25 mg/kg IV push over 1–2 min (max 10 mg per dose); repeat every 5 min until seizures stop up to 3 doses or 30 mg. MD: not applicable	40	98%	Not applicable	Not applicable	Rapid redistribution Active metabolite. IV formulation contains propylene glycol. IV solution may be administered rectally if no IV access. Preferred benzodiazepine for rectal administration.
Fosphenytoin	LD: 20 mg PE/kg IV (up to 150 mg/min); max 2000 mg. If still seizing, give additional 5 mg/kg IV (max 500 mg) MD: use phenytoin Note: fosphenytoin is dosed in phenytoin equivalents	IV: 0.25 IM: 0.5	95%–99%	Induces CYP1A2, 2B6, 2C, 3A3/4 Generally, avoid use with most CYP3A4 substrates Coadministration with valproate displaces phenytoin from protein binding sites. Induces metabolism of valproate	Consider dose reduction.	Conversion half-life to phenytoin ~15–30 min. May be administered IM if no IV access (up to 99% absorption after IM administration). Compatible in saline, dextrose, and lactated ringers solution. Nontoxic diluent; decrease cutaneous reactions with extravasation. May cause hypotension, arrhythmias. Consider obtaining peak phenytoin level 2 h post IV dose or 4 h post IM dose.

(continued on next page)

Table 4
(continued)

Drug	Dosing	Approximate Half-Life (h) in Non–Critically Ill Patients	Protein Binding	Clinically Relevant Drug-Drug Interactions with Other Drugs	Consideration for Dose Adjustments in Renal Impairment	Consideration for Dose Adjustment in Hepatic Impairment	Comments
Lacosamide	LD: 10 mg/kg IV over 5–10 min (max 500 mg). If still seizing, give an additional 5 mg/kg over 5 min (max 250 mg IV) MD: 200–600 mg/d divided q12h to q6h Note: Maximum IV push dose is 400 mg administered at a rate of 80 mg/min	13	<15%		Reduce dose in severe renal impairment (CrCl <30 mL/min); max 300 mg/d. HD: 50% removed; lower dose based on CrCl, divide q12h and add 50% of morning dose to evening dose post HD. CRRT: lower dose based on	Consider dose reduction.	May prolong PR interval or induce tachyarrhythmia, including atrial fibrillation.

| Levetiracetam | LD: 60 mg/kg over 15 min (max 4500 mg) MD: 1500–4500 mg/d divided q8h to q6h Note: Maximum IV push dose is 1500 mg administered at a rate of 500 mg/min | 6 | <10% | Reduce dose based on CrCl HD: 50% removed; lower dose based on CrCl, divide q12h, and add 50% of morning dose to the evening dose post HD CRRT: lower dose based on CrCl, then increase total daily dose by 50%, and divide q6h | CrCl, then increase total daily dose by 50% and divide q8h May cause behavioral disturbances; consider switch to brivaracetam. No added therapeutic benefit when coadministered with brivaracetam. |

(continued on next page)

Table 4
(continued)

Drug	Dosing	Approximate Half-Life (h) in Non–Critically Ill Patients	Protein Binding	Clinically Relevant Drug-Drug Interactions with Other Drugs	Consideration for Dose Adjustments in Renal Impairment	Consideration for Dose Adjustment in Hepatic Impairment	Comments
Lorazepam	LD: 4 mg IVP over 2 min; repeat every 5 min until seizures stop up to 3 doses or 12 mg MD: not applicable	12	85%–90%		Not applicable	Not applicable	Rapid redistribution. IV formulation contains 80% propylene glycol; may cause metabolic acidosis. Do not administer IM or SC (IM midazolam preferred if IV access not available).

| Phenytoin | LD: 20 mg/kg IVP (up to 50 mg/min; 25 mg/min in elderly and patients with preexisting cardiovascular conditions) MD: 200–600 mg/d divided q12h or q8h | 15 | 95%–99% | Induces CYP1A2, 2B6, 2C, 3A3/4. Generally avoid use with most CYP3A4 substrates Coadministration with valproate displaces phenytoin from protein binding sites. Induces metabolism of valproate | None | Consider dose reduction. | May cause rash, fever, hypotension, or arrhythmias IV formulation contains 40% propylene glycol; may cause metabolic acidosis. Only compatible in saline (unlike fosphenytoin). Incompatibilities include D5W, potassium, insulin, heparin, norepinephrine, cephalosporin, and dobutamine. Severe tissue injury may occur with extravasation, including rare purple glove syndrome. Consider obtaining peak phenytoin (free and total) level 2 h post IV loading dose. |

(continued on next page)

Table 4
(continued)

Drug	Dosing	Approximate Half-Life (h) in Non–Critically Ill Patients	Protein Binding	Clinically Relevant Drug-Drug Interactions with Other Drugs	Consideration for Dose Adjustments in Renal Impairment	Consideration for Dose Adjustment in Hepatic Impairment	Comments
Phenobarbital	LD: 15 mg/kg IV (up to 60 mg/min); max dose 1500 mg. If still seizing, give an additional 5–10 mg/kg. MD: 1–3 mg/kg/d given q day or divided q12h or q8h	80	50%–60%	Strong inducer of UGT, CYP 3A4, 2B6, 2C9, 2A6, 1A2; dose adjustments of drugs including phenytoin and valproate might be necessary	Consider dose reduction HD: give full daily dose in evening after hemodialysis	Consider dose reduction.	Prolonged half-life (up to 140 h). May cause hypotension IV formulation contains 70% propylene glycol; may cause metabolic acidosis.

| Valproate | LD: 40 mg/kg IV (over 5–10 min); max 4000 mg. If still seizing, give additional 20 mg/kg IV (max 2000 mg) over 5 min. MD: 2000–6000 mg divided q8h or q6h | 12 | 90% | Phenytoin and valproate may displace each other from protein binding sites Valproate markedly inhibits lamotrigine metabolism resulting in increase in lamotrigine levels and risk of side effects including rash | None | Caution in hepatic impairment. | Highly plasma protein bound (up to 90%). May cause hyperammonemic encephalopathy (treated with L-carnitine supplementation), hepatotoxicity, thrombocytopenia, and platelet dysfunction. Concurrent use with carbapenems may result in markedly decreased valproic acid plasma concentrations. Consider obtaining valproate total level 2 h post IV loading dose. Highly teratogenic and associated with other adverse fetal effects. |

(continued on next page)

Table 4
(*continued*)

Drug	Dosing	Approximate Half-Life (h) in Non–Critically Ill Patients	Protein Binding	Clinically Relevant Drug-Drug Interactions with Other Drugs	Consideration for Dose Adjustments in Renal Impairment	Consideration for Dose Adjustment in Hepatic Impairment	Comments
Enteral agents							
Cannabidiol	MD: 2.5–20 mg/kg/d divided q12h	58	>94%	CYP3A4 and CYP2C19 substrate. Phenytoin and other CYP3A4 inducers decrease levels. Valproic acid and other CYP3A4 inhibitors increase levels.	None	Consider dose reduction.	Concomitant use of higher doses of cannabidiol and valproate increases the risk of transaminase elevations and hepatocellular injury. Consider discontinuation or dose adjustment of cannabidiol and/or valproate if liver enzyme elevations occur. If AST and/or ALT >3 times ULN and total bilirubin >2 times ULN, discontinue treatment. If sustained AST and/or ALT >5 times ULN, discontinue treatment.

Drug	Dosing	Half-life	Protein binding	Drug interactions	Renal impairment	Hepatic impairment	Adverse effects
Clobazam	LD: 20–40 mg MD: 20–60 mg/d divided q12h	Clobazam: 16, N-desmethyl-clobazam: 39	80%–90%	Felbamate: increase plasma concentrations of N-desmethyl-clobazam	Caution in severe renal impairment (CrCl < 30 mL/min)	Consider dose reduction: undergoes extensive hepatic metabolism.	Decreased sedation compared with other benzodiazepines. When ordering drug levels consider ordering clobazam and active metabolite (N-desmethylclobazam) drug level.
Gabapentin	LD: 1200–3600 mg MD: 2400–4800 mg divided q8h to q12h	6	<3%		Reduce dose based on CrCl HD: dose based on CrCl, administer supplemental dose post HD	None.	Occasional peripheral edema.
Oxcarbazepine	LD: 600–1200 mg MD: 600–2400 mg/ d divided q12 hr to q6hr	5	67%	Increase concentrations of phenobarbital and phenytoin	Consider 50% dose reduction in severe renal impairment HD: IR formulations preferred	ER formulation not recommended.	Dose-dependent hyponatremia; more common in elderly.

(continued on next page)

Table 4
(continued)

Drug	Dosing	Approximate Half-Life (h) in Non–Critically Ill Patients	Protein Binding	Clinically Relevant Drug-Drug Interactions with Other Drugs	Consideration for Dose Adjustments in Renal Impairment	Consideration for Dose Adjustment in Hepatic Impairment	Comments
Perampanel	LD: 6–12 mg MD: 12 mg/d	105	95%		Use not recommended in severe renal impairment (CrCl < 30 mL/min)	Consider dose reduction in mild to moderate hepatic impairment. Use not recommended in severe hepatic impairment.	May cause behavioral issues/agitation.
Pregabalin	LD: 150–300 mg MD: 150–600 mg/ d divided q8h to q6h	6	None		Reduce dose HD: dose based on CrCl, administer supplemental dose post HD	None	Occasional peripheral edema.

Topiramate	LD: 200–400 mg MD: 200–600 (reports up to 1600) mg/d divided q12h to q6h	21	15%–41%	Use with zonisamide and other carbonic anhydrase inhibitors may worsen metabolic acidosis	Reduce dose by ~50% HD: supplemental dose may be necessary	Consider dose reduction.	May cause metabolic acidosis; caution with propofol, acetazolamide, zonisamide and metformin. May cause renal stones. May be associated with oligohidrosis, with risk of hyperthermia, mainly in pediatric patients.
Vigabatrin	LD: 1500 mg. MD: 1000–3000 mg/ d divided q12h	10 (but sustained effect for several days)	None	None	Reduce dose based on CrCl	None	Potential progressive permanent peripheral vision loss after months to years of use; regular ophthalmology examinations recommended with prolonged use. May markedly reduce liver function test (ALT/ AST) in patients with documented liver disease. It is not recommended to use plasma liver function test activity as an index of liver cell damage.

Abbreviations: ALT, alanine transaminase; AST, aspartate transaminase; CrCl, Creatinine Clearance; CYP, Cytochrome P450; D5W, dextrose 5% in water; ER, extended release; GABA, gamma-Aminobutyric acid; HD, hemodialysis; HLA, human leukocyte antigen; HR, heart rate; IM, intramuscular; IR, immediate release; IV, intravenous; LD, loading dose; MD, maintenance dose; NMDA, N-Methyl-D-aspartate; PE, phenytoin equivalent; PRIS, Propofol-related Infusion Syndrome; q, every; sBP, Systolic blood pressure; SC, subcutaneous; TEN, toxic epidermal necrolysis; UGT, uridine 5'-diphospho-glucuronosyltransferase; ULN, upper limit of normal.

Adapted from the Yale New Haven Hospital status epilepticus protocol.

Perhaps the most challenging aspect in the management of SRSE is balancing the treatment of ongoing seizure with accumulating adverse effects. Prolonged SE may be complicated by infection, acute kidney injury, or neurogenic cardiac injury, such as Takotsubo cardiomyopathy.[71] In a study of nearly 25,000 patients with SE, complications of treatment was the leading cause of death.[87] Even with persistent SE, the potential risk of treatment may outweigh the potential benefit, prompting the need for most robust decision analysis tools for risk-benefit evaluations in this setting.[67] Common scenarios in which it may be reasonable to defer increasingly aggressive treatments include focal SE, SRSE with a seizure burden less than 20% per hour, or in the setting of significant treatment-related adverse effects (eg, cardiopulmonary dysfunction, renal injury, or gastrointestinal [GI] dysfunction).

As treatments accumulate, nontraditional treatment modalities may be used to reduce the potential to exacerbate ongoing adverse effects. Adjunctive SE treatments include ketogenic diet (KDT), hypothermia, and inhalational anesthetics, which have all shown promising antiepileptic effects.[88–90] Interest in KDT has particularly grown for the potential to undermine many of the proposed mechanisms of SRSE, including receptor trafficking, mitochondrial function, and modulation of proinflammatory cytokine profiles.[91] In multiple studies of children with RSE, KDT administered enterally or parenterally achieved ketosis in 2 to 6 days and lead to seizure freedom or 50% reduction in seizure burden at 5 to 7 days, with the most common side effects being acidosis, hyperlipidemia, hypoglycemia, and GI symptoms. In adults, several case series have shown similar results with achievement of ketosis at 1 to 3 days, and seizure cessation in 73% to 100% as early as 3 days.[91] Forthcoming developments include research into the potential role of cannabinoids in SE.[92]

Specific scenarios: autoimmune and post-anoxic etiologies

Many patients with RSE remain without an identifiable etiology. In one multicenter retrospective cohort, the most commonly identified causes of NORSE included non-paraneoplastic autoimmune encephalitis (19%) and paraneoplastic autoimmune

Table 5 Autoantibodies associated with inflammatory status epilepticus		
Ach receptor ganglionic neuronal	CASPR2	LGI-1
Ach receptor binding	CRMP-5	Neuronal (V-G) K+ channel
AMPA	DPPX	N-type calcium channel
Amphiphysin	GABAA	P/Q-type calcium channel
Anti-neuronal nuclear Types 1, 2, and 3	GABAB	Purkinje cell cytoplasmic type 2 and type Tr
Anti-glial nuclear	GAD65	

Abbreviations: Ach, acetylcholine; AMPA, α-amino-3-hydroxy-5-methyl-4-isoxazolepropionic acid receptor antibody; CASPR2, contactin-associated protein-like2 IgG; CRMP-5, collapsing response-mediator protein 5 antibody; DPPX, dipeptidyl-peptidase-like protein 6 antibody; GABAA, γ-aminobutyric acid A receptor antibody; GABAB, γ-aminobutyric acid B receptor antibody; GAD65, glutamic acid decarboxylase antibody; LGI-1, leucine-rich glioma-inactivated protein 1 IgG; NMDA, N-methyl-D-aspartate receptor antibody; Neuronal (V-G) K+ channel, voltage-gated potassium channel antibody.

Adapted from (Spatola, Novy and colleagues 2015) Spatola, M., J. Novy, R. Du Pasquier, J. Dalmau and A. O. Rossetti (2015). "Status epilepticus of inflammatory etiology: a cohort study." Neurology 85(5): 464-470.

Table 6
Epidemiology-based mortality score in status epilepticus

Age	Points	Comorbidity (Score Each Disease)	Points
>80	10	AIDS, metastatic solid tumor	60
71–80	8	Moderate to severe liver disease	30
61–70	7	Moderate to severe renal disease, any tumor (includes lymphoma and leukemia), hemiplegia, diabetes with end organ damage	20
51–60	5		
41–50	3		
31–40	2	Peripheral vascular disease, connective tissue disease, diabetes, myocardial infarction, cerebrovascular disease, congestive heart failure, dementia, mild liver disease, peptic ulcer disease, chronic pulmonary disease	10
21–30	1		
Score one	–	Score each disease	–

EEG	Points	Etiology	Points
Spontaneous burst suppression	60	Anoxia	65
		Acute central nervous system infection	33
		Acute cerebrovascular disease	26
After status epilepticus ictal discharges	40	Metabolic disorders	22
		Metabolic, sodium imbalance	17
		Brain tumor	16
Lateralized periodic discharges	40	Cryptogenic	12
		Head trauma	12
		Drug overdose	11
Generalized periodic discharges	40	Alcohol abuse	10
		Hydrocephalus	8
		Remote cerebrovascular event or brain injury	7
No lateralized periodic discharges, generalized periodic discharges or ictal discharges	0	Multiple sclerosis	5
		Drug withdrawal, reduction, or poor compliance	2
		Central nervous system anomalies	2
Score only worst	–	Score one	–
Total score = sum of above scores			

Abbreviation: EEG, electroencephalogram.
Adapted from (Leitinger, Holler and colleagues 2015) Leitinger, M., Y. Holler, G. Kalss, A. Rohracher, H. F. Novak, J. Hofler, J. Dobesberger, G. Kuchukhidze and E. Trinka (2015). "Epidemiology-based mortality score in status epilepticus (EMSE)." *Neurocrit Care* 22(2): 273-282.

encephalitis (18%).[93] Roughly 50% of NORSE cases remain cryptogenic, with a proportion likely stemming from autoimmune encephalitis from yet undiscovered antibodies, or a lowered seizure threshold from a dysregulated proinflammatory central nervous system response after unknown trigger.[94,95] As such, in the setting of NORSE, it is common to administer adjunct treatment for autoimmunity or inflammation, often before confirmatory testing has resulted. **Table 5** summarizes autoantibodies that should be considered in the workup of inflammatory noninfectious SE.

Several case series have suggested benefit with high-dose steroids, plasma exchange, and/or IV immunoglobulin in cryptogenic NORSE, particularly when administered early, even in the absence of definitive immune etiology.[96–98] A study of interleukin (IL)-6 inhibition included 6 patients given tocilizumab with cessation of SE after 1 to 2 doses at a median of 3 days,[99] whereas more recent studies have suggested particular benefit in the setting of elevated IL-6 levels.[100] Additional immunotherapies commonly considered include cyclophosphamide, rituximab, and anakinra.[94,97,101] For up-to-date detailed protocols on the approach to the evaluation and management of NORSE, visit norseinstitute.org.

Postanoxic SE most commonly results after cardiac arrest, likely from overwhelming glutamatergic excitotoxicity. Although postanoxic SE is commonly interpreted as a poor prognostic marker, accumulating evidence suggests that early and aggressive treatment of selected, yet refractory, cases resulted in 54% survival, with a high proportion of survivors going on to achieve functional independence.[102] Thus, RSE may be a grave sign for some, but prolonged treatment is likely justified in patients with favorable multimodal prognostic markers, including low time to return of spontaneous circulation, preserved continuity of EEG background, preserved N20 cortical potentials on somatosensory evoked potentials, low neuron specific enolase titers, and favorable neuroimaging.[102,103] Importantly, intermittent EEG post-arrest may be noninferior to cEEG for prognostication, but is much less sensitive in detecting potentially treatable seizures, with 48 hours of cEEG conferring 95% sensitivity in this setting.[104]

A common concern during the management of prolonged SE is continued utilization of resources with uncertainty regarding the possible futility of our effort. In such cases, prognostic scores such as Status Epilepticus Severity Score (STESS) and Epidemiology and Mortality Score in Status Epilepticus-Etiology, Age, Comorbidities (EMSE-EAC) may be helpful. In a trial of 125 nonanoxic SE, STESS reliably predicted in-hospital mortality, although correlation with mortality decreased after discharge.[105] Another study of 151 episodes of SE in 137 patients revealed EMSE-EAC with a cutoff of 34, and STESS with a cutoff of 4 indicated a negative predictive value for in-hospital mortality of 97.5% and 96.7%, respectively,[106] with EMSE-EAC tending to perform slightly better across multiple studies. **Table 6** summarizes EMSE-EAC score.

SUMMARY

Seizures are frequently triggered by an inciting event and result from uninhibited excitation and/or decreased inhibition of a pool of neurons. If seizure abortive physiologic mechanisms fail, the ensuing unrestrained synchronization of neurons (SE) can be life-threatening and is associated with marked morbidity potential in survivors and high medical care costs. Prognosis in SE is intimately related to etiology of seizures and their response to therapeutic measures. In general, timely implementation of pharmacologic therapy (ie, benzodiazepines as first line, followed by loading dose of parenteral antiseizure medication as second line, and therapeutic coma with IV anesthetics as third line), while concurrently performing a stepwise workup for etiology are paramount. Neurodiagnostic testing should guide titration of pharmacologic therapies, and help determine if there is a role for immune modulation.

CLINICS CARE POINTS

- Prompt monitoring for and rescuing airway and/or hemodynamic compromise, establishing secure IV access, evaluating for, and treating hypoglycemia are the cornerstone of initial seizure management.

- First-line abortive therapy includes appropriately dosed parenteral benzodiazepines: IV lorazepam (up to 0.1 mg/kg, in divided doses), IV/intramuscular/intranasal midazolam 5 to 10 mg are most commonly used

- Second-line IV therapy should be promptly considered in patients with ongoing seizures (benzodiazepine-RSE) or at risk for recurrent seizures: 20 mg/kg of fosphenytoin, 40 mg/kg of valproate, or 60 mg/kg of levetiracetam are equivalent choices.

- Third-line therapy consists of anesthetics and requires cEEG monitoring to guide depth of therapy. Ketamine is an attractive choice due to relatively fewer hemodynamic side effects and for bypassing GABAergic resistance inherent to ongoing seizures.

- Immune modulation should be considered in cryptogenic and presumed autoimmune SE.

DISCLOSURE

Carolina B Maciel reportss receiving funding from Claude D. Pepper Older Americans Independence Center and American Heart Association for research independent from this work. All the other authors have no disclosures.

REFERENCES

1. Mei Lu MF, Aurore Bergamasco WS, Benitez A, et al. Epidemiology of status epilepticus in the United States: a systematic review. Epilepsy Behav 2020;112: 107459.
2. Kortland LM, Knake S, Rosenow F, et al. Cost of status epilepticus: a systematic review. Seizure 2015;24:17–20.
3. Beg JM, Anderson TD, Francis K, et al. Burden of illness for super-refractory status epilepticus patients. J Med Econ 2017;20(1):45–53.
4. Delaj L, Novy J, Ryvlin P, et al. Refractory and super-refractory status epilepticus in adults: a 9-year cohort study. Acta Neurol Scand 2017;135(1):92–9.
5. Rossetti AO, Hurwitz S, Logroscino G, et al. Prognosis of status epilepticus: role of aetiology, age, and consciousness impairment at presentation. J Neurol Neurosurg Psychiatry 2006;77(5):611–5.
6. Rossetti AO, Logroscino G, Milligan TA, et al. Status Epilepticus Severity Score (STESS): a tool to orient early treatment strategy. J Neurol 2008;255(10):1561–6.
7. Leitinger M, Höller Y, Kalss G, et al. Epidemiology-based mortality score in status epilepticus (EMSE). Neurocrit Care 2015;22(2):273–82.
8. Nei M, Lee JM, Shanker VL, et al. The EEG and prognosis in status epilepticus. Epilepsia 1999;40(2):157–63.
9. Legriel S, Mourvillier B, Bele N, et al. Outcomes in 140 critically ill patients with status epilepticus. Intensive Care Med 2008;34(3):476–80.
10. Strzelczyk A, Ansorge S, Hapfelmeier J, et al. Costs, length of stay, and mortality of super-refractory status epilepticus: a population-based study from Germany. Epilepsia 2017;58(9):1533–41.

11. DeLorenzo RJ, Garnett LK, Towne AR, et al. Comparison of status epilepticus with prolonged seizure episodes lasting from 10 to 29 minutes. Epilepsia 1999;40(2):164–9.

12. Towne AR, Pellock JM, Ko D, et al. Determinants of mortality in status epilepticus. Epilepsia 1994;35(1):27–34.

13. Niquet J, Baldwin R, Suchomelova L, et al. Benzodiazepine-refractory status epilepticus: pathophysiology and principles of treatment. Ann N Y Acad Sci 2016; 1378(1):166–73.

14. Reindl C, Sprügel MI, Sembill JA, et al. Influence of new versus traditional antiepileptic drugs on course and outcome of status epilepticus. Seizure 2020; 74:20–5.

15. Herman ST, Abend NS, Bleck TP, et al. Consensus statement on continuous EEG in critically ill adults and children, part I: indications. J Clin Neurophysiol 2015;32(2):87–95.

16. Kubota Y, Nakamoto H, Egawa S, et al. Continuous EEG monitoring in ICU. J Intensive Care 2018;6(1):39.

17. Lee JW, LaRoche S, Choi H, et al. Development and feasibility testing of a critical care EEG monitoring database for standardized clinical reporting and multicenter collaborative research. J Clin Neurophysiol 2016;33(2):133–40.

18. Garcia-Losarcos N, VA, Loparo K. *Continuous EEG monitoring and quantitative EEG techniques.* M. De Georgia, K. Loparo (Ed.). *Neurocritical Care Informatics.* Berlin, Germany: Springer; 2020;79-109.

19. Buday J, Albrecht J, Podgorná G, et al. Seizure threshold manipulation in electroconvulsive therapy via repetitive transcranial magnetic stimulation. A novel way of augmentation? Brain Stimul 2020;13(6):1631–8.

20. Motamedi GK, R.P, RP, et al. Therapeutic brain hypothermia, its mechanisms of action, and its prospects as a treatment for epilepsy. Epilepsia 2013;54(6): 959–70.

21. Lesser JS, Fountain NB. Pathophysiology and definitions of seizures and status epilepticus. Emerg Med Clin North Am 2011;29(1):1–13.

22. Herman ST. Epilepsy after brain insult: targeting epileptogenesis. Neurology 2002;59(9 Suppl 5):S21–6.

23. Karoly PJ, Nurse ES, Freestone DR, et al. Bursts of seizures in long-term recordings of human focal epilepsy. Epilepsia 2017;58(3):363–72.

24. Hesdorffer DC, Logroscino G, Cascino G, et al. Risk of unprovoked seizure after acute symptomatic seizure: effect of status epilepticus. Ann Neurol 1998;44(6): 908–12.

25. Ankarcrona M, Dypbukt JM, Bonfoco E, et al. Glutamate-induced neuronal death: a succession of necrosis or apoptosis depending on mitochondrial function. Neuron 1995;15(4):961–73.

26. Fontaine C, Jacq G, Perier F, et al. The role of secondary brain insults in status epilepticus: a systematic review. J Clin Monit 2020;9(8):2521.

27. Gastaut H, Roger J, Lob H. *Les états de mal épileptiques: compte rendu de la réunion européenne d'information électroencéphalographique, Xe Colloque de Marseille, 1962.* H. Gastaut (Ed.). Electroencéphalographie et neurophysiologie clinique. Paris, France: Masson et Cie,1967 (Vol 1, IV-384).

28. Treatment of convulsive status epilepticus. Recommendations of the epilepsy foundation of America's working group on status epilepticus. JAMA 1993; 270(7):854–9.

29. Meldrum BS, Horton RW. Physiology of status epilepticus in primates. Arch Neurol 1973;28(1):1–9.

30. Lowenstein DH, Alldredge BK. Status epilepticus at an urban public hospital in the 1980s. Neurology 1993;43(3 Pt 1):483–8.
31. Lowenstein DH, Bleck T, Macdonald RL. It's time to revise the definition of status epilepticus. Epilepsia 1999;40(1):120–2.
32. Theodore WH, Porter RJ, Albert P, et al. The secondarily generalized tonic-clonic seizure: a videotape analysis. Neurology 1994;44(8):1403–7.
33. Trinka E, Cock H, Hesdorffer D, et al. A definition and classification of status epilepticus–report of the ILAE task force on classification of status epilepticus. Epilepsia 2015;56(10):1515–23.
34. Samanta D, Garrity L, Arya R. Refractory and super-refractory status epilepticus. Indian Pediatr 2020;57(3):239–53.
35. Shorvon S. Super-refractory status epilepticus: an approach to therapy in this difficult clinical situation. Epilepsia 2011;52(Suppl 8):53–6.
36. Hirsch LJ, Gaspard N, van Baalen A, et al. Proposed consensus definitions for new-onset refractory status epilepticus (NORSE), febrile infection-related epilepsy syndrome (FIRES), and related conditions. Epilepsia 2018;59(4):739–44.
37. Beniczky S, Hirsch LJ, Kaplan PW, et al. Unified EEG terminology and criteria for nonconvulsive status epilepticus. Epilepsia 2013;54 Suppl 6:28–9.
38. Claassen J, Mayer SA, Kowalski RG, et al. Detection of electrographic seizures with continuous EEG monitoring in critically ill patients. Neurology 2004;62(10):1743–8.
39. Westover MB, Shafi MM, Bianchi MT, et al. The probability of seizures during EEG monitoring in critically ill adults. Clin Neurophysiol 2015;126(3):463–71.
40. Trinka E, Leitinger M. Which EEG patterns in coma are nonconvulsive status epilepticus? Epilepsy Behav 2015;49:203–22.
41. Rossetti AO, Kaspar S, Raoul S, et al. Continuous vs routine electroencephalogram in critically ill adults with altered consciousness and no recent seizure: a multicenter randomized clinical trial. JAMA Neurol 2020;77(10):1–8.
42. Hill CE, Blank LJ, Thibault D, et al. Continuous EEG is associated with favorable hospitalization outcomes for critically ill patients. Neurology 2019;92(1):e9–18.
43. Singh J, Gaurav T, Jonathan A, et al. Predictors of nonconvulsive seizure and their effect on short-term outcome. J Clin Neurophysiol 2020. https://doi.org/10.1097/WNP.0000000000000687.
44. Altindag E, Okudan ZV, Tavukcu Ozkan S, et al. Electroencephalographic patterns recorded by continuous EEG monitoring in patients with change of consciousness in the neurological intensive care unit. Noro Psikiyatr Ars 2017;54(2):168–74.
45. Cissé FA, Osman GM, Legros B, et al. Validation of an algorithm of time-dependent electro-clinical risk stratification for electrographic seizures (TERSE) in critically ill patients. Clin Neurophysiol 2020;131(8):1956–61.
46. Struck AF, Ustun B, Ruiz AR, et al. Association of an electroencephalography-based risk score with seizure probability in hospitalized patients. JAMA Neurol 2017;74(12):1419–24.
47. Struck AF, Tabaeizadeh M, Schmitt SE, et al. Assessment of the validity of the 2HELPS2B score for inpatient seizure risk prediction. JAMA Neurol 2020;77(4):500–7.
48. Moffet EW, Thanujaa S, Lawrence JH, et al. Validation of the 2HELPS2B seizure risk score in acute brain injury patients. Neurocrit Care 2020. https://doi.org/10.1007/s12028-020-00939-x.
49. Haider HA, Esteller R, Hahn CD, et al. Sensitivity of quantitative EEG for seizure identification in the intensive care unit. Neurology 2016;87(9):935–44.

50. Dericioglu N, Yetim E, Bas DF, et al. Non-expert use of quantitative EEG displays for seizure identification in the adult neuro-intensive care unit. Epilepsy Res 2015;109:48–56.
51. Benbadis SR, Allen Hauser W. An estimate of the prevalence of psychogenic non-epileptic seizures. Seizure 2000;9(4):280–1.
52. Dworetzky BA, Bubrick EJ, Szaflarski JP. Nonepileptic psychogenic status: markedly prolonged psychogenic nonepileptic seizures. Epilepsy Behav 2010;19(1):65–8.
53. Anzellotti F, Dono F, Evangelista G, et al. Psychogenic non-epileptic seizures and pseudo-refractory epilepsy, a management challenge. Front Neurol 2020; 11:461.
54. Seneviratne U, Minato E, Paul E. How reliable is ictal duration to differentiate psychogenic nonepileptic seizures from epileptic seizures? Epilepsy Behav 2017;66:127–31.
55. Kapur J, Elm J, Chamberlain JM, et al. Randomized trial of three anticonvulsant medications for status epilepticus. N Engl J Med 2019;381(22):2103–13.
56. Foldvary-Schaefer N, Wyllie E. Textbook of Clinical Neurology 3rd edition. Philadelphia: Saunders Elsevier; 2008;1213-1244.
57. Thomas M, Jankovic J. Psychogenic movement disorders: diagnosis and management. CNS Drugs 2004;18(7):437–52.
58. Dworetzky BA, Mortati KA, Rossetti AO, et al. Clinical characteristics of psychogenic nonepileptic seizure status in the long-term monitoring unit. Epilepsy Behav 2006;9(2):335–8.
59. Gedzelman ER, LaRoche SM. Long-term video EEG monitoring for diagnosis of psychogenic nonepileptic seizures. Neuropsychiatr Dis Treat 2014;10:1979–86.
60. Benbadis SR, Agrawal V, Tatum WO. How many patients with psychogenic nonepileptic seizures also have epilepsy? Neurology 2001;57(5):915–7.
61. Nightscales R, McCartney L, Auvrez C, et al. Mortality in patients with psychogenic nonepileptic seizures. Neurology 2020;95(6):e643–52.
62. Caplan LR, Berger JR. Cerebellar seizures of Hughlings Jackson. Neurology 2000;55(2):323–4.
63. McCrory PR, Bladin PF, Berkovic SF. The cerebellar seizures of Hughlings Jackson. Neurology 1999;52(9):1888–90.
64. Demel SL, Broderick JP. Basilar occlusion syndromes: an update. Neurohospitalist 2015;5(3):142–50.
65. Serino D, Caputo D, Fusco L. Cerebellar fits in the 2000s. Brain Dev 2018;40(1): 77–80.
66. Hocker SE, Britton JW, Mandrekar JN, et al. Predictors of outcome in refractory status epilepticus. JAMA Neurol 2013;70(1):72–7.
67. Amorim E, McGraw CM, Westover MB. A theoretical paradigm for evaluating risk-benefit of status epilepticus treatment. J Clin Neurophysiol 2020;37(5): 385–92.
68. Andermann F, Robb JP. Absence status. A reappraisal following review of thirty-eight patients. Epilepsia 1972;13(1):177–87.
69. Shirasaka Y. Lack of neuronal damage in atypical absence status epilepticus. Epilepsia 2002;43(12):1498–501.
70. Payne ET, Zhao XY, Frndova H, et al. Seizure burden is independently associated with short term outcome in critically ill children. Brain 2014;137(Pt 5): 1429–38.
71. Hawkes MA, Hocker SE. Systemic complications following status epilepticus. Curr Neurol Neurosci Rep 2018;18(2):7.

72. Gutiérrez-Viedma Á, Parejo-Carbonell B, Romeral-Jiménez M, et al. Therapy delay in status epilepticus extends its duration and worsens its prognosis. Acta Neurol Scand 2020;143(3):281-9.
73. Sathe AG, Tillman H, Coles LD, et al. Underdosing of benzodiazepines in patients with status epilepticus enrolled in established status epilepticus treatment trial. Acad Emerg Med 2019;26(8):940-3.
74. Alldredge BK, Gelb AM, Isaacs SM, et al. A comparison of lorazepam, diazepam, and placebo for the treatment of out-of-hospital status epilepticus. N Engl J Med 2001;345(9):631-7.
75. Spatola M, Alvarez V, Rossetti AO. Benzodiazepine overtreatment in status epilepticus is related to higher need of intubation and longer hospitalization. Epilepsia 2013;54(8):e99-102.
76. Kapur J, Macdonald RL. Rapid seizure-induced reduction of benzodiazepine and Zn2+ sensitivity of hippocampal dentate granule cell GABAA receptors. J Neurosci 1997;17(19):7532-40.
77. Naylor DE, Liu H, Wasterlain CG. Trafficking of GABA(A) receptors, loss of inhibition, and a mechanism for pharmacoresistance in status epilepticus. J Neurosci 2005;25(34):7724-33.
78. Mazarati AM, Baldwin RA, Sankar R, et al. Time-dependent decrease in the effectiveness of antiepileptic drugs during the course of self-sustaining status epilepticus. Brain Res 1998;814(1-2):179-85.
79. Mazarati AM, Wasterlain CG. N-methyl-D-asparate receptor antagonists abolish the maintenance phase of self-sustaining status epilepticus in rat. Neurosci Lett 1999;265(3):187-90.
80. Niquet J, Lumley L, Baldwin R, et al. Early polytherapy for benzodiazepine-refractory status epilepticus. Epilepsy Behav 2019;101:106367.
81. Husain AM, Lee JW, Kolls BJ, et al. Randomized trial of lacosamide versus fosphenytoin for nonconvulsive seizures. Ann Neurol 2018;83(6):1174-85.
82. Sutter R, Marsch S, Fuhr P, et al. Anesthetic drugs in status epilepticus: risk or rescue? A 6-year cohort study. Neurology 2014;82(8):656-64.
83. Ayham Alkhachroum CAD-N, Mathews E, Massad N, et al. Ketamine to treat super-refractory status epilepticus. Neurology 2020. https://doi.org/10.1212/WNL.0000000000010611.
84. Muhlhofer WG, Layfield S, Lowenstein D, et al. Duration of therapeutic coma and outcome of refractory status epilepticus. Epilepsia 2019;60(5):921-34.
85. Das AS, Lee JW, Izzy S, et al. Ultra-short burst suppression as a "reset switch" for refractory status epilepticus. Seizure 2019;64:41-4.
86. Rubin DB, Brigid A, Maryum S, et al. Electrographic predictors of successful weaning from anaesthetics in refractory status epilepticus. Brain 2020;143(4):1143-57.
87. Sirikarn P, Pattanittum P, Sawanyawisuth K, et al. Causes of death in patients with status epilepticus. Epilepsy Behav 2019;101(Pt B):106372.
88. Mahmoud SH, Ho-Huang E, Buhler J. Systematic review of ketogenic diet use in adult patients with status epilepticus. Epilepsia Open 2020;5(1):10-21.
89. Legriel S, Lemiale V, Schenck M, et al. Hypothermia for neuroprotection in convulsive status epilepticus. N Engl J Med 2016;375(25):2457-67.
90. Opić P, Sutter R. The unease when using anesthetics for treatment-refractory status epilepticus: still far too many questions. J Clin Neurophysiol 2020;37(5):399-405.
91. Mcdonald TJW, Cervenka MC. Ketogenic diet therapies for seizures and status epilepticus. Semin Neurol 2020;40(6):719-29.

92. Upadhya D, Castro OW, Upadhya R, et al. Prospects of cannabidiol for easing status epilepticus-induced epileptogenesis and related comorbidities. Mol Neurobiol 2018;55(8):6956–64.

93. Gaspard N, Foreman BP, Alvarez V, et al. New-onset refractory status epilepticus: etiology, clinical features, and outcome. Neurology 2015;85(18):1604–13.

94. Culler GW, VanHaerents S. Immunologic treatments of seizures and status epilepticus. Semin Neurol 2020;40(6):708–18.

95. Sakuma H, Tanuma N, Kuki I, et al. Intrathecal overproduction of proinflammatory cytokines and chemokines in febrile infection-related refractory status epilepticus. J Neurol Neurosurg Psychiatry 2015;86(7):820–2.

96. Gall CR, Jumma O, Mohanraj R. Five cases of new onset refractory status epilepticus (NORSE) syndrome: outcomes with early immunotherapy. Seizure 2013;22(3):217–20.

97. Khawaja AM, DeWolfe JL, Miller DW, et al. New-onset refractory status epilepticus (NORSE)–The potential role for immunotherapy. Epilepsy Behav 2015;47: 17–23.

98. Li J, Saldivar C, Maganti RK. Plasma exchange in cryptogenic new onset refractory status epilepticus. Seizure 2013;22(1):70–3.

99. Jun JS, Lee ST, Kim R, et al. Tocilizumab treatment for new onset refractory status epilepticus. Ann Neurol 2018;84(6):940–5.

100. Cantarin-Extremera V, Jiménez-Legido M, Duat-Rodríguez A, et al. Tocilizumab in pediatric refractory status epilepticus and acute epilepsy: experience in two patients. J Neuroimmunol 2020;340:577142.

101. Kadoya M, Onoue H, Kadoya A, et al. Refractory status epilepticus caused by anti-NMDA receptor encephalitis that markedly improved following combination therapy with rituximab and cyclophosphamide. Intern Med 2015;54(2):209–13.

102. Beretta S, Coppo A, Bianchi E, et al. Neurological outcome of postanoxic refractory status epilepticus after aggressive treatment. Epilepsy Behav 2019;101(Pt B):106374.

103. Lybeck A, Friberg H, Aneman A, et al. Prognostic significance of clinical seizures after cardiac arrest and target temperature management. Resuscitation 2017;114:146–51.

104. Elmer J, Patrick JC, Pawan S, et al. Sensitivity of continuous electroencephalography to detect ictal activity after cardiac arrest. JAMA Netw Open 2020;3(4): e203751.

105. Aukland P, Lando M, Vilholm O, et al. Predictive value of the status epilepticus severity score (STESS) and its components for long-term survival. BMC Neurol 2016;16(1):213.

106. Sairanen JJ, Kantanen AM, Hyppölä HT, et al. Outcome of status epilepticus and the predictive value of the EMSE and STESS scores: a prospective study. Seizure 2020;75:115–20.

Neuro-Oncologic Emergencies

Zachary D. Threlkeld, MD[a], Brian J. Scott, MD[b],*

KEYWORDS

- Ischemic stroke • Status epilepticus • Metastatic epidural spinal cord compression
- Chemotherapy side effect • Neurologic immune-related adverse events
- CAR-T cell neurotoxicity • Neuro-oncology prognosis

KEY POINTS

- Cerebral edema with herniation, cerebrovascular events, status epilepticus, and metastatic epidural spinal cord compression are neuro-oncologic emergencies requiring prompt identification and treatment.
- The expanding number of chemotherapeutic agents and targeted cancer therapies has led to a broad range of rare, but potentially serious, neurologic side effects.
- Immune checkpoint inhibitors and cancer cell therapies heighten immunologic activity that can cause specific clinical syndromes affecting the central or peripheral nervous system.
- Prognostication in critically ill individuals who have neuro-oncologic disease is challenging. Effective care requires interdisciplinary team engagement and shared decision-making, often with surrogates.

INTRODUCTION

Cancer is capable of producing neurologic dysfunction through a wide variety of mechanisms, which include direct effects of the tumor on the nervous system (mass effect, herniation, seizure, spinal cord compression), indirect effects (hypercoagulability/neurovascular complications), or autoimmune paraneoplastic conditions. Cancer therapies such as radiation therapy, chemotherapy, immune checkpoint inhibitors, and cancer cell therapeutics (such as chimeric-antigen receptor T [CAR-T] cell therapies) may also produce neurologic side effects.

Although most of the neurologic effects of cancer are not acute and severe, several may present as emergencies. An understanding of the ways that cancer and cancer

[a] Division of Neurocritical Care, Department of Neurology, Stanford University School of Medicine, 300 Pasteur Drive MC 5778, Stanford, CA 94305, USA; [b] Division of Neurohospitalist Medicine, Department of Neurology, Stanford University School of Medicine, 453 Quarry Rd, 2nd Floor, Stanford, CA 94305, USA
* Corresponding author.
E-mail address: bjscott@stanford.edu

Neurol Clin 39 (2021) 545–563
https://doi.org/10.1016/j.ncl.2021.01.012
0733-8619/21/© 2021 Elsevier Inc. All rights reserved.

therapies may affect the nervous system equips clinicians who care for patients with neurologic emergencies with a useful framework to identify, effectively diagnose, and manage these complex problems.

NEOPLASTIC EMERGENCIES
Mass Effect and Herniation

Elevated intracranial pressure (ICP), hydrocephalus, and herniation may occur as a direct result of neoplastic mass effect or as a result of meningeal involvement. In most patients with ICP elevation, onset is heralded by subacute, progressive, or new headache, which may awaken the patient from sleep and often is exacerbated by coughing, straining, or lying flat. The headache may also be associated with nausea and emesis. In the case of a gradually enlarging tumor, headache may accompany progressive focal neurologic deficits and seizure due to mass effect from the tumor itself and associated peritumoral vasogenic edema. In the case of meningeal involvement, headache results from communicating hydrocephalus and may not be accompanied by focal deficits. When present, these focal deficits most typically occur in the form of cranial neuropathies and/or radiculopathies.

Tumor-related mass effect is frequently driven largely by inflammation and vasogenic edema, which responds acutely to high-dose corticosteroid therapy. Dexamethasone is the most common first-line treatment of tumor-related edema, typically given as a single dose of 10 mg intravenously (IV) in the setting of acute symptomatic mass effect, followed by an ongoing dose of 4 mg IV every 6 hours. Asymptomatic or minimally symptomatic edema on imaging does not necessarily warrant aggressive pharmacotherapy. Although dexamethasone reliably reduces peritumoral edema, it is also thought to reduce diagnostic yield of subsequent cytology or biopsy, particularly in cases of lymphoma.[1–3] If lymphoma is suspected and biopsy can be performed expeditiously, we recommend treatment of cerebral edema with hyperosmolar therapy in lieu of corticosteroids until after the biopsy is completed. Of note, more recent observational data suggest that a short course of preoperative corticosteroid treatment may not significantly reduce diagnostic sensitivity for lymphoma,[4–6] although there have been no prospective investigations to definitively answer this question.

As ICP increases to critical thresholds, clinical signs of herniation may manifest. Herniation syndromes are described in more detail elsewhere in this edition of Neurologic Clinics but generally are associated with depression of the level of consciousness and cranial nerve abnormalities. The mainstay of treatment is hyperosmolar therapy, as also described elsewhere, although this should serve only as a bridge to more definitive surgical treatment. Tumor debulking and decompressive craniectomy are options to reduce ICP. Patients with posterior fossa lesions that impede the flow of cerebrospinal fluid by obstruction of the fourth ventricle and/or aqueduct may develop acute obstructive hydrocephalus, which demands emergent treatment with cerebrospinal fluid (CSF) diversion and posterior fossa decompression in addition to bridging osmotherapy. Consensus guidelines recommend against ventriculostomy without decompressive suboccipital craniectomy due to a theoretic concern for upward herniation,[7] although clinically relevant upward herniation is probably rare in practice.[8–10]

Neurovascular Complications of Malignancy

Patients with systemic and primary central nervous system (CNS) malignancies have an increased risk of ischemic stroke and intracerebral hemorrhage, related to both cancer-mediated and treatment-related mechanisms **(Table 1)**.[11–15]

Table 1
Cerebrovascular disease in patients with cancer comprises diverse mechanisms and may be classified as an effect of malignancy or its treatment

Stroke Type	Cause	Mechanisms
Ischemic	Direct tumor effect	Vascular compression
		Vascular infiltration
		Tumor embolism
	Systemic tumor effect	Hypercoagulability
		Disseminated intravascular coagulation
		Hyperviscosity
		Nonbacterial thrombotic endocarditis
		Septic embolism
		Infectious vasculitis
	Treatment-related effect	Radiation therapy
		Chemotherapy
		Surgical resection
Hemorrhagic	Direct tumor effect	Intratumoral hemorrhage
	Systemic tumor effect	Coagulopathy
		Disseminated intravascular coagulation
		Hyperviscosity
		Thrombocytopenia
		Neoplastic aneurysm
	Treatment-related effect	Radiation therapy
		Radiation-induced vascular malformation
		Chemotherapy
Cerebral venous sinus thrombosis	Direct tumor effect	Venous sinus compression
	Systemic tumor effect	Hypercoagulability

Ischemic stroke

In a retrospective series of patients with cancer-associated ischemic stroke, lung adenocarcinoma was the most common associated malignancy, followed by primary brain tumors.[14] The primary brain tumors most commonly associated with ischemic stroke are glioma, meningioma, and primary CNS lymphoma and associated strokes are most frequently cardioembolic or perioperative.[12]

Pathophysiologically, ischemic stroke may result from direct tumor effects, systemic coagulopathy, and infection or treatment-related effects.[13,16,17] Tumors may directly compress cerebral vessels, leptomeningeal disease may infiltrate into perivascular spaces, and malignancy may directly involve vessels as in intravascular lymphoma.[16] Head and neck tumors may induce critical arterial stenosis and stroke by compression or encasement of large vessels intra- or extracranially. Leptomeningeal disease, similar to meningitis, may induce a diffuse cerebral vasculopathy and may cause small-vessel stroke via infiltration into perivascular (Virchow-Robin) spaces. Such vasculopathy may be difficult to distinguish from intravascular lymphoma, characterized by clonal lymphocytic infiltration of vessel walls causing multifocal arterial stenosis and resultant ischemic stroke. This condition is famously difficult to diagnose, requiring a high index of suspicion and typically a brain biopsy. Rarely, stroke may also result from direct tumor embolism, in which emboli contain malignant cells. Although classically described in intracardiac tumors, tumor embolism may occur in patients with a variety of (typically metastatic) cancers.[13,16]

Cancer-associated stroke may also occur as a result of systemic hypercoagulable state. Indeed, most of the strokes in patients with cancer are associated with a hypercoagulable state.[14] In severe cases, patients may develop disseminated intravascular coagulation (DIC), which predisposes to both microvascular ischemic stroke and intracerebral hemorrhage. Typically seen in advanced cancer, nonbacterial thrombotic endocarditis may itself be a sequela of chronic DIC and is characterized by sterile valvular vegetations, negative blood cultures, and systemic embolization to multiple organs.[18] Hyperviscosity syndromes are classically associated with hematologic malignancy and may cause stroke through increased resistance to cerebral blood flow; the classic presenting clinical triad is neurologic abnormalities, vision changes, and mucosal bleeding. Finally, systemic or CNS infection may produce stroke in patients with cancer who are immunosuppressed due to malignancy or its treatment. Infectious endocarditis may produce septic embolism manifesting as multifocal ischemic stroke, often with increased risk of hemorrhagic transformation. Likewise, infectious vasculitis may result from a variety of bacterial, fungal, mycobacterial, and viral causes, particularly in the setting of immunosuppression or meningitis.

Ischemic stroke may also arise as a complication of cancer treatment, including radiation therapy, tumor resection, hematopoietic stem cell transplantation, and certain chemotherapies. Such complications are described in more detail later in this article.

Outcomes after stroke are generally poorer among patients with cancer.[19,20] Patients with cancer who suffer strokes are more likely to have associated thrombosis (myocardial infarction, venous thromboembolism) and have considerably higher in-hospital mortality.[20] Cancer status also may have an effect, as stroke patients with active cancer are younger, have more severe strokes, and are more likely to have multifocal ischemic strokes than patients with nonactive cancer.[21]

Treatment of acute stroke is described in greater detail elsewhere in this edition of Neurologic Clinics but in general should follow established guidelines.[22] Observational studies suggest that IV tissue plasminogen activator (IV-tPA) is safe to administer in patients with systemic malignancy[23] but may be contraindicated in patients who have CNS tumor, coagulopathy, or thrombocytopenia. Although intracranial mass lesions are frequently considered a relative contraindication to IV-tPA, little evidence exists to support or refine this contraindication. Case series suggest that IV-tPA may be safe in patients with extra-axial tumors at low risk of hemorrhage, such as meningiomas.[24–26] Whether or not IV-tPA is indicated, endovascular treatment should be considered in patients with large-vessel occlusion.[27,28]

Therapy directed at the underlying pathophysiology should be considered, such as anticoagulation in the case of systemic thromboembolism or atrial fibrillation or plasmapheresis in the case of a leukemic hyperviscosity syndrome. In all cases, the risks of hemorrhage from antiplatelet therapy and anticoagulation in the setting of an intracranial mass lesion must be balanced with the risk of stroke. Retrospective data suggest that anticoagulation is safe in patients with brain metastases, although risk of hemorrhage increases with comorbid thrombocytopenia, hypertension, concurrent antiplatelet use, and with certain hemorrhagic metastases (melanoma and renal cell carcinoma).[29–31]

Limited evidence exists to guide anticoagulant selection in patients with cancer-related stroke.[32,33] Warfarin dosing may be challenging due to interactions with chemotherapy and resulting labile international normalized ratio. Direct oral anticoagulants (DOACs) confer a lower risk of major hemorrhage and reduced risk of recurrent stroke compared with warfarin in the general population,[34,35] and this may also apply to patients with cancer.[36–38] Retrospective data also suggest low-molecular-weight heparin (LMWH) is superior to warfarin for secondary prevention of cancer-related stroke.[39] DOACs are noninferior to LMWH for the treatment and prevention of cancer-related venous thromboembolism[40] and the same may be true for stroke although larger studies are needed.[41] Until clinical trials clarify optimal anticoagulant choice in patients with cancer-related stroke, risks and benefits of each anticoagulant should be addressed on a case-by-case basis, with a preference to avoid warfarin.

Intracerebral hemorrhage

As ischemic stroke, intracerebral hemorrhage (ICH) may occur in patients with cancer due to direct tumor effects, systemic coagulopathy and infection, and treatment-related effects.[13,16]

Primary and metastatic brain tumors may exhibit intratumoral hemorrhage, and indeed such hemorrhage may represent the presenting finding leading to cancer diagnosis.[42] Imaging characteristics such as peripheral hematoma enhancement and pronounced perihematomal edema may suggest underlying tumor as the cause of ICH. The most common primary brain tumors associated with ICH are glioblastoma and oligodendroglioma.[43,44] The most common hemorrhagic metastases are melanoma, lung, and breast cancers.[44] Despite a known propensity, hemorrhage is less common from renal cell cancer, papillary thyroid cancer, and choriocarcinoma, probably due to lower incidence overall.[44]

The coagulopathy associated with systemic malignancy increases the risk of both ICH and ischemic stroke. Thrombocytopenia and DIC are frequently seen in patients with malignancy. For example, 22% of patients with acute myelogenous leukemia in one series were found at autopsy to have ICH.[13] Furthermore, patients with ischemic stroke related to the diverse causes described earlier may develop hemorrhagic transformation.

As patients with cancer with ischemic strokes, patients who suffer ICH related to cancer have poorer outcomes than patients without cancer.[44] Treatment is largely supportive, including correction of underlying coagulopathy and thrombocytopenia. Novel pharmacologic agents for prevention of perihematomal edema and endovascular neurosurgical hematoma evacuation techniques, areas of active research in spontaneous ICH as described elsewhere in this text, may be applicable to cancer-associated hemorrhage.

Cerebral venous sinus thrombosis

Cerebral venous sinus thrombosis (CVST) may result from hypercoagulable state or due to direct compression of the sinuses by tumor.[13,45] In the absence of tumoral compression, the most common malignancy associated with CVST is leukemia.[45] Regardless of cause, CVST may result in venous infarction, hemorrhage, seizures, intracranial hypertension, and—for CVST involving the torcula and deep venous drainage—coma. Treatment depends on the clinical context and should be directed at the underlying cause, whether mass effect from a tumor or coagulopathy from hematologic malignancy. Anticoagulation is the typical treatment of non-–cancer-associated CVST, even in the setting of intraparenchymal hemorrhage.[46]

Pituitary apoplexy

Pituitary apoplexy is rare but may result when a pituitary adenoma undergoes sudden and spontaneous infarction, hemorrhage, or both.[47] The sudden increase in the volume of the pituitary exerts mass effect on surrounding structures and further compromises blood supply to pituitary tissue. Although not always present in full, the classic symptomatology is sudden onset headache, visual disturbance, cranial neuropathies, and endocrine dysfunction—typically manifesting as acute adrenal insufficiency, which may be profound.[47,48] Management requires prompt medical treatment with intravenous corticosteroids and fluid repletion. Neurosurgical intervention may be indicated for progressive cranial neuropathies or vision loss.[48]

Seizures and Status Epilepticus

Intracranial mass lesions predispose to seizures and status epilepticus, and indeed seizure is commonly the presenting symptom of a brain tumor. Dysembrioblastic neuroepithelial tumors (DNETs) and gangliomas, pediatric tumors that commonly arise in the temporal lobes, carry the highest rates of associated seizure.[49,50] Nearly all patients with DNETs will develop seizures at some point.[29] Among adults, gliomas and meningiomas are most frequently associated with seizures, although seizure incidence declines with age.[49] Interestingly, low-grade gliomas are associated with higher seizure risk than glioblastomas,[50] probably due to cortical rather than central distribution and longer survival among patients with low-grade gliomas. Metastatic tumors also predispose to seizure, although the incidence is less than observed in primary brain tumors.[51] Despite the well-described risk of seizure among individuals with intracranial mass lesions, prophylactic therapy with antiepileptic drugs (AEDs) has not demonstrated benefit and is not recommended.[52–54] Clinicians should maintain a high index of suspicion for seizure, and a low threshold to obtain electroencephalography and initiate or escalate antiseizure treatment in individuals with intracranial mass lesions presenting with encephalopathy, spells, or fluctuating focal neurologic deficits. In a prospective cohort of individuals admitted to the neuro intensive care unit with altered mental status, a history of CNS tumor was identified as a common cause and an independent risk factor for nonconvulsive status epilepticus.[55]

Symptomatic seizures arising from an underlying mass lesion have focal onset, but they may rapidly generalize and escalate, making the focality difficult to determine by semiology. Status epilepticus, defined as a seizure with duration longer than 5 minutes or multiple consecutive seizures without interval return to neurologic baseline, is a neurologic emergency.[56] Status epilepticus carries a high mortality regardless of underlying cause, with approximately 20% of status epilepticus cases resulting in death.[56–58] Mortality is higher in those with advanced age and those with an identifiable acute seizure precipitant.[57] More specifically, mortality is similar or slightly higher when the status epilepticus precipitant is a brain tumor.[58,59]

Benzodiazepines remain the mainstay of initial treatment of status epilepticus, followed by another nonbenzodiazepine AED. Choice of AED is largely driven by side-effect profile, institutional availability, and clinician experience, as no specific AED has been demonstrated to be superior in initial treatment of status epilepticus in randomized controlled trials.[56,60,61] Typical first-line agents include fosphenytoin, levetiracetam, and valproic acid due to the availability of each in rapidly loadable intravenous formulations. Levetiracetam may be preferable in patients receiving treatment of cancer due to fewer drug–drug interactions. Cytochrome P450 pathway–inducing AEDs such as phenytoin may reduce circulating levels of dexamethasone and chemotherapeutic agents, whereas pathway inhibitors such as valproic acid may increase concentrations of chemotherapeutic agents and the likelihood of toxicity.[62] Treatment of refractory status epilepticus, defined as persistent status epilepticus despite adequate treatment with a benzodiazepine and at least one additional AED,[56] is described elsewhere in this edition of Neurologic Clinics.

In cases of medically refractory epilepsy or status epilepticus due to an intracranial mass lesion, surgical mass resection may be considered as a means of achieving seizure control, although there is little evidence to guide this approach.[63–65]

Metastatic Epidural Spinal Cord Compression

In the acute care setting, metastatic epidural spinal cord compression (MESCC) most often presents with back pain and lower extremity weakness that worsens, sometimes to the point of being unable to walk, over days to weeks. As individuals with cancer often have complex prior treatment histories, are medically ill, and may have preexisting back or other pain and/or weakness, it is essential to take a careful clinical history and assess for myelopathic signs on examination. Specifically, asking about new focal pain, a change in the character of back pain, or any new motor, sensory, or bowel/bladder dysfunction is useful. Without a heightened attentiveness for concerning signs and symptoms, the symptoms of MESCC may be incorrectly attributed to things such as deconditioning, lumbar spondylosis, bony metastasis, peripheral neuropathy, or Guillain-Barre syndrome. MESCC occurs in 3% to 5% of individuals with cancer.[66] It is evenly distributed throughout the spine based on bone volume (thoracic spine [60%], followed by lumbar [25%] and cervical [15%]).[66]

MESCC is also a consideration for individuals presenting without a cancer diagnosis, as epidural spinal cord compression is the initial manifestation of cancer in up to 20% of MESCC.[67]

It is often the task of the neurologist to identify the signs/symptoms of myelopathy, recommend spine imaging, and to engage with the oncology and surgical teams in cases where radiation or surgical decompression are a consideration. A history of new radicular or mechanical back pain, new bowel or bladder dysfunction, or examination findings of increased deep tendon reflexes and pathologic reflexes such as Babinski sign or clonus are worrisome for a compressive myelopathy (or polyradiculopathy in the case of cauda equina syndrome) and warrant spine MR imaging. In cases where symptoms worsen rapidly over hours to days, or clinical features of conus medullaris syndrome or cauda equina syndrome are present, prompt identification and emergent spine imaging are especially important, as intervention may substantially alter an individual's clinical course. When possible, immediate whole spine MR imaging with intravenous contrast is optimal, because epidural metastasis may occur at multiple levels. In the absence of MR imaging availability, spine computed tomography is a reasonable alternative, although it is less sensitive.

Initial treatment of MESCC includes corticosteroids and consideration of either radiation therapy or surgical decompression. The dosing of corticosteroids is most typically moderate (10 mg dexamethasone x 1 followed by 12–16 mg daily),[67] although for severe acute compression, some advocate for high-dose dexamethasone (96 mg daily initially and daily for 3 days).[68] Although MESCC outcomes are better with steroid treatment in those with neurologic deficits, there is insufficient evidence to support a specific dosing regimen.[67] There are 2 main treatment options for MESCC, both of which are palliative: (1) radiation therapy and (2) surgical decompression. Both therapies are performed with the goal of reducing pain and prolonging functional motor ability by delaying growth of the tumor that is causing the cord compression. As a manifestation of advanced cancer, for those with radiosensitive tumor histology (lymphoma, myeloma, seminoma), limited expected survival, multilevel epidural cord tumors, severe pretreatment motor deficits, and/or poor performance status, radiation therapy often provides symptomatic benefit and local disease control.[69] For individuals who have controlled systemic cancer, high-grade compression, and/or spine instability, surgical decompression is reasonable to consider.[70,71] For select cases, surgery followed by radiation therapy is associated with a higher probability of posttreatment ambulation and prolonged ambulatory status.[72]

TREATMENT-RELATED NEUROLOGIC EMERGENCIES

An effective approach to the patient who presents with a possible neuro-oncologic emergency is to start by understanding the individual's

1. Type of cancer and its known neurologic manifestations,
2. Extent of cancer involvement
   Stage/organ involvement for systemic malignancies
   Unifocal, multifocal ± meningeal spread for intracranial tumors
   Date of most recent systemic staging and/or neuroimaging
3. Details and timeline for what treatment they have received/are receiving
   Surgical, radiation, chemotherapy, immunotherapies, cellular therapeutics

These details aid in determining whether the cancer is actively progressing or has responded to treatment and the relative timing of neurologic symptoms to various treatments. When integrated with the presenting neurologic problems and physical/neurologic examination, this approach makes it possible to generate a relevant differential diagnosis and ascertain the likelihood that the presenting illness is related to a direct or indirect effect of the cancer itself, a cancer therapeutic side-effect, or an alternate explanation (eg, immunosuppression, hypercoagulability, immobility, or a coexisting nononcologic medical condition). Common neurologic effects of radiation, chemotherapeutic drugs, immune checkpoint inhibitors, and cellular therapeutics seen in the emergency and acute care settings are reviewed here.

Radiation Therapy

Radiation therapy induces cellular injury and death, most commonly through the delivery of photon-based gamma rays to a targeted area. It is a mainstay of treatment of primary brain tumors, brain, and meningeal metastasis. In addition to the intended effect on tumor cells, radiation therapy induces endothelial injury, which is the likely the cause for neurologic complications.

Radiation-induced vasogenic cerebral edema may occur shortly after treatment, as soon as 24 to 48 hours posttreatment in the case of stereotactic radiosurgery. Depending on the size and location of the treated area, individuals may be asymptomatic, mildly symptomatic (headache, nausea, fatigue), or rarely have severe/life-threatening symptoms due to regional brain compression and mass effect. Treatment of spinal cord tumors may also result in symptomatic edema and rapid clinical deterioration. Neuroimaging, usually contrast-enhanced MR imaging, is the diagnostic test of choice, and the treatment is corticosteroids (usually dexamethasone 4–16 mg daily) dosed to symptomatic improvement. In cases where corticosteroids are contraindicated or do not result in symptomatic improvement, bevacizumab has potent antiedema effect and is an effective alternative or second-line therapy.[73] Swelling and increased contrast enhancement following radiation therapy for intracranial tumors may also happen in a more delayed fashion. When these clinical and radiographic changes occur shortly after radiation therapy (within 3 months following treatment), it is often described as "pseudoprogression" and can be clinically and radiographically difficult to distinguish from early tumor growth.[74] Inflammation due to radiation or radiation necrosis can also occur in a more delayed fashion (from months to even several years after treatment).[75]

Radiation vasculopathy is a mechanism for ischemic stroke in ~1/3 of those who have received brain or head and neck radiation.[12,76] Strokes occur within the radiation treatment area and tend to occur years after treatment (median 3.2 years).[12] Radiation-induced leukoencephalopathy is another pathologic process related to endothelial injury that does not necessarily present with clinical strokes but may be prominent on imaging and have cumulative cognitive effects.[77]

Strokelike migraine attacks after radiation therapy (SMART syndrome) present acutely with headache and neurologic deficits. SMART syndrome may occur months to several years after cranial irradiation and has been reported even decades after treatment. The symptoms mimic acute ischemic stroke but are transient and not associated with infarction on brain MR imaging, tumor growth, or focal seizure activity. Contrast-enhanced brain MR imaging reveals increased T2 signal and gyriform enhancement within the radiation treatment field. On follow-up imaging, these abnormalities spontaneously improve or completely resolve, as do the headaches and neurologic deficits.[78] It is important to distinguish SMART syndrome from posterior reversible encephalopathy syndrome or focal seizure activity, such as aggressive blood pressure management, or escalating antiseizure medications may need to be administered in these cases respectively.

Chemotherapy

The rapidly expanding knowledge of cancer biology and therapies in oncology has led to a broadened array of treatment options, improved response to therapy, and prolonged survival for individuals with cancer. Multitargeted combination therapies are commonly used to address treatment escape mechanisms. Although the overall effect of these advances is positive, individuals may experience neurologic side effects, which rarely can be severe and require urgent identification and management.

Determining whether a particular neurologic symptom is attributable to a chemotherapeutic agent is useful diagnostically and also helps inform the oncology team as they consider ongoing treatment versus modifying or discontinuing therapy. It is useful to understand neurologic complications of cancer therapies in the specific context of the individual's disease, treatment, and time course. **Table 2** provides a summary of neurologic syndromes that may be encountered in the acute care setting, as well as associated chemotherapeutic agents.

Immune Checkpoint Inhibitor Therapy

Over the past decade, immune checkpoint inhibitor (ICI) therapies have emerged as a powerful mechanism to activate host immunity against a variety of cancers.[83] ICIs work by blocking the suppressive effects of T-cell surface proteins cytotoxic T-lymphocyte antigen 4 (ipilimumab), programmed cell death 1 (PD-1) (pembrolizumab, nivolumab), or by blocking its ligand (PD-L1) on tumor cells (atezolizumab, avelumab, durvalumab).[83] As ICIs promote T-cell activation leading to tumor cell death, they may also produce adverse events (AEs) through immunologic mechanisms. These include increased cytokine release, antibody production, T-cell activity directed at normal host cells, and complement activation.[83] Moderate-to-severe neurologic AEs occur in ~1% to 3% of individuals after a median of 3 ICI cycles.[84] Neurologic AEs often occur along with systemic AEs, such as enterocolitis, pneumonitis, myocarditis, thyroiditis, or vitiligo.[84] ICI-associated AEs may involve the central nervous system, peripheral nervous system, neuromuscular junction, or muscle (**Table 3**).[83,84]

Depending on the severity of the neurologic symptoms, holding or discontinuation of ICI therapy is indicated.[85] Treatment with corticosteroids (prednisone 40–60 mg or intravenous methylprednisolone 1 g daily for 3–5 days) often results in rapid improvement.[84] For more severe neurologic impairment ($\geq$Grade III), or in the absence of improvement with corticosteroids, other immunosuppressive therapies such as intravenous immunoglobulin or plasma exchange therapy may be indicated.[85,86] Resumption of ICI therapy after a moderate-to-severe neurologic AE is associated with a risk of AE recurrence.[84]

Immune Effector Cell Therapy

CAR-T therapy is an emerging and potentially curative treatment, approved to treat relapsed or refractory hematologic malignancies,[87,88] with potential to similarly direct

Table 2
Summary of neurologic side-effects encountered in the acute care setting and their associated chemotherapeutic agent

Neurologic Side Effect	Agent	Mechanism/Target	Risk Factors/Notes
Encephalopathy	5-Fluorouracil	Antimetabolite	
	Cytarabine (IV or IT)	Antimetabolite	IT administration may precipitate a more severe necrotizing leukoencephalopathy[79]
	Methotrexate (IV or IT)	Antimetabolite	Combined brain radiation + methotrexate increases risk for leukoencephalopathy
	Fludarabine	Antimetabolite	
	Paclitaxel	Microtubule inhibition	Occurs 1–3 wk posttreatment, may progress to coma[80]
	Ifosfamide	DNA alkylation	Occurs in 10%–15%, may be reversed with intravenous methylene blue[81]
Cerebrovascular (IS, ICH, PRES[82])	Bevacizumab	Anti-VEGF MAb	
	Sunitinib	rTKI targeting VEGFR, PDGFR	
	Sorafenib	rTKI targeting VEGFR, PDGFR, RAF	
	L-Asparaginase	Enzyme	Also associated with increased risk for CVST
Seizure[79]	Cytarabine (IV or IT)	Antimetabolite	
	5-Fluorouracil	Antimetabolite	
	Busulfan	DNA alkylation	
Aseptic meningitis	Cytarabine (IT)	Antimetabolite	
	Methotrexate (IT)	Antimetabolite	
Acute cerebellar syndrome	5-Fluorouracil	Antimetabolite	
	Cytarabine (IV)	Antimetabolite	
Acute myelopathy	Cytarabine (IT)	Antimetabolite	
	Methotrexate (IT)	Antimetabolite	

Abbreviations: CVST, cerebral venous sinus thrombosis; ICH, intracerebral hemorrhage; IS, ischemic stroke; IT, intrathecal; IV, intravenous; PDGFR, platelet-derived growth factor receptor; PRES, posterior reversible encephalopathy syndrome; rTKI, receptor tyrosine kinase inhibitor; VEGFR, vascular endothelial growth factor receptor.

T-cell activity against solid tumors. CAR-T therapy is associated with a range of neurotoxicity, from mild to severe and life threatening.[89] Neurotoxicity related to CAR-T therapy has been termed immune effector cell–associated neurotoxicity syndrome (ICANS).

Although the underlying pathophysiology is poorly understood, ICANS characteristically follows cytokine release syndrome (CRS), suggesting that a systemic inflammatory response plays a role in its development.[90] Blood-brain barrier dysfunction also may contribute, as fulminant, life-threatening cerebral edema has been described as the most severe manifestation of ICANS and has also been demonstrated post mortem.[88,90,91]

Incidence of ICANS largely depends on how ICANS is defined and measured but ranges from 15% to 60% of patients receiving CAR-T cell infusion.[87–89,91,92] Low-grade ICANS, characterized as encephalopathy and headache, seems to be quite

Table 3
The spectrum of neurologic adverse events associated with immune checkpoint inhibitor therapies ipilimumab (anti-CTLA-4), pembrolizumab, and nivolumab (anti-PD-1)

Central Nervous System	Cranial Nerve	Peripheral Nerve	Muscle/Neuromuscular Junction	Classic Paraneoplastic Neurologic Syndromes
Autoimmune encephalitis	Trigeminal neuralgia	Sensory neuropathy	MG	ANNA-1 limbic encephalitis
Meningitis	Facial palsy	Small fiber + autonomic neuropathy	Myositis	Anti-P/Q Ca++ channel LEMS
Hypophysitis	Hearing loss	Polyradiculopathy	MG/myositis overlap syndrome	
Hashimoto encephalitis		AIDP/radiculoneuropathy	Myopathy + ganglionopathy	
Temporal lobe epilepsy		Neuralgic amyotrophy		
PRES		ANCA-associated multifocal motor neuropathy		
Ataxia				
Transverse myelitis				

Abbreviations: AIDP, acute inflammatory demyelinating polyneuropathy; ANCA, antineutrophil cytoplasmic antibody; ANNA-1, antineuronal nuclear antibody-1; LEMS, Lambert-Eaton Myasthenic Syndrome; MG, myasthenia gravis.

common after CAR-T therapy. More severe ICANS is less frequent but may manifest as aphasia, seizures, status epilepticus, and diffuse cerebral edema. Interestingly, although ICANS is presumably a diffuse process, focal findings are frequently observed—most notably aphasia.[91] Advanced age, severe CRS, and early CRS (<3 days postinfusion) are clinical features predictive of subsequent ICANS in patients with lymphoma.[92]

In addition to supportive care, treatment of ICANS must paradoxically strive to suppress the brisk immune response presumably responsible for ICANS without sacrificing therapeutic efficacy, which is presumably attributable to the same brisk immune response. Tocilizumab antagonizes the interleukin-6 (IL-6) receptor and has been shown to mitigate CRS symptoms without compromising treatment efficacy.[87] However, tocilizumab is also associated with increased serum levels of IL-6, and it does not cross the blood-brain barrier to block CNS IL-6 receptors, raising concern that it may worsen ICANS by shunting excess IL-6 to the central nervous system.[93,94] Indeed, the number of doses of tocilizumab administered has been shown to be an independent predictor of neurotoxicity, although this may be a marker of more severe CRS, which is itself also a predictor of neurotoxicity.[92] Siltuximab directly binds IL-6 rather than its receptor and is being investigated as an alternative to tocilizumab.[93]

Corticosteroid therapy, typically with moderate- to high-dose dexamethasone, may be administered for ICANS refractory to treatment with IL-6 inhibition. Corticosteroid therapy has historically been avoided due to theoretic concerns that ablation of CAR-T cells could reduce response rate, durability, and overall efficacy, but this has not been borne out in clinical trials.[93] It is unclear whether earlier administration of corticosteroids or coadministration with an IL-6 inhibitor might reduce ICANS incidence and severity without affecting treatment response.

PROGNOSTICATION IN NEURO-ONCOLOGIC EMERGENCIES

In general, outcomes after acute neurologic emergencies are poorer for individuals with associated CNS or systemic malignancy. Indeed, this is the case for patients with cancer who suffer ischemic stroke, ICH, and status epilepticus, as described earlier. However, as in other neurocritical illnesses, prognostication carries considerable uncertainty, poses ethical challenges, and may be complicated by clinical nihilism and self-fulfilling prophecy.

High rates of withdrawal of life-sustaining treatment in some diseases, such as ICH, limit our understanding of the natural history of the disease and may contribute to high perceived mortality[95]; this has been called the self-fulfilling prophecy, whereby an outcome is realized "by virtue of having been predicted."[96] This phenomenon contributes to prognostic uncertainty, and it is essential that such uncertainty be communicated to patients and surrogates when discussing prognostic estimates.

Clinical prognostic scales exist for a variety of neurocritical illnesses, although no scales exist specifically to address neurocritical illness in the context of known malignancy. Therefore, existing disease-specific scales may not be generalizable to patients with neuro-oncologic disease. Even existing scales may suffer from limited accuracy, poor calibration, and lack of generalizability within the disease population for which they were developed, again highlighting the need to convey uncertainty whenever estimating prognosis.[97]

Given the uncertainty associated with prognosis in neurocritical illness, we encourage disciplined use of neurodiagnostics to provide as much clarity as possible and caution against overconfidence in prognosis. Communication with the patient's oncologist, neuro-oncologist, and/or acute care oncology team is also important to integrate the prognosis related to their oncologic disease in the context of new acute neurologic illness and ensure consistent messaging to the patient and family. The clinician caring for a patient with a neuro-oncologic emergency must be cautious to avoid an overly nihilistic prognosis, which may lead to premature withdrawal of life-sustaining treatment. Conversely, the clinician must also avoid an overly optimistic prognosis that may result in survival with an unacceptable quality of life. Ultimately, goals of care are unique to each patient, and clinicians, patients, and surrogates should together strive to realize goal-concordant care, as established through a shared decision-making model.[98,99]

SUMMARY

Cancer and cancer therapies have the potential to affect the nervous system in a host of different ways. The more severe neurologic effects may result in critical illness or be experienced by individuals who are critically ill. Acute stroke intervention, including thrombolytics and interventional stroke treatment, is appropriate when the benefit outweighs the risk of harm. Intraparenchymal hemorrhage often happens in the setting of coagulopathy among those with cancer. Intracranial radiation therapy has the potential to cause acute, subacute, and long-term neurologic side effects, including cerebral edema, ischemic stroke, and SMART syndrome. A careful cancer treatment history and investigation of agents known to have neurologic side effects is an effective strategy to identify chemotherapy-related neurologic toxicities. When delivering prognostic information for individuals with neurologic critical illness and cancer, it is important not to adopt clinical nihilism and to have a good grasp of both the oncologic and neurologic disease state, which often requires intense interdisciplinary collaboration.

CLINICS CARE POINTS

- Mass effect and herniation due to intracranial neoplasms is treated with dexamethasone to reduce vasogenic edema, surgical debulking, and rarely osmotic agents or decompressive craniotomy.

- Recent neuroimaging is required before lumbar puncture in anyone with a known history of cancer or focal neurologic deficits on examination to ensure safe CSF collection.

- Stroke in individuals with cancer occurs more often than in the general population, via distinct mechanisms and less commonly in association with classic stroke risk factors.

- Sudden onset headache, visual disturbance, cranial neuropathies, and/or acute endocrine dysfunction warrants investigation for pituitary apoplexy and acute management with replacement therapies.

- Suspicion for seizure in individuals with CNS cancer is heightened, as they have an elevated risk of seizure and status epilepticus, including nonconvulsive status epilepticus.

- Rapid identification and treatment of metastatic epidural spinal cord compression leads to better pain control and improved functional outcomes.

- Immune-checkpoint inhibitors are associated with moderate-to-severe immunologic neurologic side effects in 1% to 3% of treated individuals, many of which respond to corticosteroid treatment.

- ICANS is an immunologic complication of CAR-T cell therapy that occurs in association with cytokine release syndrome and manifests as encephalopathy, language impairment, and in more severe instances cerebral edema, seizures, and depressed level of consciousness.

DISCLOSURE

The authors have nothing to disclose.

REFERENCES

1. Deangelis LM, Hormigo A. Treatment of primary central nervous system lymphoma. Semin Oncol 2004;31(5):684–92.
2. Weller M. Glucocorticoid treatment of primary CNS lymphoma. J Neurooncol 1999;43(3):237–9.
3. Haldorsen IS, Espeland A, Larsen JL, et al. Diagnostic delay in primary central nervous system lymphoma. Acta Oncol 2005;44(7):728–34.
4. Porter AB, Giannini C, Kaufmann T, et al. Primary central nervous system lymphoma can be histologically diagnosed after previous corticosteroid use: a pilot study to determine whether corticosteroids prevent the diagnosis of primary central nervous system lymphoma. Ann Neurol 2008;63(5):662–7.
5. Bullis CL, Maldonado-Perez A, Bowden SG, et al. Diagnostic impact of preoperative corticosteroids in primary central nervous system lymphoma. J Clin Neurosci 2020;72:287–91.
6. Binnahil M, Au K, Lu JQ, et al. The Influence of Corticosteroids on Diagnostic Accuracy of Biopsy for Primary Central Nervous System Lymphoma. Can J Neurol Sci 2016;43(5):721–5.
7. Braksick SA, Himes BT, Snyder K, et al. Ventriculostomy and Risk of Upward Herniation in Patients with Obstructive Hydrocephalus from Posterior Fossa Mass Lesions. Neurocrit Care 2018;28(3):338–43.
8. Wijdicks EF, Sheth KN, Carter BS, et al. Recommendations for the management of cerebral and cerebellar infarction with swelling: a statement for healthcare professionals from the American Heart Association/American Stroke Association. Stroke 2014;45(4):1222–38.
9. Gurol ME, St Louis EK. Treatment of cerebellar masses. Curr Treat Options Neurol 2008;10(2):138–50.
10. Koenig MA. Cerebral Edema and Elevated Intracranial Pressure. Continuum (Minneap Minn) 2018;24(6):1588–602.
11. Zoller B, Ji J, Sundquist J, et al. Risk of haemorrhagic and ischaemic stroke in patients with cancer: a nationwide follow-up study from Sweden. Eur J Cancer 2012;48(12):1875–83.
12. Kreisl TN, Toothaker T, Karimi S, et al. Ischemic stroke in patients with primary brain tumors. Neurology 2008;70(24):2314–20.
13. Graus F, Rogers LR, Posner JB. Cerebrovascular complications in patients with cancer. Medicine (Baltimore) 1985;64(1):16–35.
14. Cestari DM, Weine DM, Panageas KS, et al. Stroke in patients with cancer: incidence and etiology. Neurology 2004;62(11):2025–30.
15. Jo JT, Schiff D. Management of neuro-oncologic emergencies. Handb Clin Neurol 2017;141:715–41.
16. Katz JM, Segal AZ. Incidence and etiology of cerebrovascular disease in patients with malignancy. Curr Atheroscler Rep 2005;7(4):280–8.
17. Rogers LR. Cerebrovascular complications in cancer patients. Neurol Clin 2003; 21(1):167–92.
18. Rogers LR, Cho ES, Kempin S, et al. Cerebral infarction from non-bacterial thrombotic endocarditis. Clinical and pathological study including the effects of anticoagulation. Am J Med 1987;83(4):746–56.

19. Taccone FS, Jeangette SM, Blecic SA. First-ever stroke as initial presentation of systemic cancer. J Stroke Cerebrovasc Dis 2008;17(4):169–74.

20. Zhang YY, Cordato D, Shen Q, et al. Risk factor, pattern, etiology and outcome in ischemic stroke patients with cancer: a nested case-control study. Cerebrovasc Dis 2007;23(2–3):181–7.

21. Kneihsl M, Enzinger C, Wunsch G, et al. Poor short-term outcome in patients with ischaemic stroke and active cancer. J Neurol 2016;263(1):150–6.

22. Powers WJ, Rabinstein AA, Ackerson T, et al. Guidelines for the Early Management of Patients With Acute Ischemic Stroke: 2019 Update to the 2018 Guidelines for the Early Management of Acute Ischemic Stroke: A Guideline for Healthcare Professionals From the American Heart Association/American Stroke Association. Stroke 2019;50(12):e344–418.

23. Murthy SB, Karanth S, Shah S, et al. Thrombolysis for acute ischemic stroke in patients with cancer: a population study. Stroke 2013;44(12):3573–6.

24. Jaffe R, Reichman JM, Weiss AT, et al. Thrombolysis in the presence of an intracranial meningioma. Chest 1997;111(1):258.

25. Rubinshtein R, Jaffe R, Flugelman MY, et al. Thrombolysis in patients with a brain tumour. Heart 2004;90(12):1476.

26. Etgen T, Steinich I, Gsottschneider L. Thrombolysis for ischemic stroke in patients with brain tumors. J Stroke Cerebrovasc Dis 2014;23(2):361–6.

27. Merkler AE, Marcus JR, Gupta A, et al. Endovascular therapy for acute stroke in patients with cancer. Neurohospitalist 2014;4(3):133–5.

28. Zander T, Maynar J, Lopez-Zarraga F, et al. Mechanical thrombectomy in patients with tumour-related ischaemic stroke. Interv Neuroradiol 2016;22(6):705–8.

29. Carney BJ, Uhlmann EJ, Puligandla M, et al. Intracranial hemorrhage with direct oral anticoagulants in patients with brain tumors. J Thromb Haemost 2019; 17(1):72–6.

30. Donato J, Campigotto F, Uhlmann EJ, et al. Intracranial hemorrhage in patients with brain metastases treated with therapeutic enoxaparin: a matched cohort study. Blood 2015;126(4):494–9.

31. Horstman H, Gruhl J, Smith L, et al. Safety of long-term anticoagulation in patients with brain metastases. Med Oncol 2018;35(4):43.

32. Bang OY, Chung JW, Lee MJ, et al. Cancer-Related Stroke: An Emerging Subtype of Ischemic Stroke with Unique Pathomechanisms. J Stroke 2020;22(1):1–10.

33. Sanz AP, Gomez JLZ. AF in Cancer Patients: A Different Need for Anticoagulation? Eur Cardiol 2019;14(1):65–7.

34. Ntaios G, Papavasileiou V, Diener HC, et al. Nonvitamin-K-antagonist oral anticoagulants in patients with atrial fibrillation and previous stroke or transient ischemic attack: a systematic review and meta-analysis of randomized controlled trials. Stroke 2012;43(12):3298–304.

35. Ruff CT, Giugliano RP, Braunwald E, et al. Comparison of the efficacy and safety of new oral anticoagulants with warfarin in patients with atrial fibrillation: a meta-analysis of randomised trials. Lancet 2014;383(9921):955–62.

36. Shah S, Norby FL, Datta YH, et al. Comparative effectiveness of direct oral anticoagulants and warfarin in patients with cancer and atrial fibrillation. Blood Adv 2018;2(3):200–9.

37. Melloni C, Dunning A, Granger CB, et al. Efficacy and Safety of Apixaban Versus Warfarin in Patients with Atrial Fibrillation and a History of Cancer: Insights from the ARISTOTLE Trial. Am J Med 2017;130(12):1440–1448 e1.

38. Laube ES, Yu A, Gupta D, et al. Rivaroxaban for Stroke Prevention in Patients With Nonvalvular Atrial Fibrillation and Active Cancer. Am J Cardiol 2017;120(2): 213–7.

39. Jang H, Lee JJ, Lee MJ, et al. Comparison of Enoxaparin and Warfarin for Secondary Prevention of Cancer-Associated Stroke. J Oncol 2015;2015:502089.

40. Raskob GE, van Es N, Verhamme P, et al. Edoxaban for the Treatment of Cancer-Associated Venous Thromboembolism. N Engl J Med 2017;378(7):615–24.

41. Nam KW, Kim CK, Kim TJ, et al. Treatment of Cryptogenic Stroke with Active Cancer with a New Oral Anticoagulant. J Stroke Cerebrovasc Dis 2017;26(12): 2976–80.

42. Schrader B, Barth H, Lang EW, et al. Spontaneous intracranial haematomas caused by neoplasms. Acta Neurochir (Wien) 2000;142(9):979–85.

43. Licata B, Turazzi S. Bleeding cerebral neoplasms with symptomatic hematoma. J Neurosurg Sci 2003;47(4):201–10 [discussion: 10].

44. Navi BB, Reichman JS, Berlin D, et al. Intracerebral and subarachnoid hemorrhage in patients with cancer. Neurology 2010;74(6):494–501.

45. Raizer JJ, DeAngelis LM. Cerebral sinus thrombosis diagnosed by MRI and MR venography in cancer patients. Neurology 2000;54(6):1222–6.

46. Saposnik G, Barinagarrementeria F, Brown RD Jr, et al. Diagnosis and management of cerebral venous thrombosis: a statement for healthcare professionals from the American Heart Association/American Stroke Association. Stroke 2011;42(4):1158–92.

47. Oldfield EH, Merrill MJ. Apoplexy of pituitary adenomas: the perfect storm. J Neurosurg 2015;122(6):1444–9.

48. Johnston PC, Hamrahian AH, Weil RJ, et al. Pituitary tumor apoplexy. J Clin Neurosci 2015;22(6):939–44.

49. Ruda R, Bello L, Duffau H, et al. Seizures in low-grade gliomas: natural history, pathogenesis, and outcome after treatments. Neuro Oncol 2012;14(Suppl 4): iv55–64.

50. Kerkhof M, Vecht CJ. Seizure characteristics and prognostic factors of gliomas. Epilepsia 2013;54(Suppl 9):12–7.

51. van Breemen MS, Wilms EB, Vecht CJ. Epilepsy in patients with brain tumours: epidemiology, mechanisms, and management. Lancet Neurol 2007;6(5):421–30.

52. Kong X, Guan J, Yang Y, et al. A meta-analysis: Do prophylactic antiepileptic drugs in patients with brain tumors decrease the incidence of seizures? Clin Neurol Neurosurg 2015;134:98–103.

53. Sirven JI, Wingerchuk DM, Drazkowski JF, et al. Seizure prophylaxis in patients with brain tumors: a meta-analysis. Mayo Clin Proc 2004;79(12):1489–94.

54. Glantz MJ, Cole BF, Forsyth PA, et al. Practice parameter: anticonvulsant prophylaxis in patients with newly diagnosed brain tumors. Report of the Quality Standards Subcommittee of the American Academy of Neurology. Neurology 2000; 54(10):1886–93.

55. Laccheo I, Sonmezturk H, Bhatt AB, et al. Non-convulsive status epilepticus and non-convulsive seizures in neurological ICU patients. Neurocrit Care 2015;22(2): 202–11.

56. Brophy GM, Bell R, Claassen J, et al. Guidelines for the evaluation and management of status epilepticus. Neurocrit Care 2012;17(1):3–23.

57. Claassen J, Lokin JK, Fitzsimmons BF, et al. Predictors of functional disability and mortality after status epilepticus. Neurology 2002;58(1):139–42.

58. DeLorenzo RJ, Hauser WA, Towne AR, et al. A prospective, population-based epidemiologic study of status epilepticus in Richmond, Virginia. Neurology 1996;46(4):1029–35.

59. Towne AR, Pellock JM, Ko D, et al. Determinants of mortality in status epilepticus. Epilepsia 1994;35(1):27–34.

60. Kapur J, Elm J, Chamberlain JM, et al. Randomized Trial of Three Anticonvulsant Medications for Status Epilepticus. N Engl J Med 2019;381(22):2103–13.

61. Treiman DM, Meyers PD, Walton NY, et al. A comparison of four treatments for generalized convulsive status epilepticus. Veterans Affairs Status Epilepticus Cooperative Study Group. N Engl J Med 1998;339(12):792–8.

62. Vecht CJ, Wagner GL, Wilms EB. Interactions between antiepileptic and chemotherapeutic drugs. Lancet Neurol 2003;2(7):404–9.

63. Chang EF, Potts MB, Keles GE, et al. Seizure characteristics and control following resection in 332 patients with low-grade gliomas. J Neurosurg 2008;108(2):227–35.

64. Choi JY, Chang JW, Park YG, et al. A retrospective study of the clinical outcomes and significant variables in the surgical treatment of temporal lobe tumor associated with intractable seizures. Stereotact Funct Neurosurg 2004;82(1):35–42.

65. Englot DJ, Berger MS, Barbaro NM, et al. Predictors of seizure freedom after resection of supratentorial low-grade gliomas. A review. J Neurosurg 2011;115(2):240–4.

66. Cole JS, Patchell RA. Metastatic epidural spinal cord compression. Lancet Neurol 2008;7(5):459–66.

67. Kumar A, Weber MH, Gokaslan Z, et al. Metastatic spinal cord compression and steroid treatment. Clin Spine Surg 2017;30(4):156–63.

68. Sorensen S, Helweg-Larsen S, Mouridsen H, et al. Effect of high-dose dexamethasone in carcinomatous metastatic spinal cord compression treated with radiotherapy: a randomised trial. Eur J Cancer 1994;30A(1):22–7.

69. Ropper AE, Ropper AH. Acute Spinal Cord Compression. N Engl J Med 2017;376(14):1358–69.

70. Rades D, Abrahm JL. The role of radiotherapy for metastatic epidural spinal cord compression. Nat Rev Clin Oncol 2010;7(10):590–8.

71. Tabouret E, Cauvin C, Fuentès S, et al. Reassessment of scoring systems and prognostic factors for metastatic spinal cord compression. Spine J 2015;15 5:944–50.

72. Patchell RA, Tibbs PA, Regine WF, et al. Direct decompressive surgical resection in the treatment of spinal cord compression caused by metastatic cancer: a randomised trial. Lancet 2005;366(9486):643–8.

73. Levin VA, Bidaut L, Hou P, et al. Randomized double-blind placebo-controlled trial of bevacizumab therapy for radiation necrosis of the central nervous system. Int J Radiat Oncol Biol Phys 2011;79(5):1487–95.

74. Wen PY, Macdonald DR, Reardon DA, et al. Updated response assessment criteria for high-grade gliomas: response assessment in neuro-oncology working group. J Clin Oncol 2010;28(11):1963–72.

75. Rahman R, Alexander BM, Wen PY. Neurologic Complications of Cranial Radiation Therapy and Strategies to Prevent or Reduce Radiation Toxicity. Curr Neurol Neurosci Rep 2020;20(8):34.

76. Parikh NS, Burch JE, Kamel H, et al. Recurrent Thromboembolic Events after Ischemic Stroke in Patients with Primary Brain Tumors. J Stroke Cerebrovasc Dis 2017;26(10):2396–403.

77. Bompaire F, Lahutte M, Buffat S, et al. New insights in radiation-induced leukoencephalopathy: a prospective cross-sectional study. Support Care Cancer 2018; 26(12):4217–26.

78. Kerklaan JP, Lycklama a Nijeholt GJ, Wiggenraad RG, et al. SMART syndrome: a late reversible complication after radiation therapy for brain tumours. J Neurol 2011;258(6):1098–104.

79. Baker WJ, Royer GL Jr, Weiss RB. Cytarabine and neurologic toxicity. J Clin Oncol 1991;9(4):679–93.

80. Nieto Y, Cagnoni PJ, Bearman SI, et al. Acute encephalopathy: a new toxicity associated with high-dose paclitaxel. Clin Cancer Res 1999;5(3):501–6.

81. Pelgrims J, De Vos F, Van den Brande J, et al. Methylene blue in the treatment and prevention of ifosfamide-induced encephalopathy: report of 12 cases and a review of the literature. Br J Cancer 2000;82(2):291–4.

82. Tlemsani C, Mir O, Boudou-Rouquette P, et al. Posterior reversible encephalopathy syndrome induced by anti-VEGF agents. Targeted Oncol 2011;6(4):253–8.

83. Postow MA, Sidlow R, Hellmann MD. Immune-Related Adverse Events Associated with Immune Checkpoint Blockade. N Engl J Med 2018;378(2):158–68.

84. Dubey D, David WS, Reynolds KL, et al. Severe Neurological Toxicity of Immune Checkpoint Inhibitors: Growing Spectrum. Ann Neurol 2020;87(5):659–69.

85. Brahmer JR, Lacchetti C, Schneider BJ, et al. Management of immune-related adverse events in patients treated with immune checkpoint inhibitor therapy: American Society of Clinical Oncology Clinical Practice Guideline. J Clin Oncol 2018;36(17):1714.

86. Puzanov I, Diab A, Abdallah K, et al. Managing toxicities associated with immune checkpoint inhibitors: consensus recommendations from the Society for Immunotherapy of Cancer (SITC) Toxicity Management Working Group. J Immunother Cancer 2017;5(1):95.

87. Neelapu SS, Locke FL, Bartlett NL, et al. Axicabtagene Ciloleucel CAR T-Cell Therapy in Refractory Large B-Cell Lymphoma. N Engl J Med 2017;377(26): 2531–44.

88. Schuster SJ, Svoboda J, Chong EA, et al. Chimeric Antigen Receptor T Cells in Refractory B-Cell Lymphomas. N Engl J Med 2017;377(26):2545–54.

89. Gutierrez C, McEvoy C, Mead E, et al. Management of the critically ill adult chimeric antigen receptor-T cell therapy patient: a critical care perspective. Crit Care Med 2018;46(9):1402–10.

90. Gust J, Hay KA, Hanafi LA, et al. Endothelial Activation and Blood-Brain Barrier Disruption in Neurotoxicity after Adoptive Immunotherapy with CD19 CAR-T Cells. Cancer Discov 2017;7(12):1404–19.

91. Rubin DB, Danish HH, Ali AB, et al. Neurological toxicities associated with chimeric antigen receptor T-cell therapy. Brain 2019;142(5):1334–48.

92. Rubin DB, Al Jarrah A, Li K, et al. Clinical Predictors of Neurotoxicity After Chimeric Antigen Receptor T-Cell Therapy. JAMA Neurol 2020. https://doi.org/10.1001/jamaneurol.2020.2703.

93. Neelapu SS, Tummala S, Kebriaei P, et al. Chimeric antigen receptor T-cell therapy - assessment and management of toxicities. Nat Rev Clin Oncol 2018;15(1): 47–62.

94. Lee DW, Kochenderfer JN, Stetler-Stevenson M, et al. T cells expressing CD19 chimeric antigen receptors for acute lymphoblastic leukaemia in children and young adults: a phase 1 dose-escalation trial. Lancet 2015;385(9967):517–28.

95. Becker KJ, Baxter AB, Cohen WA, et al. Withdrawal of support in intracerebral hemorrhage may lead to self-fulfilling prophecies. Neurology 2001;56(6):766–72.

96. Hemphill JC 3rd, White DB. Clinical nihilism in neuroemergencies. Emerg Med Clin North Am 2009;27(1):27–37, vii–viii.
97. Wartenberg KE, Hwang DY, Haeusler KG, et al. Gap Analysis Regarding Prognostication in Neurocritical Care: A Joint Statement from the German Neurocritical Care Society and the Neurocritical Care Society. Neurocrit Care 2019;31(2): 231–44.
98. Cai X, Robinson J, Muehlschlegel S, et al. Patient preferences and surrogate decision making in neuroscience intensive care units. Neurocrit Care 2015. https://doi.org/10.1007/s12028-015-0149-2.
99. Knies AK, Hwang DY. Palliative care practice in neurocritical care. Semin Neurol 2016;36(6):631–41. https://doi.org/10.1055/s-0036-1592358.

Neuroinfectious Disease Emergencies

Caleb R.S. McEntire, MD[a], Pria Anand, MD[b],
Anna M. Cervantes-Arslanian, MD[b,c,d],*

KEYWORDS

- Neurologic infections • Neurologic emergency • Stroke • Meningitis • Encephalitis
- Acute flaccid myelitis

KEY POINTS

- Neurologic emergencies can be caused by bacterial, viral, fungal, or parasitic infections and can affect any portion of the neuraxis.
- In most neuroinfectious emergencies, prompt antimicrobial treatment significantly improves outcomes in terms of mortality and residual neurologic disability. Corticosteroids as an adjunctive to antimicrobial therapy can decrease morbidity and mortality in some disease, but in others it can potentially worsen outcomes.
- Neuroinfectious syndromes can often be difficult to distinguish from one another, and well-validated algorithms should be used to guide effective empiric treatment.
- Neurologic infections can often be complicated by secondary neurologic emergencies, notably stroke, seizure, hydrocephalus, and intracranial hypertension.
- Close communication with neurosurgery is required for effective management of many neuroinfectious emergencies because cerebrospinal fluid diversion or decompression can improve outcomes when appropriately used.

INTRODUCTION

Infections of the central nervous system (CNS) can present emergently and heterogeneously. Many CNS infections can progress rapidly without appropriate treatment and lead to secondary neurologic emergencies; thus, it is crucial to identify and treat these diseases promptly. Fortunately, infectious diseases present one of the few opportunities in neurologic critical care to treat a patient with potential for a full or near full recovery because the outcomes can often be improved significantly with appropriate

[a] Department of Neurology, Brigham and Women's Hospital, 60 Fenwood Road, 1st Floor, Boston, MA 02115, USA; [b] Department of Neurology, Boston University School of Medicine, Boston Medical Center, 72 East Concord Street Suite C3, Boston, MA 02118, USA; [c] Neurosurgery, Boston University School of Medicine, Boston Medical Center, Boston, MA, USA; [d] Medicine (Infectious Disease), Boston University School of Medicine, Boston Medical Center, Boston, MA, USA
* Corresponding author. Department of Neurology, Boston University School of Medicine, Boston Medical Center, 72 East Concord Street Suite C3, Boston, MA 02118.
E-mail address: Anna.cervantes@bmc.org

Neurol Clin 39 (2021) 565–588
https://doi.org/10.1016/j.ncl.2021.02.003
0733-8619/21/© 2021 Elsevier Inc. All rights reserved.

neurologic.theclinics.com

antimicrobial treatment. Even in those situations where no curative agent is available, supportive therapy can decrease the risk of future death or disability. Acute care neurologists must develop familiarity with neuroinfectious pathogens, the emergent syndromes they cause, and the use of empiric treatments that could significantly change the trajectory of a patient's survival and recovery.

MENINGITIS

Meningitis is an inflammatory disease of the subarachnoid space and meninges that commonly presents with headache, fever, and meningismus. Viral pathogens are the most common cause of meningitis, but are generally less morbid than bacterial etiologies.[1,2] The most common causes of viral meningitis worldwide vary by region; enteroviruses seem to be the most common cause of the syndrome in the United States specifically,[3] and echovirus 30 in particular is a common cause in the UK,[4] whereas varicella zoster virus may be the most common in Denmark.[5] Meningitis of any cause can present subtly and may rapidly progress, leading to significant morbidity and mortality if not treated promptly.

Bacterial Meningitis

Epidemiology

The annual incidence of acute bacterial meningitis (ABM) in adults in the United States has decreased significantly with the introduction of routine immunization using the *Haemophilus influenzae*, meningococcal, 7-valent *Streptococcus pneumoniae*, and 13-valent pneumococcal vaccines since 1990. These vaccines are more than 95% effective, and have significantly decreased disease prevalence in countries where they are widely used.[6–10] Incidence in the United States is now estimated at about 1.38 cases per 100,000 individuals,[11] but in some regions of the world the incidence can be orders of magnitude higher. In the so-called meningitis belt located in the Sahel region of north Africa, meningitis epidemics (predominantly caused by serogroup A meningococcus) occur as often as every 8 to 12 years, often lasting multiple years each and affecting an estimated 100 to 800 per 100,000 individuals, or as many as 1 per 100 individuals in some more severely affected communities.[12,13] Although the diagnosis of ABM may be more or less likely depending on geographic prevalence and rates of vaccination, given the potentially devastating consequences of untreated infection, empiric therapy should be considered in all suspected cases regardless of location.

Clinical presentation and diagnosis

A 2004 prospective study of 696 individuals with community-acquired ABM found that the most common presenting signs and symptoms included headache (87%), nuchal rigidity (83%), a fever of greater than 38°C (77%), a Glasgow Coma scale of less than 14 (69%), and nausea (62%). Ninety-5% of patients had at least 2 of these findings, 4% had only 1, and only 1% of individuals had none of these signs and symptoms on presentation.[14]

Thus, the classic triad of fever, nuchal rigidity, and acutely altered mental status occurs in only a minority of patients and may vary based on both host- and pathogen-specific factors, including age and organism. Estimates of the frequency of these findings range from 36% in individuals less than 60 years of age to 58% of patients older than 60 years. The triad is significantly more likely to appear in meningococcal meningitis (58%) than in pneumococcal meningitis (27%).[15,16]

More severe manifestations of ABM can include seizures, coma, and focal neurologic deficits, and the likelihood of progression to these complications is organism dependent. Individuals with pneumococcal meningitis are more likely to develop any of the 3 of these features during the course of their illness than individuals with meningococcal meningitis.[17,18] Individuals with CNS listeriosis are less likely to present with characteristic signs of meningeal irritation, but are more likely to develop seizures and focal neurologic deficits early in the course of disease. These patients can also present with ataxia and cranial nerve palsies in the context of a rhombencephalitis.[19,20]

Listeria monocytogenes can cause meningoencephalitis or (more rarely) meningitis without parenchymal involvement primarily in pregnant women, infants less than 2 years of age, or adults more than 60 years of age.[19,21] Up to 84% of individuals with CNS listeriosis present with a syndrome of meningoencephalitis, most commonly including signs of fever and altered mental status. The characteristic rhombencephalitis syndrome often associated with CNS listeriosis may present in as few as 17% of patients according to several large-scale reviews of the disease over the past 2 decades, and absence of brainstem signs cannot reliably rule out the infection.[19,20]

The diagnosis of suspected ABM should begin with serum cell counts and blood culture, which will grow organisms in 50% to 90% of cases.[15,18] Every individual with suspected meningitis should have a cerebrospinal fluid (CSF) analysis with cell counts, protein, glucose, and culture through lumbar puncture (LP), unless there is a specific contraindication such as uncontrollable coagulopathy or concerns for a focal lesion with a mass effect. Chemistry should be drawn at the same time for comparison of serum and CSF glucose. The panel may also show other metabolic derangements that frequently accompany ABM, including hyponatremia, which is found in more than 50% of children with ABM.[22] CSF characteristics predictive of bacterial meningitis include a ratio of CSF to serum glucose of less than 0.23, a protein level of greater than 220 mg/dL, and a white cell count of greater than 2000/mm^3. At least one of these findings is present in up to 88% of individuals with bacterial meningitis. Opening pressure on LP is most often elevated, with a normal (<200 mm of water) opening pressure seen in only 20% of patients. Individuals with opening pressure of greater than 400 mm of water more often present in coma.[15,23]

Imaging has relatively low usefulness in the diagnosis of ABM. The majority of contrast-enhanced computed tomography (CT) scans are normal,[24] and one-half of contrast-enhanced MRI scans are normal.[25,26] The signs of meningitis that MRI can show, such as T2 hypointensities in subcortical white matter[27] and enhancement of the subarachnoid spaces,[28] are nonspecific.[25]

LP can be obtained in most patients, but a CT scan should be obtained first in cases with papilledema, new seizure, focal neurologic deficit, or other findings suggestive of increased intracranial pressure (ICP).[29] Herniation accounts for up to 30% of mortalities in ABM and there is a strong temporal association between LP and herniation.[30,31] Therefore, in select patients presenting with fulminant ABM with poor examination and imaging concerns for diffuse edema or hydrocephalus, there may be a role for placement of an external ventricular drain to identify an organism, determine the ICP, and therapeutically drain CSF in cases where the ICP is increased. It is important to note that individuals with severely symptomatic initial clinical presentations of ABM are particularly susceptible to rapid deterioration without prompt treatment initiation.[32] Thus, diagnostic testing should not delay the administration of antibiotic therapy and corticosteroids, and all individuals with suspected meningitis should have blood cultures drawn and empiric therapy administered as soon as possible.[33]

Management

The mainstay of treatment for ABM is prompt initiation of antibiotic therapy. The relative prevalence of different pathogens can vary by location; in the United States, S pneumoniae accounts for the majority of cases, and Neisseria meningitidis is a close second, accounting for a combined 70% to 90% of cases.[15,34] In the meningitis belt of north Africa, H influenzae is the most common pathogen, followed closely by S pneumoniae.[13,35] As noted elsewhere in this article, CNS listeriosis can affect vulnerable individuals in many climates. Empiric antibiotic regimens can thus be tailored to host factors and local antibiograms, but an initial regimen for most immunocompetent individuals with normal renal function includes a combination of vancomycin and a third-generation cephalosporin.[36] Empiric coverage for neurolisteriosis with ampicillin should also be included for appropriate patients, because a delay in treatment has been associated with worsened outcomes.[19,37,38]

Several large-scale studies have examined the efficacy of corticosteroids as an adjunct to antimicrobials in ABM, finding that the treatment does improve morbidity and mortality in some groups of patients. The European Dexamethasone in Adulthood Bacterial Meningitis Study, a double-blind, placebo-controlled study of 301 patients with bacterial meningitis, showed a significant decrease in mortality (7% vs 15%) and all unfavorable acute outcomes (15% vs 25%) in the dexamethasone versus placebo groups, although these benefits were only seen in patients with S pneumoniae meningitis.[39] In a follow-up study of these patients at a median of 8 years after the initial presentation, no significant differences were found in long-term outcomes, including persistent cognitive dysfunction or hearing loss.[40] A separate follow-up study at 13 years showed that no additional benefits in morbidity or mortality were seen after 8 weeks, suggesting that dexamethasone's beneficial effects are seen only in the initial period.[41]

A larger meta-analysis of 623 patients from other studies similarly showed a significant decrease in mortality and neurologic sequelae in S pneumoniae meningitis with corticosteroid administration, with a nonsignificant decrease in meningitis caused by N meningitidis or other pathogens.[42] Of note, although a single study of patients with bacterial meningitis did show unfavorable outcomes associated with dexamethasone administration, this study did not control for disease severity and was likely influenced by a higher frequency of steroid use in patients with concomitant clinical deterioration who were more likely to have poor outcomes.[15] Our recommendation is that dexamethasone should be administered to all adults with suspected ABM and an unknown pathogen, and that it be continued for patients with CSF or blood cultures confirming S pneumoniae infection.

Emergent complications

Stroke. Ischemic stroke in the setting of infectious vasculitis can occur in 14% to 25% of individuals with ABM, although this can range from 9% in meningococcal meningitis to 36% in pneumococcal meningitis and is associated with poor prognosis, including a higher mortality.[43–45] Aneurysm formation, intracerebral hemorrhage, and venous sinus thrombosis have all been described as well, although they are much rarer.[43,46–49] The timing of stroke is highly variable and may not be prevented by the initiation of appropriate antibiotic therapy. Advanced age at presentation, immunocompromise, having otitis media or sinusitis before diagnosis of ABM, a lower level of consciousness on admission, and a low CSF white blood cell (WBC) count have all been associated with an increased risk of stroke.[45,50,51] There are no robust studies looking at the primary or secondary prevention of stroke in ABM, although some extrapolation may be made from a small randomized study using aspirin in the context of tuberculous meningitis (TBM).[52] A small series of ABM in children suggests the use of heparin and aspirin for secondary prevention may be safe.[53] Stroke in ABM can be attributed to many causes, including a hypercoagulable state, endothelial dysfunction, immune-mediated vasospasm or thrombosis, and acute vasculitis. There is an uncertain benefit to using steroids or other immunomodulatory drugs in these cases.[54,55] Transcranial Doppler ultrasound examination is a noninvasive way to routinely assess for increased cerebral blood flow velocities as a screen for vasculitis[55] and we often use this modality to monitor patients with more severe ABM.

Seizure. Seizures complicate ABM in 17% to 27% of adults.[17,56,57] Seizures are associated with an increased risk of persistent neurologic deficits and in-hospital mortality, which occurs in 41% of ABM patients with seizures compared with 16% of those without seizures.[17] In addition, seizure during the acute phase of illness can predispose patients to a long-term risk of epilepsy, even after convalescence from acute infection.[17] Factors associated with seizure include lower CSF WBC count, elevated CSF total protein, and elevated serum erythrocyte sedimentation rate. Pneumococcal meningitis, alcohol use, diabetes, and ABM-associated stroke also increase risk of seizure development.[32,46,58] Most studies do not suggest the use of routine seizure prophylaxis in all ABM patients, but given the high morbidity of seizures when they do occur, the threshold for beginning antiepileptic drugs should be low in patients with predisposing factors or clinical evidence of seizure. We advocate for routine use of continuous electroencephalogram monitoring for any patients with a depressed mental status without clear structural explanation, because the risk of nonconvulsive status epilepticus in critically ill patients is high.[59]

Intracranial hypertension and cerebral edema. Intracranial hypertension is likely under-recognized in ABM patients and may be responsible for the persistence of poor outcomes in some patients with ABM despite early antibiotics and supportive care. Cerebral herniation occurs in up to 5% of all individuals with ABM, and has been reported at autopsy in approximately 30% of individuals who die from the condition.[30,60]

An increased ICP is more common in patients who present with a Glasgow coma scale of less than 9, and admission to the neurointensive care unit is indicated in the case of seizures or signs of brainstem dysfunction.[61–63] There have been several studies investigating the routine use of hyperosmolar therapies, most often glycerol,[64] to empirically treat potentially elevated ICP, but these have not shown benefit for all patients. Of note, a CT scan of the brain has consistently been shown to be nonpredictive of increased ICP in ABM, and a negative CT scan should not preclude the initiation of ICP monitoring when otherwise indicated.[65,66] The use of ICP monitors in selected patients with ABM for either ICP– or cerebral perfusion pressure–directed therapy has been shown to decrease mortality and neurologic sequalae, including hearing loss or disability.[62,67–70] It has been our practice to consider ICP monitoring (either through an intraparenchymal monitor or an external ventricular drain) in patients who present in a coma (Glasgow coma scale of <8).

Hydrocephalus. Hydrocephalus complicates 3% to 21% of patients with ABM and is associated with worsened neurologic outcomes and mortality.[71–73] In the majority of patients, hydrocephalus is present on hospital admission[71] and is associated with increased age and worse level of consciousness at admission.[72] Elevated CSF protein may cause communicating hydrocephalus through increased viscosity, leading to decreased absorption of CSF through the arachnoid villi. High CSF protein as well as enlarged ventricular size, even without clinically apparent hydrocephalus, are risk factors for mortality in ABM.[74] Despite the association with poor outcomes, early treatment with external ventricular drainage and eventual permanent shunting can lead to successful outcomes, with some patients achieving a near full neurologic recovery.[72]

Cryptococcal Meningitis

Epidemiology

Cryptococcosis is an infection caused by the yeast form of the basidiomycetous fungi *Cryptococcus neoformans* and *Cryptococcus gattii*, heavily encapsulated obligate aerobes that are most commonly associated with pulmonary disease, meningitis, and fungal mass lesions known as cryptococcomas. *C neoformans* causes the majority of clinical infection, accounting for up to 95% of cases, and is primarily associated with immunocompromised patients, but can also infect apparently immunocompetent hosts with CNS involvement.[75,76] *C gattii* generally infects immunocompetent hosts, although both subclinical immune defects and more clinically evident immunodeficiency both seem to be risk factors for infection in some individuals.[75,77–79]

Cryptococcal meningitis generally follows inhalation of *C neoformans* or *C gattii* spores from soil, especially near birds such as pigeons, with subsequent hematogenous spread from the lungs to the CNS.[80] The most common risk factor for the development of the disease is HIV infection, but it can occur with a variety of immunosuppressive etiologies, including solid organ transplants, hematologic malignancies, use of ibrutinib, sarcoidosis, and glucocorticoid therapies.[81]

Clinical presentation and diagnosis

The presentation of cryptococcal meningitis can be indolent with progressive worsening over months, but also can present with acute decompensation over days. The most common presenting symptoms are nonspecific, such as headache and fever, which can make prompt diagnosis challenging.[76] Seizures and focal deficits occur in greater than 10% of patients, commonly those that have cryptococcomas (discussed elsewhere in this article).

The CSF in cryptococcal meningitis typically shows an elevated WBC count with lymphocytic predominance, elevated protein, and a low ratio of CSF to serum glucose. The opening pressure is often markedly elevated. CSF should be sent for fungal culture, cryptococcal antigen testing, and India ink staining. Serum cryptococcal antigen is also recommended by the World Health Organization.[82–84]

MRI can show leptomeningeal enhancement in both immunosuppressed and immunocompetent individuals, and can additionally show dilated Virchow–Robin spaces and pseudocysts in the former and intraventricular cystic lesions in the latter.[85,86]

Management of cryptococcal infection

Treatment for cryptococcal meningitis should begin immediately with intravenous amphotericin B and flucytosine in areas where these therapies are accessible. In many resource-scarce areas, these agents may be difficult to find, in which case high-dose fluconazole plus flucytosine can be used as an oral regimen, or amphotericin B plus fluconazole can be used if intravenous therapies are feasible but flucytosine is unavailable.[87–90] The empiric use of steroids is not recommended and may be harmful.[91]

Emergent complications

Intracranial hypertension and hydrocephalus. A common notable feature of cryptococcal meningitis is persistent elevated ICP, which is most often related to hydrocephalus. As noted elsewhere in this article, the opening pressure in cryptococcal meningitis is frequently increased, and patients with cryptococcal meningitis often require daily large-volume LP for therapeutic removal of CSF until the closing pressure is within the normal range. Therapeutic LP significantly improves outcomes of morbidity and mortality, and should be performed daily as needed in individuals with clinical signs of increased ICP and persistent opening pressures of at least

25cmH2O in cryptococcal meningitis of the CSF.[92,93] Some patients may require longer term CSF diversion.[94,95] The adjunct use of hyperosmolar therapies may show benefit, but have not been studied rigorously.[96,97] Acetazolamide is not an effective agent for control of increased ICP in cryptococcal meningitis, may cause increased adverse events, and should not be used.[98]

Tuberculous Meningitis

Clinical presentation and diagnosis

TBM is a challenging entity in the acute care setting because it can be difficult to distinguish from other causes of meningitis and because of potential adverse consequences of empiric antituberculous therapy. Multiple retrospective and prospective studies have examined optimal risk stratification for TBM.[99–101] One study in a resource-limited, high-prevalence area used risk stratification data gathered from retrospective analysis of 251 adults and applied these prospectively to 75 adults presenting with signs and symptoms of meningitis, demonstrating 86% sensitivity and 79% specificity. The 5 risk factors used to risk stratify in this study were age (<36 years old), duration of symptoms ($\geq$6 days), serum WBC count (>15,000 cells/mm^3), CSF WBC count (<750 cells/mm^3), and CSF neutrophil proportion (<90%).[102]

Beyond the use of CSF cell count and differential to discriminate between TBM and non-TBM, CSF culture has little usefulness in the diagnosis of TBM in the acute setting. Even with large volumes of CSF, acid fast bacilli visualization by microscopy is approximately 15% sensitive and culture is only 50% to 60% sensitive after 2 to 4 weeks of growth.[103] The Xpert MTB/RIF quantitative polymerase chain reaction of CSF can return results in less than 24 hours from first clinical contact with a patient. This test yields sensitivity 47% with uncentrifuged CSF samples and 82% with centrifuged CSF samples as well as a specificity of 95%, and so may offer a useful rule-in test for TB in high-burden areas.[104]

In 1 study of 61 patients, only approximately 10% reported a history of pulmonary TB, and pulmonary findings cannot reliably discriminate TBM from other causes.[105] TB seems to affect the CNS in 10% of active infections.[106] This number is increased by up to 5-fold in individuals with HIV infection, and is even further increased among those with a CD4+ cell count of less than 100 cells/mL.[107]

Management

TBM should be treated promptly with 4-drug antituberculous therapy, including rifampin, isoniazid, pyrazinamide, and either ethambutol or streptomycin. Because CNS penetration of both ethambutol and streptomycin is poor[108] and no large-scale randomized studies have examined them head to head, there is no uniform consensus on which agent is more effective, although the World Health Organization recommendations are for streptomycin rather than ethambutol.[109] Corticosteroids significantly decrease death and disabling residual neurologic deficits among survivors, and in an observational study that performed serial MRIs on patients with TBM with or without dexamethasone treatment, the dexamethasone group showed a stroke rate of 27% compared with 58% in the placebo group.[110,111]

Emergent complications

Stroke. Patients with TBM are at high risk of ischemic stroke compared with the general population, whether or not they have received treatment for the underlying infection. Stroke can occur in 15% to 60% of individuals who acquire tuberculosis and is almost invariably ischemic, although hemorrhage can also rarely be seen.[112,113] The clinical syndrome seen most frequently in stroke secondary to TB involves the tubercular zone of the caudate head, anteromedial thalami, and anterior limb and genu of the internal capsule in up to 75% of patients, rarely manifesting with cortical signs such as aphasia or apraxia.[113,114] Because patients with TBM are often altered or obtunded, the recognition of more subtle focal signs can be difficult and rapid imaging is essential if there is any suspicion for a cerebrovascular event. Aspirin provides a modest decrease in the absolute mortality in individuals with TBM-associated stroke, and so our practice is to give aspirin 81 mg/d to patients with TBM.[52]

Hydrocephalus. TBM can result in obstructive or communicating hydrocephalus, the former when a tuberculoma or inflammation of the cerebral aqueduct impedes CSF flow and the latter when the inflammatory process extends to the basilar cisterns and impedes CSF circulation and resorption. This can be the presenting symptom in up to one-third of patients, although it can also occur late in the course of disease, even after the initiation of antituberculous medications.[115,116] External ventricular drains are often needed in acute management, with some patients needing definitive treatment by shunting or ventriculostomy.[117]

Encephalitis. Encephalitis refers to an inflammation of the brain parenchyma and may present with heterogenous signs and symptoms, including altered mental status, seizures, and focal neurologic signs. Some clinical features are suggestive of one or more specific pathogens: pharyngeal spasms and hyperactivity combined with opisthotonos could suggest rabies infection; behavioral dysregulation could be consistent with herpes simplex virus; and tremor of the eyelids, tongue, lips, or extremities could suggest West Nile virus. Encephalitis displays a notable seasonal variation, depending on the causative pathogen, and a causative organism is never identified in up to 40% to 60% of cases.[118] Although accurate estimates of the incidence are thus difficult to obtain, its overall incidence is lower than that of meningitis.[119] Mortality can be high owing to cerebral edema as a consequence of widespread parenchymal inflammation, and empiric therapy for potentially treatable viruses should be initiated early and continued until an alternative etiology is identified.

Herpes Simplex Virus

Clinical presentation and diagnosis
Worldwide, herpes simplex virus is the most common identified causative pathogen of encephalitis. When left untreated, herpes simplex encephalitis can have a mortality rate of up to 70%, with significant morbidity in survivors. Even with optimal treatment, mortality can approach 20%.[120,121] Presentation of the syndrome in the majority of patients is with fever in addition to a variety of neurologic findings that can include altered mentation, cranial nerve deficits, cortical signs, and seizures.

The diagnosis of herpes simplex encephalitis should made be with LP and MRI. A CSF analysis generally shows lymphocytic pleocytosis, high red blood cell count, and elevated protein. Importantly, however, a normal CSF profile can occur both early in the disease process and in some patients on tumor necrosis factor-alpha inhibitors or other immunomodulatory therapies, and empiric treatment should not be halted based solely on an unremarkable CSF analysis.[122–125] Herpes simplex virus-1 polymerase chain reaction in CSF is 98% sensitive and 94% specific compared with the gold standard of brain biopsy and can result rapidly, although empiric treatment should not be delayed while awaiting a result. The highest sensitivity for polymerase chain reaction is 2 to 10 days after the onset of illness.[126]

MRI typically shows unilateral temporal lobe lesions that can have an associated mass effect. In a study of 251 patients with temporal lobe encephalitis, bilateral temporal lobe involvement ($P = .01$) and involvement outside the temporal lobes, cingulate, or insula (P = .005) were associated with a lower odds of herpes simplex encephalitis compared with other causes.[127] Imaging may be more sensitive and specific than CSF analysis early in the disease, but can also have false negatives.[128]

Management

Early treatment of herpes simplex virus encephalitis with intravenous acyclovir decreases morbidity and mortality compared with late administration.[126,129,130] Some studies have suggested that corticosteroids may decrease morbidity and mortality in herpes simplex virus cases with significant mass effect or edema,[131,132] although no high-powered evidence exists for this. Currently, guidelines from the Infectious Diseases Society of America recommend further research on the role of corticosteroids in the treatment of herpes simplex encephalitis,[133] whereas the Association of British Neurologists and British Infection Association National Guidelines endorse that steroids may have a role in herpes simplex encephalitis treatment with class C–III evidence.[131,134] Given that all diagnostic modalities can be falsely negative early in the disease course when treatment will offer the highest benefit, acyclovir should be started in any patient with a clinical suspicion for encephalitis and intravenous corticosteroids may be considered in any patients with clinical or imaging evidence of a mass effect.

Management of intracranial hypertension and malignant edema in encephalitis

Bacterial and viral encephalitides can both cause malignant edema and life-threatening intracranial hypertension, and in these cases ICP monitoring and surgical management may improve outcomes drastically. There are little direct data on ICP monitoring in encephalitis.[135,136] One encephalitis center found that the use of ICP monitors combined with hyperosmolar therapy may have an association with lower mortality.[137] Similar to other intracranial pathologies, if a patient's examination is limited and the risk of intracranial hypertension is high, the placement of a monitor may help to tailor therapy.

A systematic review encompassing 48 patients with encephalitis owing to viral (54%), bacterial (19%), or unknown/other (27%) pathogens treated with decompressive craniectomy demonstrated a significant decrease in both mortality and residual neurologic deficits compared with similar cohorts that had not received surgical intervention. There was a significant association between viral encephalitis and a favorable outcome when compared with bacterial encephalitis. Although the data quality is limited by selection bias, it does suggest that craniectomy could improve outcomes in some patients with viral encephalitis and severe mass effect. Further research in this area could help to clarify which factors classify individuals who stand to benefit from craniectomy.[138]

Coronavirus Disease 2019

Coronavirus disease 2019 (COVID-19) has rapidly become recognized as a multisystem illness, with known effects on virtually every organ system. Neurologic manifestations of COVID-19 are broad and may include emergent presentations such a seizure, cerebrovascular events, and meningoencephalitis.[139–153] These complications may result from direct invasion of the CNS by severe acute respiratory syndrome coronavirus 2, inflammation, hypercoagulable state, or as a result of critical illness and systemic infection. No specific treatments exist for the neurologic complications of COVID-19. However, limited data suggest that tissue plasminogen activator may be safe and effective in the treatment of COVID-19–associated stroke, and infection should not preclude the acute treatment of cerebrovascular events.[154] There have also been several reports of successful treatment of a parainfectious encephalitis with steroids.[155-157] For a further discussion of the management of COVID-19 related neurologic emergencies, please see Julie G. Shulman and colleagues' article, "Neurologic Emergencies During the COVID-19 Pandemic," in this volume.

INFECTIOUS INTRACRANIAL MASS LESIONS
Clinical Presentation

Infectious mass lesions in the brain can be caused by a variety of bacterial, fungal, parasitic, or viral pathogens. Infectious abscesses of any etiology occur in up to 0.3 to 1.3 per 100,000 people per year among immunocompetent hosts, with higher rates among immunocompromised hosts.[158] Intracranial abscess can present with heterogeneous symptoms depending on the location of the lesion or lesions, but the most common presenting features are the relatively nonspecific triad of headache, fever, and focal neurologic deficit. Headache is the most common of these 3 symptoms, occurring in up to 69% of patients with a bacterial abscess. Fever and focal neurologic deficits each occur in only one-half of patients at presentation. Neck stiffness occurs in 15% of patients and usually reflects either occipital abscess or rupture of the abscess contents into the ventricles.[159] Importantly, the classic triad of headache, fever, and focal neurologic deficit is present in only about 20% of patients with intracranial infectious mass lesions.[159]

Bacterial Abscess

Diagnosis

Diagnosis should begin with cranial imaging, either a CT scan with contrast or MRI with contrast, depending on the patient's clinical stability. Diagnosis of the underlying pathogen can be determined with blood and CSF cultures in only about one-quarter of patients, and can take days to result. A CSF Gram stain can often take several hours to return results depending on the testing facility, and medical treatment should not be delayed while awaiting testing.[160] In many cases, aspiration of the abscess is the only mechanism for identifying the pathogen.

Causative pathogens for intracranial bacterial abscesses can vary depending on the route of introduction. Abscess after mechanical disruption of the skull and blood–brain barrier, as with head trauma or neurosurgery, is often caused by skin-colonizing bacteria including Staphylococcus aureus, S epidermidis, or gram-negative bacilli.[161] Abscesses secondary to parameningeal infectious sources such as the paranasal sinuses or middle ears are most often owing to streptococcus species.[159] In cases of hematogenous spread, the primary infection often determines the causative organism in the abscess. For instance, odontogenic infections can lead to abscesses with typical oral flora such as Fusobacterium, Streptococcus, and Bacillus species,[162,163] and endocarditis can seed abscesses with viridans streptococci and S aureus.[164] Nocardia asteroides can lead to intracranial abscess after inhalation of soil-dwelling spores, colonization of the lungs, and subsequent hematogenous spread to the brain.[165]

Management

Immediate initiation of antibiotic therapy for bacterial brain abscesses is crucial, because each day of treatment delay can result in up to a 50% increase in mortality.[166] In some limited cases, such as stable patients without severe disease and for whom surgery is imminent, there may be value in delaying antibiotics until after abscess drainage to maximize the yield of pathogen identification within the stereotactic aspirate.[160,166] Neurosurgery should generally be contacted at the time of the initial diagnosis of any intracranial abscess.[167] Urgent surgical intervention should be considered in patients with rapidly progressive neurologic deficits in the context of an intracranial mass effect or proximity of abscess to a ventricle.[168]

Empiric treatment for the condition usually consists of a third- or fourth-generation cephalosporin plus vancomycin and metronidazole to cover the most likely culprit bacteria. For patients with a known parameningeal focus of infection and no history of head trauma or neurosurgery, empiric treatment can comprise ceftriaxone or cefotaxime plus metronidazole, adding vancomycin only if staphylococcal infection is specifically suspected (e.g., with potential source of seeding from skin).[160]

Fungal Abscess

Fungal species are responsible for up to 90% of brain abscesses in solid organ transplant recipients, and fungal abscesses can occur in up to 5% of all allogeneic stem cell transplant recipients.[169,170] Some fungal species including both more common systemic pathogens like aspergillus[171] and cryptococcus[172,173] as well as many dematiaceous molds, most notably *Cladophialophora bantiana*,[174–176] can also cause abscesses in immunocompetent hosts, although this infection is quite rare. Regardless of host characteristics and fungal species, intracranial fungal abscesses are highly morbid.

Aspergillosis

CNS aspergillosis occurs most often in individuals with prolonged neutropenia or immunosuppression in the setting of AIDS, patients with poorly controlled diabetes, or recipients of hematopoietic stem cell or solid organ transplants, although it has also been described rarely in immunocompetent individuals.[177,178] The disease can occur in the setting of disseminated infection or secondary to direct spread from the paranasal sinuses. Fungal invasion into the lumen of the cerebral vasculature can also lead to proximal vessel thrombosis that results in large territory infarcts and intracranial hemorrhage.[179,180] The diagnosis can be assisted with detection of galactomannan antigen and $1,3-\beta$-D-glucan in CSF, although these findings are nonspecific and may also be positive in the setting of some other fungal pathogens.[181,182]

Serum galactomannan antigen is effective in the detection of invasive aspergillosis, with positive and negative predictive values ranging from 85% to 93% and 95% to 98.7%, respectively, although it does not provide discrimination between CNS and other infections.[182,183] In patients with a high susceptibility to CNS aspergillosis, such as bone marrow transplant recipients, positive serum galactomannan antigenemia can precede clinical features, and so tracking this even in asymptomatic patients is reasonable.[184]

CNS involvement of *Aspergillus* spp. can occur with or without systemic or pulmonary infection, and the disease may present with seizures or focal neurologic signs. The most effective treatment is voriconazole, which improves outcomes in terms of both morbidity and mortality.[185–187] Although combination therapy with voriconazole and an echinocandin has been successful in some case reports and case series, no large-scale prospective or retrospective studies provide evidence to support this practice.[177,188] Of note, amphotericin B has not shown any significant benefit in individuals with CNS aspergillosis, and could potentially worsen outcomes.[169,189,190]

Mucormycosis

Mucormycosis refers to any infection caused by fungi in the order Mucorales, most commonly those in the *Mucor* and *Rhizopus* genera. The most common form of neurologic mucormycosis is rhino–orbital–cerebral infection, which usually manifests as a rapidly progressive sinusitis with fever, nasal congestion and purulent discharge, headache, and sinus pain. Isolated cerebral mucormycosis can be more difficult to diagnose and manage because it presents without nasal sinus or orbital sites of infection, and can also rapidly progress to death if left untreated.[191]

Most individuals who develop rhino–orbital–cerebral mucormycosis have an underlying immune suppression, most commonly diabetes mellitus, followed by hematologic malignancy,[192,193] although some smaller studies have suggested that up to a third of patients may be immunocompetent.[194] Patients treated with deferoxamine are also at strongly increased risk of the disease, because many of the *Mucorales* fungi seem able to use the medication to augment their own supply of iron.[191,195]

The CNS invasion of mucormycosis requires prompt diagnosis and surgical management as well as initiation of amphotericin B to avoid mortality. Early tissue diagnosis followed by surgical excision of the necrotic tissue and aggressive antifungal therapy can decrease morbidity and mortality, so a low threshold for these interventions should be maintained if there is an underlying suspicion for infection (eg, presentation with diabetic ketoacidosis or an underlying hematologic malignancy).[196,197] One study of patients with hematologic malignancy who presented with mucormycosis infection showed that delay of treatment by 6 days or more doubled mortality at 12 weeks after diagnosis when compared with early treatment (82.9% vs 48.6%).[192]

NEUROTOXIN SYNDROMES
Botulism

Botulism is an uncommon but life-threatening syndrome caused by release of the botulinum neurotoxin by *Clostridium* bacterial species. Botulinum toxin inhibits the release of acetylcholine at the neuromuscular junction, leading to a rapid and potentially fatal flaccid paralysis. The syndrome of botulism was first described in relation to tainted meat consumption in the 1800s, and has since been described most commonly in infants after the consumption of honey that contains low levels of botulinum spores, or in adults after penetrating wounds or consumption of improperly canned foods, because the bacterium is heat stable at 100°C for up to 5 hours.[198]

The clinical presentation of botulism generally begins with at least 1 cranial nerve finding (most commonly dysarthria or ptosis) followed by symmetric, descending paralysis. Fever and altered mental status are absent in virtually all patients.[199] In infants, the syndrome can present with the floppy baby syndrome, including weak suck, ptosis, constipation, and decreased activity.

Definitive diagnosis of botulism is with the detection of botulinum toxin in serum, stool, wound culture, or other specimen depending on the method of exposure. However, these tests generally take at least 1 day to return results, and so are not useful in the hyperacute setting. Treatment is with antitoxin, which has been shown to decrease mortality, although with fairly heterogeneous results.[200] The administration of antitoxin within the first 24 to 48 hours of symptom onset improves mortality compared with later administration, and prompt treatment is crucial for this illness, although antitoxin may have benefits even after the acute window.[200,201]

Tetanus

Tetanus is a peripheral nervous system disorder caused by *Clostridium tetani*, a hardy, toxin-producing anaerobe that can cause severe morbidity and mortality in neonates and adults. The pathogen *C tetani* can contaminate feces, hard surfaces, or soil, where it can survive for years and still cause infection through the inhibition of glycine and GABA release at neuromuscular junctions.[202] Although the prevalence and mortality have been decreased drastically in resource-rich countries with the advent of near-universal vaccination and effective supportive therapy in intensive care units, mortality can still reach 50% in resource-limited environments. Even with effective therapy, functional disability can be present in more than one-third of patients.[203,204]

Exposure to tetanus is most often through inoculation owing to penetrating trauma, and the incubation period ranges from 3 days to 3 weeks, with an average of about 8 days.[205] The clinical presentation can be divided into 4 general phenotypes: generalized, local, cephalic, and neonatal. Generalized tetanus is by far the most common presentation of the disease, and is the most likely to be life threatening. The first symptom in 80% of patients is trismus, although some can present with autonomic activity such as hyperhidrosis and tachycardia.

Given the high morbidity and mortality of tetanus, prompt treatment with antibiotics and tetanus immunoglobulin is necessary when tetanus is suspected. Antibiotic therapy, usually with metronidazole or penicillin G, may have relatively little impact in the acute setting, but is generally recommended.[206] Immunoglobulin administration has been shown to decrease the need for and duration of mechanical ventilation and is indicated as soon as a diagnosis of tetanus is considered.[207–209]

SUMMARY

Neuroinfectious diseases can be challenging diagnostically in the acute setting given the heterogeneity of their presentation and lack of universally reliable criteria for definitive diagnosis. However, appropriate empiric treatment can drastically decrease morbidity and mortality and should be initiated in affected individuals even before a specific pathogen is determined. With proper interpretation of CSF and serum analysis, imaging, epidemiologic data, and clinical presentation, infections of the CNS can be effectively managed in the acute-care setting to improve outcomes.

There is abundant opportunity for research in the diagnosis and management of neuroinfectious emergencies. The initiation of antimicrobial therapy decreases morbidity and mortality in a wide variety of pathogens that affect the CNS, yet many patients still do poorly potentially owing to associated complications including stroke, intracranial hypertension, cerebral edema, and hydrocephalus. More research is needed to help risk stratify who is at risk for these complications, how they should be monitored, and what preventative strategies are needed. We need more specific and sensitive assays of serum and CSF to improve the time to disease diagnosis, and thus improve the end points for patients. In particular, investigation of which CNS pathogens can be diagnosed through serum assays could have a significant impact both in resource-abundant settings where LP may not be performed in patients with a lower suspicion for central disease, and in resource-scarce settings, where LP can be both logistically difficult and stigmatized by many patients.[210–212]

Although improved CSF and serum testing remains under research, clear management algorithms could also significantly alter the trajectory of many neuroinfectious emergencies. Although no set of clinical criteria will perfectly diagnose a specific pathogen at bedside, algorithms that provide reasonably accurate guidance on initial management steps (antifungal vs antibacterial medications, whether to begin corticosteroids, whether to involve neurosurgery) could improve outcomes for patients, even using the tools already available to us.

CLINICS CARE POINTS

- Treatment for ABM should include broad empiric coverage for gram-positive and gram-negative organisms. Adjunctive steroids should be given with the first doses of antibiotics and can be discontinued if the organism found in CSF is not *S pneumoniae*.

- Empiric acyclovir should be started promptly for any patient with clinical suspicion of encephalitis. MRI and LP can both be falsely negative early in the disease course, and so acyclovir can be started even if these are initially unrevealing.

- TBM can be difficult to differentiate from other nonbacterial meningitides, namely, cryptococcal meningitis. Treatment with 4-drug therapy as well as corticosteroids should be started in patients with risk factors for tuberculosis infection.

- CNS aspergillosis should be treated with voriconazole. Amphotericin B is ineffective in this syndrome and could potentially cause harm.

- Cryptococcal meningitis and cryptococcoma both require prompt systemic treatment with amphotericin B and flucytosine. Daily therapeutic LP should be performed in symptomatic patients until the closing pressure is within the normal range.

- Treatment of botulism with antitoxin decreases mortality when administered within 24 to 48 hours of symptom onset. Because confirmatory testing often takes more than 1 day to return, antitoxin should be administered immediately on clinical suspicion of the syndrome.

- Tetanus immunoglobulin can decrease time on a ventilator as well as mortality and should be administered as soon as the diagnosis is considered.

DISCLOSURE

The authors declare no conflicts of interest.

REFERENCES

1. Rotbart HA. Viral meningitis. Semin Neurol 2000;20(3):277–92.
2. Lee BE, Davies HD. Aseptic meningitis. Curr Opin Infect Dis 2007;20(3):272–7.
3. Whitley RJ, Gnann JW. Viral encephalitis: familiar infections and emerging pathogens. Lancet 2002;359(9305):507–13.
4. Holmes CW, Koo SS, Osman H, et al. Predominance of enterovirus B and echovirus 30 as cause of viral meningitis in a UK population. J Clin Virol 2016;81:90–3.
5. Bodilsen J, Storgaard M, Larsen L, et al. Infectious meningitis and encephalitis in adults in Denmark: a prospective nationwide observational cohort study (DASGIB). Clin Microbiol Infect 2018;24(10):1102.e1-5.
6. Centers for Disease Control and Prevention (CDC). Progress toward elimination of Haemophilus influenzae type b invasive disease among infants and children–United States, 1998-2000. MMWR Morb Mortal Wkly Rep 2002;51(11):234.
7. Black SB, Shinefield HR, Fireman B, et al. Efficacy in infancy of oligosaccharide conjugate Haemophilus influenzae type b (HbOC) vaccine in a United States population of 61,080 children. The Northern California Kaiser Permanente Vaccine Study Center Pediatrics Group. Pediatr Infect Dis J 1991;10(2):97–104.
8. Cowgill KD, Ndiritu M, Nyiro J, et al. Effectiveness of Haemophilus influenzae type b conjugate vaccine introduction into routine childhood immunization in Kenya. Jama 2006;296(6):671–8.
9. Maiden MC, MacLennan JM. Editorial commentary: fifteen years of protection by meningococcal C conjugate vaccines: lessons from disease surveillance. Clin Infect Dis 2014;59(9):1222.
10. Stefanelli P, Rezza G. Impact of vaccination on meningococcal epidemiology. Hum Vaccin Immunother 2016;12(4):1051–5.
11. Terry PM, Glancy GR, Graham A. Meningovascular syphilis of the spinal cord presenting with incomplete Brown-Sequard syndrome: case report. Sex Transm Infect 1989;65(3):189–91.

12. Frasch CE. Recent developments in Neisseria meningitidis group A conjugate vaccines. Expert Opin Biol Ther 2005;5(2):273–80.
13. Mohammed I, Iliyasu G, Habib AG. Emergence and control of epidemic meningococcal meningitis in sub-Saharan Africa. Pathog Glob Health 2017; 111(1):1–6.
14. Weisfelt M, van de Beek D, Spanjaard L, et al. A risk score for unfavorable outcome in adults with bacterial meningitis. Ann Neurol 2008;63(1):90–7.
15. Van de Beek D, De Gans J, Spanjaard L, et al. Clinical features and prognostic factors in adults with bacterial meningitis. N Engl J Med 2004;351(18):1849–59.
16. Weisfelt M, Van De Beek D, Spanjaard L, et al. Community-acquired bacterial meningitis in older people. J Am Geriatr Soc 2006;54(10):1500–7.
17. Zoons E, Weisfelt M, De Gans J, et al. Seizures in adults with bacterial meningitis. Neurology 2008;70(22 Part 2):2109–15.
18. Bijlsma MW, Brouwer MC, Kasanmoentalib ES, et al. Community-acquired bacterial meningitis in adults in the Netherlands, 2006-14: a prospective cohort study. Lancet Infect Dis 2016;16(3):339–47.
19. Charlier C, Perrodeau É, Leclercq A, et al. Clinical features and prognostic factors of listeriosis: the MONALISA national prospective cohort study. Lancet Infect Dis 2017;17(5):510–9.
20. Mylonakis E, Hohmann EL, Calderwood SB. Central nervous system infection with Listeria monocytogenes: 33 years' experience at a general hospital and review of 776 episodes from the literature. Medicine 1998;77(5):313–36.
21. Schuchat A, Robinson K, Wenger JD, et al. Bacterial meningitis in the United States in 1995. New Engl J Med 1997;337(14):970–6.
22. Kaplan S, Feigin RD. Treatment of meningitis in children. Pediatr Clin North Am 1983;30(2):259–69.
23. Spanos A, Harrell FE, Durack DT. Differential diagnosis of acute meningitis: an analysis of the predictive value of initial observations. Jama 1989;262(19): 2700–7.
24. Cabral DA, Flodmark O, Farrell K, et al. Prospective study of computed tomography in acute bacterial meningitis. J Pediatr 1987;111(2):201–5.
25. Hughes D, Raghavan A, Mordekar S, et al. Role of imaging in the diagnosis of acute bacterial meningitis and its complications. Postgrad Med J 2010; 86(1018):478–85.
26. Castillo M. Imaging of meningitis. Paper presented at: Seminars in Roentgenology 2004;39(4).
27. Lee JH, Na DG, Choi KH, et al. Subcortical low intensity on MR images of meningitis, viral encephalitis, and leptomeningeal metastasis. AJNR Am J Neuroradiol 2002;23(4):535–42.
28. Tsuchiya K, Inaoka S, Mizutani Y, et al. Fast fluid-attenuated inversion-recovery MR of intracranial infections. AJNR Am J Neuroradiol 1997;18(5):909–13.
29. Hasbun R, Abrahams J, Jekel J, et al. Computed tomography of the head before lumbar puncture in adults with suspected meningitis. New Engl J Med 2001; 345(24):1727–33.
30. Joffe AR. Lumbar puncture and brain herniation in acute bacterial meningitis: a review. J Intensive Care Med 2007;22(4):194–207.
31. Rennick G, Shann F, De Campo J. Cerebral herniation during bacterial meningitis in children. Br Med J 1993;306(6883):953–5.
32. Aronin SI, Peduzzi P, Quagliarello VJ. Community-acquired bacterial meningitis: risk stratification for adverse clinical outcome and effect of antibiotic timing. Ann Intern Med 1998;129(11):862–9.

33. van Crevel H, Hijdra A, de Gans J. Lumbar puncture and the risk of herniation: when should we first perform CT? J Neurol 2002;249(2):129–37.
34. Thigpen MC, Whitney CG, Messonnier NE, et al. Bacterial Meningitis in the United States, 1998–2007. N Engl J Med 2011;364(21):2016–25.
35. McIntyre PB, O'Brien KL, Greenwood B, et al. Effect of vaccines on bacterial meningitis worldwide. Lancet 2012;380(9854):1703–11.
36. Tunkel AR, Hartman BJ, Kaplan SL, et al. Practice guidelines for the management of bacterial meningitis. Clin Infect Dis 2004;39(9):1267–84.
37. Arslan F, Meynet E, Sunbul M, et al. The clinical features, diagnosis, treatment, and prognosis of neuroinvasive listeriosis: a multinational study. Eur J Clin Microbiol Infect Dis 2015;34(6):1213–21.
38. Lim S, Chung DR, Kim Y-S, et al. Predictive risk factors for Listeria monocytogenes meningitis compared to pneumococcal meningitis: a multicenter case–control study. Infection 2017;45(1):67–74.
39. de Gans J, van de Beek D. Dexamethasone in Adults with Bacterial Meningitis. N Engl J Med 2002;347(20):1549–56.
40. Weisfelt M, Hoogman M, van de Beek D, et al. Dexamethasone and long-term outcome in adults with bacterial meningitis. Ann Neurol 2006;60(4):456–68.
41. Fritz D, Brouwer MC, van de Beek D. Dexamethasone and long-term survival in bacterial meningitis. Neurology 2012;79(22):2177–9.
42. van de Beek D, de Gans J, McIntyre P, et al. Steroids in adults with acute bacterial meningitis: a systematic review. Lancet Infect Dis 2004;4(3):139–43.
43. Bodilsen J, Dalager-Pedersen M, Schønheyder HC, et al. Stroke in community-acquired bacterial meningitis: a Danish population-based study. Int J Infect Dis 2014;20:18–22.
44. Katchanov J, Heuschmann PU, Endres M, et al. Cerebral infarction in bacterial meningitis: predictive factors and outcome. J Neurol 2010;257(5):716–20.
45. Schut ES, Lucas MJ, Brouwer MC, et al. Cerebral infarction in adults with bacterial meningitis. Neurocrit Care 2012;16(3):421–7.
46. Durand ML, Calderwood SB, Weber DJ, et al. Acute bacterial meningitis in adults–A review of 493 episodes. New Engl J Med 1993;328(1):21–8.
47. Gironell A, Domingo P, Mancebo J, et al. Hemorrhagic stroke as a complication of bacterial meningitis in adults: report of three cases and review. Clin Infect Dis 1995;21(6):1488–91.
48. Pfister H-W, Feiden W, Einhäupl K-M. Spectrum of complications during bacterial meningitis in adults: results of a prospective clinical study. Arch Neurol 1993;50(6):575–81.
49. Pfister H-W, Borasio GD, Dirnagl U, et al. Cerebrovascular complications of bacterial meningitis in adults. Neurology 1992;42(8):1497.
50. Klein M, Koedel U, Pfefferkorn T, et al. Arterial cerebrovascular complications in 94 adults with acute bacterial meningitis. Crit Care 2011;15(6):R281.
51. Katchanov J, Siebert E, Klingebiel R, et al. Infectious vasculopathy of intracranial large-and medium-sized vessels in neurological intensive care unit: a clinico-radiological study. Neurocrit Care 2010;12(3):369–74.
52. Misra U, Kalita J, Nair P. Role of aspirin in tuberculous meningitis: a randomized open label placebo controlled trial. J Neurol Sci 2010;293(1–2):12–7.
53. Boelman C, Shroff M, Yau I, et al. Antithrombotic therapy for secondary stroke prevention in bacterial meningitis in children. J Pediatr 2014;165(4):799–806.
54. Czartoski T, Hallam D, Lacy J, et al. Postinfectious vasculopathy with evolution to moyamoya syndrome. J Neurol Neurosurg Psychiatry 2005;76(2):256–9.

55. Ries S, Schminke U, Fassbender K, et al. Cerebrovascular involvement in the acute phase of bacterial meningitis. J Neurol 1996;244(1):51–5.
56. Pomeroy SL, Holmes SJ, Dodge PR, et al. Seizures and other neurologic sequelae of bacterial meningitis in children. New Engl J Med 1990;323(24):1651–7.
57. Rosman NP, Peterson DB, Kaye EM, et al. Seizures in bacterial meningitis: prevalence, patterns, pathogenesis, and prognosis. Pediatr Neurol 1985;1(5):278–85.
58. Lai W-A, Chen S-F, Tsai N-W, et al. Clinical characteristics and prognosis of acute bacterial meningitis in elderly patients over 65: a hospital-based study. BMC Geriatr 2011;11(1):91.
59. Claassen J, Mayer S, Kowalski R, et al. Detection of electrographic seizures with continuous EEG monitoring in critically ill patients. Neurology 2004;62(10):1743–8.
60. Horwitz SJ, Boxerbaum B, O'Bell J. Cerebral herniation in bacterial meningitis in childhood. Ann Neurol 1980;7(6):524–8.
61. Lindvall P, Ahlm C, Ericsson M, et al. Reducing intracranial pressure may increase survival among patients with bacterial meningitis. Clin Infect Dis 2004; 38(3):384–90.
62. Glimåker M, Johansson B, Halldorsdottir H, et al. Neuro-intensive treatment targeting intracranial hypertension improves outcome in severe bacterial meningitis: an intervention-control study. PLoS One 2014;9(3):e91976.
63. Edberg M, Furebring M, Sjölin J, et al. Neurointensive care of patients with severe community-acquired meningitis. Acta Anaesthesiol Scand 2011;55(6):732–9.
64. Wall EC, Ajdukiewicz KM, Bergman H, et al. Osmotic therapies added to antibiotics for acute bacterial meningitis. Cochrane Database Syst Rev 2018;(2):CD008806.
65. Larsen L, Poulsen FR, Nielsen TH, et al. Use of intracranial pressure monitoring in bacterial meningitis: a 10-year follow up on outcome and intracranial pressure versus head CT scans. Infect Dis 2017;49(5):356–64.
66. Winkler F, Kastenbauer S, Yousry TA, et al. Discrepancies between brain CT imaging and severely raised intracranial pressure proven by ventriculostomy in adults with pneumococcal meningitis. J Neurol 2002;249(9):1292–7.
67. Abulhasan YB, Al-Jehani H, Valiquette M-A, et al. Lumbar drainage for the treatment of severe bacterial meningitis. Neurocrit Care 2013;19(2):199–205.
68. Tariq A, Aguilar-Salinas P, Hanel RA, et al. The role of ICP monitoring in meningitis. Neurosurg Focus 2017;43(5):E7.
69. Grände PO, Myhre E, Nordström CH, et al. Treatment of intracranial hypertension and aspects on lumbar dural puncture in severe bacterial meningitis. Acta Anaesthesiol Scand 2002;46(3):264–70.
70. Kumar R, Singhi S, Singhi P, et al. Randomized controlled trial comparing cerebral perfusion pressure–targeted therapy versus intracranial pressure–targeted therapy for raised intracranial pressure due to acute CNS infections in children. Crit Care Med 2014;42(8):1775–87.
71. Kasanmoentalib ES, Brouwer MC, van der Ende A, et al. Hydrocephalus in adults with community-acquired bacterial meningitis. Neurology 2010;75(10):918–23.
72. Wang K-W, Chang W-N, Chang H-W, et al. Clinical relevance of hydrocephalus in bacterial meningitis in adults. Surg Neurol 2005;64(1):61–5.
73. Bodilsen J, Schønheyder HC, Nielsen H. Hydrocephalus is a rare outcome in community-acquired bacterial meningitis in adults: a retrospective analysis. BMC Infect Dis 2013;13(1):321.
74. Sporrborn JL, Knudsen GB, Sølling M, et al. Brain ventricular dimensions and relationship to outcome in adult patients with bacterial meningitis. BMC Infect Dis 2015;15(1):367.

75. Mitchell DH, Sorrell TC, Allworth AM, et al. Cryptococcal disease of the CNS in immunocompetent hosts: influence of cryptococcal variety on clinical manifestations and outcome. Clin Infect Dis 1995;20(3):611–6.

76. Maziarz EK, Perfect JR. Cryptococcosis. Infect Dis Clin 2016;30(1):179–206.

77. Poley M, Koubek R, Walsh L, et al. Cryptococcal meningitis in an apparent immunocompetent patient. J Investig Med High Impact Case Rep 2019;7. 2324709619834578.

78. MacDougall L, Fyfe M, Romney M, et al. Risk factors for cryptococcus gattii infection, British Columbia, Canada. Emerg Infect Dis 2011;17(2):193.

79. Marr KA, Datta K, Pirofski L-a, et al. Cryptococcus gattii infection in healthy hosts: a sentinel for subclinical immunodeficiency? Clin Infect Dis 2012;54(1): 153–4.

80. Emmons CW. Saprophytic sources of Cryptococcus neoformans associated with the Pigeon (Columba livia). Am J Hyg 1955;62(3):227–32.

81. Pappas PG, Perfect JR, Cloud GA, et al. Cryptococcosis in human immunodeficiency virus-negative patients in the era of effective azole therapy. Clin Infect Dis 2001;33(5):690–9.

82. Advice WR. Diagnosis, prevention, and management of cryptococcal disease in HIV-infected adults, adolescents, and children. Geneva: WHO; 2011.

83. Wake RM, Britz E, Sriruttan C, et al. High cryptococcal antigen titers in blood are predictive of subclinical cryptococcal meningitis among human immunodeficiency virus-infected patients. Clin Infect Dis 2018;66(5):686–92.

84. Jia DT, Thakur K. Fungal infections of the central nervous system. Paper presented at: Seminars in Neurology. Thieme Medical Publishers; 2019;39(3).

85. Loyse A, Moodley A, Rich P, et al. Neurological, visual, and MRI brain scan findings in 87 South African patients with HIV-associated cryptococcal meningoencephalitis. J Infect 2015;70(6):668–75.

86. Sarkis RA, Mays M, Isada C, et al. MRI findings in cryptococcal meningitis of the non-HIV population. Neurologist 2015;19(2):40–5.

87. Larsen RA, Leal MAE, Chan LS. Fluconazole compared with amphotericin B plus flucytosine for cryptococcal meningitis in AIDS: a randomized trial. Ann Intern Med 1990;113(3):183–7.

88. Larsen RA, Bozzette SA, Jones BE, et al. Fluconazole combined with flucytosine for treatment of cryptococcal meningitis in patients with AIDS. Clin Infect Dis 1994;19(4):741–5.

89. Kizza HM, Oishi K, Mitarai S, et al. Combination therapy with fluconazole and flucytosine for cryptococcal meningitis in Ugandan patients with AIDS. Clin Infect Dis 1998;26(6):1362–6.

90. Nussbaum JC, Jackson A, Namarika D, et al. Combination flucytosine and high-dose fluconazole compared with fluconazole monotherapy for the treatment of cryptococcal meningitis: a randomized trial in Malawi. Clin Infect Dis 2010; 50(3):338–44.

91. Williamson PR, Jarvis JN, Panackal AA, et al. Cryptococcal meningitis: epidemiology, immunology, diagnosis and therapy. Nat Rev Neurol 2017;13(1):13.

92. Bicanic T, Brouwer AE, Meintjes G, et al. Relationship of cerebrospinal fluid pressure, fungal burden and outcome in patients with cryptococcal meningitis undergoing serial lumbar punctures. Aids 2009;23(6):701–6.

93. Rolfes MA, Hullsiek KH, Rhein J, et al. The effect of therapeutic lumbar punctures on acute mortality from cryptococcal meningitis. Clin Infect Dis 2014; 59(11):1607–14.

94. Park MK, Hospenthal DR, Bennett JE. Treatment of hydrocephalus secondary to cryptococcal meningitis by use of shunting. Clin Infect Dis 1999;28(3):629–33.
95. Cherian J, Atmar RL, Gopinath SP. Shunting in cryptococcal meningitis. J Neurosurg 2016;125(1):177–86.
96. Graybill JR, Sobel J, Saag M, et al. Diagnosis and management of increased intracranial pressure in patients with AIDS and cryptococcal meningitis. Clin Infect Dis 2000;30(1):47–54.
97. Jacobs CS, Etherton MR, Lyons JL. Fungal infections of the central nervous system. Curr Infect Dis Rep 2014;16(12):449.
98. Newton PN, Thai LH, Tip NQ, et al. A randomized, double-blind, placebo-controlled trial of acetazolamide for the treatment of elevated intracranial pressure in cryptococcal meningitis. Clin Infect Dis 2002;35(6):769–72.
99. Kumar R, Singh SN, Kohli N. A diagnostic rule for tuberculous meningitis. Arch Dis Child 1999;81(3):221–4.
100. Pehlivanoglu F, Yasar KK, Sengoz G. Tuberculous meningitis in adults: a review of 160 cases. ScientificWorldJournal 2012;2012:169028.
101. Thwaites GE, Tran TH. Tuberculous meningitis: many questions, too few answers. Lancet Neurol 2005;4(3):160–70.
102. Thwaites G, Chau T, Stepniewska K, et al. Diagnosis of adult tuberculous meningitis by use of clinical and laboratory features. Lancet 2002;360(9342):1287–92.
103. Bahr NC, Boulware DR. Methods of rapid diagnosis for the etiology of meningitis in adults. Biomarkers Med 2014;8(9):1085–103.
104. Patel VB, Theron G, Lenders L, et al. Diagnostic accuracy of quantitative PCR (Xpert MTB/RIF) for tuberculous meningitis in a high burden setting: a prospective study. PLoS Med 2013;10(10):e1001536.
105. Sütlaş PN, Unal A, Forta H, et al. Tuberculous meningitis in adults: review of 61 cases. Infection 2003;31(6):387–91.
106. Bourgi K, Fiske C, Sterling TR. Tuberculosis meningitis. Curr Infect Dis Rep 2017;19(11):39.
107. Leeds IL, Magee MJ, Kurbatova EV, et al. Site of extrapulmonary tuberculosis is associated with HIV infection. Clin Infect Dis 2012;55(1):75–81.
108. Donald PR. Cerebrospinal fluid concentrations of antituberculosis agents in adults and children. Tuberculosis 2010;90(5):279–92.
109. World Health O. Guidelines for treatment of drug-susceptible tuberculosis and patient care: 2017 update. Geneva, Switzerland: World Health Organization; 2017.
110. Thwaites GE, Macmullen-Price J, Tran THC, et al. Serial MRI to determine the effect of dexamethasone on the cerebral pathology of tuberculous meningitis: an observational study. Lancet Neurol 2007;6(3):230–6.
111. Jubelt B. Dexamethasone for the treatment of tuberculous meningitis in adolescents and adults. Curr Neurol Neurosci Rep 2006;6(6):451–2.
112. Kalita J, Misra UK, Nair PP. Predictors of Stroke and Its Significance in the Outcome of Tuberculous Meningitis. J Stroke Cerebrovasc Dis 2009;18(4):251–8.
113. Misra UK, Kalita J, Maurya PK. Stroke in tuberculous meningitis. J Neurol Sci 2011;303(1–2):22–30.
114. Caplan LR, Bogousslavsky J. Uncommon causes of stroke. Cambridge, UK: Cambridge University Press; 2008.
115. Chan K, Cheung R, Fong C, et al. Clinical relevance of hydrocephalus as a presenting feature of tuberculous meningitis. QJM 2003;96(9):643–8.

116. Lan SH, Chang WN, Lu CH, et al. Cerebral infarction in chronic meningitis: a comparison of tuberculous meningitis and cryptococcal meningitis. QJM 2001;94(5):247–53.

117. Rajshekhar V. Management of hydrocephalus in patients with tuberculous meningitis. Neurol India 2009;57(4):368.

118. Kennedy PG, Quan P-L, Lipkin WI. Viral encephalitis of unknown cause: current perspective and recent advances. Viruses 2017;9(6):138.

119. Gaieski DF, O'Brien NF, Hernandez R. Emergency neurologic life support: meningitis and encephalitis. Neurocrit Care 2017;27(Suppl 1):124–33.

120. Arciniegas DB, Anderson CA. Viral encephalitis: neuropsychiatric and neurobehavioral aspects. Curr Psychiatry Rep 2004;6(5):372–9.

121. Levitz RE. Herpes simplex encephalitis: a review. Heart Lung 1998;27(3):209–12.

122. Bradford RD, Pettit AC, Wright PW, et al. Herpes simplex encephalitis during treatment with tumor necrosis factor-alpha inhibitors. Clin Infect Dis 2009;49(6):924–7.

123. Nahmias AJ, Whitley RJ, Visintine AN, et al. Herpes simplex virus encephalitis: laboratory evaluations and their diagnostic significance. J Infect Dis 1982;145(6):829–36.

124. Razavi B, Razavi M. Herpes simplex encephalitis–an atypical case. Infection 2001;29(6):357–8.

125. Crusio RH, Singson SV, Haroun F, et al. Herpes simplex virus encephalitis during treatment with etanercept. Scand J Infect Dis 2014;46(2):152–4.

126. McGrath N, Anderson NE, Croxson MC, et al. Herpes simplex encephalitis treated with acyclovir: diagnosis and long term outcome. J Neurol Neurosurg Psychiatry 1997;63(3):321–6.

127. Chow FC, Glaser CA, Sheriff H, et al. Use of clinical and neuroimaging characteristics to distinguish temporal lobe herpes simplex encephalitis from its mimics. Clin Infect Dis 2015;60(9):1377–83.

128. McCabe K, Tyler K, Tanabe J. Diffusion-weighted MRI abnormalities as a clue to the diagnosis of herpes simplex encephalitis. Neurology 2003;61(7):1015–6.

129. Sköldenberg B, Forsgren M, Alestig K, et al. Acyclovir versus vidarabine in herpes simplex encephalitis. Randomised multicentre study in consecutive Swedish patients. Lancet 1984;2(8405):707–11.

130. Whitley RJ, Alford CA, Hirsch MS, et al. Vidarabine versus acyclovir therapy in herpes simplex encephalitis. N Engl J Med 1986;314(3):144–9.

131. Solomon T, Michael B, Smith P, et al. Management of suspected viral encephalitis in adults–association of British Neurologists and British Infection Association National Guidelines. J Infect 2012;64(4):347–73.

132. Kamei S, Sekizawa T, Shiota H, et al. Evaluation of combination therapy using aciclovir and corticosteroid in adult patients with herpes simplex virus encephalitis. J Neurol Neurosurg Psychiatry 2005;76(11):1544–9.

133. Tunkel AR, Glaser CA, Bloch KC, et al. The management of encephalitis: clinical practice guidelines by the Infectious Diseases Society of America. Clin Infect Dis 2008;47:303–27.

134. Bradshaw MJ, Venkatesan A. Herpes simplex virus-1 encephalitis in adults: pathophysiology, diagnosis, and management. Neurotherapeutics 2016;13(3):493–508.

135. Brain TF. Guidelines for the management of severe traumatic brain injury. VIII. Intracranial pressure thresholds. J neurotrauma 2007;24:S55.

136. Kumar G, Kalita J, Misra UK. Raised intracranial pressure in acute viral encephalitis. Clin Neurol Neurosurg 2009;111(5):399–406.
137. Thakur KT, Motta M, Asemota AO, et al. Predictors of outcome in acute encephalitis. Neurology 2013;81(9):793–800.
138. Pérez-Bovet J, Garcia-Armengol R, Buxó-Pujolràs M, et al. Decompressive craniectomy for encephalitis with brain herniation: case report and review of the literature. Acta Neurochir 2012;154(9):1717–24.
139. Greenland JR, Michelow MD, Wang L, et al. COVID-19 infection: implications for perioperative and critical care physicians. Anesthesiology 2020;132(6):1346–61.
140. Ye M, Ren Y, Lv T. Encephalitis as a clinical manifestation of COVID-19. Brain Behav Immun 2020;88:945–6.
141. Duong L, Xu P, Liu A. Meningoencephalitis without respiratory failure in a young female patient with COVID-19 infection in Downtown Los Angeles, early April 2020. Brain Behav Immun 2020;87:33.
142. Moriguchi T, Harii N, Goto J, et al. A first case of meningitis/encephalitis associated with SARS-Coronavirus-2. Int J Infect Dis 2020;94:55–8.
143. Pittock SJ, Debruyne J, Krecke KN, et al. Chronic lymphocytic inflammation with pontine perivascular enhancement responsive to steroids (CLIPPERS). Brain 2010;133(9):2626–34.
144. Anand P, Lau KV, Chung DY, et al. Posterior reversible encephalopathy syndrome in patients with coronavirus disease 2019: two cases and a review of the literature. J Stroke Cerebrovasc Dis 2020;29:105212.
145. Cariddi LP, Damavandi PT, Carimati F, et al. Reversible Encephalopathy Syndrome (PRES) in a COVID-19 patient. J Neurol 2020;267(11):3157–60.
146. Kaya Y, Kara S, Akinci C, et al. Transient cortical blindness in COVID-19 pneumonia; a PRES-like syndrome: case report. J Neurol Sci 2020;413:116858.
147. Poyiadji N, Shahin G, Noujaim D, et al. COVID-19–associated acute hemorrhagic necrotizing encephalopathy: CT and MRI features. Radiology 2020;201187.
148. Franceschi A, Ahmed O, Giliberto L, et al. Hemorrhagic posterior reversible encephalopathy syndrome as a manifestation of COVID-19 infection. AJNR Am J Neuroradiol 2020;41(7):1173–6.
149. Haddad S, Tayyar R, Risch L, et al. Encephalopathy and seizure activity in a COVID-19 well controlled HIV patient. IDCases 2020;21:e00814.
150. Koralnik IJ, Tyler KL. COVID-19: a global threat to the nervous system. Ann Neurol 2020;88(1):1–11.
151. Mao L, Jin H, Wang M, et al. Neurologic manifestations of hospitalized patients with coronavirus disease 2019 in Wuhan, China. JAMA Neurol 2020;77(6):683–90.
152. Anand P, Al-Faraj A, Sader E, et al. Seizure as the presenting symptom of COVID-19: a retrospective case series. Epilepsy Behav 2020;112:107335.
153. Nwajei F, Anand P, Abdalkader M, et al. Cerebral Venous Sinus Thromboses in Patients with SARS-CoV-2 infection: three cases and a review of the literature. J Stroke Cerebrovasc Dis 2020;105412.
154. Carneiro T, Dashkoff J, Leung LY, et al. Intravenous tPA for Acute Ischemic Stroke in Patients with COVID-19. J Stroke Cerebrovasc Dis 2020;29(11):105201.
155. Muccioli L, Pensato U, Cani I, et al. Covid-19-associated encephalopathy and cytokine-mediated neuroinflammation. Ann Neurol 2020;88(4):860–1.
156. Pilotto A, Odolini S, Stefano Masciocchi S, et al. Steroid-responsive encephalitis in Covid-19 disease. Ann Neurol 2020;88(2):423–7.

157. Delamarre L, Gollion C, Grouteau G, et al. COVID-19–associated acute necrotising encephalopathy successfully treated with steroids and polyvalent immunoglobulin with unusual IgG targeting the cerebral fibre network. J Neurol Neurosurg Psychiatry 2020;91(9):1004–6.

158. Kastenbauer S, Pfister H-W, Wispelwey B, et al. Brain abscess. Infections Cent Nervous Syst 2004;3:479–507.

159. Brouwer MC, Coutinho JM, van de Beek D. Clinical characteristics and outcome of brain abscess: systematic review and meta-analysis. Neurology 2014;82(9): 806–13.

160. Brouwer MC, Tunkel AR, van de Beek D. Brain abscess. N Engl J Med 2014; 371(18):1758.

161. Yang KY, Chang WN, Ho JT, et al. Postneurosurgical nosocomial bacterial brain abscess in adults. Infection 2006;34(5):247–51.

162. Ewald C, Kuhn S, Kalff R. Pyogenic infections of the central nervous system secondary to dental affections—a report of six cases. Neurosurg Rev 2006;29(2): 163–7.

163. Parahitiyawa N, Jin L, Leung W, et al. Microbiology of odontogenic bacteremia: beyond endocarditis. Clin Microbiol Rev 2009;22(1):46–64.

164. Arlotti M, Grossi P, Pea F, et al. Consensus document on controversial issues for the treatment of infections of the central nervous system: bacterial brain abscesses. Int J Infect Dis 2010;14:S79–92.

165. Valarezo J, Cohen J, Valarezo L, et al. Nocardial cerebral abscess: report of three cases and review of the current neurosurgical management. Neurol Res 2003;25(1):27–30.

166. Gutiérrez-Cuadra M, Ballesteros MA, Vallejo A, et al. Brain abscess in a third-level hospital: epidemiology and prognostic factors related to mortality. Rev Esp Quimioter 2009;22(4):201–6.

167. Liu C, Bayer A, Cosgrove SE, et al. Clinical practice guidelines by the Infectious Diseases Society of America for the treatment of methicillin-resistant Staphylococcus aureus infections in adults and children. Clin Infect Dis 2011;52(3): e18–55.

168. Muzumdar D, Jhawar S, Goel A. Brain abscess: an overview. Int J Surg 2011; 9(2):136–44.

169. Baddley JW, Stroud TP, Salzman D, et al. Invasive mold infections in allogeneic bone marrow transplant recipients. Clin Infect Dis 2001;32(9):1319–24.

170. Selby R, Ramirez CB, Singh R, et al. Brain abscess in solid organ transplant recipients receiving cyclosporine-based immunosuppression. Arch Surg 1997; 132(3):304–10.

171. Bhatt Y, Pahade N, Nair B. Aspergillus petrous apicitis associated with cerebral and peritubular abscesses in an immunocompetent man. J Laryngol Otol 2013; 127(4):404.

172. Al-Tawfiq J, Ghandour J. Cryptococcus neoformans abscess and osteomyelitis in an immunocompetent patient with tuberculous lymphadenitis. Infection 2007; 35(5):377–82.

173. Zheng LX, De Zhi K. Multiple cerebellar abscess and pneumonia caused by Cryptococcus in an immunocompetent adult patient. Pakistan J Med Sci 2011;27(2):448–50.

174. Borkar S, Sharma M, Rajpal G, et al. Brain abscess caused by Cladophialophora bantiana in an immunocompetent host: need for a novel cost-effective antifungal agent. Indian J Med Microbiol 2008;26(3):271.

175. Garg N, Devi IB, Vajramani GV, et al. Central nervous system cladosporiosis: an account of ten culture-proven cases. Neurol India 2007;55(3):282.
176. Revankar SG. Cladophialophora bantiana brain abscess in an immunocompetent patient. Can J Infect Dis Med Microbiol 2011;22:149–50.
177. Segal BH, Walsh TJ. Current approaches to diagnosis and treatment of invasive aspergillosis. Am J Respir Crit Care Med 2006;173(7):707–17.
178. Ruhnke M, Kofla G, Otto K, et al. CNS aspergillosis. CNS Drugs 2007;21(8): 659–76.
179. Hurst RW, Judkins A, Bolger W, et al. Mycotic aneurysm and cerebral infarction resulting from fungal sinusitis: imaging and pathologic correlation. AJNR Am J Neuroradiol 2001;22(5):858–63.
180. Ho CL, Deruytter MJ. CNS aspergillosis with mycotic aneurysm, cerebral granuloma and infarction. Acta Neurochir 2004;146(8):851–6.
181. Mikulska M, Furfaro E, Del Bono V, et al. (1-3)-β-D-glucan in cerebrospinal fluid is useful for the diagnosis of central nervous system fungal infections. Clin Infect Dis 2013;56(10):1511–2.
182. Soeffker G, Wichmann D, Loderstaedt U, et al. Aspergillus galactomannan antigen for diagnosis and treatment monitoring in cerebral aspergillosis. Prog Transplant 2013;23(1):71–4.
183. Klont RR, Mennink-Kersten MA, Verweij PE. Utility of Aspergillus antigen detection in specimens other than serum specimens. Clin Infect Dis 2004;39(10): 1467–74.
184. Maertens J, Van Eldere J, Verhaegen J, et al. Use of circulating galactomannan screening for early diagnosis of invasive aspergillosis in allogeneic stem cell transplant recipients. J Infect Dis 2002;186(9):1297–306.
185. De Lastours V, Lefort A, Zappa M, et al. Two cases of cerebral aspergillosis successfully treated with voriconazole. Eur J Clin Microbiol Infect Dis 2003;22(5): 297–9.
186. Schwartz S, Ruhnke M, Ribaud P, et al. Improved outcome in central nervous system aspergillosis, using voriconazole treatment. Blood 2005;106(8):2641–5.
187. Tattevin P, Bruneel F, Lellouche F, et al. Successful treatment of brain aspergillosis with voriconazole. Clin Microbiol Infect 2004;10(10):928–31.
188. Damaj G, Ivanov V, Le Brigand B, et al. Rapid improvement of disseminated aspergillosis with caspofungin/voriconazole combination in an adult leukemic patient. Ann Hematol 2004;83(6):390–3.
189. Denning DW, Stevens DA. Antifungal and surgical treatment of invasive aspergillosis: review of 2,121 published cases. Rev Infect Dis 1990;12(6):1147–201.
190. Walsh TJ, Anaissie EJ, Denning DW, et al. Treatment of aspergillosis: clinical practice guidelines of the Infectious Diseases Society of America. Clin Infect Dis 2008;46(3):327–60.
191. Spellberg B, Edwards J, Ibrahim A. Novel perspectives on mucormycosis: pathophysiology, presentation, and management. Clin Microbiol Rev 2005;18(3): 556–69.
192. Chamilos G, Lewis RE, Kontoyiannis DP. Delaying Amphotericin B–based frontline therapy significantly increases mortality among patients with hematologic malignancy who have zygomycosis. Clin Infect Dis 2008;47(4):503–9.
193. Roden MM, Zaoutis TE, Buchanan WL, et al. Epidemiology and outcome of zygomycosis: a review of 929 reported cases. Clin Infect Dis 2005;41(5):634–53.
194. Mohindra S, Mohindra S, Gupta R, et al. Rhinocerebral mucormycosis: the disease spectrum in 27 patients. Mycoses 2007;50(4):290–6.

195. Boelaert JR, Van Cutsem J, de Locht M, et al. Deferoxamine augments growth and pathogenicity of Rhizopus, while hydroxypyridinone chelators have no effect. Kidney Int 1994;45(3):667–71.
196. Malik AN, Bi WL, McCray B, et al. Isolated cerebral mucormycosis of the basal ganglia. Clin Neurol Neurosurg 2014;124:102–5.
197. Verma A, Brozman B, Petito CK. Isolated cerebral mucormycosis: report of a case and review of the literature. J Neurol Sci 2006;240(1–2):65–9.
198. Hatheway CL, Hauschild AHW, Dodds KL. Clostridium botulinum: ecology and control in foods. Food Science and Technology 1993;54:3–20.
199. Rao AK, Lin NH, Jackson KA, et al. Clinical Characteristics and Ancillary Test Results Among Patients With Botulism—United States, 2002–2015. Clin Infect Dis 2017;66(suppl_1):S4–10.
200. O'Horo JC, Harper EP, El Rafei A, et al. Efficacy of antitoxin therapy in treating patients with foodborne botulism: a systematic review and meta-analysis of cases, 1923-2016. Clin Infect Dis 2017;66(suppl_1):S43–56.
201. Yu PA, Lin NH, Mahon BE, et al. Safety and improved clinical outcomes in patients treated with new equine-derived heptavalent botulinum antitoxin. Clin Infect Dis 2017;66(suppl_1):S57–64.
202. Ebisawa I, Takayanagi M, Kurata M, et al. Density and distribution of Clostridium tetani in the soil. Jpn J Exp Med 1986;56(2):69–74.
203. Mahieu R, Reydel T, Maamar A, et al. Admission of tetanus patients to the ICU: a retrospective multicentre study. Ann Intensive Care 2017;7(1):112.
204. Thwaites CL, Beeching NJ, Newton CR. Maternal and neonatal tetanus. Lancet 2015;385(9965):362–70.
205. for Disease Control C, Prevention Others. Epidemiology and prevention of vaccine-preventable diseases: tetanus [Internet]. Atlanta: CDC; 2012. Accessed September 20, 2016.
206. Afshar M, Raju M, Ansell D, et al. Narrative review: tetanus—a health threat after natural disasters in developing countries. Ann Intern Med 2011;154(5):329–35.
207. American Academy of P, Pickering LK. Red Book: 2009 report of the Committee on infectious diseases. Elk Grove Village, IL: American Academy of Pediatrics; 2009.
208. Hassel B. Tetanus: pathophysiology, treatment, and the possibility of using botulinum toxin against tetanus-induced rigidity and spasms. Toxins 2013;5(1): 73–83.
209. List WF. The immediate treatment of tetanus with high doses of human tetanus antitoxin. Notfallmedizin 1981;7:731–3.
210. Birbeck GL. Barriers to care for patients with neurologic disease in rural Zambia. Arch Neurol 2000;57(3):414–7.
211. King M, Rwegerera G. An audit of consent practices and perceptions of lumbar puncture, Botswana inpatient setting experience. Afr J Emerg Med 2015; 5(2):66–9.
212. Sulaiman WAW, Saliluddin SM, Ong YJ, et al. A cross sectional study assessing the knowledge and attitudes towards lumbar puncture among the staff of a public university in Malaysia. Clin Epidemiol Glob Health 2018;6(1):29–33.

Autoimmune Neurologic Emergencies

Pooja Raibagkar, MD[a],*, Anil Ramineni, MD[b]

KEYWORDS

- Autoimmune • Neurologic emergency • Antibody • Paraneoplastic • Encephalitis
- Neurosarcoidosis • Demyelinating disease • Neuromyelitis optica

KEY POINTS

- Immune-mediated neurologic disorders include a large spectrum of heterogeneous disorders with the potential for rapid deterioration and requirement of intensive care and management.
- Early identification and appropriate management may lead to a favorable outcome.
- Reduced level of consciousness, autonomic dysfunction, seizures, and treatment-refractory movement disorders are common reasons for the intensive care unit level of care in autoimmune and paraneoplastic encephalitis.
- Demyelinating disorders such as tumefactive multiple sclerosis, Marburg variant, Balo concentric sclerosis, and acute disseminated encephalomyelitis may manifest with a tumorlike presentation and have a high risk of morbidity and mortality.
- Systemic autoimmune rheumatologic disorders may have life-threatening neurologic manifestations.

AUTOIMMUNE AND PARANEOPLASTIC ENCEPHALITIS
Introduction

Autoimmune encephalitis encompasses a range of disorders in which the body's immune system pathologically attacks the brain. This condition may occur in association with a tumor, in which case it is referred to as paraneoplastic encephalitis. The clinical syndrome depends on the regions of the brain that are affected.[1] This article focuses on the syndromes and disorders most pertinent when considering the neurologic emergency. Early recognition and management of these disorders are crucial to ensuring the best possible outcome.

Antigen targets in autoimmune encephalitis can be broadly divided into 2 categories: (1) intracellular neuronal proteins, and (2) cellular surface/synaptic proteins.

[a] Concord Hospital Neurology Associates, 246 Pleasant Street, Concord, NH 03301, USA;
[b] Lahey Hospital & Medical Center, Beth Israel Lahey Health, 41 Mall Road, Burlington, MA 01803, USA
* Corresponding author.
E-mail address: Praibagkar86@gmail.com

Neurol Clin 39 (2021) 589–614
https://doi.org/10.1016/j.ncl.2021.01.006
neurologic.theclinics.com

The first category is also referred to as onconeuronal proteins because of the strong association with cancer and involves a T cell–mediated response causing neuronal injury. The prognosis tends to be poorer in these conditions.[2] Although antibodies are a useful marker of a disease, it is unclear what role (if any) they play in the pathophysiology. The second category has a variable association with cancer and a better prognosis. The antibodies in this category are considered directly pathogenic, causing synaptic dysfunction in neurons.[2]

Patients may rapidly decline as a result of their illness and often require intensive care treatment. Reasons for intensive care unit (ICU) management include disturbance in consciousness, autonomic dysfunction, status epilepticus, treatment-refractory movement disorders, as well as mechanical ventilation.[3]

Diagnosis

When considering autoimmune and paraneoplastic encephalitis, the most important differential diagnosis is infectious encephalitis.[4] Most cases of infectious encephalitis are viral; however, bacterial and fungal causes should also be considered carefully. A detailed travel and exposure history is essential. As well, knowledge of a patient's immune system function (human immunodeficiency virus [HIV] status, transplant, cancer, rheumatologic condition, and so forth) is important.[5] In particular, herpes simplex virus (HSV) encephalitis has a significant overlap with the clinical syndromes in autoimmune and paraneoplastic encephalitis. Early treatment with acyclovir in HSV encephalitis improves the chances of survival with a good neurologic recovery. As such, treatment should be started empirically while diagnostic testing is pursued. Additional antibiotic and antiviral therapy should be started empirically depending on clinical suspicion and the patient's risk factors.[6,7]

Diagnosis of autoimmune and paraneoplastic encephalitis relies on a combination of clinical presentation with testing including neural-specific autoantibodies, neuroimaging (Magnetic Resonance Imaging [MRI] brain), electroencephalogram (EEG), and cerebrospinal fluid (CSF) evaluation (**Box 1**).[4] Results of antibody testing may be delayed but should not preclude empiric treatment, particularly in ill patients. Four distinct possibilities exist when diagnosing autoimmune or paraneoplastic encephalitis in a patient with a characteristic clinical syndrome:

1. Antibody present with underlying tumor (paraneoplastic)
2. Antibody absent with underlying tumor (paraneoplastic)
3. Antibody present without underlying tumor (autoimmune)

Box 1
Diagnostic criteria for possible autoimmune encephalitis[4]

1. Subacute onset (rapid progression of <3 months) of working memory deficits (short-term memory loss), altered mental status, or psychiatric symptoms

2. At least 1 of the following:
   - New focal central nervous system findings
   - Seizures not explained by a previously known seizure disorder
   - CSF pleocytosis (WBC>5 cells/mm^3)
   - MRI features suggestive of encephalitis

3. Reasonable exclusion of alternative causes

Abbreviation: WBC, white blood cell count.

4. Antibody and tumor absent (autoimmune, or consider alternate cause)

Given the close relationship of antibody profile to tumor type in addition to clinical presentation, ongoing tumor screening should be considered on a case-by-case basis (**Table 1**).[1,2,8,9]

Limbic encephalitis

The limbic system is an interconnected group of structures, including the amygdala, hippocampus, cingulate gyrus, anterior thalamus, hypothalamus, and mammillary bodies. This system is involved in emotion, behavior, and memory, among other functions. Understandably, pathologic inflammation of this system can lead to neuropsychiatric symptoms such as behavior and mood changes and problems with memory. Seizures are common in cases of limbic encephalitis, and patients may present with convulsive or nonconvulsive status epilepticus. EEG monitoring should be pursued in patients with alterations in mental status.[10]

The onconeuronal antibodies that occur more often with limbic encephalitis include anti-Hu, anti-Ri, and anti-Ma2 (anti-Ta), and these patients almost always have underlying cancer.[11] The neuronal cell-surface antibodies that are more frequently associated with limbic encephalitis include anti-LGI1, anti-$GABA_b$ receptor, and anti-AMPA receptor antibodies.[9] The likelihood and type of underlying cancer vary based on the particular antibody.[12] Patients with anti-LGI1 encephalitis may have faciobrachial dystonic seizures, which can precede the development of limbic encephalitis.[13]

Limbic encephalitis tends to affect bilateral temporal lobes, and caution should be exercised in the diagnosis when there is unilateral (or no) involvement of the temporal lobes on MRI (**Box 2, Fig. 1**).[4] Detection of specific antibodies can confirm the diagnosis. Alternate causes, such as HSV encephalitis and glioma, should be excluded as best as possible. The findings in HSV encephalitis tend to be less confined to the limbic system, can have hemorrhagic features, and may show diffusion restriction and contrast uptake on MRI. Human herpesvirus 6–associated encephalitis can mimic autoimmune limbic encephalitis and should be considered in immunocompromised patients in the proper clinical setting.[4]

Anti–N-methyl-D-aspartate receptor encephalitis

Anti–N-methyl-D-aspartate (NMDA) receptor encephalitis is the most common autoimmune or paraneoplastic encephalitis. There is a predisposition for anti-NMDA receptor (anti-NMDAR) encephalitis to affect young patients less than the age of 45 years and women to a much greater degree than men. This gender discrepancy is not as evident in the pediatric and elderly populations.[14]

A significant portion of patients have an underlying teratoma, which most often affects the ovary, although may be found elsewhere, including testis, head, neck, and thyroid.[1] Early detection and removal of this tumor is important in the management of anti-NMDA encephalitis. HSV encephalitis has been known to precede the development of anti-NMDAR encephalitis. There is a significantly higher prevalence of antibodies to HSV-1 in patients with anti-NMDAR encephalitis, suggesting some association between this infection and the development of anti-NMDAR encephalitis.[15]

There has been a highly characteristic syndrome described with 5 phases of clinical illness; however, patients need not follow this precise trajectory.[16]

1. Prodromal phase: nonspecific symptoms similar to a viral illness
2. Psychotic ± seizure phase: psychiatric symptoms including hallucinations, mood lability, seizures

Table 1
Antibody, associated syndromes, and cancer frequency/type[1,2,8,9]

Antibody	Clinical Syndrome	Tumor Frequency	Most Common Tumor Type
Onconeuronal			
ANNA-1 (Hu)	Encephalomyelitis, sensory neuropathy, cerebellar degeneration	>75%	Small cell lung cancer
Anti-Ma/Ta	Encephalitis, brainstem dysfunction, ophthalmoparesis	>80%	Testicular cancer (young men), small cell lung cancer, breast cancer
PCA-1 (Yo)	Cerebellar degeneration	>85%	Gynecologic cancer, breast cancer
CV2/CRMP-5-IgG	Encephalitis, hyperkinetic movements, polyneuropathy	Common	Small cell lung cancer, thymoma
GAD65	Limbic encephalitis, stiff person syndrome	Rare	—
Amphiphysin-IgG	Encephalomyelitis with rigidity, myoclonus, stiff person phenomenon	Common	Breast cancer, small cell lung cancer
ANNA-2 (Ri)	Brainstem syndrome (opsoclonus myoclonus, cranial neuropathy), cerebellar syndrome	Common	Breast cancer, small cell lung cancer
PCA-Tr	Cerebellar degeneration	Common	Hodgkin lymphoma
Cell Surface/Protein			
NMDA receptor	Encephalitis, mutism, hyperkinetic movements, catatonia	10%–50%	Ovarian teratoma
LGI1 (VGKC-complex)	Faciobrachial dystonic seizures, limbic encephalitis	<10%	Lung, thymoma
AMPA receptor	Limbic encephalitis, psychosis	70%	Lung, thymoma
GABA$_b$ receptor	Limbic encephalitis	60%	Lung, neuroendocrine
CASPR2 (VGKC-complex)	Morvan syndrome, neuromyotonia, limbic encephalitis	<30%	Lung, thymoma
Glycine receptor	PERM, stiff person syndrome	~10%	Lymphoma, thymoma
GluR5	Ophelia syndrome, limbic encephalitis		Hodgkin lymphoma
GABA$_a$ receptor	Encephalitis, seizures	~25%	Thymoma
DPPX	Encephalitis, PERM	<10%	Lymphoma

(continued on next page)

Table 1
(continued)

Antibody	Clinical Syndrome	Tumor Frequency	Most Common Tumor Type
Dopamine-2 receptor	Basal ganglia encephalitis, dyskinesias	Unknown	—
Neurexin-3 α	Encephalitis	Unknown	—
IgLON5	Sleep disorder, brainstem dysfunction	Unknown	—
GluR1	Cerebellar ataxia	Rare	Hodgkin lymphoma
Neuronal ganglionic AChR	Encephalitis, postural tachycardia syndrome	~30%	Thymoma, breast/bladder/rectal/lung cancer, lymphoma
MOG-IgG	Acute disseminated encephalomyelitis	No association	—
Adenylate-kinase 5	Memory loss	No association	—
P/Q-and N-type VGCC	Lambert-Eaton myasthenic syndrome, cerebellar degeneration, rare encephalitis	60%	Small cell lung cancer
GluR3	Rasmussen encephalitis	unknown	—

Abbreviations: AChR, acetylcholine receptor; AGNA, antiglial neuronal nuclear antibody type 1; AMPA, alpha-amino-3-hydroxy-5-methyl-4-isoxazole-propionic acid; ANNA, antineuronal nuclear antibody; CASPR, contactin-associated protein; CRMP-5, collapsin response mediator protein-5; DPPX, dipeptidyl-peptidase–like protein 6; GABA, gamma aminobutyric acid; GAD65, 65 kDa isoform of glutamic acid decarboxylase; GluR, glutamate receptor; IgG, immunoglobulin G; LGI, leucin-rich glioma inactivated protein; MOG, myelin oligodendrocyte glycoprotein; NMDA, N-methyl-ᴅ-aspartate; PERM, progressive encephalomyelitis with rigidity and myoclonus; PCA, Purkinje cell antibody; VGCC, voltage-gated calcium channel; VGKC, voltage-gated potassium channel.

3. Unresponsive and/or catatonic phase: decreased level of consciousness with central hypoventilation, which may progress to catatonia or coma
4. Hyperkinetic phase: orofacial and limb dyskinesias and dysautonomia
5. Gradual recovery phase

Diagnosis may be highly suspected based on a classic clinical presentation, particularly in association with a teratoma (**Box 3**). MRI brain may be normal in more than 50% of patients. In abnormal MRI, brain lesions often occur in the medial temporal lobe, frontal, and parietal cortex. However, lesions have also been described in the cerebellum, thalamus, basal ganglia, brainstem, and spinal cord (**Fig. 2**).[17] EEG is most often nonspecific, but, in a proportion of patients, there may be a characteristic finding of extreme delta brush. CSF typically reveals a mild-moderate lymphocytic pleocytosis, normal or mildly increased protein concentration, and greater than 50% of patients have oligoclonal bands.[18] CSF NMDAR antibodies are more sensitive than serum NMDAR antibodies, and CSF antibody titer may be useful to track response to treatment and relapse.[14]

The prognosis for recovery is generally favorable, but early recognition and aggressive treatment are necessary. Low severity of disease and early treatment is

---

Box 2

Diagnostic criteria for definite autoimmune limbic encephalitis

1. Subacute onset (rapid progression of <3 months) of working memory deficits, seizures, or psychiatric symptoms suggesting the involvement of the limbic system

2. Bilateral brain abnormalities on T2-weighted FLAIR MRI highly restricted to medial temporal lobes

3. At least 1 of the following:
   - CSF pleocytosis (WBC>5 cells/mm^3)
   - EEG with epileptic or slow-wave activity involving the temporal lobes

4. Reasonable exclusion of alternative causes

Abbreviation: FLAIR, fluid-attenuated inversion recovery.

---

associated with good outcome.[14] In patients who are not having clinical improvement or continue to clinically worsen in spite of therapy, strong consideration should be given to escalation of immunosuppression. Case reports of administration of bortezomib and prophylactic oophorectomy (with the discovery of microteratomas) exist in severe, refractory cases of anti-NMDAR encephalitis.[19–21]

Intensive care unit management in anti–N-methyl-D-aspartate receptor encephalitis

Supportive care is a cornerstone for the management of autoimmune or paraneoplastic encephalitis. Intensive care monitoring and treatment may be necessary, and this is particularly true of anti-NMDAR encephalitis. Mechanical ventilation is often required, with a median duration of 38 days, and correspondingly tracheostomy is frequently pursued to optimize patient comfort and safety. Sedatives and anesthetics are commonly required; however, agents with NMDAR antagonist properties (ie,

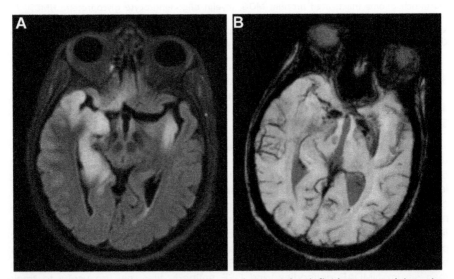

Fig. 1. Paraneoplastic limbic encephalitis. Axial T2-weighted fluid-attenuated inversion recovery (FLAIR) magnetic resonance (MR) images show bilateral temporal lobe hyperintensities, worse on right (*A*) without evidence of hemorrhage on gradient recalled echo T2-weighted image (*B*).

Box 3
Diagnostic criteria for anti–*N*-methyl-ᴅ-aspartate receptor encephalitis[4]

Probable
1. Rapid onset (<3 months) of at least 4 of the 6 following major groups of symptoms:
   - Abnormal (psychiatric) behavior or cognitive dysfunction
   - Speech dysfunction (pressured speech, verbal reduction, mutism)
   - Seizures
   - Movement disorder, dyskinesias, or rigidity/abnormal postures
   - Decreased level of consciousness
   - Autonomic dysfunction or central hypoventilation
2. At least 1 of the following:
   - Abnormal EEG (focal or diffuse slow or disorganized activity, epileptic activity, or extreme delta brush)
   - CSF with pleocytosis or oligoclonal bands
3. Reasonable exclusion of other disorders
   Diagnosis can be made in the presence of 3 of the above group symptoms accompanied by a systemic teratoma

Definite
1. Diagnosis can be made in presence of 1 or more of the 6 major group of symptoms and immunoglobulin (Ig) G anti-GluN1 antibodies, after reasonable exclusion of other disorders

---

ketamine, nitrous oxide, and volatile anesthetics) are generally avoided given the theoretic worsening of synaptic function (clinical data are lacking).[18]

Anti-NMDAR antibodies may affect the basal ganglia, resulting in hyperkinetic movement disorders, which can range from orofacial dyskinesias to ballismus. The latter is best treated with dopamine (D_2) antagonists, or, if these are inadequate, vesicular monoamine transporter type 2 (VMAT2) inhibitors such as tetrabenazine. Sedation may be required with benzodiazepines, barbiturates, or propofol.[18]

Dysautonomia may have various manifestations, including hyperthermia, bradycardia, tachycardia, hypertension, hypotension, gastrointestinal dysmotility, and/or urinary retention. Most patients who are young and healthy tolerate some degree of dysautonomia, and caution should be exercised in overtreating symptoms such as hypertension or tachycardia because this may precipitate profound hypotension or bradycardia.[18] In some patients, bradycardia may be so profound as to necessitate transient pacing or even pacemaker placement. Medications used for other forms of paroxysmal sympathetic hyperactivity may be helpful for this dysautonomia. These medications include gabapentin, α-2 agonists, β-blockers, benzodiazepines, opioids, and baclofen.[18] Attention to bowel regimen is key to avoid ileus or small bowel obstruction. Medications should be constantly reevaluated and removed as soon possible to mitigate polypharmacy and reduce sedation and other adverse side effects.

Treatment

Early recognition and initiation of treatment are critical to recovery in autoimmune and paraneoplastic encephalitis. The focus of treatment is initiation of immunosuppression and removal of tumor if present. Initial treatment is with pulse-dose methylprednisolone, although caution should be exercised if concern for infection or central nervous system (CNS) lymphoma exists (**Fig. 3**). As well, treatment with intravenous immunoglobulin (IVIg) and/or plasma exchange (PLEX) is initiated.[11,22] Early removal of the tumor is crucial for recovery, and close attention should be paid to computed tomography (CT), fludeoxyglucose (FDG)-positron emission tomography (PET), and

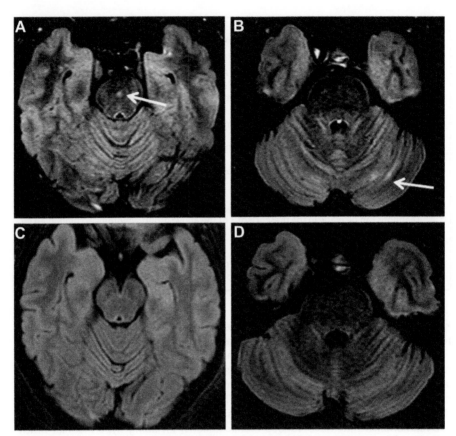

Fig. 2. Anti-NMDA receptor encephalitis. Axial T2-weighted FLAIR MR images show brain-stem and cerebellar hyperintensities (*white arrows*) (*A, B*) followed by resolution after treatment (*C, D*).

ultrasonography imaging for potential tumors. Referring to a protocol screening, such as that proposed by the European Federation of Neurological Societies Task Force, may be beneficial.[2]

In patients who are severely ill requiring ICU admission, particularly with anti-NMDAR encephalitis, then consideration should be given to the initiation of second-line therapies. These therapies include rituximab and/or cyclophospamide.[11]

Despite aggressive and adequate treatment, there is the potential for relapse, which may be as much as 10% to 20% depending on the type of autoimmune or paraneoplastic encephalitis.[14,23] Patients should be monitored for recurrence of clinical symptoms or antibodies. As well, patients should have ongoing tumor screening as deemed appropriate. Early consultation of specialists who deal with commonly associated tumor types should be considered, such as gynecology for anti-NMDAR encephalitis. Patients may benefit from steroid-sparing agents for maintenance therapy to prevent relapse, although the precise duration remains ill defined.[11]

Steroid-responsive encephalopathy with autoimmune thyroiditis

Steroid-responsive encephalopathy with autoimmune thyroiditis (SREAT) was formerly known as Hashimoto encephalopathy. This disorder primarily affects women

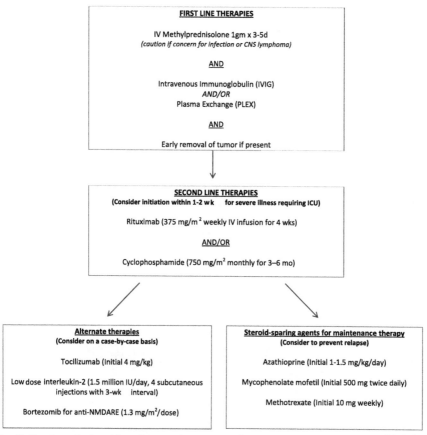

Fig. 3. Treatment algorithm for autoimmune and paraneoplastic encephalitis.[2,9,10,22] d, days; IV, intravenous; IVIg, intravenous immunoglobulin; PLEX, plasma exchange; wk, week.

in a wide age range, although it may also affect men. SREAT is associated with the presence of serum thyroid antibodies, and frequently patients also have overt or subclinical thyroid disease.[24] These antibodies are markers of autoimmunity and do not play a direct role in the pathogenesis. Clinical manifestations include encephalopathy, seizures, myoclonus, hallucinations, and strokelike episodes (**Box 4, Fig. 4**). SREAT is characterized by an excellent response to corticosteroids, although other forms of immunosuppression may be required.[25,26] It should be noted that 13% of the population has thyroid antibodies, and an exhaustive search should be pursued for other causes, including other autoimmune or paraneoplastic encephalitides.[4] Consideration should be given to rare entities such as mitochondrial disorders, including MELAS (mitochondrial encephalopathy, lactic acidosis, and strokelike episodes), which typically manifest with lactic acidosis. Although these disorders commonly manifest before the age of 20 years, genetic testing may be considered on a case-by-case basis.[27]

Bickerstaff brainstem encephalitis

Bickerstaff brainstem encephalitis is a clinical syndrome involving impairment of consciousness, ataxia, and bilateral ophthalmoparesis. This syndrome is often preceded

> **Box 4**
> **Diagnostic criteria for steroid-responsive encephalopathy with autoimmune thyroiditis (Hashimoto encephalopathy)[4]**
>
> Diagnosis can be made when all 6 of the following criteria are met:
> 1. Encephalopathy with seizures, myoclonus, hallucinations, or strokelike episodes
> 2. Subclinical or mild overt thyroid disease (usually hypothyroidism)
> 3. Brain MRI normal or with nonspecific abnormalities
> 4. Presence of serum thyroid (thyroid peroxidase, thyroglobulin) antibodies
> 5. Absence of well-characterized neuronal antibodies in serum and CSF
> 6. Reasonable exclusion of other disorders

by an infectious prodrome, and patients may have additional symptoms of pupillary abnormalities, facial palsy, bulbar dysfunction, and limb weakness.[28] Anti-GQ1b immunoglobulin G (IgG) is diagnostic of Bickerstaff encephalitis, and overlap may be present with Miller-Fisher syndrome and Guillain-Barré syndrome and its variants (**Box 5**). Most often, this syndrome has a monophasic course with a good outcome; however, it is important to exclude alternative diagnoses, particularly in the absence of GQ1b antibodies (>30% of patients may not have these antibodies).[29] Important differential diagnoses include listeria rhombencephalitis, viral or postviral rhombencephalitis, neurosarcoidosis, chronic lymphocytic inflammation with pontine perivascular enhancement responsive to steroids, and primary CNS lymphoma.[30]

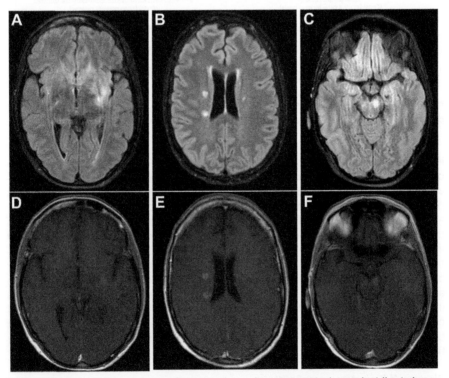

Fig. 4. SREAT at the time of disease flare. Basal ganglia, periventricular, and midbrain hyperintensities with patchy enhancement in axial T2-weighted FLAIR (*A–C*) and contrast-enhanced T1-weighted MR images (*D–F*) respectively.

Box 5
Diagnostic criteria for Bickerstaff brainstem encephalitis[4]

Probable
1. Subacute onset (rapid progression of <4 weeks) of all the following symptoms
   - Decreased level of consciousness
   - Bilateral external ophthalmoplegia
   - Ataxia
2. Reasonable exclusion of other disorders

Definite
1. Diagnosis can be made in the presence of positive IgG anti-GQ1b antibodies even if bilateral external ophthalmoplegia is not complete or ataxia cannot be assessed, or if recovery has occurred within 12 weeks after onset

---

Clinic care points

- Diagnosis of autoimmune and paraneoplastic encephalitis relies on a combination of clinical presentation with characteristic neural-specific autoantibodies (serum and/or CSF), neuroimaging, EEG, CSF profile, and comprehensive search for systemic malignancy.
- SREAT is associated with the presence of antithyroid autoantibodies, but they do not play a direct role in pathogenesis.
- Bickerstaff encephalitis is characterized by a decreased level of consciousness, bilateral external ophthalmoplegia, ataxia, and presence of anti-GQ1b antibodies.

Demyelinating Diseases

Multiple sclerosis

Multiple sclerosis (MS) is the most common inflammatory demyelinating CNS disorder with heterogeneous clinical and pathologic features. There is perivenular inflammation/demyelination manifesting as periventricular, juxtacortical, infratentorial, and spinal cord lesions on MRI of the brain and spinal cord (**Fig. 5**).[31] The 10-year cumulative incidence of ICU admission is 6% for patients with MS; young adults (<40 years old) are most commonly at risk. One-year mortality after ICU admission was as high as 26%.[32] This article focusses on the aggressive disease phenotype, which frequently causes neurologic emergencies. These emergencies include tumefactive lesions, Marburg type, and Balo concentric sclerosis. Patients often present with signs and symptoms of cerebral mass lesions, including encephalopathy, seizures, impaired consciousness, cognitive deficits, and focal neurologic signs with potential for rapid deterioration.[33]

Tumefactive lesions are typically greater than 2 cm in size. Imaging features of these lesions may mimic those of neoplasm; therefore, a high level of suspicion is required, especially when lumbar puncture is precluded because of mass effect and risk of herniation. Imaging characteristics that help distinguish these large demyelinating lesions from high-grade enhancing neoplasm include T2 hypointense rim, peripheral restricted diffusion, a paucity of perilesional edema, and open ring enhancement. Marburg variant, also called acute fulminant MS, is the most severe form and is characterized on MRI brain by confluent, disseminated, multifocal T2 hyperintense lesions in the white matter caused by inflammation, necrosis, and extensive destruction. It progresses rapidly to coma with a high risk of increased intracranial pressure (ICP) and herniation. Balo concentric sclerosis consists of demyelinating lesions with a

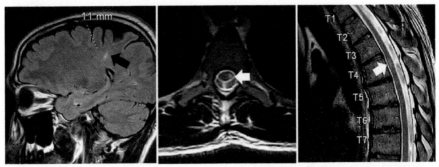

Fig. 5. MS in a 30-year-old woman. (*A*) Sagittal T2-weighted FLAIR MR image shows hyperintense perpendicular lesion (*black arrow*) in periventricular white matter along the posterior aspect of the body of the right lateral ventricle. Axial (*B*) and sagittal (*C*) T2-weighted fast spin echo MR images of thoracic spine show eccentric expansile focus at T4 level (*white arrows*).

concentric ring appearance formed by areas of demyelination alternating with relatively preserved myelin. The lesions can occur in isolation or with classic MS.[31,34] CSF may show increased protein level or mild pleocytosis, but oligoclonal bands are less frequent; when present, it may suggest overlap with MS.[35–37] Acute treatment relies on corticosteroids with a low threshold to add IVIg and PLEX. Long-term immunomodulatory treatment, such as cyclophosphamide or rituximab, can be considered for refractory cases, but data are limited. It is prudent to vigilantly monitor for signs and symptoms of increased ICP and consider invasive ICP monitoring. Neurosurgical consultation and evaluation for decompressive craniectomy should be sought early to prevent brainstem herniation.[35]

Neuromyelitis optica spectrum disorder
Neuromyelitis optica spectrum disorder (NMOSD) is an immune-mediated demyelinating disorder directed against the areas of CNS rich with aquaporin 4 (AQP4) water channels, predominantly the optic nerves and spinal cord. It is a distinct disease entity from MS. About 70% to 80% of patients have positive serum AQP4 IgG, and a subset of patients without this antibody has positive myelin oligodendrocyte glycoprotein (MOG) IgG.[38–40] Coexisting autoimmune diseases such as thyroiditis, systemic lupus erythematosus (SLE), or Sjögren syndrome are often found in NMOSD (more frequently in AQP4-positive patients).[41,42]

Cardinal features of NMOSD are transverse myelitis, optic neuritis, and area postrema syndrome. CSF analysis may show neutrophilic pleocytosis with a lesser frequency of oligoclonal bands (30%).[38] AQP4 IgG antibody testing is more sensitive in serum (sensitivity 75%–80%, specificity 99%) compared with CSF by cell-based assays.[38,43,44]

Respiratory compromise may be encountered in the setting of brain stem involvement in NMOSD. Patients with neuromyelitis optica are observed to have a shorter time from onset of symptoms to need for ventilatory support compared with those with MS (2.5 vs 19 years). The intubation can also be prolonged.[45] Respiratory failure in the setting of recurrent myelitis is the most common cause of death, with a 5-year mortality of 30%.[46–48]

Acute episode treatment includes high-dose corticosteroids (methylprednisolone 1000 mg intravenously daily for 5 days) with a low threshold to escalate to PLEX.

Prevention of future attack is key, with a variety of immunomodulatory treatment options available, including rituximab (B cell–depleting treatment), eculizumab (complement C5 inhibitor), satralizumab (interleukin-6 inhibitor), inebilizumab (B-cell lineage–depleting treatment), and older immunosuppressants such as azathioprine and mycophenolate mofetil.[49]

Acute disseminated encephalomyelitis

Acute disseminated encephalomyelitis (ADEM) is a rare, idiopathic inflammatory demyelinating condition with rapid, progressive, multifocal gray-white matter involvement. Although not always, there is typically preceding infection. The disease has a female preponderance with disease onset in the third or fourth decade of life.[50,51] The pathophysiologic mechanism is thought to be molecular mimicry, by which antiviral antibodies or a cell-mediated response to pathogens cross react with myelin autoantigens.[51] The symptoms are variable depending on the location, number, and volume of lesions. In general, it is characterized by encephalopathy, seizures, and focal neurologic deficits. Brain MRI typically shows bilateral, asymmetric, poorly marginated T2/fluid-attenuated inversion recovery (FLAIR) hyperintensities involving deep and subcortical white matter as well as gray matter such as cortex, basal ganglia, and thalamus along with brainstem, cerebellum, and spinal cord involvement (**Fig. 6**). The characteristic feature is the simultaneous presence of enhancing and nonenhancing lesions.[52] CSF results are variable, with lymphocytic pleocytosis, increased protein level, increased IgG index, and infrequent presence of oligoclonal bands (which, when present, may predict progression to MS).[51,53] Rarely, the course can be relapsing, which suggests either MS or MOG IgG-related demyelinating disease.[54]

Acute treatment is instituted with intravenous corticosteroid followed by IVIg or PLEX in refractory cases.[51,52] Patients with ADEM can deteriorate rapidly with requirement of close monitoring for increased ICP from edema and prevention of brain herniation. Up to a third of patients may require ICU-level care.[55–57] Acute hemorrhagic encephalomyelitis (also known as Hurst acute necrotizing hemorrhagic leukoencephalitis or Hurst disease) is a rare but fulminant form of ADEM with a high possibility of rapid deterioration.[35]

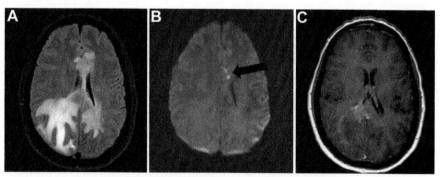

Fig. 6. Acute disseminated encephalomyelitis in a 32-year-old man. (*A*) Axial T2-weighted FLAIR MR image shows a confluent biparietal subcortical and periventricular white matter lesion. Diffusion-weighted image (*B*) shows restricted diffusion (*black arrow*) in genu and trunk of corpus callosum. Contrast-enhanced T1-weighted MR image (*C*) shows patchy enhancement within the lesion.

Acute transverse myelitis

Acute transverse myelitis (ATM) is a focal disorder of the spinal cord, specifically related to inflammation, as shown by imaging and/or spinal fluid analysis, presenting with a well-defined sensory level, and reaching clinical nadir between 4 hours and 21 days after symptom onset.[58] The main causes include MS, NMOSD, systemic rheumatologic disease (SLE, Sjögren syndrome, sarcoidosis), and infection (coxsackie virus and *Mycoplasma pneumoniae*). Up to a third of cases are idiopathic.[59,60]

After defining a clinically compatible syndrome of myelopathy, which developed in acute to subacute time frame with neurologic signs and symptoms of motor, sensory, and/or autonomic dysfunction, finding surrogate evidence of inflammation is the key to differentiating this condition from noninflammatory causes of acute/ subacute myelopathy. Evidence of inflammation is frequently found in CSF analysis (ie, pleocytosis, increased IgG index, in addition to gadolinium-enhancing lesion on MRI).[58] Once the diagnosis of ATM is confirmed, the next step is to identify the underlying cause by appropriate testing and characteristic imaging features.[61] It is important to remember that many cases of presumed idiopathic transverse myelitis often are related to an alternative specific myelopathy. The criteria proposed 18 years ago by the Transverse Myelitis Consortium Working Group relied heavily on features such as CSF pleocytosis and increased IgG index or oligoclonal bands as well as MRI gadolinium enhancement, which are nonspecific findings and seen in inflammatory and noninflammatory myelopathies. Instead, characteristic MRI gadolinium enhancement and T2 hyperintensity patterns indicate a particular cause.[58,62]

Spinal cord transverse myelitis lesions caused by MS are peripherally located and wedge shaped, covering 1 or 2 vertebral segments only. In contrast, NMOSD-related transverse myelitis has centrally located longitudinally extensive cord lesions, sometimes with extension to brainstem as well as associated evidence of optic neuritis. Longitudinally extensive transverse myelitis is also seen with SLE, Sjögren syndrome, sarcoidosis, and spinal cord ischemia. It is important to differentiate inflammatory from noninflammatory causes of myelopathy such as spinal cord ischemia, tumor, spinal dural arteriovenous fistula, compression, nutrition deficiency, and infection (especially varicella-zoster virus).[62] Paraneoplastic causes are typically linked to antiamphiphysin or CRMP-5 antibodies.[60] Sarcoidosis-related transverse myelitis has a characteristic thick dorsal subpial and trident pattern of enhancement.[62]

Treatment relies on an accurate diagnosis and understanding of the underlying cause. Although there are no randomized controlled trials, intravenous corticosteroids are the mainstay of treatment of an acute episode.[63] Additional immunotherapies in the form of PLEX can be considered, but data are limited depending on the severity and cause.

Clinics care points

- Tumefactive MS, Marburg type, and Balo concentric sclerosis may pose a grave prognosis but can be managed effectively if diagnosis and supportive care are provided early.
- Longitudinally extensive transverse myelitis, optic neuritis, and area postrema syndrome are hallmark features of neuromyelitis optica spectrum disorder.
- Fulminant demyelinating disorders require close monitoring for signs and symptoms of increased ICP and consideration of invasive ICP monitoring as well as medical and surgical therapies as necessary.

Systemic Autoimmune Disorders that Affect the Nervous System

Neurosarcoidosis

Sarcoidosis, known as the mysterious disease and a great mimicker, is a chronic immune-mediated disorder that may affect people of all racial and ethnic backgrounds and at all ages.[64,65] Systemic manifestations include anterior uveitis, cough, dyspnea, rash, and polyarthritis because of involvement of joints, lungs, skin, and eyes.[66,67] Up to 50% of patients have a neurologic sign or symptom as the presenting manifestation of sarcoidosis at the time of diagnosis.[68]

Neurologic involvement occurs in 5% to 10% of patients with systemic sarcoidosis.[68,69] Any level of the neuraxis can be affected, but the most common finding is a facial nerve palsy (25%–50%), followed by other cranial neuropathies (including optic, vestibular).[67,68] CNS involvement includes neuroendocrine dysfunction caused by hypothalamic inflammation and pituitary dysfunction, basal meningitis and radiculomyelopathy caused by perivascular granulomatous inflammation in brain and spinal cord respectively, communicating or noncommunicating hydrocephalus, encephalopathy/vasculopathy, and meningeal mass lesions (granulomas). Peripheral nervous system (PNS) involvement includes mononeuropathy, mononeuritis multiplex; generalized sensory, sensorimotor, and motor polyneuropathies; and acute or chronic proximal myopathy and muscle atrophy.[67,68,70–72]

Histopathologic evidence of noncaseating granuloma with no detectable microorganism is the gold standard for diagnosis.[65] MRI of the brain with contrast is the imaging modality of choice (**Fig. 7**). It often shows enhancement of meninges and cranial nerves, nonspecific white matter changes, hydrocephalus, and parenchymal granulomas (representing inflammation along the Virchow-Robin space).[73] Spinal cord imaging findings that strongly indicate sarcoidosis include enhancement of dorsal subpial space extending greater than 3 vertebral segments and intramedullary

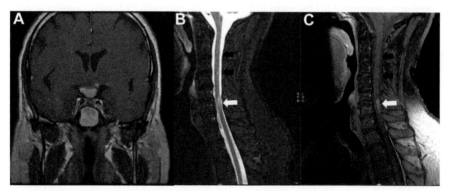

Fig. 7. Pulmonary and osseous sarcoidosis in 42-year-old man diagnosed 1 year prior, presenting with panhypopituitarism. (*A*) Coronal T1-weighted contrast-enhanced MR image shows large, homogeneously enhancing suprasellar mass (infundibulum) and a satellite lesion in the left optic tract. Sagittal T2-weighted short tau inversion recovery (*B*) and contrast-enhanced T1-weighted (*C*) MR images of cervical and thoracic spine of another 42-year-old man with ocular and pulmonary sarcoidosis diagnosed 1 year prior, now presenting with subacute ascending numbness and weakness, and sphincter dysfunction. There are multiple T2 hyperintense lesions in the cervical cord, which enhance with contrast (*black arrows*). The lesion at the C6 level (*white arrows*) is causing some mild expansion of the cord. (*Courtesy of* Dr. Sergi Martinez-Ramirez, Sarcoid Center, Boston University School of Medicine/ Boston Medical Center, Boston, MA)

enhancement often lasting greater than 2 months. These findings can help distinguish neurosarcoidosis from other demyelinating diseases.[74] CSF analysis shows increased protein level (up to 250 mg/dL) in up to two-thirds of patients, pleocytosis in 50%, increased opening pressure in 10%, and hypoglycorrhachia in 14% of patients.[71,73,75] CSF angiotensin-converting-enzyme level has low sensitivity and specificity. The possibility of increased ICP should be considered in patients with suspected neurosarcoidosis, and appropriate examination/testing should precede the lumbar puncture to safely perform this procedure (**Table 2**).[76]

First-line induction treatment is typically oral or intravenous glucocorticoids depending on disease extent and disease severity.[77] Long-term maintenance treatment is necessary and should be considered early in patients with moderate to severe disease burden, deterioration on glucocorticoid treatment, and contraindication to glucocorticoid treatment. Infliximab, a chimeric antibody blocking the effect of tumor necrosis factor alpha, has shown promising results in terms of disease burden on MRI, neurologic deficits, and symptom relief.[78] However, there are no randomized, placebo-controlled treatment trials and, depending on patient factors such as convenience, cost, and side effect profile, various options, such as mycophenolate mofetil, azathioprine, methotrexate, cyclophosphamide, rituximab, and leflunomide, can be considered.[69,79,80]

Systemic lupus erythematosus

SLE is a chronic autoimmune disease with the ability to affect essentially any organ, characterized by the production of autoantibodies against intracellular components.[81] The heterogeneous manifestations commonly include fatigue, fever, weight loss, myalgia, arthritis/arthralgia, and mucocutaneous involvement.[81] Neurologic pathophysiology includes coagulopathy leading to thromboembolic phenomenon, autoantibodies, cytokines, and cell-mediated inflammation; vasculitis is rare.[82–84]

A broad range of neurologic and psychiatric manifestations may occur at the time of diagnosis or during the first year of illness (**Box 6**).[85–87] Demyelinating disorders and myelopathy are rarely (<1%) seen in SLE. All patients with SLE with myelitis should be checked for AQP4 antibodies because most of these patients satisfy NMOSD criteria. The treatment of neuropsychiatric SLE (NPSLE) depends on the severity and underlying mechanism (inflammation vs thromboembolic) of neurologic disease. High-dose corticosteroids followed by a steroid-sparing agent such as cyclophosphamide, mycophenolate mofetil, or azathioprine is traditionally considered. Emerging therapies involve anti-CD20 monoclonal antibodies.[88,89]

Thromboembolic events in the form of arterial and venous thrombosis are present in 20% of NPSLE cases and are strongly correlated with antiphospholipid (aPL) antibodies and lupus anticoagulant.[90] Antiphospholipid antibody syndrome is characterized by thrombosis in the venous and/or arterial circulation and/or adverse pregnancy outcomes in the presence of persistently increased titers of 1 or more aPL antibodies, including lupus anticoagulant, anticardiolipin antibodies, and anti-B2-glycoprotein 1 antibodies.[91] Antiphospholipid antibodies accelerate atherosclerosis and increase the risk of stroke approximately 8-fold in individuals aged less than 50 years.[92,93] Brain infarcts can appear as large territorial infarcts, localized cortical infarcts, bilateral border zone infarcts, or anterior basal ganglia lesions. Stenotic arterial lesions may also be seen in the stem or major branches of major cerebral arteries.[93,94] Lifelong anticoagulation with warfarin with International Normalized Ratio target of 2.5 to 3 is indicated in all aPL antibody–related thrombosis events because of high risk of recurrence with less intense therapy.[82]

Catastrophic antiphospholipid syndrome involves multiorgan thrombosis, which may lead to acute renal failure, respiratory distress syndrome, diffuse alveolar hemorrhage, encephalopathy, and adrenal hemorrhage. Prompt diagnosis and intervention with a

Table 2
Systemic autoimmune disorders with characteristic systemic and neurologic clinical findings, imaging features, and neurologic presentations leading to intensive care unit care as well as factors associated with worse outcome

Clinical Syndrome	Systemic Characteristics (Most Common)	Most Common Neurologic Syndrome	Imaging Characteristics	Neurologic Presentations Requiring Critical Care Management	Factors (Systemic/ Neurologic) Associated with Worse Prognosis in ICU
Neurosarcoidosis	Lungs, mediastinal lymph nodes, cutaneous, ocular involvement	Cranial neuropathies, meningeal disease, brain parenchymal disease (hypothalamus and pituitary gland), spinal cord disease	Parenchymal granuloma: T1 isointense, variable postcontrast enhancement Spinal cord: subpial intramedullary lesion (>3 vertebral segments); trident sign of contrast enhancement	Guillain-Barré syndrome,[116] sarcoid encephalopathy with diffuse inflammation and focal hydrocephalus,[117] obstructive hydrocephalus[118,119]	Hydrocephalus, intraparenchymal mass lesions, seizures at presentation, multiple cranial nerve involvement, myelopathy, chronic meningitis[70]
Neuropsychiatric lupus	Constitutional symptoms, photosensitive skin lesions, oral/nasal ulcers, lymphadenopathy, Raynaud phenomenon, arthritis	Headache, mood disorder, cognitive dysfunction, seizure, strokes (antiphospholipid antibody syndrome)	White matter hyperintensities (periventricular/ subcortical), cortical or deep gray matter hyperintensities, cerebral atrophy, restricted diffusion pattern (acute/ subacute infarct, vasogenic edema)	Intracranial hemorrhage, seizures, venous sinus thrombosis[120]	Cytopenia, thrombocytopenia, infection, pulmonary hemorrhage[121]
Sjögren syndrome	Dry mouth, dry eyes, arthritis, Raynaud phenomenon, pulmonary involvement, interstitial nephritis, purpura, lymphoma	Peripheral: sensory neuronopathy, small fiber neuropathy Central: cranial neuropathy (V), optic neuritis and myelitis (overlap with NMOSD)	Demyelinating lesions, T2 hyperintensity of dorsal column, white matter hyperintensities, NMO-like lesions	Ascending polyneuropathy, myelitis, stroke[122]	Lymphoproliferative malignancy, hypocomplementemia, advanced age at diagnosis, vasculitis, cryoglobulinemia, and parotid enlargement[122]

Abbreviation: NMO, neuromyelitis optica.

Box 6
Neuropsychiatric systemic lupus erythematosus manifestations affecting central nervous system and peripheral nervous system

CNS	PNS
Aseptic meningitis	Acute inflammatory demyelinating polyradiculoneuropathy
Cerebrovascular disease	Autonomic disorder
Demyelinating syndrome	Mononeuropathy, single/multiplex
Headache	Myasthenia gravis
Movement disorder	Neuropathy, cranial
Myelopathy	Plexopathy
Seizure disorder	Polyneuropathy
Cognitive dysfunction	—
Mood disorder	—
Acute confusional state	—
Anxiety disorder	—
Psychosis	—

combination of anticoagulants, glucocorticoids, IVIg, and PLEX are critical (**Box 7**). Refractory cases may be benefited by consideration of rituximab or eculizumab.[91] Antiphospholipid syndrome should always be suspected in patients with SLE with stroke.[95]

Sjögren syndrome

Sjögren syndrome is a progressive autoimmune condition characterized by xerostomia and xerophthalmia caused by lymphocytic infiltration of exocrine glands (lacrimal and salivary).[96] Extraglandular inflammation leads to cutaneous, pulmonary, renal, and

Box 7
Checklist for patients with a systemic rheumatologic disease with neurologic syndrome admitted to intensive care unit[120,123–125]

Is systemic rheumatologic disease newly diagnosed in ICU?	New diagnosis may require organ support therapy as well intensification of immunosuppressive treatment in the ICU
Is there an exacerbation of systemic rheumatologic disease with an established diagnosis?	Multiorgan involvement such as pulmonary, cardiovascular, renal injury, in addition to neurologic dysfunction, should be considered
What type of immunosuppressant used?	Cyclophosphamide use before ICU admission associated with increased risk of mortality in SLE
Is there multiorgan involvement?	Cardiac involvement may account for mortality for systemic autoimmune disease (sarcoidosis); gastrointestinal hemorrhage associated with a higher risk of death in SLE
Is there evidence of infection?	Infection is the leading cause of ICU admission in patients with systemic rheumatologic disease and can coexist with neurologic compromise
Are there coexisting other autoimmune diseases or comorbidities?	Hypertension, peptic ulcer disease, chronic kidney disease, cardiac dysfunction and so forth can significantly affect the course as well as medication consideration while in the ICU
Has cytotoxic medication been used for a long time?	Consider malignancy in differential diagnosis
Was there a diagnostic or therapeutic invasive procedure recently performed?	Consider iatrogenic causes for infection

vascular involvement and hematologic abnormalities.[97] PNS involvement is seen in 5% to 15% of cases, whereas the involvement of the CNS occurs in 2% of cases and may precede the diagnosis by 2 years in 80% of patients in whom it occurs.[98–100] CNS disease may affect spinal cord, brain stem, optic nerves, cerebellum, and cerebral hemispheres and may require mechanical ventilation in selected scenarios.[101,102] Chronic B-cell stimulation makes individuals susceptible to the development of lymphoma.[103]

Neurologic syndromes may precede the onset of sicca symptoms (dry mouth and dry eyes) in 25% to 92% of patients.[104,105] A wide array of syndromes comprises Sjögren-related CNS involvement. These syndromes include transverse myelitis, optic neuritis, demyelinating disease, meningoencephalitis, cognitive changes, and asymptomatic brain MRI lesions.[100,106] There is significant overlap with NMOSD with regard to demyelinating brain and spinal cord syndromes and related clinical and imaging findings.[107–109]

Diagnosis requires a high level of suspicion and application of American-European Consensus Group Revised International Classification Criteria.[110] Serum autoantibodies (anti-Ro/SSA and anti-La/SSB) have low sensitivity, and diagnostic evaluation with salivary gland biopsy, Schirmer test, or a rose bengal test should be considered if clinical suspicion is high.[99] Lumbar puncture in the setting of CNS demyelinating disease is typically associated with 1 to 2 oligoclonal bands compared with MS, in which oligoclonal bands are greater than 2.[107] Sjögren syndrome–associated myelitis, optic neuritis, and/or brain lesions require testing for NMOSD.[95,102]

Sensory ganglionopathy, sensorimotor neuropathy, and painful small fiber neuropathy (in severe cases) require treatment with IVIg.[102,111,112] Multiple mononeuropathies or cranial neuropathies respond to corticosteroids.[104] Vasculitic features may have a favorable response to rituximab.[113] An acute treatment of demyelinating disease is intravenous methylprednisolone for 5 days and PLEX in severe cases.[114] Long-term remission treatment geared toward NMOSD is recommended in Sjögren syndrome–related myelitis with positive AQP4 antibodies in the form of eculizumab, rituximab, azathioprine, or mycophenolate mofetil.[114,115] Cyclophosphamide can be considered in refractory cases of Sjögren syndrome–related myelitis.[100]

Clinics care points

- Whole-body FDG-PET is a valuable study when sarcoidosis is suspected, and chest radiograph and CT are unrevealing because up to 90% of patients with sarcoidosis have pulmonary and mediastinal involvement.
- Neuropsychiatric lupus-related thrombotic processes require antiplatelet and anticoagulation treatment, whereas inflammatory processes are treated with corticosteroids and immunosuppression.
- Sjögren syndrome predominantly affects the peripheral nervous system in the form of sensory ganglionopathy, painful small fiber neuropathy, and trigeminal neuropathy.

SUMMARY

Autoimmune neurologic emergencies are common and may impose significant challenges in the early phases of patient management in intensive care when diagnostic test results such as serum and CSF antibodies, systemic inflammatory markers, and testing for occult malignancy may not yet be available. Knowledge of the typical neurologic manifestations of primarily nervous system disorder or secondary nervous system involvement from systemic autoimmune diseases is of paramount importance to early recognition and initiation of treatment.

DISCLOSURE

Drs P. Raibagkar and A. Ramineni have nothing to disclose.

REFERENCES

1. Newman MP, Blum S, Wong RC, et al. Autoimmune encephalitis. Intern Med J 2016;46(2):148–57.
2. Lancaster E. The Diagnosis and Treatment of Autoimmune Encephalitis. J Clin Neurol 2016;12(1):1–13.
3. Gunther A, Schubert J, Witte OW, et al. [Intensive care aspects of autoimmune encephalitis]. Med Klin Intensivmed Notfmed 2019;114(7):620–7.
4. Graus F, Titulaer MJ, Balu R, et al. A clinical approach to diagnosis of autoimmune encephalitis. Lancet Neurol 2016;15(4):391–404.
5. Dubey D, Pittock SJ, Kelly CR, et al. Autoimmune encephalitis epidemiology and a comparison to infectious encephalitis. Ann Neurol 2018;83(1):166–77.
6. Fitch MT, Abrahamian FM, Moran GJ, et al. Emergency department management of meningitis and encephalitis. Infect Dis Clin North Am 2008;22(1): 33–52, v-vi.
7. Jubelt B, Mihai C, Li TM, et al. Rhombencephalitis/brainstem encephalitis. Curr Neurol Neurosci Rep 2011;11(6):543–52.
8. Kelley BP, Patel SC, Marin HL, et al. Autoimmune Encephalitis: Pathophysiology and Imaging Review of an Overlooked Diagnosis. AJNR Am J Neuroradiol 2017; 38(6):1070–8.
9. Hermetter C, Fazekas F, Hochmeister S. Systematic review: syndromes, early diagnosis, and treatment in autoimmune encephalitis. Front Neurol 2018;9:706.
10. Moise AM, Karakis I, Herlopian A, et al. Continuous EEG findings in autoimmune encephalitis. J Clin Neurophysiol 2021;38(2):124–9.
11. Shin YW, Lee ST, Park KI, et al. Treatment strategies for autoimmune encephalitis. Ther Adv Neurol Disord 2018;11. 1756285617722347.
12. Lai M, Huijbers MG, Lancaster E, et al. Investigation of LGI1 as the antigen in limbic encephalitis previously attributed to potassium channels: a case series. Lancet Neurol 2010;9(8):776–85.
13. Irani SR, Michell AW, Lang B, et al. Faciobrachial dystonic seizures precede Lgi1 antibody limbic encephalitis. Ann Neurol 2011;69(5):892–900.
14. Titulaer MJ, McCracken L, Gabilondo I, et al. Treatment and prognostic factors for long-term outcome in patients with anti-NMDA receptor encephalitis: an observational cohort study. Lancet Neurol 2013;12(2):157–65.
15. Salovin A, Glanzman J, Roslin K, et al. Anti-NMDA receptor encephalitis and nonencephalitic HSV-1 infection. Neurol Neuroimmunol Neuroinflamm 2018; 5(4):e458.
16. Lin KL, Lin JJ. Neurocritical care for Anti-NMDA receptor encephalitis. Biomed J 2020;43(3):251–8.
17. Bacchi S, Franke K, Wewegama D, et al. Magnetic resonance imaging and positron emission tomography in anti-NMDA receptor encephalitis: A systematic review. J Clin Neurosci 2018;52:54–9.
18. Neyens RR, Gaskill GE, Chalela JA. Critical Care Management of Anti-N-Methyl-D-Aspartate Receptor Encephalitis. Crit Care Med 2018;46(9):1514–21.
19. Scheibe F, Prüss H, Mengel AM, et al. Bortezomib for treatment of therapy-refractory anti-NMDA receptor encephalitis. Neurology 2017;88(4):366–70.
20. Shin YW, Lee ST, Kim TJ, et al. Bortezomib treatment for severe refractory anti-NMDA receptor encephalitis. Ann Clin Transl Neurol 2018;5(5):598–605.

21. Anderson D, Nathoo N, Henry M, et al. Oophorectomy in NMDA receptor encephalitis and negative pelvic imaging. Pract Neurol 2020. https://doi.org/10.1136/practneurol-2020-002676.

22. Nosadini M, Mohammad SS, Ramanathan S, et al. Immune therapy in autoimmune encephalitis: a systematic review. Expert Rev Neurother 2015;15(12):1391–419.

23. Broadley J, Seneviratne U, Beech P, et al. Prognosis in autoimmune encephalitis: Database. Data Brief 2018;21:2694–703.

24. Castillo P, Woodruff B, Caselli R, et al. Steroid-responsive encephalopathy associated with autoimmune thyroiditis. Arch Neurol 2006;63(2):197–202.

25. Jiang Y, Tian X, Gu Y, et al. Application of plasma exchange in steroid-responsive encephalopathy. Front Immunol 2019;10:324.

26. Cornejo R, Venegas P, Goñi D, et al. Successful response to intravenous immunoglobulin as rescue therapy in a patient with Hashimoto's encephalopathy. BMJ Case Rep 2010;2010. bcr0920103332.

27. El-Hattab AW, Adesina AM, Jones J, et al. MELAS syndrome: Clinical manifestations, pathogenesis, and treatment options. Mol Genet Metab 2015;116(1–2):4–12.

28. Odaka M, Yuki N, Yamada M, et al. Bickerstaff's brainstem encephalitis: clinical features of 62 cases and a subgroup associated with Guillain-Barré syndrome. Brain 2003;126(Pt 10):2279–90.

29. Koga M, Kusunoki S, Kaida K, et al. Nationwide survey of patients in Japan with Bickerstaff brainstem encephalitis: epidemiological and clinical characteristics. J Neurol Neurosurg Psychiatry 2012;83(12):1210–5.

30. Moragas M, Martínez-Yélamos S, Majós C, et al. Rhombencephalitis: a series of 97 patients. Medicine (Baltimore) 2011;90(4):256–61.

31. Sarbu N, Shih RY, Jones RV, et al. White matter diseases with radiologic-pathologic correlation. Radiographics 2016;36(5):1426–47.

32. Marrie RA, Bernstein CN, Peschken CA, et al. Intensive care unit admission in multiple sclerosis: increased incidence and increased mortality. Neurology 2014;82(23):2112–9.

33. Hardy TA, Chataway J. Tumefactive demyelination: an approach to diagnosis and management. J Neurol Neurosurg Psychiatry 2013;84(9):1047–53.

34. Hardy TA, Tobin WO, Lucchinetti CF. Exploring the overlap between multiple sclerosis, tumefactive demyelination and Balo's concentric sclerosis. Mult Scler 2016;22(8):986–92.

35. Hardy TA, Reddel SW, Barnett MH, et al. Atypical inflammatory demyelinating syndromes of the CNS. Lancet Neurol 2016;15(9):967–81.

36. Altintas A, Petek B, Isik N, et al. Clinical and radiological characteristics of tumefactive demyelinating lesions: follow-up study. Mult Scler 2012;18(10):1448–53.

37. Kiriyama T, Kataoka H, Taoka T, et al. Characteristic neuroimaging in patients with tumefactive demyelinating lesions exceeding 30 mm. J Neuroimaging 2011;21(2):e69–77.

38. Wingerchuk DM, Banwell B, Bennett JL, et al. International consensus diagnostic criteria for neuromyelitis optica spectrum disorders. Neurology 2015;85(2):177–89.

39. Wingerchuk DM, Lennon VA, Lucchinetti CF, et al. The spectrum of neuromyelitis optica. Lancet Neurol 2007;6(9):805–15.

40. Jarius S, Ruprecht K, Kleiter I, et al. MOG-IgG in NMO and related disorders: a multicenter study of 50 patients. Part 2: Epidemiology, clinical presentation,

radiological and laboratory features, treatment responses, and long-term outcome. J Neuroinflammation 2016;13(1):280.

41. Jarius S, Ruprecht K, Wildemann B, et al. Contrasting disease patterns in sero-positive and seronegative neuromyelitis optica: A multicentre study of 175 patients. J Neuroinflammation 2012;9:14.

42. Wingerchuk DM, Weinshenker BG. The emerging relationship between neuro-myelitis optica and systemic rheumatologic autoimmune disease. Mult Scler 2012;18(1):5–10.

43. Majed M, Fryer JP, McKeon A, et al. Clinical utility of testing AQP4-IgG in CSF: Guidance for physicians. Neurol Neuroimmunol Neuroinflamm 2016;3(3):e231.

44. Waters PJ, McKeon A, Leite MI, et al. Serologic diagnosis of NMO: a multicenter comparison of aquaporin-4-IgG assays. Neurology 2012;78(9):665–71 [discussion: 669].

45. Pittock SJ, Weinshenker BG, Wijdicks EF. Mechanical ventilation and tracheostomy in multiple sclerosis. J Neurol Neurosurg Psychiatry 2004;75(9):1331–3.

46. Wingerchuk DM, Weinshenker BG. Neuromyelitis optica: clinical predictors of a relapsing course and survival. Neurology 2003;60(5):848–53.

47. Wingerchuk DM, Hogancamp WF, O'Brien PC, et al. The clinical course of neuromyelitis optica (Devic's syndrome). Neurology 1999;53(5):1107–14.

48. von Geldern G, McPharlin T, Becker K. Immune mediated diseases and immune modulation in the neurocritical care unit. Neurotherapeutics 2012;9(1):99–123.

49. Holroyd KB, Manzano GS, Levy M. Update on neuromyelitis optica spectrum disorder. Curr Opin Ophthalmol 2020;31(6):462–8.

50. Schwarz S, Mohr A, Knauth M, et al. Acute disseminated encephalomyelitis: a follow-up study of 40 adult patients. Neurology 2001;56(10):1313–8.

51. Guimaraes MPM, Nascimento ACB, Alvarenga RMP. CLINICAL course of acute disseminated encephalomyelitis in adults from Rio de Janeiro: Retrospective study of 23 cases and literature review. Mult Scler Relat Disord 2020;46:102424.

52. Sonneville R, Demeret S, Klein I, et al. Acute disseminated encephalomyelitisin the intensive care unit:clinical features and outcome of 20 adults. Intensive Care Med 2008;34(3):528–32.

53. Papetti L, Figa Talamanca L, Spalice A, et al. Predictors of evolution into multiple sclerosis after a first acute demyelinating syndrome in children and adolescents. Front Neurol 2018;9:1156.

54. Flanagan EP. Neuromyelitis optica spectrum disorder and other non-multiple sclerosis central nervous system inflammatory diseases. Continuum (Minneap Minn) 2019;25(3):815–44.

55. Ketelslegers IA, Visser IE, Neuteboom RF, et al. Disease course and outcome of acute disseminated encephalomyelitis is more severe in adults than in children. Mult Scler 2011;17(4):441–8.

56. Dombrowski KE, Mehta AI, Turner DA, et al. Life-saving hemicraniectomy for fulminant acute disseminated encephalomyelitis. Br J Neurosurg 2011;25(2): 249–52.

57. Bourke D, Woon K. Craniectomy for acute disseminated encephalomyelitis. Pract Neurol 2020.

58. Transverse Myelitis Consortium Working Group. Proposed diagnostic criteria and nosology of acute transverse myelitis. Neurology 2002;59(4):499–505.

59. Bhat A, Naguwa S, Cheema G, et al. The epidemiology of transverse myelitis. Autoimmun Rev 2010;9(5):A395–9.

60. Cho TA, Bhattacharyya S. Approach to Myelopathy. Continuum (Minneap Minn) 2018;24(2, Spinal Cord Disorders):386–406.

61. Greenberg BM, Thomas KP, Krishnan C, et al. Idiopathic transverse myelitis: corticosteroids, plasma exchange, or cyclophosphamide. Neurology 2007; 68(19):1614–7.
62. Zalewski NL, Flanagan EP, Keegan BM. Evaluation of idiopathic transverse myelitis revealing specific myelopathy diagnoses. Neurology 2018;90(2): e96–102.
63. Kerr DA, Ayetey H. Immunopathogenesis of acute transverse myelitis. Curr Opin Neurol 2002;15(3):339–47.
64. Rybicki BA, Major M, Popovich J Jr, et al. Racial differences in sarcoidosis incidence: a 5-year study in a health maintenance organization. Am J Epidemiol 1997;145(3):234–41.
65. Iannuzzi MC, Rybicki BA, Teirstein AS. Sarcoidosis. N Engl J Med 2007;357(21): 2153–65.
66. Crouser ED, Maier LA, Wilson KC, et al. Diagnosis and detection of sarcoidosis. an official american thoracic society clinical practice guideline. Am J Respir Crit Care Med 2020;201(8):e26–51.
67. Joseph FG, Scolding NJ. Neurosarcoidosis: a study of 30 new cases. J Neurol Neurosurg Psychiatry 2009;80(3):297–304.
68. Stern BJ, Krumholz A, Johns C, et al. Sarcoidosis and its neurological manifestations. Arch Neurol 1985;42(9):909–17.
69. Lower EE, Broderick JP, Brott TG, et al. Diagnosis and management of neurological sarcoidosis. Arch Intern Med 1997;157(16):1864–8.
70. Culver DA, Ribeiro Neto ML, Moss BP, et al. Neurosarcoidosis. Semin Respir Crit Care Med 2017;38(4):499–513.
71. Pawate S, Moses H, Sriram S. Presentations and outcomes of neurosarcoidosis: a study of 54 cases. QJM 2009;102(7):449–60.
72. Bihan H, Christozova V, Dumas JL, et al. Sarcoidosis: clinical, hormonal, and magnetic resonance imaging (MRI) manifestations of hypothalamic-pituitary disease in 9 patients and review of the literature. Medicine (Baltimore) 2007;86(5): 259–68.
73. Fritz D, van de Beek D, Brouwer MC. Clinical features, treatment and outcome in neurosarcoidosis: systematic review and meta-analysis. BMC Neurol 2016; 16(1):220.
74. Flanagan EP, Kaufmann TJ, Krecke KN, et al. Discriminating long myelitis of neuromyelitis optica from sarcoidosis. Ann Neurol 2016;79(3):437–47.
75. Bruandet A, Richard F, Bombois S, et al. Alzheimer disease with cerebrovascular disease and vascular dementia: clinical features and course compared with Alzheimer disease. J Neurol Neurosurg Psychiatry 2009;80(2):133–9.
76. Scott TF. Cerebral herniation after lumbar puncture in sarcoid meningitis. Clin Neurol Neurosurg 2000;102(1):26–8.
77. Statement on sarcoidosis. Joint Statement of the American Thoracic Society (ATS), the European Respiratory Society (ERS) and the World Association of Sarcoidosis and Other Granulomatous Disorders (WASOG) adopted by the ATS Board of Directors and by the ERS Executive Committee, February 1999. Am J Respir Crit Care Med 1999;160(2):736–55.
78. Lord J, Paz Soldan MM, Galli J, et al. Neurosarcoidosis: Longitudinal experience in a single-center, academic healthcare system. Neurol Neuroimmunol Neuroinflamm 2020;7(4):e743.
79. Scott TF, Yandora K, Valeri A, et al. Aggressive therapy for neurosarcoidosis: long-term follow-up of 48 treated patients. Arch Neurol 2007;64(5):691–6.

80. Doty JD, Mazur JE, Judson MA. Treatment of corticosteroid-resistant neurosarcoidosis with a short-course cyclophosphamide regimen. Chest 2003;124(5):2023–6.

81. Kaul A, Gordon C, Crow MK, et al. Systemic lupus erythematosus. Nat Rev Dis Primers 2016;2:16039.

82. Schwartz N, Stock AD, Putterman C. Neuropsychiatric lupus: new mechanistic insights and future treatment directions. Nat Rev Rheumatol 2019;15(3):137–52.

83. Calle-Botero E, Abril A. Lupus Vasculitis. Curr Rheumatol Rep 2020;22(10):71.

84. Steup-Beekman GM, Zirkzee EJ, Cohen D, et al. Neuropsychiatric manifestations in patients with systemic lupus erythematosus: epidemiology and radiology pointing to an immune-mediated cause. Ann Rheum Dis 2013;72(Suppl 2):ii76–9.

85. Hanly JG, Urowitz MB, Siannis F, et al. Autoantibodies and neuropsychiatric events at the time of systemic lupus erythematosus diagnosis: results from an international inception cohort study. Arthritis Rheum 2008;58(3):843–53.

86. Hanly JG, Urowitz MB, Sanchez-Guerrero J, et al. Neuropsychiatric events at the time of diagnosis of systemic lupus erythematosus: an international inception cohort study. Arthritis Rheum 2007;56(1):265–73.

87. Unterman A, Nolte JE, Boaz M, et al. Neuropsychiatric syndromes in systemic lupus erythematosus: a meta-analysis. Semin Arthritis Rheum 2011;41(1):1–11.

88. Neuwelt CM, Lacks S, Kaye BR, et al. Role of intravenous cyclophosphamide in the treatment of severe neuropsychiatric systemic lupus erythematosus. Am J Med 1995;98(1):32–41.

89. Bertsias GK, Boumpas DT. Pathogenesis, diagnosis and management of neuropsychiatric SLE manifestations. Nat Rev Rheumatol 2010;6(6):358–67.

90. Mok CC, Lau CS, Wong RW. Neuropsychiatric manifestations and their clinical associations in southern Chinese patients with systemic lupus erythematosus. J Rheumatol 2001;28(4):766–71.

91. Garcia D, Erkan D. Diagnosis and Management of the Antiphospholipid Syndrome. N Engl J Med 2018;378(21):2010–21.

92. Narshi CB, Giles IP, Rahman A. The endothelium: an interface between autoimmunity and atherosclerosis in systemic lupus erythematosus? Lupus 2011;20(1):5–13.

93. Kittner SJ, Gorelick PB. Antiphospholipid antibodies and stroke: an epidemiological perspective. Stroke 1992;23(2 Suppl):I19–22.

94. Christodoulou C, Sangle S, D'Cruz DP. Vasculopathy and arterial stenotic lesions in the antiphospholipid syndrome. Rheumatology (Oxford) 2007;46(6):907–10.

95. Bhattacharyya S, Helfgott SM. Neurologic complications of systemic lupus erythematosus, sjogren syndrome, and rheumatoid arthritis. Semin Neurol 2014;34(4):425–36.

96. Brito-Zeron P, Baldini C, Bootsma H, et al. Sjogren syndrome. Nat Rev Dis Primers 2016;2:16047.

97. Ramos-Casals M, Tzioufas AG, Font J. Primary Sjogren's syndrome: new clinical and therapeutic concepts. Ann Rheum Dis 2005;64(3):347–54.

98. Birnbaum J. Peripheral nervous system manifestations of Sjogren syndrome: clinical patterns, diagnostic paradigms, etiopathogenesis, and therapeutic strategies. Neurologist 2010;16(5):287–97.

99. Ramos-Casals M, Solans R, Rosas J, et al. Primary Sjogren syndrome in Spain: clinical and immunologic expression in 1010 patients. Medicine (Baltimore) 2008;87(4):210–9.

100. Delalande S, de Seze J, Fauchais AL, et al. Neurologic manifestations in primary Sjogren syndrome: a study of 82 patients. Medicine (Baltimore) 2004;83(5): 280–91.
101. Ramos-Casals M, Brito-Zeron P, Font J. The overlap of Sjogren's syndrome with other systemic autoimmune diseases. Semin Arthritis Rheum 2007;36(4): 246–55.
102. Berkowitz AL, Samuels MA. The neurology of Sjogren's syndrome and the rheumatology of peripheral neuropathy and myelitis. Pract Neurol 2014;14(1):14–22.
103. Nocturne G, Mariette X. Sjogren Syndrome-associated lymphomas: an update on pathogenesis and management. Br J Haematol 2015;168(3):317–27.
104. Mori K, Iijima M, Koike H, et al. The wide spectrum of clinical manifestations in Sjogren's syndrome-associated neuropathy. Brain 2005;128(Pt 11):2518–34.
105. Gono T, Kawaguchi Y, Katsumata Y, et al. Clinical manifestations of neurological involvement in primary Sjogren's syndrome. Clin Rheumatol 2011;30(4):485–90.
106. Alexander EL, Alexander GE. Aseptic meningoencephalitis in primary Sjogren's syndrome. Neurology 1983;33(5):593–8.
107. Alexander EL, Malinow K, Lejewski JE, et al. Primary Sjogren's syndrome with central nervous system disease mimicking multiple sclerosis. Ann Intern Med 1986;104(3):323–30.
108. Maggi P, Absinta M, Grammatico M, et al. Central vein sign differentiates Multiple Sclerosis from central nervous system inflammatory vasculopathies. Ann Neurol 2018;83(2):283–94.
109. Kahlenberg JM. Neuromyelitis optica spectrum disorder as an initial presentation of primary Sjogren's syndrome. Semin Arthritis Rheum 2011;40(4):343–8.
110. Vitali C, Bombardieri S, Jonsson R, et al. Classification criteria for Sjogren's syndrome: a revised version of the European criteria proposed by the American-European Consensus Group. Ann Rheum Dis 2002;61(6):554–8.
111. Wakasugi D, Kato T, Gono T, et al. Extreme efficacy of intravenous immunoglobulin therapy for severe burning pain in a patient with small fiber neuropathy associated with primary Sjogren's syndrome. Mod Rheumatol 2009;19(4): 437–40.
112. Morozumi S, Kawagashira Y, Iijima M, et al. Intravenous immunoglobulin treatment for painful sensory neuropathy associated with Sjogren's syndrome. J Neurol Sci 2009;279(1–2):57–61.
113. Mekinian A, Ravaud P, Hatron PY, et al. Efficacy of rituximab in primary Sjogren's syndrome with peripheral nervous system involvement: results from the AIR registry. Ann Rheum Dis 2012;71(1):84–7.
114. Sellner J, Boggild M, Clanet M, et al. EFNS guidelines on diagnosis and management of neuromyelitis optica. Eur J Neurol 2010;17(8):1019–32.
115. Trebst C, Jarius S, Berthele A, et al. Update on the diagnosis and treatment of neuromyelitis optica: recommendations of the Neuromyelitis Optica Study Group (NEMOS). J Neurol 2014;261(1):1–16.
116. Sarada PP, Sundararajan K. The devil is in the detail: Acute Guillain-Barre syndrome camouflaged as neurosarcoidosis in a critically ill patient admitted to an Intensive Care Unit. Indian J Crit Care Med 2016;20(4):238–41.
117. Ho SU, Berenberg RA, Kim KS, et al. Sarcoid encephalopathy with diffuse inflammation and focal hydrocephalus shown by sequential CT. Neurology 1979;29(8):1161–5.
118. Kimura H, Takeuchi J, Tsutada T, et al. [A case of neurosarcoidosis with recurrent brainstem infarction, obstructive hydrocephalus and brainstem atrophy]. Rinsho Shinkeigaku 2018;58(7):445–50.

119. Schlitt M, Duvall ER, Bonnin J, et al. Neurosarcoidosis causing ventricular loculation, hydrocephalus, and death. Surg Neurol 1986;26(1):67–71.
120. Janssen NM, Karnad DR, Guntupalli KK. Rheumatologic diseases in the intensive care unit: epidemiology, clinical approach, management, and outcome. Crit Care Clin 2002;18(4):729–48.
121. Keysser G. [Epidemiology and outcome of patients with rheumatic diseases in the intensive care unit]. Z Rheumatol 2019;78(10):925–31.
122. Ruiz-Ordonez I, Aragon CC, Padilla-Guzman A, et al. Sjogren Syndrome in the Intensive Care Unit: An Observational Study. J Clin Rheumatol 2020;26(7S Suppl 2):S174–9.
123. Brunnler T, Susewind M, Hoffmann U, et al. Outcomes and prognostic factors in patients with rheumatologic diseases admitted to the ICU. Intern Med 2015; 54(16):1981–7.
124. Mustafa M, Gladston Chelliah E, Hughes M. Patients with systemic rheumatic diseases admitted to the intensive care unit: what the rheumatologist needs to know. Rheumatol Int 2018;38(7):1163–8.
125. Dumas G, Geri G, Montlahuc C, et al. Outcomes in critically ill patients with systemic rheumatic disease: a multicenter study. Chest 2015;148(4):927–35.

Movement Disorder Emergencies

Diana Apetauerova, MD[a,b], Pritika A. Patel, NP[a], Joseph D. Burns, MD[a,b,c], David P. Lerner, MD[a,b],*

KEYWORDS

- Parkinson disease • Encephalopathy • Psychosis • Hyperpyrexia • Dystonia
- Serotonin syndrome • Neuroleptic malignant syndrome • Malignant catatonia

KEY POINTS

- Although chronic progressive worsening is expected in Parkinson disease, there are multiple ways in which acute decompensation can occur. Acute psychosis in Parkinson disease is a common nonmotor complication and defined as illusions, false sense of presence, hallucinations, and/or delusions. Abrupt withdrawal of dopaminergic agents in patients who have chronically taken them can result in the Parkinson-hyperpyrexia syndrome, which is nearly identical clinically to neuroleptic malignant syndrome.
- Status dystonicus, characterized by severe, generalized, continuous dystonic spasm, can result in rhabdomyolysis and renal failure and has an associated mortality rate of up to 10%.
- The triad of serotonin syndrome includes altered mental status, neuromuscular excitability, and autonomic instability. Early identification, withdrawal of potential precipitant medications, and early use of benzodiazepine are the cornerstones of treatment.
- Neuroleptic malignant syndrome and malignant catatonia comprise a spectrum of diseases defined by encephalopathy, rigidity, hyperthermia, and autonomic instability. Early identification, withdrawal of potential precipitant medications, and early use of benzodiazepines are the cornerstones of treatment.

SEVERE NEUROLOGIC DECOMPENSATION IN THE SETTING OF NONNEUROLOGICAL ILLNESS IN PATIENTS WITH SYNUCLEINOPATHIES
Acute Psychosis

Parkinson disease psychosis
Case 1: a 68-year-old right-handed man with a 12-year history of Parkinson disease (PD), complicated by motor fluctuation and impulse control behavior, was undergoing evaluation for deep brain stimulation (DBS) and subsequently admitted for worsening visual hallucinations. His daily medication regimen consisted of levodopa, 1200 mg; entacapone, 200 mg; amantadine, 100 mg; and rasagiline, 1 mg. He had experienced

[a] Division of Neurology, Lahey Hospital and Medical Center, Burlington, MA 01805, USA;
[b] Department of Neurology, Tufts University School of Medicine, Boston, MA 02111, USA;
[c] Department of Neurosurgery, Tufts University School of Medicine, Boston, MA 02111, USA
* Corresponding author. 41 Mall Road, Burlington, MA 01805.
E-mail address: david.lerner@lahey.org

Neurol Clin 39 (2021) 615–630
https://doi.org/10.1016/j.ncl.2021.01.005
0733-8619/21/© 2021 Elsevier Inc. All rights reserved.

neurologic.theclinics.com

mild visual hallucinations for about 3 years, and they worsened about 3 weeks before admission. At the same time, he started to have delusions, believing that various people were "Satan" and that they were trying to hurt him. He was admitted initially to the inpatient neurology service and was found to have pneumonia complicated by hyponatremia (Na = 119 mEq/L). Within days he developed a neuroleptic malignant-like syndrome (rigidity, fluctuating level of alertness, elevated creatine kinase (CK) greater than 2000 U/L, labile tachycardia, and hypertension) that was complicated by hypoxia and required intubation. During his 1-month intensive care unit (ICU) stay the psychotic features worsened. Therefore, amantadine, rasagiline, and entacapone were gradually discontinued. In addition, his levodopa dosage was gradually decreased to 750 mg daily. He was treated with dexmedetomidine and quetiapine without benefit. A single dose of olanzapine for severe agitation worsened the hyperpyrexia syndrome. Then clozapine was initiated, which gradually improved his psychotic symptoms. Clozapine, 25 mg, 5 times a day before each levodopa dose, became part of his daily medication regimen. Although his psychotic features subsided with this therapy, he continued to be unable to tolerate higher than 900 mg levodopa daily due to akesthesias. Ultimately, 2 years later, he was found to be an appropriate candidate for enteral suspended levodopa therapy, which improved his severe motor fluctuations. Of note, his cognitive testing revealed mild cognitive impairment but no signs of dementia.

Definition. Parkinson disease psychosis (PDP) is a common nonmotor phenomenon in patients with PD treated with dopaminergic drugs and is associated with high morbidity and mortality. According to the National Institute of Neurological Disorders-National Institute of Mental Health (NIND-NIMH) criteria, the diagnosis of PDP requires at least one of the following: illusions, false sense of presence, hallucinations, or delusions. These features should occur following PD onset and should be present for at least 1 month, either as recurrent or continuous symptoms, excluding other causes (dementia or other psychiatric disorders such as schizophrenia or bipolar disorder) and noting associated features, such as the presence or absence of insight, dementia, and PD treatments.[1] PDP can be associated with other psychiatric diagnoses, including depression and dementia. PDP is a source of considerable caregiver stress and burnout.[2] Illusions or hallucinations occur in 15% to 40% of treated patients with PD.[3–6] Up to 10% of patients experience delusions, usually in addition to hallucinations.

Psychosis can also occur in other alpha synucleinopathies, including dementia with lewy bodies (DLB) and multisystem atrophy (MSA). In contrast to PD, core features of DLB are recurrent visual and other types of hallucinations, as well as systematized delusions.[7] Thus, psychosis may occur in DLB regardless of treatment with dopamine replacement therapies or other antiparkinsonian treatments. Approximately 75% of patients with DLB experience hallucinations, and more than 50% have delusions.[8] Psychotic symptoms occur in around 20% of patients with MSA, most of whom have cerebellar type, one form of MSA with predominant cerebellar features including gait and limb ataxia, dysarthria, and oculomotor dysfunction. Severe refractory psychotic symptoms seem to be associated with poor prognosis.[9]

Visual hallucinations can be common in the normal PD disease process but differ depending on the stage of the disease. In early stages, visual hallucinations occur with preserved insight. However, in later stages patients might not recognize the misperceptions. In early stages, patients may experience passive hallucinations (eg, brief visions of a person, or more commonly an animal, passing in peripheral vision) or presence hallucinations (the sensation of somebody's presence when, in fact, no person is there).[10] As the disease progresses, more complex visual hallucinations can occur. These may consist of one or more people, who may or may not be familiar, and may be living or deceased. The visual hallucinations can also be of animals, children, or objects. In PDP visual hallucinations are commonly formed, and patients also experience illusions. *Illusions*, in contrast, are misinterpretations of a real, typically visual, stimulus (eg, seeing a tree as a person). *Auditory hallucinations* are most common in primary psychotic disorders. However, in later stages of PD, when patients are more cognitively impaired, auditory hallucinations can occur and are typically described as indistinct sounds (eg, radio playing in the room).[11]

Delusions are false interpretations of experienced misperceptions, which often involve the topics of persecution, imposters, or grandiosity. The content of delusions is commonly paranoid, often centered on beliefs of infidelity and abandonment. Delusions may involve family members, which can be very stressful for the surrounding family. *Capgras syndrome* (a delusion that someone has been replaced by an identical-looking impostor) and *Fregoli syndrome* (a delusion that multiple different people are in fact a single person who changes their appearance or is in disguise) can also present in PDP, commonly seen in patients with dementia.[12]

Clinical features. PDP is typically progressive over time, both in frequency and severity. Early symptoms of PDP are considered benign, because insight is often retained, and treatment is not an urgent need. However, insight is often lost as PD progresses.[13] As PDP progresses, delusions and paranoia can emerge, and these symptoms may become more troublesome, especially if agitation occurs. Patients and their caregivers should be educated about PDP, and clinicians need to monitor for symptoms during each visit. In an acute setting, sudden onset of psychotic symptoms must be regarded as an emergency.[14]

Common precipitating factors of psychosis are medical conditions such as dehydration, infections (eg, urinary tract infection, pneumonia), metabolic dysfunction, psychosocial factors (poor sleep and limited nutrition), psychological factors (stress and hospital admissions), and medication changes (offending agents may include: amantadine, anticholinergics, dopaminergics, pain medications etc.). Patients with PD with dementia, and most of the patients with DLB, experience complex psychotic symptoms, including hallucinations and persecutory delusions in the context of dementia. Sometimes this is complicated by delirium. These patients typically do not have insight into their psychosis, often finding their hallucinations frightening. They may display behavioral changes (including "sundowning" and other forms of agitation) and typically require treatment. Often, patients experience rapid eye movement (REM) sleep behavior disorder with vivid perceptions and illogical thinking. Clinically, distinguishing nocturnal psychotic symptoms from sleep-related and perceptual disturbances, particularly in patients with hallucinations, can be difficult.

Psychosis in MSA is much less common than psychosis seen in PD or DLB. Visual and auditory hallucinations as well as persecutory and jealousy delusions have been described.

Pathophysiology. The exact pathophysiology of PDP has not yet been determined. Extrinsic (drug-related) and intrinsic (neurotransmitter dysfunction–related) causes of PDP have been suggested.[15] Theories involving the neurotransmitters dopamine, acetylcholine, and serotonin are being studied.

In contrast to PD, where dopaminergic medications are believed to be the major cause of PDP, DLB psychosis often happens in patients who are not treated with dopaminergic medications. The association between psychosis in DLB and cognitive impairment suggests more widespread brain involvement including other neurotransmitter systems and neural pathways. Cholinergic deficits and Lewy body pathology in acetylcholine-producing neurons in the brain are common in both PD with dementia and DLB. These deficits may be associated with the occurrence of psychosis in both disorders.[16] In addition, increased numbers of Lewy bodies in the temporal lobe and the amygdala, areas implicated in the generation of complex visual images, have been found to be associated with the onset and presence of visual hallucinations.[17]

Psychotic symptoms in MSA are not associated with levodopa or other antiparkinsonian medication treatment, visual acuity, cognitive and/or depression scores, or even disease duration. Similar to PD and DLB, the exact mechanism of psychosis in MSA is not well understood.

Diagnosis. At this time there are no rating scales validated for the measurement of PDP or psychosis in other alpha synucleinopathies. Thus, diagnosis of psychosis is based on clinical presentation. A detailed history, preferably from a caregiver, is essential. In the case of a patient with well-established idiopathic PD, acute onset of psychotic symptoms is suggestive of PDP. However, in a patient with acute onset of psychotic symptoms in early stages of parkinsonism, this is more suggestive of DLB.

Management. Management of acute psychosis should first start with reviewing recent changes in PD medications and evaluation for acute precipitating conditions that can be treated: dehydration, infection, and metabolic disorders are common. Other less common, but serious, causes must be considered: cerebral infarction, intracranial hemorrhage, or central nervous system (CNS) infection. In addition, the following should also be evaluated: visual acuity, sleep deprivation, irregular nutrition, psychosocial stress, deprivation or overload of sensory inputs, recent surgery (eg, deep brain stimulation) with or without anesthesia, as well as changes to other nonparkinsonian drugs (eg, anticholinergics, β-blockers, corticosteroids, benzodiazepines).

When considering reducing PD medications for management of PDP, adjustment should be based on the potential of each medication to worsen psychosis. In general, reductions should first be made to adjunctive agents (anticholinergics, monoamine oxidase B inhibitors, amantadine) and then dopamine agonists and catechol-O-methyltransferase inhibitors. Reductions in levodopa should be made only if reductions of other antiparkinsonian agents have failed to be effective. Care must be taken not to avoid removal of all dopaminergic medications, especially suddenly, because this can cause significant worsening of parkinsonism symptoms and lead to the Parkinson-hyperpyrexia syndrome. There are no guidelines on how quickly one should reduce the dose of these medications, but changes have to be implemented cautiously and gradually, as motor symptoms can deteriorate significantly. It is always important to reduce polypharmacy first and then reduce levodopa gradually and based on the individual patient's needs. Generally, do not reduce by more than 20% to 30% of levodopa in one interval.

When all other causes of PDP have been addressed and the cause is therefore thought to be related to disease progression, then medication management with atypical antipsychotics (clozapine, pimavanserin, quetiapine) and/or cholinesterase inhibitors (donepezil, rivastigmine) is appropriate. Antidepressants (eg, selective serotonin reuptake inhibitors, mirtazapine) can also be helpful in patients with PDP who also are experiencing depression and/or insomnia symptoms. Benzodiazepines should be avoided in this population.

Cholinesterase inhibitors are the recommended first-line treatment of DLB because of their benefit for cognitive symptoms and relative lack of toxicity compared with antipsychotic medications.[18] Atypical neuroleptics (eg, olanzapine, quetiapine, clozapine) must be used with caution, as patients with DLB can develop sensitivity to these medications and they generally have a worse side-effect profile.[19] Patients with psychosis in MSA are typically treated with the same strategy as patients with PD.

Parkinson Hyperpyrexia Syndrome

Case 2: a 77-year-old woman with PD and prior abdominal surgeries for diverticulosis and diverticulitis was admitted for a small bowel obstruction. Her relevant home medications included carbidopa/levodopa, 25 to 250 mg, 5 times a day and amantadine, 100 mg, twice a day. Because of her small bowel obstruction and initial conservative management, the patient had a nasogastric tube that was on low wall suction. Although medications were administered via nasogastric tube followed by clamping, on reopening the tube there was large output, between 900 mL and 2600 mL every 24 hours. On hospital day 3, she developed abrupt onset depressed level of consciousness, rigidity, tremulousness, tachycardia, tachypnea, and fever to 41.7°C (107°F). Because of her rapid clinical decompensation and poor airway protection, she was intubated. Because of her poor gastrointestinal absorption, there was concern for Parkinson hyperpyrexia syndrome. There were no nonenteral dopamine agonists available in the acute setting, so the patient was treated with dantrolene, midazolam infusion for sedation, acetaminophen, and external cooling with ice packs and cooling blanket. Over the course of 8 hours her temperature returned to normal, her mental status improved, and she was started on transdermal dopamine agonist, rotigotine. Within 24 hours of initiation of rotigotine, her rigidity and tremulousness resolved.

Definition: Parkinsonism-hyperpyrexia syndrome (PHS) is rare but potentially life-threatening in patients with PD and other forms of parkinsonism. It most often occurs after rapidly reducing or discontinuing antiparkinson medications and therefore is something patients and clinicians must be mindful of when making medication adjustments. The clinical presentation is similar to neuroleptic malignant syndrome (NMS) with altered mental status, fever, rigidity, elevated serum creatinine kinase, and autonomic dysfunction. Notably, a similar presentation may develop in patients whose DBS is abruptly stopped or malfunctions.[20] Therefore, in patients with DBS who show signs of PHS, the device should immediately be interrogated. Mortality is reported as 4%, and one-third of patients experience long-term sequelae.[21] Patients with PHS require management in an intensive care setting for close monitoring.[22] Management in the ICU includes intravenous fluids, electrolyte replacement, antipyretics and cooling measures, judicious use of benzodiazepines, and gradual reintroduction of previous antiparkinson medication regimen.[22] In patients experiencing dysphagia, a nasogastric tube can help with providing dopaminergic therapy. If this fails, other therapeutic options are intramuscular or intravenous apomorphine and transdermal rotigotine. Close monitoring of not only vital signs but also routine checking of serum muscle enzymes, renal function, and clotting function is necessary.[22]

ACUTE MOVEMENT DISORDERS
Status Dystonicus

Case 3: a 17-year-old boy with cerebral palsy with dystonic features was hospitalized for tendon release surgery, after which he developed significant nausea treated with several doses of intravenous metoclopramide. On the third day after administration of metoclopramide, he started to develop severe worsening of dystonia in all extremities and started to have repetitive flailing movements of his body and facial grimacing. Over the next 4 months these abnormal movements continued, and he was trialed on several medications without benefit (baclofen, trihexyphenidyl, diazepam, lorazepam, tetrabenazine, and risperidone). He required several hospitalizations including a 4-week ICU stay with intubation and propofol sedation to treat the movements. Four months after onset, bilateral globus pallidus internus DBS surgery was performed. All antidystonia medications were discontinued 2 weeks later, and he returned to pretendon surgery status.

Definition

Status dystonicus, or dystonic storm, is another rare but life-threatening movement disorder emergency. It is characterized by generalized, continuous, and severe dystonic spasms. Typically it develops gradually in patients with preexisting generalized primary or secondary dystonia. It is often triggered by a precipitating event such as medication adjustment/withdrawal, deep brain stimulator device failure, infection, hyperthermia, dehydration, trauma, or penicillamine therapy in the setting of Wilson disease.

Clinical features

The clinical presentation is most commonly sustained muscle spasm characterized by dystonic muscle contractions or postures. Status dystonicus can present as tonic (sustained contractions and abnormal postures) or phasic (rapid and repetitive dystonic contractures). The movements of status dystonicus commonly overlap with additional hypekinetic movements such as chorea or myoclonus. Without treatment, hyperpyrexia, dehydration, rhabdomyolysis associated with renal failure, aspiration pneumonia, respiratory failure, and ultimately multiorgan failure can occur.[23] The mortality rate is up to 10%, with most deaths secondary to renal failure from rhabdomyolysis and respiratory failure.[23,24]

Management

Status dystonicus is often refractory to standard antidystonia pharmacotherapy alone. Treatment of the precipitating event, when possible, is therefore essential and is usually effective. Supportive management similar to that described in this article for NMS is also key. However, when these do not work, more aggressive management with a combination of high-dose anticholinergics (eg, trihexyphenidyl), dopamine receptor antagonists (eg, risperidone), and/or dopamine depleting agents (eg, tetrabenazine) is needed. Clonidine, clonazepam, and baclofen may also be beneficial. Early transfer to an ICU is recommended, as monitoring of respiratory and airway status is critical. Some patients may require endotracheal intubation, mechanical ventilation, and sedation with intravenous midazolam and propofol.[24,25] In refractory cases, intrathecal baclofen, pallidotomy, or bilateral deep-brain stimulation of the globus pallidus pars interna may be considered.[26] Botulinum toxin is not effective in the acute setting. Clinicians should also be mindful that functional dystonia can mimic status dystonicus. Therefore, in patients without preexisting dystonia, clinicians should look for positive features (eg, distractibility) of a functional movement disorder.[27]

Serotonin Syndrome

Case 4: a 68-year-old woman with anxiety, depression, and neuropathic pain presented to a community hospital with a sudden change in mental status. Minutes after having last been seen well, she was found agitated, rummaging through bedroom drawers, and not answering questions. Home medications included gabapentin, hydroxyzine, ondansetron, tramadol, and sertraline. On arrival to the emergency department her agitation was severe enough that she was intubated. Her initial evaluation was notable for tachycardia, low-grade fever, toxicology screen positive for opioids (not prescribed), and an unremarkable CT head and CT angiography (CTA) of the head and neck. Empirical antimicrobials for possible CNS infection were started. Three days later she was transferred to the medical ICU of a tertiary care hospital. Her initial neurologic examination, performed 5 minutes after stopping infusions of propofol, fentanyl, and dexmedetomidine, was notable for spontaneous eye opening and visual orientation but she was not following commands. Her pupils were 5 mm and briskly reactive with other brainstem reflexes intact. She had normal tone, no adventitious movements, localized to pain with both arms, and had diffuse hyperreflexia including the jaw jerk and sustained ankle clonus. She developed intermittent fevers to as high as 103 F. Continuous electroencephalogram (EEG) did not show seizures, lumbar puncture revealed normal cerebral spinal fluid (CSF), and MR imaging of the brain was unremarkable. Three days after transfer, serotonin syndrome was suspected. Accordingly, fentanyl infusion was changed to hydromorphone, and enteral cyproheptadine was started as a 12 mg load followed by 8 mg every 6 hours. Midazolam, propofol, and dexmedetomidine infusions were continued. Two days after starting cyproheptadine the hyperreflexia resolved, and within 4 days she was following commands. Her subsequent course was complicated by severe pneumonia with sepsis and ARDS, during which cyproheptadine was weaned. Signs of recurrent serotonin syndrome in the form of hyperreflexia with ankle clonus, asterixis, myoclonus, and chorea were apparent after deep sedation for ARDS was weaned. Cyproheptadine was restarted with rapid resolution of these abnormalities over 2 days, then weaned off over the course of a week. Despite a 2-month hospitalization that required tracheostomy and percutaneous gastrostomy, the patient fully recovered within 1 month after discharge.

Definition
Serotonin syndrome is an acute onset, severe toxic syndrome caused by a sudden pathologic increase in CNS serotonergic transmission. In the CNS, serotonin acts on 7 groups of serotonin receptor families (5-HT1–5-HT7), and it is hypothesized the neurologic manifestations of serotonin syndrome occur largely via activation of the postsynaptic 5-HT1a receptor system.[28–30] Many cases of serotonin syndrome occur in patients taking multiple serotonergic medications (reported in 16.1%) or large doses of a single drug (15.4%).[31]

Clinical features
Onset of serotonin syndrome is typically rapid, less than 13 hours from ingestion of the culprit serotonergic drug, but can present in a delayed fashion over the course of days.[32–34] The typical syndrome is a triad of altered mental status including coma, neuromuscular excitability, and autonomic hyperactivity.[29] Neuromuscular excitability includes rigidity, tremor, hyperreflexia, and clonus, with a predilection for the lower extremities.[33] Autonomic dysfunction largely takes the form of sympathetic hyperactivity, including diaphoresis, hyperthermia, diarrhea, and hemodynamic instability.[35]

Although there are clinical grading tools for the assessment of possible serotonin syndrome (**Table 1**), there is no combination of radiographic or laboratory tests that identify serotonin syndrome with high specificity.[35] Therefore, one must use a combination of history, imaging, laboratory testing including toxicology testing, and a reasonable index of suspicion to make the diagnosis.

Management
As with management of other medical emergencies, management of severe non-neurologic organ dysfunction including, but not limited to, respiratory failure, cardiac dysrhythmias and hemodynamic instability, hypovolemia, renal dysfunction, and electrolyte abnormalities comes first. After stabilization, removal of all proserotonergic

Table 1
Diagnosis of serotonin syndrome: the Hunter serotonin toxicity criteria

Use of at least one proserotonergic medication AND	At least ONE of the following clinical findings:
	Spontaneous clonus
	Inducible clonus AND agitation *or* diaphoresis
	Ocular clonus AND agitation *or* diaphoresis
	Inducible clonus AND increase muscle tone AND hyperthermia (temp >38oC)
	Ocular clonus AND increase muscle tone AND hyperthermia (temp >38oC)
	Tremor and hyperreflexia

Adapted from Lerner DP, Tadevosyan A, Burns JD. Neurol Clin. 2020.

drugs (**Table 2**) should occur. It is crucial to avoid inadvertent administration of new proserotonergic medications, especially fentanyl for analgesia in the ICU. Benzodiazepines are an essential component of management of the neurologic hyperactivity and cardiovascular instability. If patients do not respond to administration of intravenous benzodiazepines, cyproheptadine, a 5-HT-1a and 5-HT-2a receptor antagonist should be added.[36] It is also important to consider the possibility of coingestion with other potential medications and toxins, and it is not uncommon that inadvertent and intentional overdose involves polypharmacy. Reintroduction of serotonergic medications should be avoided even once the signs and symptoms of serotonin syndrome resolve. Considerations of the risks and benefits of reintroduction of these agents should occur before restarting any serotonergic medications in the future, and this reintroduction should occur slowly, with close follow-up, and in conjunction with the patient's neurologist.[36]

The autonomic hyperactivity can be striking, and there are limited data to guide management of severe autonomic dysfunction.[37] Administration of benzodiazepine and cyproheptadine can improve blood pressure. Reasonable strategies in addition to benzodiazepines for management of the hemodynamic dysfunction include carefully avoiding hypovolemia (which has the tendency to exacerbate hypotension and tachycardia) and the use of intravenous opiates such as hydromorphone and propofol for sustained, severe hypersympathetic features. "Traditional" antihypertensive medications may be required.[37] Intravenous calcium channel blockers, including diltiazem, nicardipine, and clevidipine, can be effective.[37,38] Adrenergic blockade with α- and/or β-blockers also has anecdotal evidence but seem to have slow blood pressure control.[37,39,40] There are even less data on nitrate administration, but this class of medication seems to have appropriate effect on hypertension management.[37,41,42]

Neuroleptic Malignant Syndrome

Definition

NMS, occurring in 0.02% to 3% of all patients taking antipsychotic medications, is the most serious and life-threatening adverse reaction of these widely used medications.[43–45] In-hospital mortality associated with NMS is reported as 3% to 20%.[46,47] The exact neuropharmacologic pathophysiology is unknown, but there is clearly an association between decreased activity of dopamine D2 receptors and subsequent severe sympathetic and neuromuscular hyperactivity.[48] Although antipsychotic

Table 2
Summary of drugs associated with serotonin syndrome and hypothesized pathophysiology

Mechanism of Action	Drug/Medication
Promotion of synthesis of serotonin in the serotonergic presynaptic cells	L-tryptophan
Inhibition of serotonin degradation in the presynaptic cells (inhibition of monoamine oxidase)	MAOIs Methylene blue Linezolid
Stimulation of serotonin release from vesicles in the presynaptic cells	Amphetamines Mirtazapine Dextromethorphan MDMA Opioids (oxycodone, meperidine) Tramadol
Inhibition of serotonin reuptake transporter (SERT) on the presynaptic cells (leading to increase of serotonin in synaptic cleft)	SSRI/SNRI TCA Opiates (meperidine, methadone) Tramadol Trazodone Bupropion MDMA Cocaine/Amphetamines St. John's wort
Direct serotonin agonism (activation of postsynaptic 5-HT$_{1A}$ receptor)	Buspirone LSD Triptan class of medications Ergot class of medication Fentanyl Lithium Metoclopramide
Indirect serotonin agonism	Cytochrome p450 modulators • Altered drug metabolism and clearance Opioids (morphine) • Activation of GABA and glutamate receptors and indirect stimulation or proserotonergic cells.

Abbreviations: GABA, gamma aminobutyric acid; LSD, lysergic acid diethylamide; MAOI, monoamine oxidase inhibitors; MDMA, 3,4-methylenedioxy-N-methylamphetamine; SNRI, serotonin and norepinephrine reuptake inhibitor; SSRI, selective serotonin reuptake inhibitor; TCA, tricyclic antidepressant.
Adapted from Lerner DP, Tadevosyan A, Burns JD. Neurol Clin. 2020.

medications are most commonly implicated, antiemetic drugs (eg, metoclopramide and promethazine) can also cause NMS.[45,49]

Although NMS will usually develop during the initiation phases, and can happen after a single dose, the syndrome is idiosyncratic.[50]

Clinical features

The tetrad of encephalopathy, rigidity, fever, and dysautonomia commonly evolves over one to 3 days.[48] Most cases of NMS begin with encephalopathy, which can present as a multitude of phenotypes including agitation, catatonia (see the later section on Malignant Catatonia), and even coma.[48] Fever can become severe and may result in hemodynamic collapse if severe enough. Dysautonomia, as noted in the SS section, can be difficult to control and commonly presents as tachycardia, marked hypertension, and potentially dysrhythmias.

The motor manifestation of NMS is commonly a striking feature. Rigidity is generalized and often severe. Nearly 75% of all patients with NMS will have elevation of serum creatinine kinase, and rhabdomyolysis is present in almost 33% of patients.[51] Respiratory failure, which is commonly multifactorial, is present in 12% to 19% of all hospitalized cases.[38,52]

The classic tetrad of symptoms is most commonly associated with typical antipsychotics, whereas NMS associated with the atypical antipsychotics and antiemetics can often have absence of hyperpyrexia and severe rigidity.[45,48,53] In fact, the NMS-like syndrome occurring in association with atypical antipsychotics and antiemetics frequently seems similar to malignant catatonia (MC), suggesting that the 2 disorders lie in different locations along the spectrum of disorders associated with dopamine-predominant dysregulated monoaminergic neurotransmission.[54]

Management

As always, ABCs (airway, breathing, circulation), are the first priority. Identification and removal of the inciting agent is essential. Benzodiazepines and bromocriptine are commonly used to manage agitation, hyperpyrexia, and muscle rigidity.[55] Other dopaminergic agents including amantadine and levodopa can be considered as adjuvant therapy in refractory cases.[55]

As with malignant hyperthermia, dantrolene (dose of 1–2.5 mg/kg with maximum daily dose of 10 mg/kg/d) should be considered when rigidity and hyperthermia are immediately life-threatening.[54] Although dantrolene will treat these symptoms, it fails to treat the underlying dysautonomia and encephalopathy and therefore is best considered as adjunctive therapy. The mean recovery time is 7 to 11 days.[45,49]

It is also important to consider coingestion with other potential medications and toxins, and it is not uncommon that inadvertent and intentional overdose involves polypharmacy.

In most cases, atypical antipsychotics can be restarted safely approximately 4 weeks after resolution of symptoms, but there should be close follow-up, as recurrence can be as high as 10% to 20%.[56]

Malignant Catatonia

Case 5: a 72-year-old woman with bipolar disorder, secondary progressive multiple sclerosis, and rheumatoid arthritis was admitted to a community hospital with sudden-onset confusion, marked mainly by a paucity of spontaneous behavior and slowness of responses. Her initial evaluation revealed fever, hypotension, and leukopenia. Neurologic examination on admission was notable for significantly increased latency of response with relatively preserved response accuracy and moderate, diffusely increased tone most consistent with rigidity. Hypotension and fever improved within a day with intravenous fluids and antibiotics for a concurrent Staphylococcus aureus pneumonia, yet her mental status worsened and by hospital day 3 she had developed bihemispheric coma with diffusely significantly increased muscle tone, recurrent fevers, and mildly elevated CK (800 IU/L). CSF obtained by lumbar puncture was normal. NMS was suspected, prompting initiation of dantrolene and bromocriptine and transfer to the ICU of a tertiary care hospital. Her neurologic examination on transfer was notable for absent eye opening yet moderately strong resistance to passive eye opening and present blink to threat from both sides, intact brainstem reflexes, no spontaneous movements, prominent palmar grasp reflexes, and diffuse severe increase in tone most consistent with rigidity with some element of paratonia and normal muscle stretch reflexes. CT head, CTA head and neck, MR imaging of brain, continuous EEG, and extensive serum and CSF evaluation for autoimmune encephalopathy did not reveal an underlying cause. Despite increasing the dose of bromocriptine and adding standing lorazepam and amantadine, only the tone improved but not the mental status, and intermittent noninfectious fevers continued. Because of her persistently depressed level of consciousness she could not be extubated and a tracheostomy was performed. Five weeks after admission, in the face of no substantial improvement, carbidopa/levodopa was started. By the next day she began to show signs of improvement with spontaneous eye opening, tracking, and returning efforts to shake hands. Within days she was fully alert and speaking with a speaking tracheostomy valve. Two weeks later she was discharged to acute rehabilitation.

Definition

Patients with major depression disorder, bipolar disorder, and schizophrenia are most likely to experience MC. However, MC can occur in patients without such a history, often in association with acute nonneurological illness.[54] Catatonia is a spectrum disorder that includes some combination of mutism, hypophonia, reduced interaction with the environment, negativism, increased tone, posturing, posturing, automatic obedience, echolalia, stereotypy, and echopraxia. Severe forms closely resemble NMS with autonomic instability, severe muscle rigidity, and hyperthermia, which can lead to rhabdomyolysis, coma, and death.[54,57,58] Mutism, withdrawn or hypoactive catatonia, is much more common than severe psychomotor agitation.[54] When MC is associated with use of neuroleptic medications it is commonly referred to as NMS (see earlier discussion).[57,59] It is difficult to ascertain the true incidence of catatonia due to multiple nomenclatures, but retrospective and prospective studies of inpatient psychiatry consultations report 1.6% to 5.5% of inpatient psychiatry consultations are diagnosed with catatonia.[60–63] Although these studies were observational, there is a trend toward patients older than 65 years having slightly higher incidence (6.3% vs 2.4%).[63]

Catatonia can occur as a feature of multiple other disorders, including primary anti-N-methyl-D-aspartate receptor encephalitis, paraneoplastic limbic encephalitis, viral encephalitis, ictal catatonia, brain tumor, multiple sclerosis, ischemic stroke, systemic lupus erythematous, hyponatremia, B12 deficiency, and Wilson disease.[54] Finally, several medications have been reported to be associated with catatonia (**Table 3**).

Table 3
Drugs associated with catatonia

Immunosuppressive Medications	Illicit Drugs
Tacrolimus	3,4-Methylenedioxy-N-methylamphetamine (MDMA)
Cyclosporine	Cocaine withdrawal
Steroids	Phencyclidine (PCP)
Miscellaneous	Antibiotics
Baclofen	Fluoroquinolones
Dopamine agonists	Cephalosporins
Methoxetamine	Azithromycin
Disulfiram	

Clinical features

Catatonia associated with psychiatric disorders and catatonia associated with acute medical conditions present similarly. The most common signs are immobility (97%), mutism (97%), withdrawal and refusal to eat (91%), and staring (87%).[64] Motor symptoms occur in 27% to 58% of cases.[64]

Both withdrawn/hypoactive catatonia and psychomotor-agitated catatonia can be difficult to diagnose, as the patient will be unable to provide history, and its features often suggest the much more common septic encephalopathy. Reduced interactivity with the environment and mutism, particularly when some higher functions such as blinking to threat and localizing painful stimuli are preserved, should raise suspicion of catatonia. Relevant psychiatric history can also raise the suspicion of catatonia, as it is associated with mood disorders and schizophrenia.[64]

Management

Management of catatonia associated with acute medical conditions requires a multitiered approach. Treatment should be directed at the underlying medical conditions, removal of potential causative and/or perpetuating medications, and abating the catatonic features.[54] The mainstay treatment of abatement of catatonic features is low-dose benzodiazepines (less than 8 mg/d of lorazepam), which have been reported to be successful in 59% to 97% of cases.[64] Although there are limited supporting data, additional medications that can be considered include levodopa, memantine, amantadine, dextromethorphan/quinidine, minocycline, and atypical antipsychotics.[54] Care should be given when using antipsychotics, as progression to MC/NMS has been reported.[65]

Immobility and refusal to eat can lead to life-threatening medical complications including dehydration, pressure ulcers, deep vein thrombosis, and pneumonia.[64] Those with MC should receive therapies similar to NMS including dantrolene for severe, intractable rigidity and hyperthermia, and short-acting antihypertensive medications for dysautonomia.[54]

Electroconvulsive therapy can be considered in refractory malignant cases. The conventional course consists of daily treatment of up to 5 days followed by 3 times a week until improvement occurs.[54]

CLINICS CARE POINTS

- Acute decompensation of patients with chronic PD can occur due to rapid titration or omission of dopaminergic medications, which can be seen following deep brain stimulator implantation, admission for surgical procedures, protracted nil per os status, and common infections. This can result in severe psychosis or life-threatening hyperpyrexia that will require ICU admission, supportive care, and reintroduction of dopaminergic medications.

- Serotonin syndrome and NMS exist as a spectrum of disorders and may overlap. Patients will commonly ingest multiple medications and can present with features of both SS and NMS. Mainstay of treatment is removal of the offending agent, supportive care, and early benzodiazepine administration. Although benzodiazepines will treat the agitation, the autonomic instability will require close vital sign monitoring.

- Catatonia is a not rare acute psychiatric and movement disorder condition that can have a wide spectrum of presentation. MC can seem nearly identical to NMS with marked hyperthermia, rigidity, and encephalopathy and is treated in similar fashion.

DISCLOSURE

The authors have nothing to disclose.

REFERENCES

1. Ravina B, Marder K, Fernandez HH, et al. Diagnostic criteria for psychosis in Parkinson's disease: report of an NINDS, NIMH work group. Mov Disord 2007;22: 1061–8.

2. Thanvi BR, Lo TC, Harsh DP. Psychosis in Parkinson's disease. Postgrad Med J 2005;81(960):644–6.

3. Fénelon G, Mahieux F, Huon R, et al. Hallucinations in Parkinson's disease: prevalence, phenomenology, and risk factors. Brain 2000;123:733–45.

4. Marsh L, Williams JR, Rocco M, et al. Psychiatric comorbidities in patients with Parkinson disease and psychosis. Neurology 2004;63:293–300.

5. Giladi N, Treves TA, Paleacu D, et al. Risk factors for dementia, depression, and psychosis in long-standing Parkinson's disease. J Neural Transm 2000;10: 759–71.

6. Aarsland D, Larsen JP, Cummings JL, et al. Prevalence and clinical correlates of psychotic symptoms in Parkinson disease: a community-based study. Arch Neurol 1999;56:595–601.

7. McKeith IG, Dickson DW, Lowe J, et al. Consortium on DLB: Diagnosis and management of dementia with Lewy bodies: third report of the DLB consortium. Neurology 2005;65:1863–72.

8. Aarsland D, Ballard C, Larsen JP, et al. A comparative study of psychiatric symptoms in dementia with Lewy bodies and Parkinson's disease with and without dementia. Int J Geriatr Psychiatry 2001;16:528–36.

9. Palma JA, Martinez J, Norcliffe-Kaufman L, et al. 28th International Symposium on the autnomic system: Psychosis in Multiple System Atrophy. Clin Auton Ress 2017;27(5):319–20.

10. Friedman JH. Parkinson's disease psychosis update. Behav Neurol 2013;27(4): 469–77.

11. Chaudhury S. Hallucinations: Clinical aspects and managements'. Ind Psychiatry J 2000;10(1):5.

12. Moro A, Munhoz RP, Moscovich M, et al. Delusional misidentification syndrome and other unusual delusions in advanced Parkinson's disease. Parkinsonism Relat Disord 2013;19:751–4.

13. Josephs KA. Capgras syndrome and its relationship to neurodegenerative disease. Arch Neurol 2007;64(12):1762–6.

14. Muller T, Baas J, Kassubek, et al. Laboratory assessments in the course of Parkinson's disease: a clinician's perspective". J Neural Transm 2016;123(1):65–71.

15. Samudra N, Patel N, Womack KB, et al. Psychosis in Parkinson disease: a review of etiology, phenomenology, and management. Drugs Aging 2016;33(12): 855–63.

16. Perry EK, McKeith I, Thompson P, et al. Topography, extent, and clinical relevance of neurochemical deficits in dementia of Lewy body type, Parkinson's disease, and Alzheimer's disease. Ann N Y Acad Sci 1991;640:197–202.

17. Harding AJ, Broe GA, Halliday GM. Visual hallucinations in Lewy body disease relate to Lewy bodies in the temporal lobe. Brain 2002;125:391–403.

18. Wesnes KA, McKeith IG, Ferrara R, et al. Effects of rivastigmine on cognitive function in dementia with Lewy bodies: a randomised placebo-controlled international study using the Cognitive Drug Research computerized assessment system. Dement Geriatr Cogn Disord 2002;13:183–92.

19. Takahashi H, Yoshida K, Sugita T, et al. Quetiapine treatment of psychotic symptoms and aggressive behavior in patients with dementia with Lewy bodies: a case series. Prog Neuropsychopharmacol Biol Psychiatry 2003;27:549–53.
20. Artusi CA, Merola A, Espay AJ, et al. Parkinsonism–hyperpyrexia syndrome and deep brain stimulation. J Neurol 2015;262(12):2780–2.
21. Takubo H, Harada T, Hashimoto T, et al. A collaborative study on the malignant syndrome in Parkinson's disease and related disorders. Parkinsonism Relat Disord 2003;9(Suppl 1):S31–41.
22. Simonet C, Tolosa E, Camara A, et al. Emergencies and critical issues in Parkinson's disease. Pract Neurol 2020;20(1):15–25.
23. Manji H, Howard RS, Miller DH, et al. Status dystonicus: the syndrome and its management. Brain 1998;121(2):243–52.
24. Chang FCF, Frucht SJ. "ICU Intensive Care Unit Movement Disorder Emergencies." Non-Parkinsonian Movement Disorders 2017;150–60.
25. Termsarasab P, Steven J. Frucht. "Dystonic storm: a practical clinical and video review. J Clin Movement Disord 2017;4(1):10.
26. Zorzi G, Marras C, Nardocci N, et al. Stimulation of the globus pallidus internus for childhood-onset dystonia. Movement Disord 2005;20(9):1194–200.
27. Gandhi SE, Newman EJ, Marshall VL. Emergency presentations of movement disorders. Pract Neurol 2020. https://doi.org/10.1136/practneurol-2019-002277.
28. Barnes NM, Sharp T. A review of central 5-HT receptors and their function. Neuropharmacology 1999;38(8):1083–152.
29. Boyer EW, Shannon M. The serotonin syndrome. NEJM 2005;352(11):1112–20.
30. Francescangeli J, Karamchandani K, Powell M, et al. The serotonin syndrome: from molecular mechanisms to clinical practice. Int J Mol Sci 2019;20(9):2288.
31. Werneke U, Jamshidi F, Taylor DM, et al. Conundrums in neurology: diagnosing serotonin syndrome â€" a meta-analysis of cases. BMC Neurol 2016;16:97.
32. Nelson LS, Erdman AR, Booze LL, et al. Selective serotonin reuptake inhibitor poisoning: An evidence-based consensus guideline for out-of-hospital management. Clin Toxicol 2007;45(4):315–32.
33. Birmes P, Coppin D, Schmitt L, et al. Serotonin syndrome: a brief review. Can Med Assoc J 2003;168(11):1439–42.
34. Little K, Lin CM, Reynolds PM. Delayed Serotonin Syndrome in the Setting of Mixed Fluoxetine and Serotonin Antagonist Overdose. Am J Case Rep. 2018;19:604–7.
35. Dunkley EJ, Isbister GK, Sibbritt D, et al. The Hunter Serotonin Toxicity Criteria: simple and accurate diagnostic decision rules for serotonin toxicity. QJM 2003; 96(9):635–42.
36. Lerner DP, Tadevosyan A, Burns JD. Toxin-Induced Subacute Encephalopathy. Neurol Clin 2020;38(4):799–824.
37. Ott M, Mannchen JK, Jamshidi F, et al. Management of severe arterial hypertension associated with serotonin syndrome: a case report analysis based on systematic review techniques. Ther Adv Psychopharmacol 2019;9:1–32.
38. Levine M, Truitt CA, O'Connor AD. Cariotoxicity and serotonin syndrome complicating a milnacipran overdose. J Med Toxicol 2011;7:312–6.
39. Moseson E, Nichols D. The clinical roller coaster severe serotonin syndrome. Crit Care Med 2013;41(12):A348.
40. Beatty NC, Nicholson WT, Langman LJ, et al. Pharmacogenetic workup of perioperative serotonin syndrome. J Clin Anesth 2013;25:662–5.
41. Villar JM, Lopez AC. Serotoninergic syndrome after the administration of clomipramine tablet in a critical patient. Med Intesniva 2007;31:343–4.

42. Choudhury M, Hote MP, Verma Y. Serotonin syndrome in a postoperative patient. J Anesthesiol Ciln Pharmacol 2011;27:233–5.

43. 38Velamoor VR. Neuroleptic malignant syndrome. Recognition, prevention and management. Drug Saf 1998;1:73–82.

44. Levenson JL. Neuroleptic malignant syndrome. Am J Psychiatry 1985;142(10): 1137–45.

45. Caroff SN, Mann SC. Neuroleptic malignant syndrome. Med Clin North Am 1993; 77(1):185–202.

46. Caroff SN. The neuroleptic malignant syndrome. J Clin Psychiatry 1980;41(3): 79–83.

47. Shalev A, Hermesh H, Munitz H. Mortality from neuroleptic malignant syndrome. J Clin Psychiatry 1989;50(1):18–25.

48. Rosebush PI, Anglin RE, Richards C, et al. Neuroleptic malignant syndrome and the acute phase response. J Clin Psychopharmacol 2008;28(4):459–61.

49. Kogoj, Velikonja I. Olanzapine induced neuroleptic malignant syndrome-a care review. Hum Psychopharmacol 2003;18:301.

50. Pope HG Jr, Aisle HG, Keck PE Jr, et al. Neuroleptic malignant syndrome: long-term follow-up of 20 cases. J Clin Psychiatry 1991;52:208.

51. Lang FU, Lang S, Becker T, et al. Neuroleptic malignant syndrome or catatonia? Trying to solve the catatonic dilemma. Psychopharmacology 2015;232(1):1–5.

52. Nakamura M, Yasunaga H, Miyata H, et al. Mortality of neuroleptic malignant syndrome induced by typical and atypical antipsychotic drugs: a propensity-matched analysis from the Japanese Diagnosis Procedure Combination database. J Clin Psychiatry 2012;73(4):427–30.

53. Caroff SN, Mann SC. Neuroleptic malignant syndrome and malignant hyperthermia. Anaesth Intensive Care 1993;21(4):477–8.

54. Denysenko L, Freudenreich O, Philbrick K, et al. "Catatonia in Medically Ill Patients An Evidence-Based Medicine (EBM) Monograph for Psychosomatic Medicine Practice." (2015). Available at: https://www.eapm.eu.com/wp-content/uploads/2018/06/Catatonia_APM-EAPM_2015-04-17.pdf.

55. Carbone JR. The neuroleptic malignant and serotonin syndromes. Emerg Med Clin North Am 2000;18(2):317–25.

56. Ananth J1, Parameswaran S, Gunatilake S, et al. Neuroleptic malignant syndrome and atypical antipsychotic drugs. J Clin Psychiatry 2004;65(4):464–70.

57. Mann SC, Caroff SN, Ungvari GS, et al. Catatonia, malignant cataonia and neuroleptic malignant syndrome. Curr Psychiatry Rev 2013;9:111–9.

58. Philbrick KL, Rummans TA. Malignant Catatonia. J Neuropsychiatry Clin Neurosci 1994;6:1–13.

59. Fink M. Neuroleptic malignant syndrome and catatonia: one entity or two? Biol Psychiatry 1996;39:1–4.

60. Zarr ML, Now T. Catatonia and burns. Burns 1990;16:133–4.

61. Carroll BT, Spetie L. Catatonia on the consultation-liaison service: a replication study. Int J Psychiatry Med 1994;24:329–37.

62. Cottencin O, Warembourg F, de Chouly de Enclave MB, et al. Catatonia and consultaiton-liasion psychiatry study of 12 cases. Prog Neuro-psychopharmacol Biol Psychiatry 2007;31:1170–6.

63. Jaimes-Albornoz W, Serra-Mestres J. Prevelance and clinical correlations of catatonia in older adults referred to a liaison psychiatry service in a general hospital. Ger Hosp Psychiatry 2013;35:512–6.

64. Rassmussen SA, Mazurek MF, Rosebush PI. Catatonia: our current understanding of its diagnosis, treatment and pathophysiology. World J Psychiatry 2016;6: 391–8.

65. Jacob A, Francis A. Neuroleptic malignant syndrome induced by atypical neuroleptics and responsive to lorazepam. Neuropsychiatry Dis Treat 2006;15: 302–4.

Neuro-Ophthalmic Emergencies

Samuel J. Spiegel, MD[a], Heather E. Moss, MD, PHD[a,b],*

KEYWORDS

- Neuro-ophthalmology • Emergency • Giant cell arteritis • Pituitary apoplexy
- Central retinal artery occlusion • Papilledema • Cavernous sinus syndrome
- Rhino-orbital-cerebral mucositis

KEY POINTS

- Sudden monocular vision loss is the most common ocular presenting symptom of giant cell arteritis.
- Pituitary apoplexy causes the sudden enlargement of the pituitary gland, and the risk of acute secondary adrenal insufficiency warrants empiric corticosteroid supplementation.
- Patients with acute branch retinal artery occlusion, central artery occlusion, or monocular transient vision loss thought to be due to ischemia should be emergently referred to a stroke center for evaluation.
- Rhino-orbital-cerebral mucormycosis is typically fatal without urgent therapy, and treatment includes emergent antifungal therapy.
- Cavernous sinus thrombosis is a life-threatening condition; for suspected infectious causes, antibiotic therapy directed at the primary infection is recommended.

INTRODUCTION

Emergencies are patient presentations that, if not identified and treated promptly, may lead to significant morbidity or mortality. Accordingly, neuro-ophthalmic emergencies are those presenting with neuro-ophthalmic signs and symptoms. In determining what topics to review in this article, consideration was given to the differentiation of conditions needing emergent versus urgent management. For the purposes of this article, we define an emergency as any condition requiring evaluation within 24 hours, often through emergency department referral. For example, the differential diagnosis for a patient presenting with retrobulbar optic neuropathy is broad including, in increasing

[a] Department of Neurology and Neurological Sciences, Stanford University, 300 Pasteur Drive, Palo Alto, CA 94305, USA; [b] Department of Ophthalmology, Stanford University, 2370 Watson Court, Palo Alto, CA 94303, USA
* Corresponding author. Spencer Center for Vision Research, 2370 Watson Court MC 5353, Palo Alto, CA 94303.
E-mail address: Hemoss@stanford.edu

Neurol Clin 39 (2021) 631–647
https://doi.org/10.1016/j.ncl.2021.01.004
0733-8619/21/© 2021 Elsevier Inc. All rights reserved.
neurologic.theclinics.com

order of urgency, optic nerve sheath meningioma, optic neuritis, and giant cell arteritis (GCA), with the latter constituting an emergency.

Additionally, most patients do not present with an emergent diagnosis, rather with symptoms and signs suggesting this condition. Thus, organization by diagnosis may not be as useful to the clinician. Therefore, we frame our discussion around acute vision loss, and diplopia. Within these categories, we discuss important considerations when assessing these symptoms and highlight the emergent conditions that cause them, their evaluation, and their management. Owing to the myriad ways that many neuro-ophthalmic diseases present, it is impossible to be all encompassing, but we hope that our presentation helps students, practicing physicians, and other health care providers to build and begin to fill in their own framework for approaching patients with neuro-ophthalmic emergencies.

ACUTE VISION LOSS
Approach to the History and Examination

As in most neurologic conditions, localization is an important first step in diagnosing a patient. For visual complaints, both ophthalmic and neurologic structures need to be considered (**Box 1**). History questions that can provide insight include the severity of vision loss (what can the patient see or not see?), the nature of the vision loss (eg, positive [bright], negative [dark or dim], distortion), binocularity (right eye, left eye, both eyes together or separately), and location (central or peripheral visual field). A comparison of vision loss between eyes is particularly helpful to localize vision loss anterior to, within, or posterior to the chiasm. It should be noted that many people with bilateral homonymous visual field deficits can misinterpret these as monocular in origin.[1] If the symptom persists, an active comparison of vision between the eyes is instructive. If the symptom has resolved, questioning the patient regarding symptom change if they closed one eye or the other when symptomatic can provide clues.

Box 1

Approach to history and examination in a patient with vision loss owing to afferent visual pathway dysfunction

History
- What can the patient see or not see?
- What is the nature of vision loss (eg, positive [bright], negative [dark or dim], distortion)?
- Is the vision loss monocular or binocularity (right eye, left eye, both eyes together or separately)?
  ○ Did the patient compare 1 eye with the other eye?
- Where in the visual field is there vision loss (central or peripheral visual field)?

Examination
- Visual acuity in each eye separately
  ○ Snellen eye chart, ability to count fingers, identify hand motion or light perception
- Color vision comparison between eyes
  ○ Red desaturation
- Confrontation visual fields in each eye separately
  ○ Typically count fingers in 4 quadrants
- Pupillary examination
  ○ Direct response, relative afferent pupillary defect (anisocoria is not caused by afferent visual pathway dysfunction)
- Fundoscopic examination
  ○ Disc margin and color, cup:disc ratio, caliber of arteries/veins, and spontaneous venous pulsations

The physical examination should include visual acuity, color vision (red desaturation), confrontation visual fields, pupillary examination, and fundoscopic examination in addition to a targeted neurologic examination. Visual acuity should be checked using a patient's habitual refractive correction for testing distance and/or pinhole. If large text cannot be discerned, the ability to count fingers, identify hand motion, or see light should be determined. Visual acuity that improves 2 or more lines on Snellen when using a pinhole is likely optical in origin, related to refractive error or cataract. Red desaturation can be tested by having the patient cover each aye alternately, while asking them to compare the brightness or hue of a red object or stimulus. If the color is perceived differently between eyes, usually described as a lighter red or pink in the affected eye, this finding is positive. Bedside testing of confrontation visual fields has poor sensitivity; however, specificity of finger counting is reasonable.[2] Central (visual acuity) and/or peripheral (confrontation visual fields) testing demonstrating vision loss in 1 eye localizes anterior to the optic chiasm; in the temporal aspect of both eyes, localizes to the chiasm; or on the same side of both eyes (ie, homonymous defects) localizes to the visual pathways behind the chiasm or to the same problem on both sides anterior to the chiasm. In a patient with symmetric pupils, a comparison of the direct and indirect responses to light is helpful to detect asymmetric optic nerve disease. This can be visualized using the swinging flashlight test, looking for dilation when moving to the worse eye and constriction when moving to the better eye (a relative afferent pupillary defect). The anterior ophthalmic and funduscopic examinations will identify most ophthalmic causes of vision loss and are also important for the identification of optic nerve head abnormalities, such as swelling or pallor and retinal vascular changes.

Particular attention should be paid to symptoms and signs localizing to near the afferent visual pathway or suggesting neurologic syndromes that can involve vision loss. Associated signs and symptoms that can help to localize an optic neuropathy include the following.

- Orbit: proptosis, orbital pain, extraocular movement limitations
- Orbital apex: ipsilateral cranial nerves III, IV, VI, or V1 dysfunction
- Skull base/pituitary: cranial nerves III, IV, VI, V1, or V2, sympathetic pathway dysfunction
- Cerebral hemispheres: sensorimotor deficit, aphasia, cognitive dysfunction

Some emergent neuro-ophthalmic causes of vision loss are GCA, pituitary apoplexy, retinal arterial occlusion, papilledema, and cerebral ischemic or hemorrhagic stroke. With the exception of pituitary apoplexy, these diseases can present in transient form (eg, transient ischemic attacks) and are thus important differential considerations in the patient with transient or fixed vision loss.

Giant Cell Arteritis

Background and presentation

GCA is a medium and large vessel vasculitis that almost exclusively affects those older than the age of 50.[3] Its prevalence in the general population is less than 1%, estimated to be 0.36 per 100,000.[4,5] Owing to its vision-threatening, as well as life-threatening, complications, its early recognition is crucial. Sudden monocular vision loss due to optic neuropathy (anterior or posterior) caused by arteritis of the branches of the ciliary or ophthalmic arteries is the most common presenting visual symptom of GCA. Often this is preceded by transient episodes of vision loss. Without treatment about one-half of patients will have arteritic optic neuropathy in the fellow eye and such double eye involvement is commonly blinding. Stroke, aortic dissection, aortitis, and myocardial infarction are notable, yet less common, life-threatening complications of GCA.

Although sudden monocular vision loss owing to ischemic optic neuropathy is the most common ocular presenting symptom, GCA can present with other causes of acute vision loss. including ophthalmic artery occlusion or posterior circulation ischemic stroke.[6] Cranial nerve or orbital involvement can cause diplopia.[7] Although visual manifestations may be intermittent initially, persistent visual deficits are usually irreversible once they occur. An estimated 4% to 20% of patients will present with primary visual symptoms; however, 50% will experience visual symptoms over the course of the disease. GCA is associated with many systemic symptoms caused by systemic inflammation and focal ischemia (**Table 1**).[8] Careful questioning regarding pain anywhere in the distribution of the external carotid artery (lateral face/temple, neck, ear, jaw, occipital, or scalp) should be performed. However, a minority of patients do not have any systemic symptoms.

Examination

When the symptoms are transient, it is common for the neuro-ophthalmic examination to be normal between episodes, so a high clinical suspicion and careful history are necessary to make this diagnosis. If there is persistent vision loss the clinician should be able to measure this in the ways described elsewhere in this article. Relative afferent pupillary defect and fundoscopic examination showing pallid disc edema suggest arteritic anterior optic neuropathy, whereas relative afferent pupillary defect and a normal anterior optic nerve suggest posterior ischemic optic neuropathy.

Laboratory evaluation

The erythrocyte sedimentation rate and C-reactive protein should be drawn given the high sensitivity (approximately 86.9% and 84.1%, respectively) in patients with temporal artery biopsy-proven GCA.[9] Implicit in this imperfect sensitivity is that GCA can occur without elevation of systemic inflammatory blood tests. A complete blood count can be helpful in evaluating for thrombocytosis, anemia, and leukocytosis, but this modality has a significantly lower sensitivity.

Imaging

Retinal fluorescein angiography, available in many ophthalmology clinics, can demonstrate the choroidal perfusion deficits and delayed choroidal filling that are suggestive

Table 1 Systemic symptoms in GCA[4]	
Symptom	Prevalence (%)
Headache	57
Polymyalgia rheumatica	50
Jaw claudication	48
Weight loss	40
Malaise	37
Anorexia	31
Myalgias	28
Scalp tenderness	20
Neck pain	17
No systemic symptoms	20

of GCA. MRI or ultrasound examination of the temporal artery can demonstrate arteritis. Ultrasound examination is in widespread use in Europe, where it is used as a substitute for temporal artery biopsy if the case presents typically. However, in the United States, ultrasound examination is not widely available. In about one-third of patients, the temporal arteries are not involved, and a computed tomography (CT) scan, MRI, and PET scan of the chest can be helpful in diagnosing aortitis or the involvement of other large arteries by GCA.[10] The aorta should be routinely assessed in all GCA patients at diagnosis and at follow-up.

Diagnosis
A temporal artery biopsy demonstrating multinucleated giant cell and inflammatory infiltrate (giant cells do not need to be present) is diagnostic of GCA and this is pursued for diagnostic confirmation in patients in whom there is high clinical suspicion owing to a combination of ischemic presentation, systemic symptoms, and/or elevated systemic inflammatory markers. One may need to look for healed arteritis (this entity may be described as a focal disruption of the internal elastic lamina) if there is a delay in biopsy by more than 2 weeks after initiation of steroids. If the first biopsy is negative (seen in 4%–10% of cases), a second site should be considered in high-risk patients. In some geographic regions, a temporal artery ultrasound examination showing findings consistent with arteritis is diagnostic in lieu of a temporal artery biopsy.

Treatment
In patients with acute vision loss suspected due to GCA, the emergent initiation of steroids before temporal artery biopsy is appropriate to prevent further ischemic episodes. Three days of high-dose intravenous methylprednisolone (1000 mg/d) followed by a slow prednisone taper over 1 year is a common regimen, although oral-only regimens are also used. Intravenous therapy may diminish the likelihood of fellow eye involvement and was associated with a slightly better prognosis for visual improvement.[11] In regard to the frequent ischemic events seen in GCA at sites other than the eye, such as myocardial infarction and stroke, some evidence supports the use of low-dose daily aspirin.[12] Chronic therapy for GCA is beyond the scope of this review, but is often done in coordination with rheumatology.[9]

Clinics care points
- Up to 20% of patients who present with visual symptoms from GCA may not have systemic manifestations.
- Patients with visual symptoms from suspected GCA should be urgently evaluated by an eye care provider, yet this should not delay empiric treatment.
- The erythrocyte sedimentation rate and C-reactive protein are most sensitive for GCA, but can be nonspecific and negative in up to 10% of patients.
- Temporal artery biopsy remains the gold standard for diagnosis in the United States, but arranging this procedure should not delay treatment because the pathologic findings can still be seen within 2 weeks of initiation of steroids.
- Initiation of GCA treatment is emergent, because untreated GCA is associated with recurrent ischemic events, particularly in those with visual presentations.

Pituitary Apoplexy

Background and presentation
Pituitary apoplexy is a life-threatening condition that results from a sudden enlargement of the pituitary gland as a result of hemorrhage or infarction. It is a rare

complication of pituitary adenomas, occurring in 0.6% to 9.0% of pituitary adenomas, although up to 81% of affected patients are unaware that they have a pituitary tumor before experiencing apoplexy.[13] It is a neurosurgical emergency. Associated disruptions in endocrine function can be fatal if not treated promptly. Corticotropic deficiency, occurring in 50% to 80% of cases, can be life threatening, potentially causing severe hemodynamic problems and hyponatremia owing to acute secondary adrenal insufficiency.

Common symptoms are sudden onset severe headache; neck stiffness; vision loss owing to chiasm, optic nerve, or optic tract compression; and diplopia owing to cavernous sinus invasion (**Table 2**). There may also be symptoms of pituitary hormone imbalance. Most cases present spontaneously, although a minority are precipitated by malignant hypertension, anticoagulation, or dopamine agonists.[14]

Examination
Observation of the patient's mental status is imperative because brainstem or hypothalamic compression can lead to depressed consciousness and cardiopulmonary dysfunction. In regard to neuro-ophthalmologic examination in the emergent setting, one should check for cranial nerve palsies as well as central and peripheral vision loss. Variable patterns of visual field impairment may be observed, with bitemporal hemianopsia owing to compression of the optic chiasm being most common.

Laboratory evaluation
Endocrine evaluation at presentation should include random cortisol, free thyroxine, thyroid-stimulating hormone, growth hormone (insulin-like growth factor-1), prolactin, a complete blood count, and a metabolic panel. Anterior pituitary hormonal dysfunction is present in 80% of patients upon presentation.[15] Evaluation of the hypothalamic pituitary axis function should not delay treatment with glucocorticoids.

Imaging and diagnosis
A standard noncontrast head CT scan has a low sensitivity for pituitary apoplexy because it can be difficult to observe on axial images at standard spacing. A CT scan protocolled for visualization of the pituitary or MRI are preferred. MRI in particular is superior for evaluation of hemorrhage, tumor burden, and compression of surrounding structures (**Fig. 1**).

Management
The risk of acute secondary adrenal insufficiency warrants empiric corticosteroid supplementation (preferably preceded by blood draw for serum cortisol determination) before confirmatory imaging.[16] Therapy should consist of hydrocortisone 50 mg every 6 hours or a bolus of 100 to 200 mg followed by 50 to 100 mg every 6 hours.[16] These patients should be admitted for close monitoring to a neurologic intensive care unit.

Table 2	
Presenting findings in pituitary apoplexy[13]	
Symptom, Sign, or Condition	**Prevalence (%)**
Headache	87
Panhypopituitarism	73
Decreased visual acuity	56
Bitemporal hemianopsia	34
Diabetes Insipidus	8

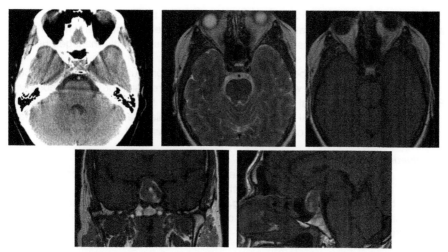

Fig. 1. Neuroimaging features of pituitary apoplexy. Noncontrast axial CT scan (*top left*) with normal appearing sella. Axial T2 weighted MRI (*top center*) and axial T1-weighted MRI without contrast (*top right*) from the same patient demonstrating layer layering hemorrhage in the sella. Coronal (*bottom left*) and sagittal (*bottom right*) T1 MRI without contrast (*bottom left*) from a different patient, showing a well-circumscribed sellar mass with suprasellar extension and mass effect on the optic chiasm, containing central and peripheral rim T1 hyperintense signal suggestive of areas of hemorrhage. (Images Courtesy Bryan Lanzman, MD, Department of Radiology, Stanford University.)

Endocrinology input for the management of pituitary dysfunction as well as neurosurgery input for tumor management are important. Although some patients can be managed successfully with close observation and medical treatment, surgical decompression improves visual acuity and visual fields in the majority of cases (76% and 79%, respectively).[13]

Clinics care points

- MRI is the imaging modality of choice for pituitary apoplexy; a pituitary protocol CT scan is preferred over a noncontrast CT scan of the head.
- Pituitary apoplexy is a neurosurgical emergency, warranting emergent consultation of neurosurgery, neurocritical care, and endocrinology.
- The initiation of empiric steroids is critical for the treatment of secondary adrenal insufficiency.
- Surgical decompression is most useful in patients with clinical signs of compression of structures underlying visual or other vital functions.

Ocular Vascular Events: Central Retinal Artery Occlusion, Branch Retinal Artery Occlusion, and Amaurosis Fugax

Background and presentation

Central retinal artery occlusion (CRAO), branch retinal artery occlusion (BRAO), and amaurosis fugax (transient vision loss from retinal or optic nerve ischemia) etiologies include large artery occlusive disease (atherothrombosis, embolus, dissection), arterial emboli, hypercoagulable disorders, and calcific emboli. The final common pathway for these disorders is ischemia to the retina, the optic nerve, or both. In 1 study, 24% of patients with monocular ischemic vision loss had concurrent cerebral infarcts on MRI, reinforcing that these are strokes of the eye. This includes 9% of patients with transient monocular vision loss owing to ocular transient ischemic attack.[17,18] Emergent evaluation is essential owing to the high short-term risk of a second event owing to the presence of undiagnosed or insufficiently managed risk factors, such as carotid artery stenosis or atrial fibrillation.

Patients with a CRAO experience acute, painless, monocular vision loss, with 80% of affected patients having visual acuity of count fingers vision or worse. Those with BRAO will experience visual field loss in the territory of the occluded artery, often an altitudinal monocular visual field defect.[19] A monocular transient ischemic attack (amaurosis fugax) typically causes severe vision loss lasting 1 to 15 minutes.[20]

Examination
Ischemic retina can seem normal in the hyperacute stage, before becoming pale owing to edema. In CRAO, there is a cherry red spot in the macula, which is not perfused by the central retinal artery (**Fig. 2**). In CRAO, BRAO, and amaurosis fugax, the examiner may be able to identify a cholesterol or calcium plaque in one of the retinal arteries.

Testing
In patients presenting less than 72 hours after symptom onset, emergent evaluation is recommended, preferably at a stroke center. The workup should include standard of care for stroke, including a lipid panel, hemoglobin A1c, electrocardiogram, cardiac telemetry, transthoracic echocardiogram, and an MRI of the brain with the addition

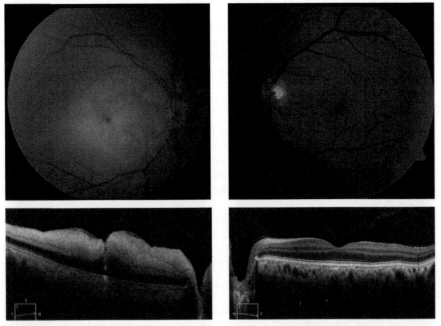

Fig. 2. Ophthalmic imaging features of acute central artery occlusion. Widefield retinal images (*top*) show a retinal whitening owing to edema in the affected (*left*) compared with unaffected eye (*right*). The edema spares the macula leaving a "cherry red spot." Optical coherence tomography cross-sectional images through the macula and optic nerve (*bottom*) show the retinal edema in the affected eye (*left*) that is not seen in the unaffected eye (*right*).

of vessel imaging (CT angiography or MR angiography). Updated guidelines are published regularly by the American Heart Association.[21]

Management
There is heterogeneity in acute treatment among academic institutions for treatment of CRAO.[22] Some interventions aim to increase perfusion by decreasing the intraocular pressure (eg, via intraocular paracentesis, intravenous acetazolamide, or topical glaucoma drops). Studies examining the usefulness of systemic thrombolysis using alteplase suggest that the time window for successful intervention is likely to be less than approximately 6 hours.[23,24] There have been mixed data in regard to the efficacy of intra-arterial thrombolysis, with some case series and at least 1 meta-analysis showing a benefit; however, a more recent randomized control study failing to show improvement in visual acuity with intra-arterial thrombolysis.[19,25]

Monitoring during the early period when risk for second eye or brain events is highest is essential. This practice offers the opportunity to identify and intervene on secondary risk factors. For noncardioembolic events, the use of antiplatelet agents is recommended to decrease the risk of recurrent stroke or cardiovascular events. Prevention should include the initiation of an antiplatelet or anticoagulant, depending on the clinical situation.[21]

Clinics care points

- Patients with acute BRAO, CRAO, or monocular transient vision loss thought to be due to ischemia should be referred emergently to a stroke center for evaluation.
- Emergent evaluation should include lipid panel, hemoglobin A1c, electrocardiogram, and cardiac telemetry, transthoracic echocardiogram, and MRI of the brain with the addition of vessel imaging (CT angiography or MR angiography).
- Acute treatment aimed at improving retinal perfusion may include lowering the intraocular pressure and systemic and/or directed endovascular thrombolysis.

Ischemic and Hemorrhagic Stroke

Background and presentation
Cerebral infarction and hemorrhage impacting the optic radiations or visual cortex cause acute vision loss with homonymous visual field loss. Lateral geniculate nucleus lesions are associated with wedge-shaped homonymous contralateral visual field loss in both eyes. Isolated visual symptoms are rare, but can occur from either anterior circulation (anterior choroidal artery) or posterior circulation (posterior choroidal artery) strokes. Dysfunction of the optic radiations is associated with incongruous visual field loss in the opposite field in both eyes. Owing to the distributed nature of the radiations, it is rare for an injury to them to cause isolated visual symptoms and it is typical to have other symptoms or signs that localize to the relevant parietal or temporal lobe. Occipital lobe dysfunction is associated with congruous visual field loss in the opposite field in both eyes. Unlike visual field defects localizing to the optic radiations, those from occipital lobe dysfunction commonly occur in the absence of other neurologic dysfunction. Central vision may be spared owing to dual arterial supply from both anterior and posterior circulations to the occipital poles.

Diagnosis and management
CT and MRI are helpful for the diagnosis of acute cerebral ischemic stroke or hemorrhage. The reader is referred to excellent reviews on diagnosis and management of acute stroke for further details.[21]

Papilledema Owing to Increased Intracranial Pressure

Background and presentation

High intracranial pressure causes optic nerve head swelling owing to compression of the optic nerve by the high-pressure cerebrospinal fluid in the optic nerve sheath. Papilledema is an emergency to prevent vision loss from high ICP and neurologic deterioration from any underlying secondary cause. The former occurs in about one-half of affected people and is severe in 10%. If not treated promptly, this vision loss can be permanent.

Common symptoms of a high intracranial pressure include headache and pulsatile tinnitus. When papilledema causes vision loss, it typically impacts the periphery and the central vision is spared. Transient visual obscurations, described as blacking or graying out of vision in 1 or both eyes for seconds provoked by head movements, might be a marker of borderline optic nerve head perfusion. Diplopia owing to sixth nerve palsy is a false localizing sign of high intracranial pressure.

Examination

Optic nerve swelling is typically bilateral, but can be asymmetric. Retinal hemorrhages or cotton wool spots suggest acute and severe injury. In late stages, the swelling can reduce and become pale owing to atrophy.

Imaging

Neuroimaging to exclude a mass lesion or venous sinus thrombosis as a cause of high intracranial pressure should be pursued emergently. Additionally, ultrasound examination demonstrating an enlarged optic nerve sheath diameter and change in diameter with eye movement may allow for the early diagnosis of intracranial hypertension when direct intracranial pressure measurement is not feasible or delayed. In 1 meta-analysis, consisting of primarily patients with traumatic brain injury and intracranial hemorrhage with intracranial pressure monitoring, a positive ultrasound examination was found to be associated with a 51-fold higher risk of an elevated intracranial pressure and was shown to have a sensitivity of 90% and specificity of 85%.[26]

Diagnosis

If a secondary cause is not found on imaging, lumbar puncture with measurement of opening pressure in the lateral decubitus position is important to identify cerebrospinal fluid inflammation or infection, confirm high intracranial pressure, and provide temporary treatment.

Management

Primary management is directed at any underlying cause. In patients with vision loss, regardless of whether intracranial pressure elevation is primary or secondary, intracranial pressure–directed therapy is important. Medications (acetazolamide, furosemide, topiramate) are first line with surgical interventions (optic nerve sheath fenestration, cerebrospinal fluid diversion shunt, venous sinus stenting) reserved for progression or severe vision loss cases.[27] Surgical procedure selection varies across institutions. Many times, the decision is often based on local expertise and surgeon availability with predominant symptom and patient preference being taken into consideration.[28]

DIPLOPIA
Approach to the History and Examination

The first thing a clinician should establish when evaluating a patient with diplopia is whether they are experiencing monocular or binocular diplopia. Binocular diplopia owing to ocular misalignment will resolve with covering either eye. If diplopia persists with either eye covered, this is unlikely to be a neurologic problem and likely owing to a problem with the optics of the anterior visual pathway. It is important to note that, in a minority of people (eg, those with poor vision in one eye or poor integration of the eyes), ocular misalignment does not cause diplopia.

The goal of a comprehensive eye movement examination is to facilitate pattern identification to localize the lesion. Examination of the extent of eye movements may be sufficient to characterize the eye movement disorder causing diplopia. If there are any limitations, evaluation of eye movements induced by reflex maneuvers (eg, vestibulo-ocular reflex using dolls eyes or caloric tests) can be helpful to localize any eye limitation to a supranuclear or cranial nerve/nuclear origin. However, it is important to recognize that full extraocular movements do not exclude a neurologic disorder causing diplopia, because very small degrees of ocular misalignment not apparent on examination can cause diplopia. The patient can help to characterize this by describing if the images are horizontally, vertically, or obliquely oriented with respect to each other and if the images change in orientation or separation distance in different directions of gaze. Methods of eye alignment testing include examining the reflection of light in the pupils for relative displacement off of the center of the pupil (eg, if the light reflects off the inner iris of 1 eye, this finding suggests the eyes are relatively turned out). Alternately, covering each eye while the patient fixates on an object is an easy bedside test. If there is ocular misalignment, the newly uncovered eye will saccade to regain fixation. The eye movement examination is a small part of the cranial nerve examination and must be interpreted in the context of a full neurologic examination and history.

Patterns of ocular motility disorders and their emergent causes are discussed below. After this is a discussion of 2 diseases causing complex ocular misalignment patterns necessitating emergent intervention.

Ocular Motility Disorder Patterns and Emergent Causes

Cranial nerve III palsy

A non-nuclear third nerve palsy in isolation affects the superior rectus, inferior rectus, medical rectus, and inferior oblique (ie, all extraocular movement, except the superior oblique and lateral rectus). Additional localizing signs are a larger and less reactive ipsilateral pupil and ptosis. A nuclear third nerve palsy additionally causes bilateral ptosis and bilateral upgaze deficits.

Emergent causes of third nerve palsy include the following.

- Aneurysm compressing the ipsilateral nerve (discussed elsewhere in this article).
- Uncal herniation (typically associated with altered mental status).
- Brainstem parenchymal event (stroke, demyelination, tumor) including:
  - Benedikt syndrome (with contralateral movement disorder owing to involvement of the red nucleus)
  - Claude syndrome (with contralateral ataxia owing to involvement of the superior cerebellar peduncle)
  - Weber syndrome (with contralateral hemiparesis owing to involvement of the cerebral peduncle)

Cranial nerve IV palsy

A non-nuclear fourth nerve palsy in isolation affects the superior oblique muscle, causing vertical diplopia that is worse in downgaze, contralateral gaze, and ipsilateral head tilt. Owing to the torsional action of the superior oblique, the image in the affected eye can appear tilted. Patients may adopt a compensatory head tilt away from the affected eye. A nuclear fourth nerve palsy causes contralateral superior oblique dysfunction owing to the fact that the fourth cranial nerve crosses before innervating the superior oblique. The eye movements often appear full. An isolated fourth nerve palsy is rarely from an emergent cause. However, it is easy to confuse a fourth nerve palsy with a skew deviation (discussed elsewhere in this article).

Cranial nerve VI palsy
A non-nuclear sixth nerve palsy in isolation affects the lateral rectus muscle to cause horizontal diplopia in ipsilateral gaze that resolves in contralateral gaze. Usually, but not always, there is an obvious abduction deficit on the affected side. A nuclear sixth nerve palsy causes an ipsilateral gaze palsy (ie, affecting both eyes and therefore without diplopia).

Emergent causes of sixth nerve palsy include the following.
- Elevated intracranial pressure (eg, tumor, venous sinus thrombosis, meningitis) causing sixth nerve palsy as a false localizing sign.
- Cavernous sinus syndrome: The sixth nerve floats freely within the cavernous sinus and can be affected in isolation by pathologies in this region (discussed elsewhere in this article).
- Gradenigo syndrome (with retro-orbital pain owing to V1 involvement) and otitis media (owing to petrous apicitis).
- Brainstem parenchymal event (stroke, demyelination, tumor).

Horizontal gaze palsy
A devastating impairment of horizontal gaze results from pontine lesions that affect the horizontal gaze center and sixth cranial nerve nucleus, with stroke being a common cause. In palsies owing to stroke, the eyes will not move as either a voluntary or vestibular reflexive response. Another common cause of horizontal gaze palsy is a contralateral cerebral hemisphere insult to the frontal eye fields (also typically caused by a stroke). The conjugate gaze palsy resulting from a supratentorial lesion will inhibit voluntary eye movement but vestibular eye movement is intact (eg, response to cold caloric testing and vestibulo-ocular reflex).

Internuclear ophthalmoplegia
Internuclear ophthalmoplegia is caused by a lesion of the medial longitudinal fasciculus and is characterized by horizontal diplopia that is present in contralateral gaze only. Often there is nystagmus of the abducting (normal) eye and slowed adducting saccade of the affected eye. Adduction of the affected eye is often better during convergence, because this does not use the medial longitudinal fasciculus. An emergent cause is focal brainstem infarct.

Skew deviation
Skew deviation is a supranuclear disorder characterized by vertical diplopia with tilting of images in both eyes. Typically, it is associated with other vestibular or cerebellar symptoms and signs. Emergent causes include stroke involving the brainstem and/or cerebellum.

Orbital Apex Syndrome from Rhino–Orbital–Cerebral Mucositis

Background and presentation
Rhino–orbital–cerebral mucormycosis is typically fatal without urgent therapy. This opportunistic fungal infection arising in the paranasal sinuses is seen in patients with diabetes mellitus, diabetic ketoacidosis, hematologic malignancies, those who are chronically immunosuppressed, and those with an elevated serum iron.[29] Extension into the orbit can cause blindness and subsequent extension into the

cavernous sinus can be fatal owing to invasion of the cavernous segment of the carotid artery, promoting intracranial thrombosis or mycotic aneurysm formation, infarction, or subarachnoid hemorrhage.[30,31] Rapid diagnosis and treatment is important at the time of recognition of orbital symptoms owing to the risk of mortality.[31] Late diagnosis, bilateral sinusitis, immunosuppression, presence of hemiplegia or hemiparesis, and the extent of invasion are correlated with a worse prognosis, despite treatment.[32] Mortality remains extremely high, even with treatment, and has been reported up to 50%.[33]

Typical symptoms of mucormycosis invading the orbital apex include pain, vision loss from optic neuropathy, diplopia, ptosis, and decreased corneal sensation (**Table 3**).

Imaging
Orbit protocol imaging can be helpful to identify bone erosion (CT scan), cavernous sinus involvement (MRI), and soft tissue changes in the nasal sinuses and orbit. Fungi can appear dark on T2 sequences of MRI, which adds a diagnostic challenge. Imaging is insensitive; thus, negative imaging does not exclude this entity.[31]

Diagnosis
Endoscopic evaluation of the paranasal sinuses for eschar and biopsy should be considered for definite diagnosis. If sinus biopsy histopathology is unrevealing, then an orbital apex biopsy can be considered.[30,31]

Treatment
Rhino–orbital mucor treatment consists of immediate antifungal therapy with amphotericin B (5–10 mg/kg/d, the latter if central nervous system involvement). Surgical debridement of the infected areas should be performed if possible.

Clinics care points

- Negative imaging does not exclude rhino–orbital–cerebral mucormycosis and nasal endoscopy with biopsy or orbital biopsy may be necessary.
- Treatment with immediate antifungal therapy and surgical debridement improves outcomes, but mortality remains high.
- Emergent ophthalmology, otorhinolaryngology, and infectious disease consultations are indicated.

Table 3 Early findings in mucormycosis[30]	
Symptom or Sign	**Prevalence (%)**
Fever	44
Nasal mucosal ulceration/necrosis	38
Periorbital and facial swelling	34
Decreased vision	30
Ophthalmoplegia	29
Sinusitis	26
Headache	25
Black eschar of skin, nasal mucosa, or palate	20

Cavernous Sinus Thrombosis

Background and presentation

Cavernous sinus thrombosis is a life-threatening condition that should be considered when evaluating patients with combinations of cranial nerve III, IV, and VI palsies; Horner syndrome; and sensory changes in the distribution of the ophthalmic and/or maxillary divisions of the trigeminal nerve. When the underlying etiology may be due to a septic sinus thrombosis, morbidity and mortality remain high even in the modern era of antibiotic treatment (30%).[34] The most common pathogen causing septic cavernous sinus thrombosis is *Staphylococcus aureus* (66%), with *Streptococcus pneumoniae*, gram-negative bacilli, and anaerobic bacteria being less frequently identified.[35] Infection typically spreads to the cavernous sinus through the venous system from a primary site in the sphenoid and ethmoid sinuses, mouth, ear, or orbital regions. Aseptic cavernous sinus thrombosis occurs in the setting of prothrombotic disorders (polycythemia, pregnancy oral contraceptive pills), as well as extrinsic damage to the cavernous sinus (surgery, compression from tumor, trauma).

The presenting features of these patients are directly related to the anatomic structures involved, mass effect, infection, and impaired venous outflow. Therefore, patients will present with some combination of fever, proptosis, and cranial nerve palsies. Any process that elevates venous pressure in the cavernous sinus can transmit this pressure to the orbit to cause significant orbital signs, including proptosis and red eyes. Vision can be affected if the process extends superiorly to the optic chiasm or if blood flow to the eye is impaired. Overall, 50% to 80% of patients will present with periorbital edema, headache, lethargy, altered sensorium, optic disc edema, and retinal venous engorgement. Eye findings are nearly universal (90%). Less than 50% of patients have decreased visual acuity, sluggish or dilated pupils, periorbital and corneal sensory loss, and meningismus. Rarely, seizures and hemiparesis may occur, typically owing to cerebral venous infarction. Owing to the intercavernous sinus, spread to the opposite site is common in the first days.[34,35]

Laboratory evaluation

Blood cultures should be obtained routinely and are frequently positive. Lumbar puncture is important to exclude meningitis and may show elevated opening pressure and pleocytosis, even in culture-negative samples. Blood cultures are more sensitive than cerebrospinal fluid cultures (70% vs 20%).[34] Screening for thrombophilia may give false results if anticoagulation therapy has been started and should be delayed until after treatment is completed.[36]

Imaging

High-resolution contrast-enhanced head CT scans typically show cavernous sinus expansion and irregular filling defects, in addition to dilated superior ophthalmic veins, soft tissue edema, proptosis, and concurrent thrombosis of the tributary veins.[37] High-resolution head MRI, is helpful to access the extension of infection.[32] A CT venogram and contrast-enhanced MR venogram are highly sensitive, whereas noncontrast CT scans and time-of-flight MR venogram may miss the diagnosis.[36]

Treatment and management

Empiric antibiotic therapy with vancomycin, a third- or fourth-generation cephalosporin, and metronidazole should be started as soon as the diagnosis is suspected and before the return of culture results.[38] This regimen can later be tailored to culture and sensitivity results. Prolonged duration of intravenous antibiotic therapy is recommended—typically 3 to 4 weeks—or at least 2 weeks beyond clinical resolution. Anticoagulation is controversial and has not been convincingly shown to decrease mortality; however, there is a trend toward decreased morbidity. Current evidence favors the use of anticoagulation along with antibiotics early in the course.[38–41] Corticosteroids are often given but without demonstrated efficacy.[36]

Clinics care points

- A CT venogram and contrast-enhanced MR venogram are highly sensitive, whereas noncontrast CT and time-of-flight MR venogram may miss the diagnosis of cavernous sinus thrombosis.
- Because the distinction between aseptic and septic cavernous sinus thrombosis may not be initially known, management with broad antibiotics is recommended, until a septic etiology is ruled out.
- Anticoagulation with unfractionated heparin or low-molecular-weight heparin is definitely indicated in aseptic cases and probably beneficial in septic etiologies.

SUMMARY

This article aimed to provide the clinician with a framework for approaching patients with potentially vision- and life-threatening neuro-ophthalmologic conditions as well as review the presentation, evaluation, and emergency treatment of select conditions. There is a much broader differential diagnosis for each presentation than presented herein. We hope that guidance on clinical approach to patients who present with acute vision loss or diplopia will help the reader to localize the presentation to direct further investigations and institute vision and life-saving therapies in a timely fashion.

DISCLOSURE

No commercial or financial conflicts of interests to disclose. National Institutes of Health P30 026877, Research to Prevent Blindness Unrestricted Grant.

REFERENCES

1. Trobe JD. The neurology of vision. Oxford university press; 2001. p. 488.
2. Kerr NM, Chew SSL, Eady EK, et al. Diagnostic accuracy of confrontation visual field tests. Neurology 2010;74(15):1184–90.
3. Weyand CM, Goronzy JJ. Giant-cell arteritis and polymyalgia rheumatica. Ann Intern Med 2003;139(6):505–15.
4. Smetana GW, Shmerling RH. Does this patient have temporal arteritis? JAMA 2002;287(1):92–101.
5. Johnson LN, Arnold AC. Incidence of nonarteritic and arteritic anterior ischemic optic neuropathy: population-based study in the state of Missouri and Los Angeles County, California. J Neuroophthalmol 1994;14(1):38–44.
6. Vodopivec I, Rizzo JF III. Ophthalmic manifestations of giant cell arteritis. Rheumatology 2018;57(suppl_2):ii63–72.
7. Soriano A, Muratore F, Pipitone N, et al. Visual loss and other cranial ischaemic complications in giant cell arteritis. Nat Rev Rheumatol 2017;13(8):476.
8. Buttgereit F, Dejaco C, Matteson EL, et al. Polymyalgia rheumatica and giant cell arteritis: a systematic review. JAMA 2016;315(22):2442–58.
9. Kermani TA, Schmidt J, Crowson CS, et al. Utility of erythrocyte sedimentation rate and C-reactive protein for the diagnosis of giant cell arteritis. Semin Arthritis Rheum 2012;41:866–71. Elsevier.

10. Berger CT, Sommer G, Aschwanden M, et al. The clinical benefit of imaging in the diagnosis and treatment of giant cell arteritis. Swiss Med Wkly 2018;148(3334): w14661.
11. Liu GT, Glaser JS, Schatz NJ, et al. Visual morbidity in giant cell arteritis: clinical characteristics and prognosis for vision. Ophthalmology 1994;101(11):1779–85.
12. Fraser JA, Weyand CM, Newman NJ, et al. The treatment of giant cell arteritis. Rev Neurol Dis 2008;5(3):140.
13. Semple PL, Webb MK, de Villiers JC, et al. Pituitary apoplexy. Neurosurgery 2005;56(1):65–73.
14. Biousse V, Newman NJ, Oyesiku NM. Precipitating factors in pituitary apoplexy. J Neurol Neurosurg Psychiatry 2001;71(4):542–5.
15. Johnston PC, Hamrahian AH, Weil RJ, et al. Pituitary tumor apoplexy. J Clin Neurosci 2015;22(6):939–44.
16. Briet C, Salenave S, Bonneville J-F, et al. Pituitary apoplexy. Endocr Rev 2015; 36(6):622–45.
17. Biousse V, Nahab F, Newman NJ. Management of acute retinal ischemia: follow the guidelines! Ophthalmology 2018;125(10):1597–607.
18. Helenius J, Arsava EM, Goldstein JN, et al. Concurrent acute brain infarcts in patients with monocular visual loss. Ann Neurol 2012;72(2):286–93.
19. Cugati S, Varma DD, Chen CS, et al. Treatment options for central retinal artery occlusion. Curr Treat Options Neurol 2013;15(1):63–77.
20. Donders R. Clinical features of transient monocular blindness and the likelihood of atherosclerotic lesions of the internal carotid artery. J Neurol Neurosurg Psychiatry 2001;71(2):247–9.
21. Powers WJ, Rabinstein AA, Ackerson T, et al. Guidelines for the early management of patients with acute ischemic stroke: 2019 update to the 2018 guidelines for the early management of acute ischemic stroke: a guideline for healthcare professionals from the American Heart Association/American Stroke Association. Stroke 2019;50(12):e344–418.
22. Youn TS, Lavin P, Patrylo M, et al. Current treatment of central retinal artery occlusion: a national survey. J Neurol 2018;265(2):330–5.
23. Chen CS, Lee AW, Campbell B, et al. Efficacy of intravenous tissue-type plasminogen activator in central retinal artery occlusion: report from a randomized, controlled trial. Stroke 2011;42(8):2229–34.
24. Tobalem S, Schutz JS, Chronopoulos A. Central retinal artery occlusion–Rethinking retinal survival time. BMC Ophthalmol 2018;18(1):101.
25. Arnold M, Koerner U, Remonda L, et al. Comparison of intra-arterial thrombolysis with conventional treatment in patients with acute central retinal artery occlusion. J Neurol Neurosurg Psychiatry 2005;76(2):196–9.
26. Dubourg J, Javouhey E, Geeraerts T, et al. Ultrasonography of optic nerve sheath diameter for detection of raised intracranial pressure: a systematic review and meta-analysis. Intensive Care Med 2011;37(7):1059–68.
27. Ahmad SR, Moss HE. Update on the diagnosis and treatment of Idiopathic Intracranial Hypertension. Semin Neurol 2019;39:682–91. Thieme Medical Publishers.
28. Spitze A, Malik A, Al-Zubidi N, et al. Optic nerve sheath fenestration vs cerebrospinal diversion procedures: what is the preferred surgical procedure for the treatment of idiopathic intracranial hypertension failing maximum medical therapy? J Neuroophthalmol 2013;33(2):183–8.
29. Binder U, Maurer E, Lass-Flörl C. Mucormycosis–from the pathogens to the disease. Clin Microbiol Infect 2014;20:60–6.

30. Yohai RA, Bullock JD, Aziz AA, et al. Survival factors in rhino-orbital-cerebral mucormycosis. Surv Ophthalmol 1994;39(1):3–22.
31. Thurtell MJ, Chiu AL, Goold LA, et al. Neuro-ophthalmology of invasive fungal sinusitis: 14 consecutive patients and a review of the literature. Clin Exp Ophthalmol 2013;41(6):567–76.
32. Prabhu RM, Patel R. Mucormycosis and entomophthoramycosis: a review of the clinical manifestations, diagnosis and treatment. Clin Microbiol Infect 2004;10: 31–47.
33. Kalin-Hajdu E, Hirabayashi KE, Vagefi MR, et al. Invasive fungal sinusitis: treatment of the orbit. Curr Opin Ophthalmol 2017;28(5):522–33.
34. DiNubile MJ. Septic thrombosis of the cavernous sinuses. Arch Neurol 1988; 45(5):567–72.
35. Southwick FS, Richardson EP Jr, Swartz MN. Septic thrombosis of the dural venous sinuses. Medicine (Baltimore) 1986;65(2):82–106.
36. Plewa MC, Tadi P, Gupta M. Cavernous Sinus Thrombosis. 2020 Jul 8. In: StatPearls [Internet]. Treasure Island (FL): StatPearls Publishing; 2020. PMID: 28846357.
37. Schuknecht B, Simmen D, Yüksel C, et al. Tributary venosinus occlusion and septic cavernous sinus thrombosis: CT and MR findings. Am J Neuroradiol 1998; 19(4):617–26.
38. Desa V, Green R. Cavernous sinus thrombosis: current therapy. J Oral Maxillofac Surg 2012;70(9):2085–91.
39. Bhatia K, Jones NS. Septic cavernous sinus thrombosis secondary to sinusitis: are anticoagulants indicated? A review of the literature. J Laryngol Otol 2002; 116(9):667.
40. Levine SR, Twyman RE, Gilman S. The role of anticoagulation in cavernous sinus thrombosis. Neurology 1988;38(4):517.
41. Khatri IA, Wasay M. Septic cerebral venous sinus thrombosis. J Neurol Sci 2016; 362:221–7.

Neurological Emergencies During Pregnancy

Elizabeth Macri, MD[a], Diana Greene-Chandos, MD, FNCS[b],*

KEYWORDS

- Neurocritical care in pregnancy • Stroke in pregnancy • Seizures in pregnancy
- Intracerebral hemorrhage in pregnancy • Cerebral venous sinus thrombosis
- Posterior reversible encephalopathy syndrome
- Neuroimmune disorders in pregnancy • Brain death in pregnancy

KEY POINTS

- Neurologic emergencies in pregnant patients create unique clinical scenarios. The presentation ranges from a subtle headache to focal neurologic deficits and seizures. Following a clinical algorithm assists in differentiating underlying neuroemergencies from tension or migraine headaches.
- Management of neurovascular disorders in pregnant patients is reviewed, including ischemic stroke; intracerebral hemorrhage and subarachnoid hemorrhage; posterior reversible encephalopathy syndrome; and reversible cerebral vasoconstrictive syndrome.
- Seizure and status epilepticus management in pregnant patients is reviewed, including pregnancy-specific risks, such as preeclampsia; changes in antiepileptic drug levels for those with known seizures; and teratogenicity of certain of antiepileptic drugs.
- Management of neuroimmunologic disorders, such as myasthenia gravis and multiple sclerosis, and the safety of exacerbation medications, with special considerations during delivery are reviewed.
- Brain death (death by neurologic criteria) is discussed with a detailed description of support for the patient's body to reach fetal viability for delivery as well as the ethical considerations associated.

INTRODUCTION

Neurologic emergencies during pregnancy often present initially to nonneurologists and include exacerbation of preexisting conditions, new neurologic diagnoses, and neurologic complications of pregnancy. The postpartum period, or puerperium, is also an altered physiologic state because of recovery from pregnancy, and vigilance

[a] Department of Neurology, University of New Mexico, MSC10 5620, 1 University of New Mexico, Albuquerque, NM 87131, USA; [b] Neurosciences Critical Care Fellowship, Department of Neurology, University of New Mexico; MSC10 5620, 1 University of New Mexico, Albuquerque, NM 87131, USA
* Corresponding author.
E-mail address: DGreeneChandos@salud.unm.edu
Twitter: @Macrimd (E.M.); @dianagcmd (D.G.-C.)

Neurol Clin 39 (2021) 649–670
https://doi.org/10.1016/j.ncl.2021.02.008
0733-8619/21/© 2021 Elsevier Inc. All rights reserved.

for acute neurologic disorders related to pregnancy during the first 6 weeks after delivery is warranted. Early recognition of more ominous neurologic diagnoses can be challenging, as they can present with common symptoms like headache and have subtle neurologic findings if there are any at all. In addition, diagnostic evaluations and management decisions each need to be carefully considered for pregnant patients given potential effects on the fetus. Similar consideration needs to occur for the postpartum mother who is breastfeeding. In this article, the following are discussed in relation to neurologic emergencies in pregnancy: common presenting symptoms and decision algorithms; neurovascular diseases; seizures and status epilepticus; autoimmune disorders; uncommon diseases; and special circumstances of cardiac arrest with hypoxic brain injury and death by neurologic criteria.

APPROACH TO NEUROLOGIC SYMPTOMS IN PREGNANCY

The most common presenting neurologic symptom in pregnancy is headache. **Fig. 1** provides a decision tree that can guide medical professionals in the differential diagnosis and management of neurologic symptoms in pregnancy. Most transient neurologic deficits in pregnancy are due to migraine with aura.[1] These symptoms begin gradually, start with positive symptoms (ie, scintillating scotoma), followed by negative symptoms (visual field cut, hemiparesis, or hemisensory defect), and may or may not be associated with headache. If a patient has had the same deficits in the setting of a known migraine with aura before pregnancy, then the patient can be observed carefully. If there is a new headache or a change of character compared with typical headaches before pregnancy, then the diagnosis can range from worsening of migraine headaches related to pregnancy hormones, to preeclampsia, to cerebral venous sinus thrombosis (CST), or to aneurysmal subarachnoid hemorrhage (SAH). Preeclampsia can be ruled out clinically with physical examination, blood pressure measurement, and urinalysis. Preeclampsia is defined as hypertension associated with proteinuria. Hypertension is defined as a systolic blood pressure of greater than 140 mm Hg or diastolic blood pressure greater than 90 mm Hg at least twice, more than 4 hours apart after the 20th week of gestation in a previously normotensive woman and proteinuria is $\geq$300 mg in 24 hours or $\geq$1+ on a dipstick on 2 urine samples greater than 4 hours apart.[2] If preeclampsia is not the cause of a new (or new in character) headache, a noncontrast computed tomographic (CT) scan of the head is warranted urgently, as a start. Further imaging may be warranted particularly if there are new neurologic deficits and the noncontrasted head CT scan is unrevealing.

CT head may be considered because of the relatively low fetal exposure to radiation (1.0–10 mGy) when using a low radiation technique, as this is below the threshold for adverse effect to the fetus (>50 mGy).[3] Emergent CT head is fast and sensitive for acute hemorrhage. In less acute situations, MRI without contrast is the imaging modality of choice for pregnant patients because of the absence of radiation.

NEUROVASCULAR DISORDERS

Because pregnancy is a hypercoagulable state,[4] women who are pregnant or postpartum are at an increased risk of venous sinus thromboses and acute ischemic strokes. Pregnancy is associated with increased clotting factors, including factors VII, VIII, and X, von Willebrand factor, and fibrinogen. Functional Protein S levels are decreased in pregnancy because of the presence of increased binding protein, and plasminogen activator inhibitor type 1 (PAI-1) levels increase 5-fold. PAI-2 is produced by the placenta and increases most significantly in the third trimester. These hypercoagulable changes, and the associated risk of thrombosis, begin at conception and

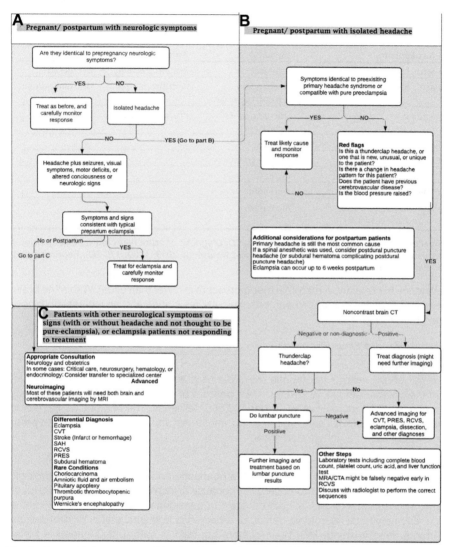

Fig. 1. Approach to a pregnant/postpartum patient. (*A*) Initial approach to a patient with neurologic symptoms (*yellow*). (*B*) The approach to a patient with headache only (*green*). (*C*) The approach when there are neurologic symptoms, with or without headache (not initially attributed to eclampsia), but does include those with severe/uncontrolled eclampsia (*blue*).[1] CTA, ; CVT, ; MRA, . (*Adapted from* Edlow JA, Caplan LR, O'Brien K, Tibbles, CD: Diagnosis of acute neurological emergencies in pregnant and post-partum women. The Lancet Neurology 2013; 12(2): 175-185.)

may not return to baseline until more than 8 weeks postpartum.[4] **Table 1** provides physiologic alterations in coagulation and fibrinolytic factors during pregnancy.

Regarding hemodynamic states in pregnancy, blood volume increases by 50%, with the largest increase of that volume in the first trimester. As such, the cardiac output must increase as well and does so by up to 30% to 50%, reaching its maximum by the end of the second trimester. Because there is decreased systemic vascular

Table 1
Alterations in coagulation and fibrinolytic factors during pregnancy[4]

Procoagulants	(Activity)	Anticoagulants	(Activity)
Factor I (fibrinogen)	Increased	Protein S activity	Decreased
Factor II	Unchanged/ insufficient data	Antithrombin III	Unchanged/mild decrease
Factor V	Unchanged/mild increase	Protein C activity	Unchanged
Factors VII, VIII, IX, X, XII, XIII	Increased		
Factor XI	Mild decrease		
von Willebrand factor	Increased		
D-Dimer	Increased		
Plasminogen activator 1 and 2 (PA-1/PA-2)	Increased		

From Edlow JA, Caplan LR, O'Brien K, Tibbles, CD: Diagnosis of acute neurological emergencies in pregnant and post-partum women. The Lancet Neurology 2013; 12(2): 175-185. Reprinted with permission from Elsevier.

resistance in pregnancy, maternal blood pressure is lower than usual. Within the brain, pregnancy causes decreased cerebral vascular resistance and an increase in blood-brain barrier permeability.[5]

Cerebral Venous Sinus Thrombosis

Epidemiology
The risk of any venous thrombotic event during pregnancy is increased 4- to 5-fold, and the postpartum risk is 20-fold.[6] Two percent of all strokes related to pregnancy are due to CST, approximately 12 per 100,000 deliveries. The risk of CST increased with increased maternal age, hypertension, infections, and excessive vomiting in pregnancy because of a dehydrated state.[7]

Presentation
Patients with CST typically present with a headache and may have focal neurologic deficits, encephalopathy, and/or seizures because of increased venous pressure leading to venous infarcts and/or hemorrhage.[8] In a pregnant woman, a new headache type, any new focal neurologic deficit, or a decrease in mental status or new seizure warrants head imaging. MRI brain without contrast is safe, but CT head is faster and should be considered in patients with significant deficits or if the patient worsens while awaiting an MRI. Given the relatively high frequency of CST in pregnant patients, if an MRI is ordered, an Magnetic Resonance Venogram (MRV) without contrast is typically done at the same time. Gadolinium contrast is avoided during pregnancy, as the risk to the fetus is unclear. CT angiogram is usually avoided because of the need for intravenous (IV) iodine contrast and the radiation exposure; however, there are no proven risks to the fetus from either, and CT angiogram of the veins may be used if MRV cannot be obtained.[9] Intracranial hemorrhage (ICH) is common in CST, present in 30% to 40% at the time of initial imaging, and may be bilateral. Infarcts, if present, are unlikely to conform to arterial territories, increasing the suspicion of underlying venous pathologic condition.

Treatment
Anticoagulant therapy with heparin (unfractionated heparin [UFH]) drip titrated to therapeutic Xa level should be initiated as soon as the diagnosis of venous sinus

thrombosis is confirmed. Anticoagulation is warranted even if there is evidence of venous hemorrhage on imaging, as the hemorrhage size will increase unless the clot burden is decreased. UFH may be transitioned to low-molecular-weight heparin (LMWH) for the duration of the pregnancy and postpartum period once stability of the patient has been ascertained. A patient who does not have significant abnormalities, such as hemorrhage or edema, on imaging other than venous thrombosis and who has a mild clinical presentation may be considered for initiation of anticoagulation therapy with LMWH without intervening UFH. In any case, once the patient is out of the critical period, anticoagulation is continued as LMWH until at least 6 weeks after delivery.[7]

Overall, 23% of CST patients will worsen despite initiation of anticoagulation. Worsening may present as a decrease in the level of consciousness, seizures, increased or new focal neurologic deficit, or increased headache. One-third of these patients will have new parenchymal pathologic condition on repeat imaging. Patients who worsen despite UFH or LMWH may be considered for interventional therapy, including mechanical clot disruption and direct injection of thrombolytic.[7] Significant cerebral edema can occur because of venous infarct with vasogenic edema, arterial infarct with cytotoxic edema, venous hemorrhage, intraventricular hemorrhage with obstructive hydrocephalus, and obstruction of cerebrospinal fluid (CSF) outflow at the arachnoid granulations in the lateral and/or sagittal sinus. Management of increased intracranial pressure (ICP) with acetazolamide[7] has been used in CST but is avoided in pregnancy because of the risk of teratogenicity. Hypertonic therapy, decompressive hemicraniectomy, surgical resection of hematomas, and/or external ventricular drain placement may be considered in the appropriate clinical and imaging context, but one must be judicious in the use hypertonic saline, as there are not enough safety data in pregnant women to assign it a pregnancy class risk. However, use has been described, with titrating solutions of 2% to 23.4% NaCl for a sodium goal up to 150 to 155. Hypertonic saline use should be reserved for life-saving circumstances only.[10–13]

It is reasonable to evaluate for an underlying hypercoagulable disorder, such as antiphospholipid antibody syndrome, factor V Leiden deficiency, prothrombin (factor II) 20210 gene mutation, antithrombin III deficiency, and protein S and/or C deficiencies.

A history of CST is not a contraindication to future pregnancies, but LMWH prophylaxis may be considered.[7]

Forty percent of patients with CST will have seizures. Treatment with antiepileptic therapy (please see later discussion, Seizure section, for specific therapies) is reasonable following a single seizure in the setting of CST. Determination of how long a patient should remain on antiepileptic therapy will depend on imaging, the number of seizures, whether the patient has had a seizure more than 2 weeks after onset of CST, and clinical presentation. Overall, 5% of patients (including those not related to pregnancy) will develop epilepsy related to CST. The decision to discontinue antiepileptic therapy should be made in conjunction with consultation with an epileptologist when possible. Prophylactic initiation of antiepileptic therapy in patients with CST is not indicated.[14]

Acute Ischemic Stroke

Epidemiology
The risk of stroke in women during child-bearing years ranges from 10.7 to 25 per 100,000 annually, with significant variation depending on the upper age limit used during retrospective studies.[1] There is conclusive evidence of increased stroke risk in the postpartum period, ranging up to 6 weeks after giving birth. The relative risk of ischemic stroke in this population is 8.7.[15]

Initial assessment

Any patient with an acute neurologic injury must have a rapid assessment for stability, including the ABC's (airway, breathing, circulation). Determining the time of onset of symptoms or time when the patient was last seen normal is of utmost importance if acute ischemic stroke is suspected. Patients may be a candidate for tissue plasminogen activator (tPA) and/or thrombectomy depending on the time of symptom onset or its surrogate, time last seen normal. Hemorrhagic and ischemic strokes can present in a similar fashion, and therefore, treatment of presumed acute ischemic stroke cannot be initiated until emergent imaging has ruled out hemorrhage. Emergent CT head is the test of choice if a patient may be a candidate for acute intervention, as this is available in most centers, can be completed rapidly, and is a very sensitive test for acute ICH. Some centers may have access to rapid MRI and may choose this option to minimize the risk of radiation to an embryo or fetus. However, administration of tPA should not be delayed to obtain an MRI if the CT head can be obtained faster. If the patient has significant neurologic deficits suggesting a large vessel occlusion, such as a National Institutes of Health Stroke Scale of 6 or greater, cervical and cerebral vascular imaging should be emergently performed. Iodine contrast is considered safe in pregnancy, as it does not cross the placenta, and a Computerized tomography angiogram (CTA) head and neck to rule out a large vessel occlusion may be considered,[16] particularly if Magnetic resonance angiogram (MRA) is not available or cannot be done emergently. With the notable exception of blood glucose measurement, laboratory studies need not be done in the emergency assessment of a patient with suspected acute ischemic stroke unless there is a reason to suspect there will be an abnormality.[17]

Treatment

Although pregnant women were excluded from the tPA trials, current expert consensus opinion is to treat with IV tPA and/or thrombectomy if indicated if the patient has moderate to severe deficits and the potential benefit outweighs the risk.[17] Thrombectomy should be done with minimal fluoroscopy and with fetal shielding. There is a trend toward increased hemorrhage in pregnant patients versus nonpregnant patients treated with tPA, but no statistical significance was achieved in the small sample size.[18] Reperfusion rates in pregnant patients were similar to nonpregnant patients.[19] There is limited experience giving tPA to pregnant women. A review of the largest stroke database in the United States, Get With The Guidelines, found that 1.5% of women who received tPA over a 5-year period were pregnant, a total of 40 women. This low number is likely due to pregnancy being listed as a relative contraindication to tPA.[19] There is limited experience with thrombectomy in pregnancy, in part because of the fear of radiation exposure to the fetus. However, a recent review of multiple small case series shows good maternal and fetal outcomes for thrombectomy in pregnancy.[20,21] In a "Get With The Guidelines" database review from 2016, there was a trend toward increased symptomatic ICH post-tPA in pregnant and postpartum patients but no major systemic bleeding.[19] There is a theoretic postpartum uterine hemorrhage risk that has not been quantified in the literature and is not listed as a contraindication to tPA.

Post-tPA and/or thrombectomy monitoring should be done in a dedicated neuroscience intensive care unit (ICU) setting. Should a large vessel occlusion result in a large ischemic stroke at risk for malignant cerebral edema, early hemicraniectomy should be considered as it is for nonpregnant patients. Typical precautions should be practiced to minimize ICP and cerebral edema, including keeping the head of the bed elevated to 30° to 45° and maintaining a neutral head and neck posture with no pressure in the region of the jugular veins to optimize cerebral venous drainage. Osmotic agents must be used judiciously in the pregnant patient. Mannitol is listed as a pregnancy category C risk. The issue with mannitol is that although it reduces cerebral edema through its osmotic diuretic effects, it also decreases amniotic fluid volumes. There is not much literature reported on mannitol use in pregnancy except 1 case report in 2015 by Handlogten and colleagues,[22] whereby they did an awake craniotomy for tumor resection in a pregnant woman. They used 0.25 g/kg of mannitol in the case and found a 30% reduction in uterine volume as a result that recovered in 48 hours. There were no negative effects to fetus from this. Mannitol has also been shown to create fetal hypoxia and acid-base disturbance.[10] Hypertonic saline is another medication used more commonly than mannitol, particularly in ischemic stroke–related edema, but in pregnancy there are little to no data. Nearly all studies of osmotic agents have excluded pregnant patients. In fact, there are not enough data to assign hypertonic saline a pregnancy category risk. However, Frontera and colleagues[10] in 2014 discuss using hypertonic saline in forms of 2% to 23.4% for cerebral edema in pregnant patients titrating to a serum sodium level of 150 to 155 with the risks being pulmonary edema and fluid overload. Caution and pause should be exercised before use of hypertonic saline in the pregnant mother as a life-saving attempt, as there are no clear data for safety regarding the fetus and pregnancy.

One item to consider that may first reveal itself as an embolic ischemic stroke is pregnancy and postpartum-related cardiomyopathy. In a study by Mogos and colleagues,[23] more than 50 million pregnancy-related hospitalizations were analyzed between 2001 and 2011. The overall rate of heart failure (HF) was 112 cases per 100,000 pregnancy-related hospitalizations. Although postpartum encounters represented only 1.5% of pregnancy-related hospitalizations, ≈60% of HF cases occurred postpartum, followed by delivery (27.3%) and antepartum (13.2%). The adjusted odds ratio between those with HF and those with ischemic stroke comparing women with and without HF in this study was 5.0 (confidence interval [CI], 2.6–9.8) for those antepartum; 8.8 (CI, 3.2–24.4) for those during delivery; and 1.0 (CI, 0.8–1.2) for those postpartum.

Finally, drugs of abuse as an underlying cause need to be considered in the pregnant patient as well with methamphetamine or cocaine related stroke or endocarditis related strokes for IV drug use.

Postpartum Angiopathy

Postpartum angiopathy is a type of reversible cerebral vasoconstriction syndrome (RCVS). RCVS presents with a sudden onset, severe (thunderclap) headache associated with diffuse cerebral vasospasm.[24] Focal neurologic deficits and/or seizures may occur.[25] There may be an overlap between postpartum angiopathy/RCVS and preeclampsia/eclampsia.[26]

RCVS can cause cortical SAH, intraparenchymal hemorrhage, ischemic stroke, and cerebral edema. As with RCVS and with other triggers, there is the potential for overlap between postpartum angiopathy and posterior reversible encephalopathy syndrome (PRES).

Postpartum angiopathy is usually fully reversible with no lasting deficits following spontaneous resolution of vasospasm and symptoms within 12 weeks. Rarely, a fulminant course can occur warranting close observation and accurate diagnosis, particularly if the patient presents with encephalopathy, seizures, and/or focal neurologic deficits.

Any patient who presents with a thunderclap headache should have SAH ruled out, and pregnant women are no different in this regard. If there is no acute blood on imaging (CT head or MRI brain), then a lumbar puncture should be done. Post-partum angiopathy can present with nontraumatic cortical SAH, which will show up in the CSF; however, the imaging will demonstrate convexal sulcal subarachnoid blood rather than cisternal hemorrhage. CSF studies will be normal, and MRI brain imaging is often normal, which helps to differentiate postpartum angiopathy from primary central nervous system (CNS) angiitis, which will have abnormalities on MRI and CSF.[27]

Treatment

Treatment is supportive with pain management that often includes opioids, because of the intense pain. Blood pressure goals are largely permissive with a systolic range of 90 to 180 mm Hg unless there is associated PRES, in which case a lower upper limit goal of approximately 160 mm Hg is often used. Avoidance of vasoconstrictive medications and maintenance of a minimum systolic blood pressure of 90 mm Hg are recommended to reduce the risk of ischemic stroke.[28] Seizures usually only occur on presentation and tend not to recur, making long-term antiepileptic therapy unnecessary. Antiepileptic drugs are typically discontinued when PRES is resolved.[29] Short-term treatment with antiepileptics is warranted if a patient has a seizure in the setting of RCVS, but seizure prophylaxis is not indicated. Steroids are contraindicated and should not be administered while a work up is in progress to differentiate between RCVS and primary CNS angiitis, as their use in patients with RCVS has been associated with worse outcomes.[30] This must be balanced against the clear potential benefits to a fetus at risk of premature delivery and the use of steroids in this situation.[31]

Posterior Reversible Encephalopathy Syndrome

PRES, also known as reversible posterior leukoencephalopathy syndrome, involves cerebral autoregulation dysfunction and endothelial malfunction. It is most often a manifestation of eclampsia when it occurs during pregnancy, and the relationship between the 2 indicates the likelihood of a common underlying pathophysiology. A rapid change in blood pressure can exceed the cerebral vasculature ability to autoregulate, leading to passive transference of systemic blood pressure to the cerebrovascular system, causing blood-brain barrier breakdown with subsequent fluid and blood extravasation outside the intracranial blood vessels.[32] This leads to edema that is typically reversible but may lead to intraparenchymal hemorrhage or ischemia, which can cause long-lasting neurologic deficits. PRES can also be due to nonhypertensive causes, including immunosuppressive or antineoplastic medications as well as renal disease.

Elevated estrogen levels in pregnancy raise total blood volume, which increases the risk of hypertension. As progesterone leads to decreased vascular tone, average blood pressures are decreased in pregnancy compared with prepregnancy baseline, making a relative increase in blood pressure more difficult to detect. In nonpregnant patients, PRES is most often associated with significantly elevated blood pressures, in the range of systolic 180 to 220+ mm Hg. However, the relative hypotension seen in pregnancy can lead to PRES in the systolic range of 140 mm Hg, particularly if there is a rapid rate of change. PRES in pregnancy can be associated with other pregnancy-related disorders of endothelial function, including eclampsia and thrombotic thrombocytopenic purpura/hemolytic uremic syndrome (TTP/HUS).

Patients with PRES present with headaches, encephalopathy, visual disturbances, and seizures and may have focal decreased sensation or strength. A CT head may show early ischemia, edema, or hemorrhage or may be unremarkable. Edema in PRES is commonly found in the occipital poles, bilaterally and asymmetrically. More advanced cases may have edema in the watershed territories between the Posterior Cerebral Artery (PCA) and Middle Cerebral Artery (MCA) territories and the Anterior Cerebral Artery (ACA) and MCA territories. PRES edema can also be seen in the bilateral cerebellar hemispheres as well as the pons. In rare cases, the edema in the pons and/or cerebellar may occur without supratentorial involvement. Occipital edema does not respect arterial distribution territories and frequently involves the posterior parietal cortices and spares the medial occipital cortices, helping differentiate this from PCA territory ischemic strokes.[33] MRI without contrast confirms the diagnosis.

Treatment involves blood pressure control, treatment of preeclampsia or eclampsia if present, and seizure management, as applicable. If blood pressure is higher than the patient's baseline, antihypertensive therapy to decrease mean arterial pressure by 10% to 25% carefully and incrementally, while monitoring for signs of hypoperfusion of the brain, kidneys, heart, and fetus, is a reasonable initial approach. If the patient has eclampsia, magnesium is used to manage seizures. Management of blood pressure and seizures should be done with the patient's obstetric team. Oral antihypertensive therapy can include the first-line drugs labetalol and nifedipine. Second-line drugs are associated with an increased risk of adverse effects but may be considered; this includes methyldopa and hydralazine. Appropriate IV antihypertensives include labetalol and nicardipine. Nitroprusside, angiotensin-converting enzyme inhibitors/angiotensin-receptor blockers, and atenolol should be avoided.[34]

PRES is fully reversible in most cases.

Intracranial Hemorrhage

The relative risk of ICH during pregnancy in women aged 15 to 44 years is 2.5. The greatest risk of SAH occurs in the third trimester, whereas the risk of intraparenchymal hemorrhage remains constant throughout pregnancy. The risk of a hemorrhagic stroke in the postpartum period is extremely high, with an estimated relative risk of 28.3 compared with non-pregnant, non- post-partum individuals. As an indication of the prominent role of ICH as a neurologic complication of pregnancy, despite being generally uncommon in pregnant and postpartum women, ICH accounts for 7.1% of all maternal mortality.[35] The various of forms of ICH that may occur in pregnancy are discussed later.

Intraparenchymal Hemorrhage

In a nonpregnant patient, the most common cause of an intraparenchymal hemorrhage is hypertension. Such hemorrhages are typically located in the basal ganglia, thalamus, cerebellum, and pons and may occur in pregnant patients with underlying traditional risk factors, such as non-pregnancy-related diabetes, prepregnancy hypertension, and/or chronic tobacco abuse. However, in the pregnant patient, the most common cause is eclampsia-related PRES as previously described. The next most common cause is CST, followed by aneurysmal SAH, arteriovenous malformations (AVM), and cerebral cavernous malformations (CCM). SAH and AVMs are further discussed later because of the increased risks during pregnancy. CCM, both sporadic and familial, have not been shown to have a significant increased risk of bleeding during pregnancy as compared with during nonpregnancy. Pregnancy has a 1.15% risk of bleeding per person per year, and nonpregnant patients have a 1.01% risk of bleeding per person per year, a nonsignificant difference. However, should they bleed, the severity of symptoms and risk of recurrent hemorrhage need to be weighed against the risks of surgical intervention at that point in the pregnancy.[36] Most CCM patients do well during pregnancy and deliver vaginally.[36] Those with family or personal history of CCM will face the decision of whether to obtain genetic testing for the condition on their fetus and can get support from the Angioma Alliance (https://www.angioma.org/) and local genetic counselors.[37]

In the pregnant patient with a new intraparenchymal hemorrhage, parenchymal and neurovascular imaging with contrast aimed at identifying a macrovascular culprit lesion, underlying mass, or evidence of PRES is imperative.

Subarachnoid Hemorrhage

SAH is commonly seen in the third trimester, and the risk is 5 times greater during pregnancy. Most spontaneous SAHs are due to aneurysm rupture, but 9% are due to AVMs in general.

Intracranial aneurysm rupture typically presents with a "thunderclap" headache, a sudden onset headache that escalates to maximum severity within seconds of onset, although the peak may be delayed for several minutes. Although there are other causes of thunderclap headaches, aneurysm rupture causing an SAH is the one most feared, most lethal, and not to be missed. Patients should undergo immediate cerebral imaging, CT head or MRI brain, to evaluate for cisternal SAH. If found, vascular imaging, time-of-flight MRA without contrast or CT angiogram, needs to follow to find the source of bleeding and facilitate planning to secure the aneurysm to prevent repeat hemorrhage. If initial imaging is negative for hemorrhage, a lumbar puncture must be done to assess for hemorrhage in the CSF. If a patient has an acute SAH, emergent neurosurgical consultation and admission to a neuroscience ICU are indicated. Strict blood pressure control to less than 140/90 mm Hg is recommended. There may be increased ICP, often because of hydrocephalus with or without intraventricular hemorrhage, necessitating the use of an external ventricular drain with a goal of normalizing ICP and reducing the degree of hydrocephalus. The method of aneurysm repair is typically guided by the anatomy of the aneurysm, and treatment of neurosurgical emergencies during pregnancy is made on a case-by-case basis because of the paucity of specific guidelines. The Neurocritical Care Society and American Heart Association aneurysmal subarachnoid guidelines do not specifically address the lower baseline blood pressures seen in pregnancy with respect to unsecured ruptured aneurysm blood pressure goals; however, as long as cerebral perfusion pressures are maintained, the mean arterial blood pressure (MAP) goal may be decreased.[38,39]

Arteriovenous Malformation

AVMs are direct arterial-to-venous blood vessel malformations without intervening capillaries. They may be part of a syndrome (eg, hereditary hemorrhagic telangiectasia), may arise de novo, or are congenital. AVMs occur in 0.1% of the population and usually present with ICH or seizure.

The risk of AVM rupture during pregnancy is thought to probably be elevated, but conflicting data about this have been published.[40,41] If true, the increased rupture risk likely occurs as a result of progesterone-mediated increases in blood volume, which places increasing hemodynamic stress on the AVM.[42] AVM rupture is commonly seen during a first pregnancy. Similar to other causes of ICH, AVM hemorrhage presents with headache and may have associated acute focal neurologic deficits, seizure, and/or altered consciousness on presentation.

Initial imaging in the form or CT head or MRI brain, depending on the severity of the clinical presentation, should be done. ICH seen on either modality with suspicion of underlying vascular abnormality should be followed up with MRA angiogram without contrast or CT angiogram. Acute management of ICH, monitoring for stability, and blood pressure control should occur in a dedicated neuroscience ICU if possible. Neurosurgical consultation for AVM management should be requested.

SEIZURES

Seizures in pregnancy may be due to eclampsia, breakthrough seizures in a patient with known epilepsy, new-onset seizure disorder unmasked during pregnancy, or other disorder associated with seizures, such as RCVS, PRES, TTP-HUS, ICH, or symptomatic seizures. Other typical causes of symptomatic seizures to be considered include toxic ingestion, withdrawal of a medication or alcohol, adverse effect of medication, acute trauma (within the past week), acute metabolic derangement, or intracranial infection.

Preeclampsia is defined as a blood pressure of greater than 140/90 mm Hg with proteinuria and occurs in 2% to 8% of all pregnancies.[1] Eclampsia is preeclampsia plus a generalized seizure without alternate cause for the seizure. Of eclamptic women, 0.6% to 3% will develop eclampsia.[1] Seizure control in eclampsia is achieved using magnesium.

Women with a preexisting seizure disorder may be at increased risk of breakthrough seizures during pregnancy because of changes in antiepileptic drug levels. Although a large trial showed no benefit to increased antiepileptic monitoring during pregnancy,[43] the pharmacokinetic changes of some antiepileptic drugs during pregnancy warrant frequent blood level monitoring, including lamotrigine, levetiracetam, oxcarbazepine, topiramate, and zonisamide.[44] Lamotrigine levels are affected by estrogen. Progesterone levels increase as the pregnancy progresses, leading to decreased lamotrigine levels, warranting increased blood level monitoring and dose increases. Other antiepileptic drug levels should be checked at least once a trimester and adjusted accordingly.[45]

New-onset seizures can occur during pregnancy in those with a predisposition for seizures because of an underlying epilepsy syndrome, mesial temporal sclerosis, history of trauma, or others. First-time seizure evaluation in a noneclamptic pregnant patient is the same as for a nonpregnant patient. A careful history to rule out previous seizures, possible secondary causes, and detailed seizure semiology is necessary. Although focal seizures and seizures arising from sleep have a greater tendency to recur, initiation of antiseizure medication is not typically initiated for those reasons alone. Initial head imaging choice will depend on the patient presentation. A patient who has failed to return to their neurologic baseline, has persistent focal neurologic deficits, has had multiple seizures acutely at time of presentation, or is in status epilepticus should get a CT head as soon as she is stabilized. A patient who has had a single seizure, is back to neurologic baseline, and is otherwise stable may be able to get an MRI brain without contrast as first-line imaging. An electroencephalogram (EEG) is warranted if there is a suspicion that the patient has failed to return to neurologic baseline because of ongoing seizures or to help assess the risk of recurrent seizures via detection of interictal epileptiform discharges. A patient with an unprovoked seizure with an abnormality on MRI or EEG that suggests an increased risk of subsequent seizure should be started on antiepileptic therapy. First-line antiepileptic therapies for pregnant women are lamotrigine and levetiracetam owing to the low risk of teratogenicity. **Tables 2** and **3** show the Food and Drug Administration (FDA) fetal risk category for common antiepileptic medications.

Finally, it is worth noting that epilepsy is not a contraindication to pregnancy. It was in the past, but data negate that historical advice.

Table 2
Antiepileptics in pregnancy: Food and Drug Administration fetus risk categories

Antiepileptic	Pregnancy Category
Carbamazepine	D
Clonazepam	D
Lacosamide	C
Lamotrigine	C
Levetiracetam	C
Topiramate	D
Valproate	D
Phenytoin	D
Phenobarbital	D
Oxcarbazepine	D
Ethosuximide	C
Everolimus	C
Felbamate	C
Gabapentin	B
Methsuximide	C
Perampanel	C
Pregabalin	C
Primidone	D
Rufinamide	C
Tiagabine	C
Zonisamide	C
Clorazepate	D
Estazolam	X
Brivaracetam	C

Definition of FDA fetal risk categories.

Category B: Animal reproduction studies have failed to demonstrate a risk to the fetus, and there are no adequate and well-controlled studies in pregnant women.

Category C: Animal reproduction studies have shown an adverse effect on the fetus, and there are no adequate and well-controlled studies in humans; however, potential benefits may warrant use of the drug in pregnant women despite potential risks.

Category D: There is positive evidence of human fetal risk based on adverse reaction data from investigational or marketing experience or studies in humans, but potential benefits may warrant use of the drug in pregnant women despite potential risks.

Category X: Studies in animals or humans have demonstrated fetal abnormalities, and/or there is positive evidence of human fetal risk based on adverse reaction data from investigational or marketing experience; the risks involved in the use of the drug in pregnant women clearly outweigh potential benefits.

STATUS EPILEPTICUS

Seizures that last 5 minutes or more or 2 or more recurrent seizures with failure to return to neurologic baseline between events meet the current definition of status epilepticus.[50] In eclamptic patients, management is with magnesium.

Management of status epilepticus involves rapid assessment and stabilization. Airway, breathing, and circulation with resuscitation and airway management as indicated should be done first. Blood glucose measurement emergently to rule out

Table 3
Antiepileptics and risk of major congenital malformation[46-493]

Antiepileptic	Rate of Major Congenital Malformation, %
Carbamazepine	5.5
Clonazepam	3, limited data
Lamotrigine	2.9 (2.3%–3.7%)
Levetiracetam	2.8 (1.7%–4.5%)
Topiramate	3.9 (1.4%–5.4%)
Valproate	10.3 (8.8%–12%)
Phenytoin	6.4 (2.8%–12.2%)
Phenobarbital	6.5 (4.2%–9.9%)
Oxcarbazepine	3.0 (1.4%–5.4%)
Gabapentin	0.7 (0.02%–3.8%)
Zonisamide	0 (0%–3.3%)

Rate of major congenital malformation (MCM) in the general population, 1.2% to 2.2%; rate of MCM in untreated epileptics, 2.8%.

Table 4
Antiepileptics used in status epilepticus with Food and Drug Administration fetus risk category

Antiepileptic	Category
Levetiracetam	C
Phenytoin	D
Valproic acid	D
Lorazepam	D
Midazolam	C
Ketamine	N
Pentobarbital	D
Phenobarbital	D
Propofol	B

Abbreviation: N, not assigned, not recommended.

Ketamine rat reproduction studies have seen hypoplasia of skeletal muscles and developmental delays.

Definition of FDA fetal risk categories.

Category B: Animal reproduction studies have failed to demonstrate a risk to the fetus, and there are no adequate and well-controlled studies in pregnant women.

Category C: Animal reproduction studies have shown an adverse effect on the fetus, and there are no adequate and well-controlled studies in humans. However, potential benefits may warrant use of the drug in pregnant women despite potential risks.

Category D: There is positive evidence of human fetal risk based on adverse reaction data from investigational or marketing experience or studies in humans, but potential benefits may warrant use of the drug in pregnant women despite potential risks.

Category X: Studies in animals or humans have demonstrated fetal abnormalities, and/or there is positive evidence of human fetal risk based on adverse reaction data from investigational or marketing experience; the risks involved in the use of the drug in pregnant women clearly outweigh potential benefits.

hypoglycemic seizures as well as for obtaining access for emergent antiepileptic medication administration should be done concomitantly if possible. Lorazepam 0.1 mg/kg or 4 mg total should be given via IV (or intraosseous [IO] if necessary) at a rate of 2 mg/min with repeat dose in 3 to 5 minutes if the patient is still seizing. Subsequent dosing with IV (or IO if necessary) levetiracetam 60 mg/kg should be infused over 15 minutes. Other first-line status epilepticus medications, such a phenytoin and valproic acid, are avoided in pregnancy because of potential teratogenicity.[51] **Table 4** shows the antiepileptic medications used in status epilepticus with their FDA fetus risk category for reference.

If no IV access is available, intramuscular (IM) midazolam 10 mg may be given.[52]

Patients who present with convulsive seizures who stop clinically seizing but fail to awaken may have transitioned to nonconvulsive status epilepticus. EEG should be performed to investigate this possibility and guide further treatment.

AUTOIMMUNE
Multiple Sclerosis

For most patients with multiple sclerosis (MS), pregnancy is a time of reduced MS activity. Disease activity may be reduced as much as 70% in the third trimester. Glucocorticoids may be used during pregnancy for disabling MS attacks. Epidural anesthesia or diazepam may be used during labor in MS patients with spasticity.[53]

Neuromyelitis Optica

Neuromyelitis optica (NMO) may be exacerbated by pregnancy and may even have onset during pregnancy. Aquaporin-4 is the target antigen in NMO and is expressed in the placenta, leading to increased risk of fetal loss. NMO treatment with azathioprine, rituximab, eculizumab, and glucocorticoids can be used in pregnancy. Severe NMO spectrum disorder during pregnancy may be treated with tocilizumab.[54]

Myasthenia Gravis

Pregnant women with myasthenia gravis generally have a good outcome, but 20% to 30% will have an exacerbation or crisis. This exacerbation or crisis typically occurs in the first trimester. Plasma exchange, IV immune globulin, and corticosteroids have a class C rating in pregnancy and are all used to treat exacerbations as they usually would for nonpregnant patients. Pyridostigmine has a class B rating in pregnancy. Weakness can occur during the second stage of labor, putting the mother at risk for protracted labor and the fetus at risk for distress. An IM dose of 1.5 mg neostigmine or 0.5 mg IV is equivalent to 60 mg of pyridostigmine and can assist through this stage of labor. Should an urgent cesarean section be required, the patient will be at greater risk for an exacerbation. If a pregnant patient with myasthenia gravis develops preeclampsia or eclampsia, magnesium should be used with significant caution, and careful observation for development of myasthenic crisis, as maternal deaths have occurred.[55] Once the infant is delivered, transient myasthenia gravis may occur in the newborn causing diffuse weakness ("floppy baby") and potentially neuromuscular respiratory weakness/failure for up to a month after delivery.[55]

RARE CAUSES OF NEUROLOGIC EMERGENCIES RELATED TO PREGNANCY
Thrombotic Thrombocytopenic Purpura

TTP presents with some or all of the classic pentad: thrombocytopenia, microangiopathic hemolytic anemia, fever, neurologic dysfunction, and renal dysfunction.

Neurologic dysfunction can have a relatively rapid or indolent course. It can present with mild encephalopathy, seizures, focal neurologic deficits, and headache. This can be associated with PRES. TTP-HUS tends to present in the second and third trimester and can be difficult to differentiate from HELLP (hemolysis, elevated liver enzymes and low platelet count) syndrome. The treatment for TTP is plasma exchange, versus the treatment for HELLP, which involves delivering the baby; therefore, ensuring the correct diagnosis rapidly is warranted.[56]

Amniotic Fluid Embolism

Amniotic fluid embolism (AFE) is rare with an incidence of 1.9 to 6.1 per 100,000 deliveries. Introduction of amniotic fluid into the maternal circulation by an unclear mechanism triggers a response similar to systemic inflammatory response syndrome. This tends to occur during labor or within 30 minutes of placental delivery. Patients may have a prodrome of agitation, anxiety, or change in mental status preceding cardiorespiratory collapse. Seizures and stroke are uncommon complications of AFE.[57,58] Management involves emergent resuscitation and stabilization of the patient. Nitric oxide or epoprostenol can be used for the pulmonary hypertension caused by AFE.[10] Extracorporeal membrane oxygenation may also be considered for refractory hypoxemia. Use of cryoprecipitate may assist in the removal of debris from amniotic fluid in the blood. If AFE does not occur during a delivery, but rather during the pregnancy, urgent delivery is recommended. AFE maternal mortality is 20%, and neonatal mortality is 20% to 60%. Of the mothers that survive AFE, 85% will have neurologic injury because of hypoxic brain injury.[10]

Metastatic Choriocarcinoma

Rarely, trophoblastic tissue will give rise to choriocarcinoma, which has a 20% incidence of metastasis to the brain. This can cause hemorrhage, invasion of cerebral blood vessels, and mass effect. If the brain is involved, there is a high likelihood that the lung is also involved, with its 80% risk of metastasis. Chemotherapy is the treatment of choice, and choriocarcinoma is very sensitive to chemotherapy with a high cure rate. There is a greater than 50% chance of cure in an isolated brain metastasis.[10] Management of high-risk lesions involves multiagent chemotherapy and may involve surgery or radiation therapy. The first-line chemotherapy regimen is EMA/CO (etoposide, methotrexate, and dactinomycin alternating with cyclophosphamide and vincristine) given on alternating weeks, although other regimens have been used.[59]

SPECIAL CIRCUMSTANCES IN PREGNANCY
Cardiac Arrest and Hypoxic Brain Injury in the Pregnant Patient

Cardiac arrest during pregnancy occurs in approximately 1/30,000 patients. Advanced cardiac life support (ACLS) is adjusted for the pregnant patient. Early airway control is recommended given reduced maternal functional residual capacity, increased oxygen consumption, and increased risk of aspiration of gastric contents owing to maternal delayed gastric emptying and decreased lower esophageal sphincter tone. During CPR, manual displacement of the uterus to the left and upward while elevating the right hip with a pillow or with the knees of a person if a pillow is not available is recommended to decompress the inferior vena cava and improve venous return to the heart. Defibrillation and medication doses used in ACLS protocols are not different for the pregnant patient. When resuscitation efforts are failing, the decision must be rapidly made to perform a cesarean section in cases whereby the fetus' gestational age is greater than 24 weeks (or the uterine size by fundus evaluation is greater than or equal to 20 weeks) to optimize neurologic outcome in the 2 patients. In fact, although this certainly will improve the viability of the fetus if performed within 5 minutes of loss of circulation, it has been shown to improve maternal viability by improving cardiac output by relieving aortocaval compression.[60,61]

If return of spontaneous circulation is achieved, then the patient should be closely monitored in the intensive care unit and placed in the left lateral decubitus position whenever possible to optimize maternal hemodynamics. Targeted temperature management has an uncertain benefit in pregnant patients. Hypothermia may add to the coagulation disturbances pregnancy already brings. During hypothermia, fetal monitoring shows decreased variability and low baseline. These issues are amplified when the patient is cooled to 32°C but less so at 36°C. For neurologic prognostication, typical neurophysiologic testing and neuroimaging should proceed as it would in a nonpregnant patient.[61]

Death by Neurologic Criteria

Pronouncing the pregnant patient dead by neurologic criteria (DNC), although exceedingly rare, presents an ethical quandary as to how to proceed for the fetus. This is particularly true if the fetus appears to be unharmed (through ultrasonic examination and cardiotocography evaluation) from the event that led to maternal DNC. If there is fetal viability and maturity to 28 to 32 weeks and beyond, the fetus would be most likely be delivered by cesarean section shortly after declaration of DNC, as the likelihood of survival is 80% at a gestational age of 28 weeks and 98% at 32 weeks.[62] However, should the fetus be less than 28 weeks in gestational age, the mother would require "somatic" or "corporeal" support to optimize chances of fetal viability. There is no mandatory lower gestational age limit set for somatic support based on the International Federation of Gynecology and Obstetrics Committee for Ethical Aspects of Human Reproduction and Women's Health.[62] Some would argue that the approach of not setting a lower limit of fetus age for which somatic support of the of the mother declared with DNC denies the mother an ability to die with dignity, desacralizes her body, and destroys her bodily integrity.[63] Others would argue that there is no reason to believe that if the mother had continued the pregnancy that she would have been opposed to continuation of corporeal support and that the fetus' rights could take precedence in these circumstances.[63] To date, there are 43 published cases since 2017 whereby corporeal support for a mother declared DNC was maintained to allow maturation to fetal viability.[63] In these cases, there was a mean of 38.3 days (range 2–107 days) of corporeal support.[62] Reports of infants delivered to these mothers resulted in children with mean APGAR scores of 7 and 8, at 1 and 5 minutes, respectively, and a mean birth weight of 1384 g (range 815–2083 g).[62] Postnatal follow-up to the age 2 years in 6 of the infants showed normal development.[62]

Maintaining corporeal support in the mother with DNC is much like supporting any patient with DNC who is donating organs while organ viability and tissue typing is being evaluated, except that the length of support is far greater. There will also need to be a perinatology physician involved in the daily care plan, continuous cardiotocography, and a readily available perinatology nurse. Although the numbers in the above paragraph show that corporeal support of DNC mothers to delivery can be successful, what is unknown is the number of unsuccessful attempts at corporeal support in pregnant DNC patients. These numbers are not reported, which is why some have called for a registry for this clinical scenario. There are predictable changes in supporting the DNC mother, and the recommendations for each are discussed.[60]

Cardiovascular

Vasomotor instability is common after DNC, and hemodynamic support is critical for maintaining adequate uteroplacental flow. The autoregulation of the uterus is also damaged, so periods of hypotension place the fetus at greater risk. Support should include maintaining the mother in the left lateral recumbent position; volume expansion with a combination of crystalloid and colloid solutions; and inotropic plus vasopressor support, if necessary, in order to maintain adequate maternal perfusion based on a minimum MAP of 65 but adjusted higher should fetal heart rate monitoring indicate a need. Dobutamine and norepinephrine is the combination more commonly used. Low-dose vasopressin has also been used, but concern regarding the effect of uterine vasoconstriction that has been demonstrated in nonpregnant patients has limited its use to treatment of diabetes insipidus.[60]

Pulmonary

The goals of the ongoing mechanical ventilatory support should be to allow for a CO_2 diffusion gradient from the fetus to mother; therefore, it is recommended to maintain CO_2 between 30 and 35. The normal Pao_2 during pregnancy is 105 mm Hg and should be considered when providing oxygen support.[60]

Endocrine

Panhypopituitarism is common. Central diabetes insipidus is seen in greater than 70% of cases, and fluid status must be maintained. Vasopressin in intermittent low doses can be used. Adrenal insufficiency may also occur, but before starting corticosteroids, maternal cortisol levels should be measured. Minimizing fetal exposure to steroids is ideal in these cases, as there is a small increase in cleft lip with or without cleft palate.[64] Thyroid function testing should also be measured, and levothyroxine only provided if indicated by the results of the thyroid panel.[60]

Temperature regulation

Given the loss of hypothalamic function in these mothers with DNC, poikilothermia is often described. Passive warming to more than 36°C is ideal, and use of acetaminophen and passive cooling to less than 38.5°C is recommended.[60]

Nutritional support

Given the increased nutritional needs of pregnancy, the DNC mother requires more support, with typically a 15% increase, given the additional energy expenditures. Daily weights and indirect calorimetry intermittently help define the caloric goals. Protein needs are greater than the typical 0.8 g/kg/d with an additional 1.3, 6.1, and 10.7 g/d needed in the first, second, and third trimesters, respectively. In addition, essential fatty acids should be 20% to 25% of the protein calories, and trace elements will all need to be increased beyond what is in standard tube feeding formulas.[60]

Infections

The mother with DNC is at high risk for urinary tract infections and ventilator-associated pneumonias. The infections are typically associated with gram-negative and gram-positive organisms, but fungal pathogens have also been supported, particularly given that daily steroids are given for panhypopituitarism. Choice of antibiotics will depend on the safety profile in pregnancy.[60]

SUMMARY

Neurologic emergencies in pregnant patients require special considerations for early acute resuscitative care, diagnostic evaluations, treatment regimens, and ethics. In these settings, the care of both the mother and the fetus are to be considered and balanced as much as possible. This article has provided a comprehensive review of the issues that occur in pregnant patients as well as of how to support a mother with DNC, so that her fetus can grow to optimum viability. There is still much more to understand on how to best manage the pregnant patient as the science and fields of acute care neurology and neurocritical care are advanced.

CLINICS CARE POINTS

- The most common presenting neurologic symptom in pregnancy is headache.
- Most transient neurologic deficits in pregnancy are due to migraine with aura.
- If a pregnant patient has a new headache and preeclampsia is ruled out using its well-established clinical criteria, urgent neuroimaging is warranted.
- CT head without contrast, using a low radiation technique (1.0–10.0 mGy), is below the threshold (>50.0 mGy) for adverse effects to the fetus.
- MRI head without contrast is the preferred neuroimaging modality in pregnancy, but can be limited by its urgent availability.
- Two percent of all strokes in pregnancy are due to cerebral venous sinus thrombosis.
- IV heparin drip should be started immediately upon diagnosis of cerebral venous sinus thrombosis and transitioned to low-molecular-weight heparin, to continue until at least 6 weeks after delivery.
- Although pregnant patients were excluded from the tissue plasminogen activator trials in acute ischemic strokes, current expert opinion is to treat with IV tissue plasminogen activator and/or thrombectomy, if indicated, for those with moderate to severe deficits; the potential benefit outweighs the risk.
- Thrombectomy in acute ischemic stroke should be done with minimal fluoroscopy and with fetal shielding.
- Large-vessel strokes with malignant cerebral edema should be considered for early hemicraniectomy.
- Mannitol is a pregnancy category C risk, as it decreases amniotic fluid volumes.
- Hypertonic saline has no pregnancy category risk assigned because of a lack of data but has been used for life-saving measures in cerebral edema without effects to the fetus.
- Posterior reversible encephalopathy syndrome (PRES) in pregnancy is most often a manifestation of eclampsia.
- Although PRES is often associated with significantly elevated blood pressures in the systolic range of 180 to 220+ mm Hg, given the relative hypotension in pregnancy, systolic blood pressures in the range of 140 mm Hg can lead to PRES.
- Nontraumatic subarachnoid hemorrhage is commonly seen in the third trimester, and the risk is 5 times greater during pregnancy.
- New-onset seizures in pregnancy most commonly occur with eclampsia, but in the noneclamptic patient, the workup should proceed as it would for the nonpregnant patient with metabolic, infectious, neuroimaging, and electroencephalogram evaluations.
- Status epilepticus in pregnancy can be safely managed with lorazepam and levetiracetam, but phenytoin and valproic acid are avoided because of potential teratogenicity.

- Multiple sclerosis disease activity is reduced throughout pregnancy.
- Aquaporin-4 is the target antigen in neuromyelitis optica and is expressed in the placenta, leading to increased risk of fetal loss.
- Of pregnant patients with myasthenia gravis, 20% to 30% will have an exacerbation or crisis.
- Pyridostigmine has a pregnancy category B risk and is useful during the second stage of labor, whereby weakness is most likely to occur in the patient with myasthenia gravis.
- Caution should be taken in patients with myasthenia gravis who develop preeclampsia/eclampsia when using magnesium, as this can precipitate an exacerbation.
- If a pregnant patient sustains such a devastating neurologic injury that death by neurologic criteria is pronounced, and the fetus is less than 28 weeks in gestational age, corporeal support can be provided successfully in order for fetal maturation to 28 to 32 weeks to occur.

DISCLOSURE

The authors have nothing to disclose.

REFERENCES

1. Edlow JA, Caplan LR, O'Brien K, et al. Diagnosis of acute neurological emergencies in pregnant and post-partum women. Lancet Neurol 2013;12(2):175–85.
2. Sibai B, Dekker G, Kupferminc M. Pre-eclampsia. Lancet 2005;365(9461): 785–99. https://doi.org/10.1016/s0140-6736(05)17987-2.
3. van Alebeek ME, de Heus R, Tuladhar AM, et al. Pregnancy and ischemic stroke: a practical guide to management. Curr Opin Neurol 2018;3(1):44–51.
4. James AH. Venous thromboembolism in pregnancy. Arterioscler Thromb Vasc Biol 2009;29:326–31.
5. Thornburg KL, Jacobson S-L, Giraud GD, et al. Hemodynamic changes in pregnancy. Semin Perinatol 2000;24(1):11–4.
6. Heit JA, Kobbervig CE, James AH, et al. Trends in the incidence of venous thromboembolism during pregnancy or postpartum: a 30-year population-based study. Ann Intern Med 2005;143:697–706.
7. Saposnik G, Barinagarrementeria F, Brown RD, et al. Diagnosis and Management of Cerebral Venous Thrombosis. A Statement for Healthcare Professionals from the American Heart Association/American Stroke Association. Stroke 2011;42: 1158–92.
8. Lu A, Shen PY, Dahlin BC, et al. Cerebral venous thrombosis and infarct: Review of imaging manifestations. Appl Radiol 2016;45(3):9–17.
9. ACOG Committee Opinion – Interim Update. Number 723. e210, October 2017, Vol 130, No 4
10. Frontera J, Ahmed W. Neurocritical Care Complications of Pregnancy and Puerperum. J Crit Care 2014;29:1069–81.
11. Vilela P, Rowley HA. Brain ischemia: CT and MRI techniques in acute ischemic stroke. Eur J Radiol 2017;96:162–72.
12. Skeik N, Porten B, Kadkhodayan Y, et al. Postpartum reversible cerebral vasoconstriction syndrome: Review and analysis of the current data. Vasc Med 2015;20(3):256–65.
13. Anand P, Lua KHV, Chung DY, et al. Posterior reversible encephalopathy syndrome in patients with coronavirus disease 2019: two cases and a review of the literature. J Stroke Cerebrovasc Dis 2020;29(11):1–7.

14. Habibabadi JM, Saadatnia M, Tabrizi N. Seizure in cerebral venous and sinus thrombosis. Epilepsia Open 2018;3(3):316–22.

15. Sells CM, Feske SK. Stroke in Pregnancy. Semin Neurol 2017;37:669–78.

16. Sadro CT, Dubinsky TJ. CT in pregnancy: risks and benefits. Applied Radiology; 2013. p. 6–16.

17. Powers WJ, Rabinstein AA, Ackerson T, et al. Guidelines for the Early Management of Patients With Acute Ischemic Stroke: 2019 Update to the 2018 Guidelines for the Early Management of Acute Ischemic Stroke: A Guideline for Healthcare Professionals From the American Heart Association/American Stroke Association. Stroke 2019;50:e344–418.

18. Cauldwell M, Rudd A, Nelson-Piercy C. Management of stroke and pregnancy. Eur Stroke J 2018;3(3):227–36.

19. Leffert LR, Clancy CR, Bateman BT, et al. Treatment patterns and short-term outcomes in ischemic stroke in pregnancy or postpartum period. Am J Obstet Gynecol 2016;214(6):723.e1–11.

20. Kular S, Ram R, Balian V, et al. Mechanical thrombectomy for acute stroke in pregnancy. Neuroradiol J 2020;33(2):134–9.

21. Bhogal P, Aguilar M, AlMatter M, et al. Mechanical thrombectomy in pregnancy: report of 2 cases and review of the literature. Intervent Neurol 2017;6:49–56.

22. Handlogten K, Sharpe EE, Brost BC, et al. Dexmedetomidine and Mannitol for Awake Craniotomy in a Pregnant Patient. Anesth Analg 2015;120(5):1099–103.

23. Mogos MF, Piano MR, McFarlin BL, et al. Heart failure in pregnant women: a concern across the pregnancy continuum. Circ Heart Fail 2018;11(1):e004005.

24. Singhal AB. Bernstein RA Postpartum angiopathy and other cerebral vasoconstriction syndromes. Neurocrit Care 2005;3(1):91.

25. Fugate JE, Ameriso SF, Ortiz G, et al. Rabinstein AA Variable presentations of postpartum angiopathy. Stroke 2012;43(3):670–6.

26. Singhal AB. Postpartum angiopathy with reversible posterior leukoencephalopathy. Arch Neurol 2004;61(3):411.

27. Godasi R, Pang G, Chauhan S, et al. Primary Central Nervous System Vasculitis. In: StatPearls. Treasure Island (FL): StatPearls Publishing; 2020.

28. Rosenbloom MH, Singhal AB. CT angiography and diffusion-perfusion MR imaging in a patient with ipsilateral reversible cerebral vasoconstriction after carotid endarterectomy. AJNR Am J Neuroradiol 2007;28(5):920.

29. Datar S, Singh T, Rabinstein AA, et al. Long-term risk of seizures and epilepsy in patients with posterior reversible encephalopathy syndrome. Epilepsia 2015; 56(4):564–8.

30. Qubty W, Irwin SL, Fox CK. Review on the diagnosis and treatment of reversible cerebral vasoconstriction syndrome in children and adolescents. Semin Neurol 2020;40(3):294–302.

31. Travers CP, Clark RH, Spitzer AR, et al. Exposure to any antenatal corticosteroids and outcomes in preterm infants by gestational age: prospective cohort study. BMJ 2017;j1039. https://doi.org/10.1136/bmj.j1039.

32. Strandgaard S, Paulson OB. Cerebral autoregulation. Stroke 1984;15(3):413.

33. Fugate JE, Claassen DO, Cloft HJ, et al. Posterior reversible encephalopathy syndrome: associated clinical and radiologic findings. Mayo Clin Proc 2010; 85(5):427.

34. Tinawi M. Hypertension in pregnancy. Arch Intern Med Res 2020;3(1):010–7.

35. Toossi S, Moheet A. Intracerebral hemorrhage in women: a review with special attention to pregnancy and the post-partum period. Neurocrit Care 2019;31: 390–8.

36. Akers A, Al-Shahi Salman R, A Awad I, et al. Synopsis of guidelines for the clinical management of cerebral cavernous malformations: consensus recommendations based on systematic literature review by the angioma alliance scientific advisory board clinical experts panel. Neurosurgery 2017;80(5):665–80.

37. Scimone C, Bramanti P, Alafaci C, et al. Update on novel ccm gene mutations in patients with cerebral cavernous malformations. J Mol Neurosci 2016;61(2): 189–98.

38. Diringer MN, Bleck TP, Hempill JC, et al. Critical care management of patients following aneurysmal subarachnoid hemorrhage: recommendations from the Neurocritical Care Society's multidisciplinary consensus conference. Neurocrit Care 2011;15:211–40.

39. Connolly EA, Rabinstein AA, Carhuapoma JR, et al. Guidelines for the management of aneurysmal subarachnoid hemorrhage: a guideline for healthcare professionals from the American Heart Association/American Stroke Association. Stroke 2012;43:1711–37.

40. Liu XJ, Wang S, Zhao YL, et al. Risk of cerebral arteriovenous malformation rupture during pregnancy and puerperium. Neurology 2014;82(20):1798.

41. Dias MS, Sekhar LN. Intracranial hemorrhage from aneurysms and arteriovenous malformations during pregnancy and the puerperium. Neurosurgery 1990;27(6): 855–65.

42. Porras JL, Yang W, Philadelphia E, et al. Hemorrhage risk of brain arteriovenous malformations during pregnancy and puerperium in a North American Cohort. Stroke 2017;48(6):1507–13.

43. Thangaratinam S, Marlin N, Newton S, et al. AntiEpileptic drug Monitoring in PREgnancy (EMPiRE): a double-blind randomised trial on effectiveness and acceptability of monitoring strategies. Health Technol Assess 2018 May;22(23): 1–152.

44. Arfman IJ, Wammes-van der Heijden EA, ter Horst PGJ, et al. Therapeutic drug monitoring of antiepileptic drugs in women with epilepsy before, during, and after pregnancy. Clin Pharmacokinet 2020;59:427–45.

45. Pennel PB, Peng L, Newport DJ, et al. Lamotrigine in pregnancy: clearance, therapeutic drug monitoring, and seizure frequency. Neurology 2008;70:2130–6.

46. Babtain FA. Management of women with epilepsy. Practical issues faced when dealing with women with epilepsy. *Neurosciences* (Riyadh) 2012;17(2):115–20.

47. Vossler DG, Weingarten M, Gidal BE, et al. Summary of Antiepileptic Drugs Available in the United States of America: working toward a world without epilepsy. Epilepsy Currents 2018;18(4 Suppl 1):1–26.

48. Vossler D. Comparative risk of major congenital malformations with 8 different antiepileptic drugs: a prospective cohort study of the EURAP registry. Epilepsy Currents 2019;19:83–5.

49. Tomson T, Batino D, Bonizzoni E, et al. Comparative risk of major congenital malformations with eight different antiepileptic drugs: a prospective cohort study of the EURAP registry. Lancet Neurol 2018;17:530–8.

50. Trinka E, Cock H, Hesdorffer D, et al. A definition and classification of status epilepticus–Report of the ILAE Task Force on Classification of Status Epilepticus. Epilepsia 2015;56(10):1515.

51. Brophy GM, Bell R, Claassen J, et al. Neurocritical Care Society Status Epilepticus Guideline Writing Committee. Guidelines for the evaluation and management of status epilepticus. Neurocrit Care 2012;17(1):3–23.

52. Silbergleit R, Durkalski V, Lowenstein D, et al, NETT Investigators. Intramuscular versus intravenous therapy for prehospital status epilepticus. N Engl J Med 2012; 366(7):591–600.
53. Dobson R, Dassan P, Roberts M, et al. UK consensus on pregnancy in multiple sclerosis: 'Association of British Neurologists' guidelines. Pract Neurol 2019;19: 106–14.
54. Mao-Draayer Y, Thiel S, Mills EA, et al. Neuromyelitis optica spectrum disorders and pregnancy: therapeutic considerations. Nat Rev Neurol 2020;16:154–70.
55. Cialfaloni E, Massey J. The management of myasthenia gravis in pregnancy. Semin Neurol 2004;24:95–100.
56. McMinn JR, George JN. Evaluation of women with clinically suspected thrombotic thrombocytopenic purpura-hemolytic uremic syndrome during pregnancy. J Clin Apher 2001;16(4):202.
57. Woo YS, Hong SC, Park SM, et al. Ischemic stroke related to an amniotic fluid embolism during labor. J Clin Neurosci 2015;22(4):767.
58. Price TM, Baker VV, Cefalo RC. Amniotic fluid embolism. Three case reports with a review of the literature. Obstet Gynecol Surv 1985;40(7):462.
59. Abu-Rustum NR, Yashar CM, Bean S, et al. Gestational Trophoblastic Neoplasia, Version 2. 2019, NCCN Clinical Practice Guidelines in Oncology. J Natl Compr Cancer Netw 2019;17(11):1374–91.
60. Mallampalli A, Guy E. Cardiac arrest in pregnancy and somatic support after brain death. Crit Care Med 2005;33(10S):S325–31.
61. Zelop C, Einav S, Mhyre JM, et al. Cardiac arrest during pregnancy: ongoing clinical conundrum. Am J Obstet Gynecol 2018;219:52–61.
62. Lewis A, Varelas P, Greer D, et al. Pregnancy and brain death: lack of guidance in US Hospital Policies. Am J Perinatology 2016;33:1382–7.
63. Cartolovni A, Dubravko H. Guidelines for the management of the social and ethical challenges in brain death during pregnancy. Int J Gynecol Obstet 2019; 146:149–56.
64. Bandoli G, Palmsten K, Forbess Smith CJ, et al. A review of systemic corticosteroid use in pregnancy and the risk of select pregnancy and birth outcomes. Rheum Dis Clin North Am 2017;43(3):489–502.

Neurologic Emergencies during the Coronavirus Disease 2019 Pandemic

Julie G. Shulman, MD[a],*, Thomas Ford, MD[a],
Anna M. Cervantes-Arslanian, MD[a,b,c]

KEYWORDS

- COVID-19 • Neurologic emergencies • Cerebrovascular disease • Thrombolysis
- Seizure

KEY POINTS

- Institutions should create protocols for managing neurologic emergencies during the pandemic that allow for rapid and thorough evaluation of patients while also minimizing viral exposure to other patients and staff.
- Less than 5% of patients with coronavirus disease 2019 will have cerebrovascular complications and these typically occur in patients who are critically ill.
- Persons with epilepsy may face significant challenges with regards to care and prevention of seizures, although there does not seem to be an increase in emergency department presentations with seizure.
- Seizure is a rare complication of coronavirus disease 2019 with antiepileptic drug selection impacted by concurrent organ failure, drug–drug interactions with coronavirus disease 2019 therapies, and ongoing drug shortages.

As the coronavirus disease 2019 (COVID-19) pandemic continues, the scientific community is working diligently to rapidly expand knowledge of the disease and disseminate this knowledge worldwide. As of January 2021, there have been more than 90,000 scientific publications relating to COVID-19.[1] The rapid expansion of data on this topic has led to novel means of interpretation and dissemination, including expedited reviews for publication in peer-reviewed journals, open source platforms for review of article preprints, widespread use of social media, and protocol sharing among academic institutions.[2] The literature regarding neurologic features of COVID-19 specifically has been primarily in the form of case reports and a few case series, limiting

[a] Department of Neurology, Boston University School of Medicine, 72 East Concord Street, Suite C3, Boston, MA 02118, USA; [b] Department of Neurosurgery, Boston University School of Medicine, 725 Albany St, Suite 7C, Boston, MA 02118, USA; [c] Department of Medicine (Infectious Diseases), Boston University School of Medicine, 801 Massachusetts Avenue, Crosstown, 2nd floor, Boston MA 02118, USA
* Corresponding author.
E-mail address: Julie.Shulman@bmc.org

Neurol Clin 39 (2021) 671–687
https://doi.org/10.1016/j.ncl.2021.02.007
0733-8619/21/© 2021 Elsevier Inc. All rights reserved.

the generalizability of this information owing to the inherent heterogeneity of these studies and patients.[3] Here, we review what has thus far been published about the intersection of COVID-19 and neurology with particular attention to cerebrovascular disease and seizure. Considerations in managing the acute presentations of these conditions in the context of the pandemic can serve as a model for management of other neurologic emergencies.

CONSIDERATIONS FOR MANAGING ACUTE STROKE DURING THE PANDEMIC
Initial Evaluation

Given the rapid sequence of events that unfold upon the activation of a stroke alert, it is critical that hospitals have standardized measures in place to protect staff from potential exposure when patients are known or suspected to be infected with severe acute respiratory syndrome novel coronavirus 2(SARS-CoV-2). Many groups have proposed adjustments to institutional stroke protocols to continue to offer timely stroke care while preserving personal protective equipment (PPE) and limiting provider exposure.[4–6] For regions with high community prevalence of COVID-19, it is reasonable to consider all patients undergoing stroke alerts to be persons under investigation. A surgical mask should be placed on the patient and 1 member of the stroke team should be designated to don PPE and enter the patient's room for the evaluation. This provider, who is charged with interviewing the patient and performing the initial examination, is then able to communicate with other members of the team (either by phone or tablet computer already placed within the room) to facilitate joint decision-making on eligibility for acute intervention. Although it is common practice at many institutions for the stroke team to accompany patients to neuroimaging studies, it is recommended that, in the case of patients with suspected or confirmed COVID-19, the initial evaluator remain in the patient's room with PPE donned to limit PPE use and accidental exposure while doffing. Upon the patient's return to their room, further examination by the designated team member can be used to guide decision-making on thrombolysis and mechanical thrombectomy.

Mechanical Thrombectomy

Unfortunately, a number of centers have seen significant delays in the delivery of mechanical thrombectomy during the pandemic, particularly for those patients arriving from another facility.[7,8] As a result, measures that simultaneously conserve PPE and maintain provider safety while still providing timely interventional therapy during the ongoing pandemic are necessary. In a recent consensus statement, the Society of Vascular and Interventional Neurology outlined several recommendations on the periprocedural management of patients who are deemed candidates for mechanical thrombectomy.[9] Before mechanical thrombectomy, it is recommended that all patients undergo screening (and testing if feasible) for COVID-19 and be placed in negative-pressure isolation if warranted. The Society of Vascular and Interventional Neurology also recommends that the number of involved personnel be limited and endotracheal intubation be avoided if possible to conserve ventilator capacity and decrease the risk of ventilator-associated injury in patients who may be managed with conscious sedation. For those requiring intubation, centers have adapted techniques (such as the use of negative-pressure rooms and barrier enclosure) to minimize the circulation of respiratory droplets.[10,11] After completion of the procedure, the Society of Vascular and Interventional Neurology recommends that initial neurologic and puncture site evaluations take place in the interventional suite while the patient awaits bed placement elsewhere in the hospital to limit donning and doffing of PPE.

Postacute Stroke Care

For acute ischemic stroke patients not meeting criteria for intervention with intravenous (IV) tissue plasminogen activator (tPA) or mechanical thrombectomy, priorities generally shift to postevent monitoring for clinical progression, as well as workup of potential etiologies and initiation of secondary prevention measures. Some institutions have moved toward the use of video evaluation by nursing staff and/or the stroke team to decrease PPE use and limit provider exposure, as well as deferring diagnostic testing that is not thought to impact inpatient management.[4] An example of a modified approach to monitoring poststroke patients who do not undergo thrombolysis or mechanical thrombectomy is shown in **Fig. 1**.

For patients undergoing acute intervention with IV tPA and/or mechanical thrombectomy, postintervention monitoring before the pandemic was largely centered around frequent examination by both bedside nursing and members of the stroke team.[12] A recent study (albeit one conducted before the pandemic) evaluated the safety of a low-intensity monitoring protocol for patients meeting a predefined threshold for low risk for neurologic decompensation and found that selected patients who underwent less frequent neurologic and vital sign checks in the 24 hours after the administration of IV tPA did not see an increased incidence of clinical worsening requiring transfer to an intensive care unit.[13] Similarly, investigations questioning the usefulness of routine surveillance neuroimaging in otherwise stable postintervention patients have called into question their necessity.[14,15] These findings have been extrapolated to inform policy about post-thrombolysis and post-thrombectomy care in the COVID-19 pandemic, when intensive care unit beds have been in short supply and frequent evaluations by providers increase the risk of exposure.[4,16,17] Examples of this process of risk stratification and disposition decision-making are shown in **Figs. 2 and 3**.

Impact on Stroke-Related Outcomes

Hospitals across the world have reported significant reductions in admissions for all types of stroke patients during the pandemic, with the most impact usually occurring during times of local government restrictions on activities and in patients with a transient ischemic attack or minor stroke. Specifically, this phenomenon has been reported in the United States,[18–22] Canada,[23] China,[24] Spain,[25] Amsterdam,[26] Brazil,[27] Bangladesh,[28]

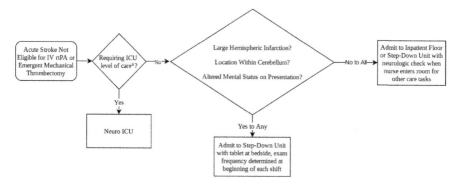

Fig. 1. Neurologic monitoring frequency in patients not receiving IV tPA or emergent mechanical thrombectomy. [a]Indications including (but not limited to) vasoactive medications, insulin drip for hyperglycemia, need for mechanical ventilation. ICU, intensive care unit. (*Adapted from* Optimization of Resources and Modifications in Acute Ischemic Stroke Care in Response to the Global COVID-19 Pandemic. J Stroke Cerebrovas Dis 2020 Aug;29(8):104980, with permission.)

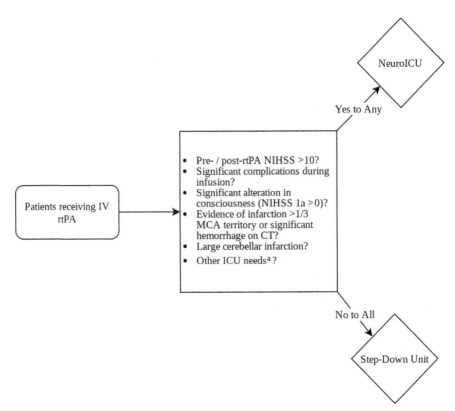

Fig. 2. Disposition determination algorithm after the administration of IV tPA. [a]Indications including (but not limited to) vasoactive medications, insulin drip for hyperglycemia, need for mechanical ventilation. CT, computed tomography; ICU, intensive care unit; MCA, middle cerebral artery; NIHSS, National Institutes of Health Stroke Scale. (*Adapted from* Optimization of Resources and Modifications in Acute Ischemic Stroke Care in Response to the Global COVID-19 Pandemic. J Stroke Cerebrovas Dis 2020 Aug;29(8):104980, with permission.)

Singapore,[29] and Norway,[30] among others. These data suggest that a large number of patients with symptoms of ischemic stroke chose not to seek medical care, a decision that, in many cases, could have a significant impact on their long-term functional status. In addition to a decrease in acute stroke presentations, delays in hospital arrival after symptom onset have been reported for those patients who do seek care,[21] likely owing to the fear of exposure to COVID-19 in a hospital setting. Upon arrival to the emergency department (ED), patients met further delays in arrival time to computed tomography scan,[21] door-to-needle time for IV tPA,[31] and door-to-groin time for mechanical thrombectomy.[8] These in-hospital delays are suspected to be due to the need for donning of PPE and sanitization procedures between patients. Delays in stroke treatment have been shown to significantly increase the risk of poor functional outcomes.[32]

CORONAVIRUS DISEASE 19–ASSOCIATED CEREBROVASCULAR DISEASE
Epidemiology

Infection with SARS-CoV-2 has been associated with a myriad of neurologic complications (**Table 1**) and the presence of neurologic symptoms seem to be quite

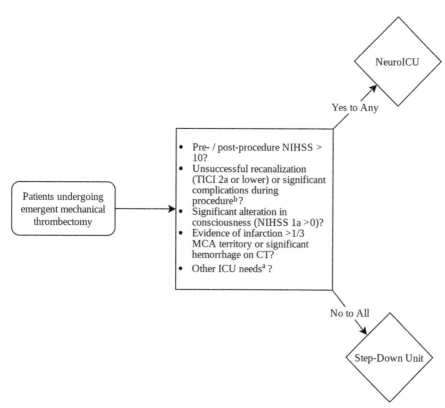

Fig. 3. Disposition determination algorithm after emergent mechanical thrombectomy. [a] Indications including (but not limited to) vasoactive medications, insulin drip for hyperglycemia, need for mechanical ventilation. [b] including (but not limited to) dissection, hemodynamic instability, and respiratory decompensation requiring intubation. CT, computed tomography; ICU, intensive care unit; MCA, middle cerebral artery; NIHSS, National Institutes of Health Stroke Scale; TICI, thrombolysis in cerebral infarction. (*Adapted from* Optimization of Resources and Modifications in Acute Ischemic Stroke Care in Response to the Global COVID-19 Pandemic. J Stroke Cerebrovas Dis 2020 Aug;29(8):104980, with permission.)

common, occurring in up to 84% of those with critical illness.[33] The majority of acute cerebrovascular disease associated with COVID-19 infection is acute ischemic stroke, but there have been reports of intracerebral hemorrhage,[34] venous sinus thrombosis,[35] posterior reversible encephalopathy syndrome (PRES),[36] reversible cerebral vasoconstriction syndrome,[37] and endotheliitis without parenchymal infarction.[38]

Ischemic stroke has been reported in 1% to 5% of patients hospitalized with COVID-19, with the higher end of that range coming from very early reports out of Wuhan, China, in predominantly critically ill patients.[39–45] Although nonspecific neurologic symptoms (such as headache, dizziness, and fatigue) are frequently reported early in the course of infection,[3] there is a suggestion that cerebrovascular disease tends to occur an average of 10 days (range, 0–33 days) after the onset of respiratory illness.[39] Most studies report that COVID-19–associated cerebrovascular disease occurs in predominantly male patients who are more than 60 years of age and have known vascular risk factors.[40,41,43–45] However, several studies reported out of New

Table 1
Neurologic complications of COVID-19

Acute Complications	Parainfectious and Postinfectious Complications
Encephalopathy	Acute disseminated encephalomyelitis
Myalgias	Acute necrotizing hemorrhagic encephalopathy
Anosmia/dysgeusia	Steroid responsive (autoimmune) encephalopathy
Headache	Myositis
Cerebrovascular complications	Critical illness neuromyopathy
Seizures	Guillain-Barre syndrome
Meningoencephalitis	Transverse myelitis
Cranial and peripheral neuropathies	Myalgic encephalomyelitis, with or without dysautonomia
Myoclonus	Sudden sensorineural hearing loss
Movement disorders	Unknown late neurologic complications
Psychosis	

York City[42,46] found strokes, particularly large vessel occlusion (LVO) strokes, occurring in younger patients. The majority of strokes reported are attributed to cardioembolism, many considered cryptogenic.[43–47] In the United States, cerebrovascular disease seems to be a complication of COVID-19 seen more commonly in racial minorities (Blacks and Hispanics),[42–44] but this may be due to more data coming from larger urban hospitals and the disproportionate effect COVID-19 has had on minority communities overall.

The mortality of ischemic stroke in COVID-19 is high (25%–44%),[40–45] leading to some speculation that stroke is predominantly associated with preexisting critical illness. Patients admitted with COVID-19 and neurologic disease have been found to have a higher in-hospital mortality (37.5% vs 4.3%) and greater disability at discharge (modified Rankin Scale of 5 vs 2) compared with patients admitted with the same neurologic diagnoses without COVID-19.[48] Similarly, when patients with COVID-19–associated ischemic stroke were compared with propensity score matched patients with stroke alone, they were found to have greater stroke severity (National Institutes of Health Stroke Scale 10 vs 6), higher risk for severe disability (modified Rankin Scale 4 vs 2; $P<.001$), and higher mortality (odds ratio, 4.3).[49] These findings suggest that COVID-19–associated cerebrovascular disease is more severe with worse functional outcomes and higher mortality than non-COVID-19–associated cerebrovascular disease.

Intracerebral hemorrhage occurs less commonly in patients with COVID-19 than acute ischemic stroke. Several reports in the spring in the United States noted that hemorrhage occurred predominantly in hospitalized patients on anticoagulation, often prescribed for elevated D-dimer levels.[34,44,50,51] Other risk factors associated with intracerebral hemorrhage include a prolonged international normalized ratio and partial thromboplastin time independent of anticoagulation use, thrombocytopenia, older age, non-White race, and mechanical ventilation.[34,50,51] Patients with COVID-19 and intracerebral hemorrhage experienced very high in-hospital mortality, up to 84.6% in 1 center.[51]

Cerebral venous sinus thromboses have been infrequently reported despite an abundance of evidence reporting deep vein thromboses elsewhere. Unlike other cerebrovascular complications, cerebral venous sinus thromboses seems to occur more often in females, with a wide age range reported. This finding is similar to patterns seen in non–COVID-associated cerebral venous sinus thromboses. It seems that cerebral venous sinus thromboses associated with COVID-19 may occur at the same time as typical respiratory or gastrointestinal symptoms, but may also occur in a delayed fashion, up to weeks after initial infection.[35]

Thirteen cases of PRES in the setting of COVID-19 have been reported as of June 30, 2020.[36] Unlike the majority of patients with PRES outside of COVID-19, these patients had only modest fluctuations in blood pressure. Risk factors for COVID-19–associated PRES include an underlying infection or immunomodulatory agents with endothelial effects. In general, as with other associated etiologies, the neurologic prognosis for COVID-19–associated PRES is favorable.[36]

Pathophysiology

Several mechanisms may lead to ischemic stroke in patients with COVID-19 (**Box 1**). One of the more widely accepted hypotheses is that SARS-CoV-2 causes damage to endothelial cells, which leads to activation of inflammatory and thrombotic pathways, microvascular and macrovascular injury, and ultimately coagulopathy similar to that seen in sepsis, characterized by elevated fibrinogen, partial thromboplastin time, D-dimer, and sometimes thrombocytopenia.[3,39] Some studies have also noted a high prevalence of antiphospholipid antibodies[52,53] in critically ill patients with COVID-19. SARS-CoV-2 can also trigger a hyperinflammatory state and cytokine storm similar to that which occurs in hemophagocytic lymphohistiocytosis.[54,55] Cellular entry of SARS-CoV-2 via the angiotensin-converting enzyme 2 receptor leads to the downregulation of receptors with consequent overactivation of the classic renin–angiotensin system axis causing vasoconstriction and a prothrombotic state.[56] Other investigators have suggested a possible direct endothelial invasion and replication within the arterial wall,[57] a process previously described in varicella zoster virus.[58] Finally, the inherent increased risk of stroke in all critically ill patients can also apply to patients with COVID-19, with potential mechanisms including destabilization of atherosclerotic plaque, triggering of atrial fibrillation, or increasing thrombus formation in conditions of hypoxia.[3]

Acute Stroke Treatment for Coronavirus Disease 19–Associated Stroke

In light of the finding that patients with COVID-19 are at risk of mixed hematologic complications,[59–61] the efficacy and safety of administration of IV tPA in this subset of acute ischemic stroke patients has been a topic of debate. Although the efficacy of thrombolysis outside of the context of the COVID-19 pandemic in decreasing

---

Box 1
Mechanisms of stroke in COVID-19

- Exacerbation of underlying risk factors
- Viral mediated hematologic derangement/hypercoagulable state
- Effects on the renin–angiotensin system
- Hyperinflammatory condition (cytokine storm)
- Complication of COVID treatments
- General critical illness, hypoxia, hypotension
- Myocarditis, stress cardiomyopathy
- Atrial fibrillation
- Endotheliitis/vasculitis

long-term disability from acute ischemic stroke has been demonstrated clearly,[62,63] there are limited data that address whether this specific patient population is at an increased risk of clinically significant hemorrhagic transformation compared with the general population, thereby altering the risk:benefit relationship. Data on this topic are limited in quality and provide mixed results. One review found that 10.3% of patients with COVID-19 (3/29) receiving IV tPA had clinically significant hemorrhagic transformation,[64] although another did not report any instances (0/13).[65] In the absence of a true consensus regarding the risk of symptomatic hemorrhage in patients with COVID-19 with suspected acute ischemic stroke, the decision to administer tPA is provider-dependent and should be made with consideration of non–COVID-specific contraindications to thrombolysis and other patient-specific factors.

In addition to increased severity of stroke, presentation with LVO stroke has been observed in patients infected with COVID-19.[42,64,66,67] Although emergent mechanical thrombectomy in a patient with confirmed COVID-19 is feasible[11] with appropriate modifications as described elsewhere in this article,[9] the limited data available thus far have unfortunately shown poor outcomes with increased mortality in patients with LVO stroke and COVID-19 compared with LVO stroke alone.[68,69] Specifically, there have been reports of increased procedural complications including clot fragmentation, downstream emboli, and distal emboli to a new vascular territory.[70] An increase in postprocedural complications, including early cerebral reocclusion[69] and deep venous thrombosis and/or pulmonary emboli,[68] has also been reported. Despite these risks, mechanical thrombectomy is recommended in patients with COVID-19 and LVO stroke, with appropriate precautions.

CONSIDERATIONS FOR MANAGING EPILEPSY DURING THE PANDEMIC

Like many chronic illnesses, medical care for persons with epilepsy (PWE) has been impacted by the pandemic. With the shutdowns seen in many countries, there has been a dramatic reduction in the availability of outpatient care such as visits with a neurologist/epileptologist and electroencephalograms (EEGs). Even when in-person visits have been available, many patients chose to defer medical care owing to the fear of viral exposure in the clinic. The advent of widely available telehealth has improved access to care but cannot entirely replicate an in-person evaluation or EEG monitoring. With overcrowding and concerns about infection control, many hospitals have canceled elective admissions and surgeries, delaying care for those awaiting characterization of epileptic spells in epilepsy monitoring units or epilepsy surgery.

The American Epilepsy Society has reported survey data of their membership indicating that 10% of PWE have noted worsening in seizure frequency unrelated to COVID-19 infection during the pandemic, with increased stress, sleep deprivation, and decreased access to medical care and pharmacies cited as potential contributors.[71] This phenomenon has been seen in previous coronavirus outbreaks as well. During the 2003 SARS epidemic in Taiwan, 1 epilepsy center noted that 22% of PWE experienced inability to access antiepileptic drugs (AEDs) owing to lack of access to health care providers and/or pharmacies, leading to increased seizure frequency in 12% (including 2 patients with status epilepticus [SE] who required intensive care unit admission).[72]

However, not all reports about epilepsy care during the pandemic have been negative. Some epileptologists have noted improvement in seizure control in PWE during the pandemic owing to better medication adherence and increased sleep.[71] Despite concerns that ED visits for seizures would increase if patients were not accessing outpatient care, 1 health system in Italy actually observed a decrease in visits for seizures during the height of the pandemic in their country.[73] Limited evidence has also suggested that PWE without other comorbidities are not at higher risk for acquiring COVID-19 or suffering from more severe complications,[74] unlike patients with a history of cerebrovascular disease.[75,76]

Approach to Managing Seizures and Status Epilepticus During the Pandemic

For the most part, the evaluation and treatment of patients with seizures and/or SE during the pandemic should be unchanged with regard to general management principles, such as those outlined in the Neurocritical Care Society Guidelines.[77] However, there are some key, novel considerations regarding infection control, medications, and resource use.

Convulsive SE should be considered aerosol generating and appropriate PPE should be used for all treating staff. This point is most critical for physicians performing endotracheal intubation. Although debate exists about whether early versus delayed intubation is superior for patient outcomes in severe COVID-19 infection,[78,79] infection control may be considered in some centers. Some centers advocate for earlier intubation in respiratory failure given the potential for increased aerosolization associated with the use of noninvasive ventilation (bilevel or continuous positive airway pressure) and to a lesser extent high-flow nasal cannula, especially in the context of lack of negative pressure rooms and sufficient PPE.[80,81] These factors may influence decision-making for patients with mild respiratory distress after a seizure.

During the pandemic, there have been several shortages of medications frequently used for continuous sedation (IV midazolam, propofol) and AEDs (valproic acid, levetiracetam) that have impacted the care of hospitalized epilepsy patients and in the emergent management of seizures and SE. The main driver for these drug shortages has been the massive increase in simultaneous worldwide need; up to one-third of hospitalized patients with COVID-19 have severe respiratory distress requiring prolonged intubation and sedation.[82] In addition, manufacturing shutdowns in China and closure of exportation from India interrupted the usual supply chain to the United States.[83] Thus, it is important for health care systems to develop alternative sedation and SE treatment protocols to account for potential shortages. In particular, ketamine has experienced a recent resurgence for use in sedation as well as seizures and SE. There may be a particular role in SARS-CoV-2 infection, because ketamine has an anti-inflammatory effect, in particular lowering levels of IL-6, which are often increased in COVID-19 infection.[84,85]

Some patients may present to the ED with seizure or SE as the presenting feature of COVID-19.[86,87] Therefore, it may be reasonable to consider all patients with seizure or SE presenting to the ED as persons under investigation. Irrespective of COVID-19 status, a typical diagnostic work-up for new seizure involves obtaining MRI and EEG. Many investigators suggest the postponement of these studies during the pandemic unless they might provide urgent information that would change management.[74] Because seizure in COVID-19 may occur secondary to conditions like stroke, cerebral venous sinus thromboses, or meningoencephalitis, in our center we advocate for obtaining these studies during admission for a new seizure diagnosis, especially if there are no other provoking factors present.

Electroencephalography

Many health care systems decreased the use of EEG during the initial surge for all patients or modified indications and restricted access. Some eliminated the use of EEG for inpatients suspected to have COVID-19 altogether or created treatment algorithms which modified the standard of care for typical evaluations such as myoclonus, encephalopathy, and nonconvulsive SE.[88]

Pursuing EEG for patients with COVID-19 requires consideration of the risk:benefit ratio, given the risk of potential viral transmission to the technologist. If the study is unlikely to change management decisions for the patient, strong consideration should be given to foregoing the study. Most studies require prolonged set-up times and close proximity to patients' faces, which increase the risk of viral transmission (which may be lessened by proper use of PPE). Although an EEG in itself is not an aerosolizing procedure, the patient population requiring EEG may have behavioral unpredictability with the potential for yelling or coughing. For this reason, we recommend the use of N95 respirators, face shields, gowns, and gloves for all technologists during EEG lead placement and adjustment of all patients. Other infection control measures may include having a dedicated machine exclusively for patients with COVID-19 or using only disposable electrodes and cables.[89]

We recommend obtaining an EEG in cases of known SE who remain encephalopathic or comatose after the initial treatment of the seizure, for myoclonus and encephalopathy that has not responded to an empiric trial of an AED,[88] and for encephalopathy or coma evaluation when other explanations have been excluded. If EEG is pursued, a standard 10 to 20 EEG complement of electrodes with electrocardiogram should be used. Expedited studies with simplified montages to screen for SE (generalized and most regional or focal types), encephalopathy, and reactivity may be helpful in the intensive care unit setting if there are concerns about resource use.[90] The interpretation of specific patterns on the intensive care unit EEG suggestive of encephalopathy, nonconvulsive SE, focal slowing (suggestive of a lesion, such as a stroke), and postanoxic changes are beyond the scope of this article, but we recommend EEG scoring as per the American Clinical Neurophysiology Society guidance.[91] We suggest continuous video EEG monitoring to limit technologist active hands-on time in the room as well as to allow the electroencephalographer to make clinical correlations with the EEG findings. With reduced montages, however, there may be difficulty in identifying artifacts and a failure to identify lateralized periodic discharges. Most societies have recommended against the use of hyperventilation during EEG to decrease the risk of viral transmission.[89,90]

Because patients with COVID-19 are often intubated (sometimes with less common ventilation strategies), the electroencephalographer may be aided in interpretation of the study if the mode and rate of ventilation is recorded. There is no reason why EEG cannot be used for patients requiring the prone position, but experience with interpretation is very limited. When prone, the typical artifacts that are usually seen in the occipital leads (representing contact with bedding for supine patients) would instead be in the frontopolar leads.[90] Furthermore, positioning affects the cerebrospinal fluid (CSF) layer surrounding the brain parenchyma and shifts from supine to prone will redistribute CSF by up to 30% owing to gravity. As CSF is more conductive than brain parenchyma, and this factor will change the scalp potentials with thicker CSF layers associated with a decreased EEG signal.[92]

CORONAVIRUS DISEASE 19–ASSOCIATED SEIZURES AND STATUS EPILEPTICUS

Seizures seem to be an infrequent complication in patients with COVID-19, with a reported incidence of less than 1.6% in single health system studies[40,93–95] There are many mechanisms by which seizures may occur in COVID-19 (**Box 2**). PWE may be at greater risk of seizure during COVID-19 (similar to other common

---

Box 2
Mechanisms of seizure in COVID-19

- Exacerbation of underlying epilepsy
- Metabolic derangements
- Hypoxia
- Hyperinflammatory condition (cytokine storm)
- Complication of COVID treatments
- General critical illness
- Meningoencephalitis, infectious, or parainfectious
- Secondary consequence of cerebrovascular disease

---

infections), although the American Epilepsy Society reported survey data indicating that most PWE (>80%) did not experience worsening of seizure frequency, although they had symptoms of COVID-19 infection.[71] Metabolic derangements, organ failure, hypoglycemia, hypoxia, and some medications used during critical illness may all lower the seizure threshold. Moreover, subclinical seizures or nonconvulsive SE are common in patients with other forms of critical illness and depressed mental status.[96] There have been reports of new-onset epilepsy in COVID-19, most of which have been described in patients with a preexisting risk factor that lowered their seizure threshold. However, not all patients have a history of epilepsy, identified preexisting risk factor, or current metabolic derangement to explain new-onset seizures.[86,97] Some of these patients have been determined to have meningoencephalitis either from SARS-CoV-2 infection or as a parainfectious process.[88,97–99] Finally, COVID-related cerebrovascular complications may also lead to seizures.

The management of seizures and SE in COVID-19 may have some notable differences with regard to AED selection. In general, we advocate for the use of an IV AED formulation to avoid concerns of malabsorption. Critically ill patients with COVID-19 are at risk for multiple organ system failures. Cardiac complications in COVID-19 may be exacerbated by the combined effects of both COVID treatments and AEDs that lead to PR and/or QT prolongation (such as hydroxychloroquine and phenytoin). Hepatic injury and potential anticoagulation use may limit the use of phenytoin, valproate, and carbamazepine. Acute kidney injury leading to the need for renal replacement therapy or placement of patients on extracorporeal membrane oxygenation may require dose adjustments to maintain therapeutic concentrations of AEDs in serum.[100] Finally, as noted elsewhere in this article, key drug shortages may influence management decisions.

SUMMARY

Significant attention must be paid to the logistical challenges of managing neurologic emergencies in the setting of the COVID-19 pandemic. Thoughtful modifications of protocols allow for efficient delivery of high-quality care for all patients while protecting health care providers from viral exposure during the pandemic. Although the percentage of SARS-CoV-2 infections associated with neurologic emergencies is small, the large and still growing number of total infected individuals will likely result in a high burden of COVID-19 associated neurologic disease.[39] COVID-19–associated cerebrovascular disease and seizure are areas of active research that require further investigation to clarify their pathophysiology and determine optimal treatment measures.

CLINICS CARE POINTS

- Institutions should create protocols for managing neurologic emergencies during the pandemic that allow for rapid and thorough evaluation of patients while also minimizing viral exposure to other patients and staff.

- Less than 5% of patients with COVID-19 will have cerebrovascular complications and these typically occur in patients who are critically ill.

- PWE may face significant challenges with regards to care and prevention of seizures, but thus far there does not seem to be an increase in ED presentations with seizure

- Seizure is a rare complication of COVID-19 with AED selection impacted by concurrent organ failure, drug–drug interactions with COVID therapies, and ongoing drug shortages.

DISCLOSURE

The authors have nothing to disclose.

REFERENCES

1. LitCovid. Available at: https://www.ncbi.nlm.nih.gov/research/coronavirus/. Accessed November 10, 2020.
2. Cervantes-Arslanian A, Lau KHV, Anand P, et al. Rapid dissemination of protocols for managing neurology inpatients with COVID-19. Ann Neurol 2020; 88(2):211–4.
3. Pezzini A, Padovani A. Lifting the mask on neurological manifestations of COVID-19. Nat Rev Neurol 2020. https://doi.org/10.1038/s41582-020-0398-3.
4. Ford T, Curiale G, Nguyen TN, et al. Optimization of resources and modifications in acute ischemic stroke care in response to the global COVID-19 pandemic. J Stroke Cerebrovasc Dis 2020. https://doi.org/10.1016/j.jstrokecerebrovasdis. 2020.104980.
5. Khosravani H, Rajendram P, Notario L, et al. Protected code stroke: hyperacute stroke management during the coronavirus disease 2019 (COVID-19) pandemic. Stroke 2020. https://doi.org/10.1161/STROKEAHA.120.029838.
6. On Behalf of the AHA/ASA Stroke Council Leadership. Temporary emergency guidance to US stroke centers during the coronavirus disease 2019 (COVID-19) pandemic: on behalf of the American Heart Association/American Stroke Association Stroke Council Leadership. Stroke 2020;51(6):1910–2.
7. Yang B, Wang T, Chen J, et al. Impact of the COVID-19 pandemic on the process and outcome of thrombectomy for acute ischemic stroke. J Neurointerv Surg 2020. https://doi.org/10.1136/neurintsurg-2020-016177.
8. Kerleroux B, Fabacher T, Bricout N, et al. Mechanical thrombectomy for acute ischemic stroke amid the COVID-19 outbreak: decreased activity, and increased care delays. Stroke 2020. https://doi.org/10.1161/STROKEAHA.120. 030373.
9. Nguyen T, Abdalkader M, Jovin T. Mechanical thrombectomy in the era of COVID-19. Emergency preparedness for the neuroscience teams. Stroke 2020;51(6):1896–901.

10. Canelli R, Connor CW, Gonzalez M, et al. Barrier enclosure during endotracheal intubation. N Engl J Med 2020;382(20):1957–8.
11. Mansour OY, Malik AM, Linfante I. Mechanical Thrombectomy of COVID-19 positive acute ischemic stroke patient: a case report and call for preparedness. BMC Neurol 2020. https://doi.org/10.1186/s12883-020-01930-x.
12. Powers WJ, Rabinstein AA, Ackerson T, et al. Guidelines for the Early Management of Patients With Acute Ischemic Stroke: 2019 Update to the 2018 Guidelines for the Early Management of Acute Ischemic Stroke: a guideline for healthcare professionals from the American Heart Association/American Stroke Association. Stroke 2019;50(12). https://doi.org/10.1161/STR.0000000000000211.
13. Faigle R, Butler J, Carhuapoma JR, et al. Safety trial of low-intensity monitoring after thrombolysis: optimal post tpa-iv monitoring in ischemic STroke (OPTIMIST). Neurohospitalist 2020;10(1):11–5.
14. George AJ, Boehme AK, Dunn CR, et al. Trimming the fat in acute ischemic stroke: an assessment of 24-h CT Scans in tPA Patients. Int J Stroke 2015; 10(1):37–41.
15. Guhwe M, Utley-Smith Q, Blessing R, et al. Routine 24-hour computed tomography brain scan is not useful in stable patients post intravenous tissue plasminogen activator. J Stroke Cerebrovasc Dis 2016;25(3):540–2.
16. Dafer RM, Osteraas ND, Biller J. Acute stroke care in the coronavirus disease 2019 pandemic. J Stroke Cerebrovasc Dis 2020. https://doi.org/10.1016/j.jstrokecerebrovasdis.2020.104881.
17. Gioia LC, Poppe AY, Laroche R, et al. Streamlined Poststroke Treatment Order Sets During the SARS-CoV-2 pandemic: simplifying while not compromising care. Stroke 2020. https://doi.org/10.1161/STROKEAHA.120.031008.
18. Esenwa C, Parides MK, Labovitz DL. The effect of COVID-19 on stroke hospitalizations in New York City. J Stroke Cerebrovasc Dis 2020. https://doi.org/10.1016/j.jstrokecerebrovasdis.2020.105114.
19. Cummings C, Almallouhi E, Al Kasab S, et al. Blacks are less likely to present with strokes during the COVID-19 pandemic: observations from the buckle of the stroke belt. Stroke 2020. https://doi.org/10.1161/STROKEAHA.120.031121.
20. de Havenon A, Ney J, Callaghan B, et al. A Rapid Decrease in Stroke, Acute Coronary Syndrome, and Corresponding Interventions at 65 United States Hospitals Following Emergence of COVID-19. medRxiv 2020. https://doi.org/10.1101/2020.05.07.20083386.
21. Ghanchi H, Takayanagi A, Savla P, et al. Effects of the COVID-19 pandemic on stroke patients. Cureus 2020. https://doi.org/10.7759/cureus.9995.
22. Sharma M, Lioutas V-A, Madsen T, et al. Decline in stroke alerts and hospitalisations during the COVID-19 pandemic. Stroke Vasc Neurol 2020. https://doi.org/10.1136/svn-2020-000441.
23. Bres Bullrich M, Fridman S, Mandzia JL, et al. COVID-19: stroke admissions, emergency department visits, and prevention clinic referrals. Can J Neurol Sci 2020. https://doi.org/10.1017/cjn.2020.101.
24. Wang J, Chaudhry SA, Tahsili-Fahadan P, et al. The impact of COVID-19 on acute ischemic stroke admissions: analysis from a community-based tertiary care center. J Stroke Cerebrovasc Dis 2020. https://doi.org/10.1016/j.jstrokecerebrovasdis.2020.105344.
25. Meza HT, Lambea GÁ, Saldaña AS, et al. Impact of COVID-19 outbreak on ischemic stroke admissions and in-hospital mortality in North-West Spain. Int J Stroke 2020;15(7):755–62.

26. Rinkel LA, Prick JCM, Slot RER, et al. Impact of the COVID-19 outbreak on acute stroke care. J Neurol 2020. https://doi.org/10.1007/s00415-020-10069-1.

27. Diegoli H, Magalhães PSC, Martins SCO, et al. Decrease in hospital admissions for transient ischemic attack, mild, and moderate stroke during the COVID-19 era. Stroke 2020. https://doi.org/10.1161/STROKEAHA.120.030481.

28. Hasan ATMH, Das SC, Islam MS, et al. Impact of COVID-19 on hospital admission of acute stroke patients in Bangladesh. PLoS One 2020. https://doi.org/10.1101/2020.09.28.316448.

29. Paliwal PR, Tan BYQ, Leow AST, et al. Impact of the COVID-19 pandemic on hyperacute stroke treatment: experience from a comprehensive stroke centre in Singapore. J Thromb Thrombolysis 2020. https://doi.org/10.1007/s11239-020-02225-1.

30. Saxhaug Kristoffersen E, Holt Jahr S, Thommessen B, et al. Effect of COVID-19 pandemic on stroke admission rates in a Norwegian population. Acta Neurol Scand 2020. https://doi.org/10.1111/ane.13307.

31. Neves Briard J, Ducroux C, Jacquin G, et al. Early impact of the COVID-19 pandemic on acute stroke treatment delays. Can J Neurol Sci 2020. https://doi.org/10.1017/cjn.2020.160.

32. Darehed D, Blom M, Glader E-L, et al. In-hospital delays in stroke thrombolysis: every minute counts. Stroke 2020;51(8):2536–9.

33. Helms J, Kremer S, Merdji H, et al. Neurologic Features in Severe SARS-CoV-2 Infection. N Engl J Med 2020;382(23):2268–70.

34. Melmed KR, Cao M, Dogra S, et al. Risk factors for intracerebral hemorrhage in patients with COVID-19. J Thromb Thrombolysis 2020. https://doi.org/10.1007/s11239-020-02288-0.

35. Nwajei F, Anand P, Abdalkader M, et al. Cerebral Venous Sinus Thromboses in Patients with SARS-CoV-2 infection: three cases and a review of the literature. J Stroke Cerebrovasc Dis 2020. https://doi.org/10.1016/j.jstrokecerebrovasdis.2020.105412.

36. Anand P, Lau KHV, Chung DY, et al. Posterior reversible encephalopathy syndrome in patients with coronavirus disease 2019: two cases and a review of the literature. J Stroke Cerebrovasc Dis 2020;29(11):105212.

37. Dakay K, Kaur G, Gulko E, et al. Reversible cerebral vasoconstriction syndrome and dissection in the setting of COVID-19 infection. J Stroke Cerebrovasc Dis 2020;29(9):105011.

38. Pugin D, Vargas M-I, Thieffry C, et al. COVID-19–related encephalopathy responsive to high-dose glucocorticoids. Neurology 2020;95(12):543–6.

39. Ellul MA, Benjamin L, Singh B, et al. Neurological associations of COVID-19. Lancet Neurol 2020;19(9):767–83.

40. Mao L, Jin H, Wang M, et al. Neurologic manifestations of hospitalized patients with coronavirus disease 2019 in Wuhan, China. JAMA Neurol 2020. https://doi.org/10.1001/jamaneurol.2020.1127.

41. Li Y, Li M, Wang M, et al. Acute cerebrovascular disease following COVID-19: a single center, retrospective, observational study. Stroke Vasc Neurol 2020;5(3):279–84.

42. Majidi S, Fifi JT, Ladner TR, et al. Emergent large vessel occlusion stroke during New York City's COVID-19 outbreak: clinical characteristics and paraclinical findings. Stroke 2020. https://doi.org/10.1161/STROKEAHA.120.030397.

43. Kihira S, Schefflein J, Mahmoudi K, et al. Association of Coronavirus Disease (COVID-19) with large vessel occlusion strokes: a case-control study. AJR Am J Roentgenol 2020;29:1–6.

44. Rothstein A, Oldridge O, Schwennesen H, et al. Acute cerebrovascular events in hospitalized COVID-19 patients. Stroke 2020. https://doi.org/10.1161/STROKEAHA.120.030995.

45. Jillella DV, Janocko NJ, Nahab F, et al. Ischemic stroke in COVID-19: an urgent need for early identification and management. PLoS One 2020. https://doi.org/10.1371/journal.pone.0239443.

46. Yaghi S, Ishida K, Torres J, et al. SARS-CoV-2 and Stroke in a New York Healthcare System. Stroke 2020;51(7):2002–11.

47. Siegler JE, Cardona P, Arenillas JF, et al. Cerebrovascular events and outcomes in hospitalized patients with COVID-19: the SVIN COVID-19 Multinational Registry. Int J Stroke 2020. https://doi.org/10.1177/1747493020959216. 174749302095921.

48. Benussi A, Pilotto A, Premi E, et al. Clinical characteristics and outcomes of inpatients with neurologic disease and COVID-19 in Brescia, Lombardy, Italy. Neurology 2020;95(7):e910–20.

49. Ntaios G, Michel P, Georgiopoulos G, et al. Characteristics and outcomes in patients with COVID-19 and acute ischemic stroke: the Global COVID-19 Stroke Registry. Stroke 2020. https://doi.org/10.1161/STROKEAHA.120.031208.

50. Dogra S, Jain R, Cao M, et al. Hemorrhagic stroke and anticoagulation in COVID-19. J Stroke Cerebrovasc Dis 2020;29(8):104984.

51. Kvernland A, Kumar A, Yaghi S, et al. Anticoagulation use and Hemorrhagic Stroke in SARS-CoV-2 Patients Treated at a New York Healthcare System. Neurocrit Care 2020. https://doi.org/10.1007/s12028-020-01077-0.

52. Beyrouti R, Adams ME, Benjamin L, et al. Characteristics of ischaemic stroke associated with COVID-19. J Neurol Neurosurg Psychiatry 2020;91(8):889–91.

53. Zhang Y, Xiao M, Zhang S, et al. Coagulopathy and antiphospholipid antibodies in patients with Covid-19. N Engl J Med 2020;382(17):e38.

54. Bhaskar S, Sinha A, Banach M, et al. Cytokine storm in COVID-19-immunopathological mechanisms, clinical considerations, and therapeutic approaches: the REPROGRAM Consortium position paper. Front Immunol 2020;11:1648.

55. Divani AA, Andalib S, Di Napoli M, et al. Coronavirus disease 2019 and stroke: clinical manifestations and pathophysiological insights. J Stroke Cerebrovasc Dis 2020;29(8):104941.

56. South AM, Tomlinson L, Edmonston D, et al. Controversies of renin-angiotensin system inhibition during the COVID-19 pandemic. Nat Rev Nephrol 2020;16(6):305–7.

57. Gulko E, Overby P, Ali S, et al. Vessel Wall Enhancement and Focal Cerebral Arteriopathy in a Pediatric Patient with Acute Infarct and COVID-19 Infection. AJNR Am J Neuroradiol 2020;41(12):2348–50.

58. Shulman JG, Cervantes-Arslanian AM. Infectious Etiologies of Stroke. Semin Neurol 2019;39(4):482–94.

59. Bhattacharjee S, Banerjee M. Immune thrombocytopenia secondary to COVID-19: a systematic review. SN Compr Clin Med 2020;1–11. https://doi.org/10.1007/s42399-020-00521-8.

60. Tang N, Li D, Wang X, et al. Abnormal coagulation parameters are associated with poor prognosis in patients with novel coronavirus pneumonia. J Thromb Haemost 2020;18(4):844–7.

61. Thachil J, Tang N, Gando S, et al. ISTH interim guidance on recognition and management of coagulopathy in COVID-19. J Thromb Haemost 2020;18(5):1023–6.

62. National Institute of Neurological Disorders and Stroke rt-PA Stroke Study Group. Tissue plasminogen activator for acute ischemic stroke. N Engl J Med 1995;333(24):1581–7.
63. Hacke W, Kaste M, Bluhmki E, et al. Thrombolysis with alteplase 3 to 4.5 hours after acute ischemic stroke. N Engl J Med 2008;359(13):1317–29.
64. Tan Y-K, Goh C, Leow AST, et al. COVID-19 and ischemic stroke: a systematic review and meta-summary of the literature. J Thromb Thrombolysis 2020. https://doi.org/10.1007/s11239-020-02228-y.
65. Carneiro T, Dashkoff J, Leung LY, et al. Intravenous tPA for Acute Ischemic Stroke in Patients with COVID-19. J Stroke Cerebrovasc Dis 2020. https://doi.org/10.1016/j.jstrokecerebrovasdis.2020.105201.
66. Oxley TJ, Mocco J, Majidi S, et al. Large-vessel stroke as a presenting feature of Covid-19 in the young. N Engl J Med 2020;382(20):e60.
67. Baracchini C, Pieroni A, Viaro F, et al. Acute Stroke Management Pathway During Coronavirus-19 Pandemic. Neurol Sci 2020;41:1003–5.
68. Pop R, Hasiu A, Bolognini F, et al. Stroke thrombectomy in patients with COVID-19: initial experience in 13 cases. AJNR Am J Neuroradiol 2020. https://doi.org/10.3174/ajnr.A6750. ajnr;ajnr.A6750v1.
69. Escalard S, Maïer B, Redjem H, et al. Treatment of acute ischemic stroke due to large vessel occlusion with COVID-19: experience from Paris. Stroke 2020;51(8):2540–3.
70. Wang A, Mandigo GK, Yim PD, et al. Stroke and mechanical thrombectomy in patients with COVID-19: technical observations and patient characteristics. J Neurointerv Surg 2020;12(7):648–53.
71. Albert DVF, Das RR, Acharya JN, et al. The Impact of COVID-19 on epilepsy care: a survey of the American Epilepsy Society membership. Epilepsy Curr 2020;20(5):316–24.
72. Lai S-L, Hsu M-T, Chen S-S. The impact of SARS on epilepsy: the experience of drug withdrawal in epileptic patients. Seizure 2005;14(8):557–61.
73. Cheli M, Dinoto A, Olivo S, et al. SARS-CoV-2 pandemic and epilepsy: the impact on emergency department attendances for seizures. Seizure 2020;82:23–6.
74. French JA, Brodie MJ, Caraballo R, et al. Keeping people with epilepsy safe during the COVID-19 pandemic. Neurology 2020;94(23):1032–7.
75. Florez-Perdomo WA, Serrato-Vargas SA, Bosque-Varela P, et al. Relationship between the history of cerebrovascular disease and mortality in COVID-19 patients: a systematic review and meta-analysis. Clin Neurol Neurosurg 2020;197:106183.
76. Pranata R, Huang I, Lim MA, et al. Impact of cerebrovascular and cardiovascular diseases on mortality and severity of COVID-19-systematic review, meta-analysis, and meta-regression. J Stroke Cerebrovasc Dis 2020;29(8):104949.
77. Brophy GM, Bell R, Claassen J, et al. Guidelines for the evaluation and management of status epilepticus. Neurocrit Care 2012;17(1):3–23.
78. Rola P, Farkas J, Spiegel R, et al. Rethinking the early intubation paradigm of COVID-19: time to change gears? Clin Exp Emerg Med 2020;7(2):78–80.
79. Matta A, Chaudhary S, Bryan Lo K, et al. Timing of Intubation and Its Implications on Outcomes in Critically Ill Patients With Coronavirus Disease 2019 Infection. Crit Care Explorations 2020;2(10):e0262.
80. Tran K, Cimon K, Severn M, et al. Aerosol generating procedures and risk of transmission of acute respiratory infections to healthcare workers: a systematic review. PLoS One 2012;7(4):e35797.

81. Schünemann HJ, Khabsa J, Solo K, et al. Ventilation techniques and risk for transmission of coronavirus disease, including COVID-19: a living systematic review of multiple streams of evidence. Ann Intern Med 2020;173(3):204–16.
82. Wunsch H. Mechanical ventilation in COVID-19: interpreting the current epidemiology. Am J Respir Crit Care Med 2020;202(1):1–4.
83. Choo EK, Rajkumar SV. Medication shortages during the COVID-19 crisis: what we must do. Mayo Clin Proc 2020;95(6):1112–5.
84. Ortoleva J. Consider Adjunctive Ketamine in Mechanically Ventilated Coronavirus Disease-2019 Patients. J Cardiothorac Vasc Anesth 2020;34(10):2580.
85. Dale O, Somogyi AA, Li Y, et al. Does intraoperative ketamine attenuate inflammatory reactivity following surgery? A systematic review and meta-analysis. Anesth Analg 2012;115(4):934–43.
86. Anand P, Al-Faraj A, Sader E, et al. Seizure as the presenting symptom of COVID-19: a retrospective case series. Epilepsy Behav 2020;112:107335.
87. Vollono C, Rollo E, Romozzi M, et al. Focal status epilepticus as unique clinical feature of COVID-19: a case report. Seizure 2020;78:109–12.
88. Anand P, Zakaria A, Benameur K, et al. Myoclonus in patients with coronavirus disease 2019: a multicenter case series. Crit Care Med 2020. https://doi.org/10.1097/CCM.0000000000004570.
89. Alotaibi F, Althani Z, Aljaafari D, et al. Saudi Epilepsy Society consensus on epilepsy management during the COVID-19 Pandemic. Neurosciences (Riyadh) 2020;25(3):222–5.
90. Gélisse P, Rossetti AO, Genton P, et al. How to carry out and interpret EEG recordings in COVID-19 patients in ICU? Clin Neurophysiol 2020;131(8):2023–31.
91. Hirsch LJ, LaRoche SM, Gaspard N, et al. American Clinical Neurophysiology Society's Standardized Critical Care EEG Terminology: 2012 version. J Clin Neurophysiol 2013;30(1):1–27.
92. Rice JK, Rorden C, Little JS, et al. Subject position affects EEG magnitudes. Neuroimage 2013;64:476–84.
93. Lu L, Xiong W, Liu D, et al. New onset acute symptomatic seizure and risk factors in coronavirus disease 2019: a retrospective multicenter study. Epilepsia 2020;(6):61. https://doi.org/10.1111/epi.16524.
94. Narula N, Joseph R, Katyal N, et al. Seizure and COVID-19: association and review of potential mechanism. Neurol Psychiatry Brain Res 2020;38:49–53.
95. Anand P, Zhou L, Bhadelia N, et al. Neurologic findings among inpatients with COVID-19 at a safety-net US hospital. Neurol Clin Pract 2020. https://doi.org/10.1212/CPJ.0000000000001031.
96. Claassen J, Mayer SA, Kowalski RG, et al. Detection of electrographic seizures with continuous EEG monitoring in critically ill patients. Neurology 2004;62(10):1743–8.
97. Sohal S, Mansur M. COVID-19 presenting with seizures. IDCases 2020;20:e00782.
98. Moriguchi T, Harii N, Goto J, et al. A first case of meningitis/encephalitis associated with SARS-Coronavirus-2. Int J Infect Dis 2020;94:55–8.
99. Karimi N, Sharifi Razavi A, Rouhani N. Frequent convulsive seizures in an adult patient with COVID-19: a case report. Iranian Red Crescent Med J 2020;22(3). https://doi.org/10.5812/ircmj.102828.
100. Asadi-Pooya AA, Attar A, Moghadami M, et al. Management of COVID-19 in people with epilepsy: drug considerations. Neurol Sci 2020;41(8):2005–11.

Moving?

Make sure your subscription moves with you!

To notify us of your new address, find your **Clinics Account Number** (located on your mailing label above your name), and contact customer service at:

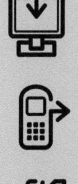

Email: **journalscustomerservice-usa@elsevier.com**

800-654-2452 (subscribers in the U.S. & Canada)
314-447-8871 (subscribers outside of the U.S. & Canada)

Fax number: **314-447-8029**

Elsevier Health Sciences Division
Subscription Customer Service
3251 Riverport Lane
Maryland Heights, MO 63043

*To ensure uninterrupted delivery of your subscription, please notify us at least 4 weeks in advance of move.

ELSEVIER